SURGERY
MINITEXT

John S.P. Lumley MS FRCS FMMA(Hon) FGA
Director of the Ernest Cooke Vascular and
Microvascular Unit, Department of Clinical
Physics, St Bartholomew's Hospital, and
Honorary Consultant Surgeon at
St Bartholomew's Hospital and the Hospital for
Sick Children, Great Ormond Street, London, UK

Paul Srodon MD FRCS
Specialist Registrar in Surgery,
St Bartholomew's and Royal London Hospitals,
London, UK

Ramanathan Visvanathan BM FRCS ILTM
Consultant Surgeon, Bronglais General Hospital
Aberystwyth
and Breast Test Wales Swansea
Honorary Lecturer, University of Wales
College of Medicine
Surgical Tutor, Royal College of Surgeons
of England, UK

A member of the Hodder Headline Group
LONDON

First published in Great Britain in 2004 by
Arnold, a member of the Hodder Headline Group,
338 Euston Road, London NW1 3BH

http://www.arnoldpublishers.com

Distributed in the United States of America by
Oxford University Press Inc.,
198 Madison Avenue, New York, NY10016
Oxford is a registered trademark of Oxford University Press

Whilst the advice and information in this book are believed to be true
and accurate at the date of going to press, neither the authors nor the
publisher can accept any legal responsibility or liability for any errors
or omissions that may be made. In particular (but without limiting the
generality of the preceding disclaimer) every effort has been made to
check drug dosages; however, it is still possible that errors have been
missed. Furthermore, dosage schedules are constantly being revised
and new side-effects recognized. For these reasons the reader is
strongly urged to consult the drug companies' printed instructions
before administering any of the drugs recommended in this book.

British Library Cataloguing in Publication Data
A catalogue record for this book is available from the British Library

Library of Congress Cataloging-in-Publication Data
A catalog record for this book is available from the Library of Congress

ISBN 0 340 80977 9
ISBN 0 340 81591 4 (International Students' Edition, restricted
territorial availability)

1 2 3 4 5 6 7 8 9 10

Commissioning Editor: Georgina Bentliff
Development Editor: Heather Smith
Project Editor: Wendy Rooke
Production Controller: Jane Lawrence
Cover Design: Amina Dudhia

Typeset in 8.5/10 pt Plantin by Charon Tec Pvt. Ltd, Chennai, India
Printed and bound in Italy

What do you think about this book? Or any other Arnold title?
Please send your comments to feedback.arnold@hodder.co.uk

CONTENTS

Contributors   ix

Preface   xi

Abbreviations   xiii

1 Principles of surgery   1
Principles of surgery   2

2 Surgery in practice   7
Admission to hospital   8
Day case surgery   8
Pre-operative assessment   11
Peri-operative drug management   12
Clinical consent   20
Anaesthesia   24
Haemostasis   32
Blood transfusion   35
Surgical procedures   41
Postoperative care   43

3 Postoperative complications   53
Postoperative complications   54
    Haemorrhage   54
    Disturbance of fluid and electrolyte balance   55
    Diabetes insipidus   61
    Acid–base balance   62
    Cardiac problems   64
    Respiratory problems   65
    Alimentary problems   68
    Neurological problems   70
    Fever   72
    Wound problems   73
    Cannula problems   74
    Venous thromboembolism   75
Nutrition   77
    Parenteral nutrition   82

4 Systems management 87

Management of systemic disease 88
Intensive care unit 88
High dependency unit 99
Brainstem death 100
Obesity 102
The elderly patient 104
Palliative care 105
The dying patient 110

5 Management of surgical disease 113

Sepsis 114
HIV and AIDS 118
    Clinical manifestations/classification 119
    Symptomatic HIV disease/AIDS 120
    Antiretroviral therapy 129
Tropical and subtropical diseases 130
    Cancers of the tropics 130
    Infections of the tropics 134
    Superficial mycoses 145
    Protozoa 147
    Flukes (trematodes) 151
    Round worms (nematodes) 154
    Tapeworms (cestodes) 161
    Poisoning by animals 164
    Ainhum 168
Anaemias 168
    Normocytic and microcytic anaemias 170
    Macrocytic anaemias 172
    Haemolytic anaemias 176
    Inherited haemolytic anaemias 176
    Blood transfusion in the treatment of severe
    anaemia 181
    Anaemias in the tropics 182
Oncology 182
Skin 188
    Lumps, ulcers, sinuses and fistulae 204

Head   207
    Cranial nerves   207
    Scalp   217
    Skull   218
    Intracranial conditions   221
    Head injury   226
    Face and jaws   231
    Ear   236
    Orbit   247
    Mouth   271
    Tongue   276
    Palate   277
    Nose   277
    Pharynx   284
    Larynx   289
    Salivary glands   293
    Neck   298
    Thyroid   307
    Thyroglossal tract   317
    Parathyroids   318

Breast diseases   320
    Benign conditions   320
    Breast cancer   329
    Axilla   336

Thorax   337
    Pulmonary disease and thoracic trauma   337
    Cardiac conditions   364

Abdomen   390
    Abdominal wall   390
    Abdominal hernias   392
    Diaphragm   394
    Acute abdomen   395
    Abdominal trauma   405
    Gynaecological emergencies   409
    Oesophagus   413
    Stomach and duodenum   423
    Bowel   434
    Stomas   452
    Abdominal sarcomas   453
    Liver   454
    Biliary tree   464

Spleen   473
Pancreas   475
Adrenal gland   486
Genitourinary system and genitalia   **492**
    Kidney and ureter   492
    Bladder and prostate   508
    Penis   527
    Scrotum and testes   533
    Sexually transmitted disease 542
Vascular   **544**
    Arteries   544
    Veins and lymphatics   580
Transplantation   **592**
Management of the multiply injured patient   **599**
    Ballistic trauma   605
    Burns   610
    Paediatric trauma   614
    Trauma in pregnancy   616
Orthopaedics   **618**
    Bones and fractures   618
    Joints and muscles   648
Upper limb   **674**
    Shoulder joint and pectoral girdle 674
    Arm   682
    Hand   694
Lower limb   **699**
    Pelvis, hip joint and thigh 699
    Knee   714
    Leg and ankle   725
    Foot   732
Spine   **740**
    Spinal injuries   749
Peripheral nerves   **759**
    Peripheral nerve injuries 759
    Neuropathy   773

6 Personal development   **777**
Personal development   **778**

Index   787

CONTRIBUTORS

Phil Hornick (Thorax: Pulmonary; Cardiac)
BSc (Hons), MBBChir, PhD, FRCS (Eng)
Specialist Registrar and Honorary Lecturer in
Cardiothoracic Surgery, Hammersmith Hospital,
London, UK

Dr Maurice Murphy (HIV and AIDS)
BSc, MB, MRCP (Ireland)
Consultant Clinical Immunology and HIV,
St Bartholomew's Hospital, London, UK

Dr Lynn A. Riddell (HIV and AIDS)
BSc, MBChB, MRCP (England)
Consultant HIV and Genitourinary Medicine,
Northampton General Hospital, Northampton, UK

L.K. Kristine Teoh (Thorax: Pulmonary; Cardiac)
MBBChir, MA, FRCS (Eng)
Specialist Registrar in Cardiothoracic Surgery,
Hammersmith Hospital, London, UK

PREFACE

The text is a concise guide to the management of the
surgical patient. It provides comprehensive coverage of the
generality of surgery, written for both the final MB student
and the basic surgical trainee preparing for the MRCS
examination. The essential knowledge for the management
of the surgical patient is included, avoiding omissions that
could lull the reader into a false sense of security on the
ward or in the examination. Examinations generally
require the same information that is needed for the ward
management of a patient, and this book, with its emphasis
on the application of surgical knowledge in the clinical
setting, is a companion to both.

The design of the book ensures that it is portable and
can be used as a ward handbook, being either carried in a
coat pocket, or left at the nursing station to be available
where and when it is needed. The style is concise (mainly
bullet points) while retaining clarity, the aim being to
provide a readable and easily understood textbook.

The text commences with an outline of the **Principles
of Surgery**, defining the stages of clinical management, the
importance of documentation and the workings of the
clinical team. Account is taken of the increasing importance
of the multidisciplinary team in the management of disease.
Surgery in Practice follows a patient's progress from the
presentation, through their preparation, and their surgical
management, including complications. The sections on
Systems Management consider co-morbidity, and
management of the elderly and terminally ill patient. This
section also includes the management of sepsis and the
seriously ill patient in the Intensive Care Unit.

The main body of the text is directed at infection and
the presentation and **management of surgical disease**,
under the five headings of definition, signs and symptoms,
investigations, management and complications. These areas
are identified within the innovative design, making use of
tables and other pedagogic features to highlight and
differentiate important and pertinent information. Detailed
management includes national guidelines and protocols
where these are evidence-based. Where conflicting opinions

exist, or management is changing, an attempt is made at consensus, but at all times practical advice on management issues is given, indicating what to do in the ward situation, including relevant medication. The final section on **Personal Development** considers the educational needs, and the knowledge, clinical skills and disciplinary requirements both of the medical student and the surgical trainee in their professional development, together with its assessment.

The format is intended to provide user-friendly access for quick retrieval of relevant information. The structure enables the student and trainee to dip in both for the initial study of the condition and for later revision at the time of an examination. The emphasis on management provides the house officer and surgical trainee with a valuable companion in the clinical environment.

The book includes a list of abbreviations, tables of normal values and a comprehensive index. No space has been given to illustrations, as these are included in complementary volumes, such as the extensively illustrated Hamilton Bailey's Physical Signs. Nevertheless, this concise surgical volume is a stand-alone text for the study and subsequent revision of surgical topics.

ABBREVIATIONS

2,3-DPG	2,3-diphosphoglycerate
AAFB	acid alcohol-fast bacillus
ACE	angiotensin-converting enzyme
ACTH	adrenocorticotropic hormone
ADH	antidiuretic hormone
AF	atrial fibrillation
AIDS	acquired immunodeficiency syndrome
ANCA	antineutrophil cytoplasmic antibody
APCs	antigen-producing cells
APTT	activated partial thromboplastin time
AR	aortic regurgitation
ARDS	acute respiratory distress syndrome
ASA	American Society of Anesthetists (ASA I, II, III)
ASD	atrial septal defect
ATLS	Advanced Trauma Life Support
AV	arteriovenous
AVR	aortic valve replacement
AZT	azidothymidine (zidovudine)
BAL	bronchoalveolar lavage
BCG	bacille Calmette–Guérin
BHIVA	British HIV Association
CABG	coronary artery bypass graft surgery
CCS	Canadian Cardiovascular Society (grading CCS0–CCS4)
CIS	carcinoma-in-situ
CMCT	central motor conduction time
CMV	cytomegalovirus
CNS	central nervous system
COX-1	cyclo-oxygenase-1
CPAP	continuous positive airway pressure
CRF	corticotropin-releasing factors
CRP	C-reactive protein
CSF	cerebrospinal fluid
CT	computerized tomography
CVA	cerebrovascular accident
CVP	central venous pressure
DCIS	ductal carcinoma-in-situ
DI	diabetes insipidus
DIC	disseminated intravascular coagulation

DVT	deep vein thrombosis
ECG	electrocardiograph
EEG	electroencephalograph
EF	ejection fraction
ELISA	enzyme-linked immunosorbent assay
ENT	ear, nose and throat
ERCP	endoscopic retrograde cholangiopancreatography
ESR	erythrocyte sedimentation rate
EUA	examination under anaesthesia
FBC	full blood count
FFP	fresh frozen plasma
FNA	fine-needle aspiration
GA	general anaesthesia
G-6-PD	glucose-6 phosphate dehydrogenase
GCSE	generalized convulsive status epilepticus
GTN	glyceryl trinitrate
GVH	graft versus host
HAART	highly active antiretroviral therapy
HAV	hepatitis A virus (also HBV, HCV)
HBS	haemoglobin S (sickle)
HCG	human chorionic gonadotrophin
HDU	high dependency unit
HHV-8	human herpes virus 8
HIDA	hepatic iminodiacetic acid
HIV	human immunodeficiency virus
HLA	human leukocyte antigen
HPV	human papilloma virus
HSV	herpes simplex virus
HTIG	tetanus immunoglobulin
ICU	intensive care unit
Ig	immunoglobulin (IgA, IgG)
IL	interleukin (-1, -6)
INR	international normalized ratio
i.m.	intramuscular
i.v.	intravenous
IVU	intravenous urography/urogram
JVP	jugular venous pulse/pressure
KS	Kaposi's sarcoma
LA	left atrium/left atrial
LCIS	lobular carcinoma in situ
LDH	lactate dehydrogenase

LFTs	liver function tests
LMA	laryngeal mask airway
LV	left ventricular
LVESD	left ventricular end systolic dimension
MAC	*Mycobacterium avium* complex
MALT	mucosa associated lymphoid tissue
MAOIs	monoamine-oxidase inhibitors
MCH	mean cell haemoglobin
MCHC	mean cell haemoglobin concentration
MCV	mean cell volume
MDT	multidisciplinary team
MEN	multiple endocrine neoplasia
MHC	major histocompatibility complex
MI	myocardial infarction
MIBG	meta-iodobenzyl-guanidine
MMPI	Minnesota Multiphasic Personality Inventory
MODS	multiple organ dysfunction syndrome
MR	mitral regurgitation
MRA	magnetic resonance angiography
MRI	magnetic resonance imaging
MRSA	methicillin-resistant *Staphylococcus aureus*
MS	mitral stenosis
MUGA scan	multigated acquisition scanning
MV	mitral valve
MVR	mitral valve replacement
NAC	nipple–areolar complex
NADP	nicotinamide adenine dinucleotide phosphate
NK	natural killer (cells)
NRTI	nucleoside reverse-transcriptase inhibitors
NNRTI	non-nucleoside reverse transcriptase inhibitor
NSAIDs	non-steroidal anti-inflammatory drugs
NSCLC	non-small-cell lung cancer
NSTEMI	non-ST-elevation myocardial infarction
NYHA	New York Heart Association (grading NYHA I–NYHA IV)
PA	pulmonary artery
PAF	platelet activating factor
PAMPs	pathogen-associated molecular patterns
PCA	patient-controlled analgesia
PCI	percutaneous intervention

PCP	*Pneumocystis carinii* pneumonia
PCR	polymerase chain reaction
PCV	packed cell volume
PDA	patent ductus arteriosus
PE	pulmonary embolism
PEEP	positive end-expiratory pressure
PEG	percutaneous endoscopic gastrostomy
PET	positron emission tomography
PFO	patent foramen ovale
PI	protease inhibitor
PMETB	Postgraduate Medical Education Training Board
POSSUM	physiological and operative severity score for the enumeration of mortality and morbidity
PPD	purified protein derivative
PSA	prostate-specific antigen
PTH	parathyroid hormone
PTT	partial thromboplastin time
PUSIL	primary upper small intestinal lymphoma
RA	right atrium/atrial
RCC	red cell count
rFVIIa	recombinant activated factor VII
RIPE	rifampicin, isoniazid, pyrizinamide and ethambutol
RV	right ventricular
SAG-M	saline, adenine, glucose-mannitol
SBE	bicarbonate and base excess
SCLC	small-cell lung cancer
SHOT	Serious Hazards of Transfusion Group
SIADH	syndrome of inappropriate ADH secretion
SIRS	systemic inflammatory response syndrome
SLE	systemic lupus erythematosus
SVC	superior vena cava
T_3	tri-iodothyronine
T_4	thyroxine
TB	tuberculosis
TENS	transcutaneous electrical nerve stimulation
Th	T-helper (cells)
TIA	transient ischaemic attack
TNF	tumour necrosis factor
TNM	tumour, nodes, metastases
TOCS	thoracic outlet compression syndrome

TPA	tissue plasminogen activator
TRALI	transfusion related acute lung injury
TSH	thyroid-stimulating hormone
TTA	to take away (e.g. drugs)
TURP	transurethral resection of the prostate
UNAIDS	Joint United Nations Programme on HIV and AIDS
VAP	ventilator-associated pneumonia
VATS	video-assisted thorascopic surgery
vCJD	variant Creutzfeld–Jakob disease
VIP	vasoactive intestinal peptide
VSD	ventricular septal defect
WHO	World Health Organization
WCC	white cell count

1

Principles of
surgery

PRINCIPLES OF SURGERY

- A doctor sets out to cure a patient's ailments. This may involve one or more therapeutic measures, such as medication, surgery, nursing care or a conservative approach (i.e. no treatment at all); above all, it should do no harm.
- The **differential diagnosis** is the most likely cause, or possible causes, of a patient's problems. This can be determined by: taking a **history**, **examining** the patient and undertaking **investigations**.
- In order to apply these skills, the doctor must communicate with the patient, their relatives and carers, in an empathetic manner that inspires confidence, and ensures that they fully understand the disease and are involved with its management.
- Investigations usually involve taking blood and radiological examinations. They may also include taking a biopsy, such as of a lymph node, and this may identify the spread of a malignant disease, and the staging of its severity.
- The doctor is also able to **assess the severity** of a patient's disease and any associated co-morbidity (other problems). Severity scores have been established for some diseases (e.g. pancreatitis) and disease states (e.g. the Glasgow Coma Score for head injuries and the American Society of Anesthesiologists (ASA) score for patients undergoing anaesthesia).
- **Management** is the processes of diagnosis, assessment and treatment. The preparation and initiation of a **management plan** is based on current medical knowledge of a patient's disease and associated problems. It must deliver safe effective care, taking into account social, ethical and cultural issues, and developing an ongoing patient–doctor partnership.
- There are often **local protocols** for managing specific conditions; these should be **evidence based**, and adhere to **national guidelines**.
- The **management plan** evolves during a patient's hospital stay, and includes further investigations and therapeutic procedures. Risks and benefits of therapeutic measures should be balanced against a conservative approach.

- A patient's **discharge plan** should consider where they should go, the help they will need, drugs TTA (to take away) and instructions on all future proposals, including a follow-up appointment.
- If a patient's condition deteriorates, protocols should be available on whether **resuscitation** is indicated and what form it should take. If a patient **dies in hospital**, institutional and national protocols must be followed for confirmation and **certification of death**, the requirement for a post-mortem or **reporting to the coroner**, and where **organ donation** may be appropriate.

Documentation

- Good documentation is essential. **Case notes** must include the patient identification on all pages (name, date of birth, gender, hospital number), history, examination, investigations, results, management decisions and the drugs prescribed. They must be clear, accurate and contemporaneous. Regular progress reports should include opinions with dates and times of each visiting clinician, and all clinical procedures, such as anaesthetics and operations, and what the patient and next-of-kin have been told.
- The notes should always be readily available so that clinical findings and management decisions can be reviewed; they are a legal requirement and serve as evidence to support or refute any subsequent complaint or medico-legal actions.
- **Discharge summaries** and **letters** should be sent to all those involved in management, including the patient's general practitioner, and copies retained in the hospital notes.
- Full use should be made of **information technology (IT)**, in order to facilitate record keeping and data retrieval. There are statutory requirements for retaining NHS notes, usually for 8 years, but for children until they are 25 years old and maternity notes should be kept for 25 years.
- With the increase in computerized records, there has been increased concern for confidentiality and the

importance of information being only available to those who have authority. Trusts are responsible for **confidentiality**, and must ensure that the use of identifiable information is justified.

- **Integrity** relates to the presentation of information and how it is recorded; incomplete data may be as harmful as is fraudulent alteration. Methods of coding vary in the number of terms used (some being in excess of 800 000); the problem-orientated record has the advantage of being directly linked to patient management.
- The documentation system must ensure rapid **availability** without compromising confidentiality or security. The systems include restriction on access, passwords being required at various levels.

Teamwork

- Good healthcare is delivered by a **multidisciplinary team**. Excellent communication within and between teams is essential for effective patient handover and continuity of care.
- Good teams have an identified leader, each member should have a specific role, and there should be clear lines of accountability.
- Regular **meetings** facilitate good working professional relationships, regular communication, allow the contribution of each member to be appreciated, and overcome personality difficulties and the isolation of individuals.
- Meetings should cover all aspects of management, taking into account the clinical governance of the unit. They allow critical appraisal of clinical practice, for questions to be raised and conflicting opinions to be aired, and the strengths and weaknesses of the unit to be identified.
- Specialist meetings may take many forms: they include radiology, pathology, audit, morbidity and mortality, and continuing education.
- **Clinical governance** is the system through which NHS Trusts and other organizations are accountable for continuously improving the quality of their services and safeguarding high standards of care, by creating an

environment in which excellence in clinical care can flourish.
- The Trust chief executive is responsible for clinical governance, and every clinician is required to take part; the process is open to public scrutiny. It involves participation in such activities as audit, training and education, research and development, and risk management.
- No healthcare delivery can be without risk, and this may be to the patients, practitioners and the organization providing the service. **Evidence-based practice** uses the results of critically appraised research, linked with clinical experience and patient values. There may be accepted protocols, guidelines, recommendations or codes of practice for many conditions the unit manages, but the team has to relate these to local circumstances and provide the best available patient care.
- The unit policy must be to create an environment in which excellence can flourish, and, through audit and feedback, it must continually monitor and improve its practice.
- **Risk management** is the process by which patient safety is protected. Therapeutic risk is analysed by monitoring treatment processes and outcomes. Where remedial risk is identified, this must be eliminated; unavoidable risk must be minimized, with contingency plans in place for its management.
- Incidents and near-misses must be documented and debated; where appropriate, they must be used to effect behavioural and policy changes within the unit. These quality assurance measures serve to reduce the vulnerability of the unit to both incidents and medico-legal challenge.

2

Surgery in practice

ADMISSION TO HOSPITAL

- Patients admitted to hospital for routine surgery usually arrive by private or public transport, accompanied by relatives or friends, who can take away excess baggage and who can confirm contact details and other information.
- Admissions types:
  - **Minor surgery** – where small procedures of short duration are carried out under local anaesthesia, and the patient is in a fit condition to leave immediately afterwards
  - **Day case** – where surgery or procedures are undertaken in a day-unit, the patient arriving and leaving on the same day
  - **In-patient** – where management of the patient requires staying overnight and for as long as is required.
- Emergency admissions may be through the out-patient or accident and emergency departments, or be transferred by ambulance from home, from the GP surgery or from another hospital.

DAY CASE SURGERY

- Day case surgery has advantages for both patient and hospital.
- Benefits for the patient:
  - Avoids an overnight stay in hospital so:
  - Does not have to bring nightclothes or undergo routine admission
  - Sleeps in their own bed postoperatively
  - Avoids an unusual and potentially disruptive hospital environment
  - Avoids an extra day in hospital with further disruption of work and other activities
  - Reduced exposure to infection from in-patient organisms.
- Benefits for the hospital:
  - Can provide a self-sufficient cost-effective day-care unit, with appropriate facilities

- Reduces costs of overnight stay
- Less disruption to in-patient services and unjustified use of scarce resources
- Rapid management and turnover of minor operations that might otherwise not get into hospital
- Shortened waiting lists
- Releases beds for more complex procedures.
- To be successful, there must be clear local guidelines ensuring appropriate choice of patient and procedure.

Choice of patient

The patient must:

- Be happy with the approach
- Fully understand, and be capable and willing to comply with, the instructions
- Be likely to attend
- Have been fully assessed in the out-patient department, including blood pressure, urine analysis and appropriate investigation
- Be usually American Society of Anesthesiologists (ASA) grade I (page 25) but for short minor procedures such as an examination under anaesthesia (EUA), grade II and even grade III may be appropriate
- Have no previous problems with general anaesthesia, where this is proposed
- Have no need for premedication or demonstrate indications of this (page 25)
- Be able to come having starved for 6 hours, children for 4 hours
- Have a responsible carer available, even if the patient usually lives alone
- Live within easy access of a hospital with transport available, should a night return be required.

Avoid:

- Babies, the disabled and the elderly, type I diabetics, moderate to severe hypertensives and patients with known coagulation problems.

Choice of procedure

- These should be short, usually less than an hour.
- GA is possible but full recovery time must be available.
- Short incisions, not laparotomy.
- Low complication rate, and low risk of bleeding.
- Pain must be controlled with simple analgesia.
- Only routine monitoring must be needed.
- No specialized nursing, such as for drains or catheter.

- Typical procedures include:
  - Excision and biopsy of superficial lesions, hernias, veins, laparoscopy with or without additional minor procedures, examination under anaesthesia, arthroscopy with or without minor procedures, minor ear, nose and throat (ENT) procedures, minimally invasive radiological and cardiological procedures.
- Ensure that:
  - The patient arrives starved, having taken their routine drugs
  - The patient is not suffering from any new problems, such as an upper respiratory tract infection
  - Recovery from general anaesthetic is complete prior to discharge
  - The patient receives full instructions
  - The patient is collected by a responsible adult and accompanied home
  - That a responsible adult is available for overnight stay, to give analgesia and any other medication, and any dressing
  - A telephone is available and that the contact number of whom and when to call is known, including a follow-up progress report the next day
  - The patient does not drive or work with heavy machinery for 24 hours.

Disadvantages

- Senior anaesthetists and surgeons must be involved, to deliver a safe and efficient service.

- There is loss of ideal training opportunities on minor procedures for trainees.
- If the patient does require overnight admission, this is as an emergency with disruption of other services.

PRE-OPERATIVE ASSESSMENT

- Pre-operative assessment quantifies the severity of the primary disease and any co-morbidity. This enables the high-risk patient to be identified and, where possible, their condition to be improved prior to surgery.
- Although age is not an independent predictive outcome, the increased incidence of associated disease is, and 70% of peri-operative deaths occur in patients over 70 years of age (although this group comprises only 25% of operations); mortality is increased eightfold in patients over the age of 80 years.
- Trauma is a major cause of death in the young, severe sepsis in all ages, and cardiorespiratory disease with increasing age. Operative mortality increases sharply with failure of more than one organ system.
- Some indication of cardiorespiratory function is given by a patient's ability to get out of bed, walk around it and climb a flight of stairs.
- More refined measures of tissue oxygen availability are the calculation of cardiac index, global oxygen delivery index and oxygen consumption index, although these require pulmonary artery catheterization. Cardiac output can be measured non-invasively with transoesophageal Doppler and indirect markers of abnormal oxygen delivery are an increased base excess, raised serum lactate, and a reduced mixed venous oxygen saturation.
- A number of objective peri-operative risk scoring systems have been developed [e.g. by the ASA (page 25) and the physiological and operative severity score for the enumeration of mortality and morbidity (POSSUM)]. Urgent and emergency surgery increase operative risk, indicating both the severity of the presenting disease and the lack of time to treat its co-morbidity.

- Assessment may indicate that surgery should not be undertaken without initial improvement of the patient's condition. When this is not possible, use of extensive resources for an inevitably poor outcome may be inappropriate. Consideration must also be given to the distress caused by such procedures both to relatives and the surgical team.

- Pre-operative **optimizing strategies** ensure that high-risk patients receive appropriate resuscitation prior to major surgery. They may include a period of pre-operative hospitalization to improve pre-morbid disease states and to control existing or newly introduced medication for cardiac and respiratory disease, diabetes, antibiotics and analgesics (page 44).

- Anaemia may require transfusion and intravascular volume must be returned to normal. This may require the judicious use of inotropes to improve stroke volume where cardiac function permits.

- Prophylaxis against peri-operative myocardial ischaemia in high-risk patients includes beta blockers and alpha 2 antagonists, to reduce blood pressure and heart rate and minimize myocardial workload. Additional oxygen may be required in both respiratory and cardiac disease. This can be delivered nasally or by mask and severe sepsis may require mechanical ventilation.

- Close liaison between surgeons, physicians and anaesthetists is important in all high-risk patients. Failure to improve cardiac function and oxygen delivery by these various manoeuvres is an indicator of poor outcome and alternatives to major surgery may be more appropriate.

PERI-OPERATIVE DRUG MANAGEMENT

- The majority of patients undergoing major surgery are already on some form of medication. This regimen is likely to be affected by anaesthesia and during the immediate postoperative phase, and new medication may be added and previous regimens revised.

- Medication should be discussed with the anaesthetic department and, preferably, the anaesthetist concerned.

Also, discussions with the pharmacy or visiting their website are likely to provide guidelines on peri-operative drug management.

- Non-essential medication may be omitted, but it is desirable to continue effective drugs and present a well-controlled patient for anaesthesia. Administration of essential oral medication can be made with up to 30 mL of water up to the time of surgery.
- Some drugs may be already prescribed intravenously and, if gastric stasis or alimentary absorption is in question, intravenous forms of the same or an equivalent medication should be considered, this being discussed with the responsible medical team.
- A few drugs, such as anticoagulants, insulin and steroids, may have to be modified over the peri-operative period (see below).
- **Pain** medication is considered on page 44.
- Pre-operative analgesia can be given orally or by suppository (diclofenac) or, for severe pain, intravenous morphine by a patient-controlled device. Discussion with the anaesthetist can provide continuity of pre- and postoperative pain management.
- In **cardiac** medication, beta blockers and digoxin are available as intravenous preparations, but note that digoxin given intravenously requires a 30% smaller dose than that given orally. Sublingual nitrates can be taken up to the time of anaesthesia. Most anti-arrhythmics are available for intravenous dosing and in the management of hypertension, angiotensin-converting enzyme (ACE) inhibitors and calcium blockers can be taken orally until the time of surgery. Potassium-sparing diuretics are omitted on the day of surgery. Frusemide and bumetanide are available in intravenous forms.
- For bronchodilators, inhalers may be used up to the time of surgery and aminophylline is available as an intravenous preparation.
- Of the various psychotherapeutic drugs, monoamine-oxidase inhibitors (MAOIs) should be withdrawn slowly over a 2 week pre-operative period. Tricyclics should be discussed with the anaesthetist, and lithium is best stopped, in the case of major surgery, 3 days pre-operatively.

Diabetes

- Diabetic patients should be managed using local guidelines, reviewing the patient's current medication and efficiency of control, and any prior surgery and its outcome. The blood sugar levels should be less than 13 mmol/L at the commencement of an elective procedure, and maintained between 8 and 11 mmol/L during the peri-operative phase, monitoring blood sugar and potassium levels hourly during the operation.
- Type I diabetic patients are brought into hospital 3 days pre-operatively and their insulin requirements prescribed as short- and intermediate-acting insulin. The patient is scheduled for the first operation of the day, the early morning dose of insulin is omitted, but an insulin/glucose infusion is commenced of 15 units in 500 mL of 5% or 10% dextrose, with 10 mmol of potassium chloride added. An hourly infusion of 100 mL delivers 3 units of insulin.
- If the blood sugar level falls below 5 mmol/L, insulin is decreased by 4 units/500 mL. If it falls below 3 mmol/L, the infusion is stopped for 1 hour. If the blood sugar rises above 10 mmol, a further 4 units of insulin is added to the initial concentration. Sensitivity of the patient to insulin is known within a few hours; the determined concentration, with regular monitoring, is continued through the postoperative phase, until the patient is feeding and their usual dose can be reinstated.
- Alternatively, a sliding scale of an infusion of insulin 1 unit/mL in 0.9% saline is prescribed as below, balanced with 5% dextrose infusion at 125 mL/hour (NB checking blood sugar hourly whatever the regimen).

Blood glucose (BM)	Infusion rate
<4 mmol/L	0.5 units/hour
4–15 mmol/L	2 units/hour
>15–20 mmol/L	4 units/hour
>20 mmol/L	Review

- Type II diabetic patients are converted to treatment with short-acting sulphonylureas, 2–3 days pre-operatively;

operative management is as for type I. When eating commences, the previous regimen of oral hypoglycaemic agents is reintroduced, but additional temporary subcutaneous insulin may be required for effective control of blood sugar levels.

- Patients are placed on **steroids** for adrenal replacement as in Addison's disease or Cushing's syndrome, for immunosuppression, and in the treatment of a number of diseases, including connective tissue disorders, allergies and malignancy. Side-effects of the drug include hyperglycaemia, fluid retention, osteoporosis, muscle wasting, hypokalaemia, hypertension, centripetal obesity, striae, fragile skin and acne.
- For the peri-operative period, medication is with intramuscular (i.m.) hydrocortisone 100 mg four times a day. The patient is converted back onto their pre-operative therapy 1–2 days after major complications have subsided.

Anticoagulation

- Anticoagulants are prescribed for proven venous thromboembolism (3–6 months after the initial episode but long-term for recurrent problems and pulmonary emboli), uncontrolled atrial fibrillation, cardiomyopathy, and long-term for mechanical cardiac valves and in bio-prosthetic valves where rhythm abnormalities persist. Also for recurrent thromboembolic problems, in grafts and vascular disease.
- The level of anticoagulation for warfarin medication is an international normalized ratio (INR) of two to three times the normal range. Severe bleeding problems can be treated with vitamin K 1 mg, which can be repeated, and fresh frozen plasma (FFP). When major surgery is to be undertaken, warfarin is stopped 2–3 days pre-operatively and, if there is high risk, such as of recurrent pulmonary emboli and embolization from auricular fibrillation, the patient is treated with intra-venous heparin; commence with 5000 international units and continue with 1000–2000 international units per hour. The dosage is monitored by an activated partial thromboplastin time (APTT).

- Aspirin is stopped 3–4 days pre-operatively and oestrogen-based contraceptive medication 4 weeks pre-operatively.
- Pre- and postoperative prophylaxis against deep vein thrombosis (DVT) (in high-risk patients, including those with a history of previous DVT, malignancy, obesity and those aged over 40 years) is with subcutaneous low molecular weight heparin daily; the dose depends on the chosen preparation and is higher with major surgery; no coagulation monitoring is used in this regimen. It is continued until full mobility has returned, usually at the time of discharge.
- Supportive compression stockings are also effective in DVT reduction and may be used routinely, or given as an additional therapy to the high-risk group postoperatively.
- Intermittent pneumatic calf compression may be used during surgery.

Jaundice

- Patients with obstructive jaundice may require surgery to relieve biliary obstruction by gallstones, cholangiocarcinoma or carcinoma of the pancreas.
- The jaundiced patient undergoing surgery is at risk from renal failure (the hepatorenal syndrome), bleeding from depleted vitamin K-dependent clotting factors (II, V, VII, IX, X), increased susceptibility to infection, and poor wound healing and recovery, as the underlying conditions often lead to malnourishment, and the surgery and its complications may necessitate long periods when the patient receives 'nil by mouth'.
- The need for such surgery is reduced by minimally invasive techniques, such as the placement of biliary stents at endoscopic retrograde cholangio-pancreatography (ERCP) or by a radiologically guided percutaneous transhepatic route. When possible, these techniques should be used to drain the biliary tree prior to any surgical procedure.
- Vitamin K 10 mg i.m. is given, and clotting studies are checked prior to surgery (oral vitamin K is not well absorbed in these cases, as it is a fat-soluble vitamin – fat absorption is impaired in biliary obstruction, because of the lack of bile salts). International

normalized ratio should be less than 1.5 to avoid excessive operative bleeding, and, if urgent surgery is required, FFP should be administered immediately before and during the procedure, as required.

- Accurate hourly fluid balance must be established pre-operatively, and intravenous (i.v.) fluids must be given, to ensure adequate urine output. Patients with cardiac disease or sepsis should undergo central venous monitoring, and, in some cases, dopamine infusions and mannitol may be required.
- Antibiotic prophylaxis is essential, ciprofloxacin 400 mg i.v. twice daily (bd) being a common choice.
- Total parenteral nutrition is often required, and place-ment of a feeding jejunostomy tube for distal enteral nutrition should be considered at surgery.

Antibiotics

- Antibiotics play an essential role in the management of infection. Their choice relates to the organism and its sensitivities, when these are known. At other times the site of infection, the clinical picture and where the patient is situated, provide a guide to the likely organism. Blood cultures are sometimes positive in the absence of an obvious source, and indicate the appropriate antibiotic.
- Other decisions to be made are the route of admin-istration, the dose and the duration of antibiotic therapy. The majority of antibiotics are taken orally, but in the hospital environment, when a rapid response is usually needed such as in the intensive care unit (ICU) environ-ment, intravenous administration is common. Some antibiotics, such as gentamicin, are given by injection only. Intramuscular injection, even when possible, should be avoided in children. In the hospital environment, the dose given is usually the highest that it is safe to use.
- The duration of antibiotic treatment for severe infections is at least 1 week, but single or combination antibiotics should be reviewed at least at 5-day intervals. When no progress is being made, consideration should be given to stopping for 12 hours and reassessing antibiotic management.

- A major problem in antibiotic management is the appearance of resistant organisms, particularly methicillin-resistant *Staphylococcus aureus* (MRSA; methicillin has been withdrawn, although the name has persisted). Resistant organisms have led to the introduction of combination antibiotic regimens and more powerful broad-spectrum antibiotics. Combinations are used if the cause of the infection is unknown, when multiple organisms are present, with resistant organisms, and when specific organisms are found to respond to tried combinations.

- Resistant organisms have led to a wide search for broad-spectrum antibiotics, but they carry the danger of destroying natural flora, particularly in the gut, where *Clostridium difficile* and fungi can colonize, producing antibiotic-associated colitis (pseudomembranous colitis), together with vaginitis and pruritus ani.

- Antibiotics have a wide range of complications, particularly when used in high intravenous doses. There are sometimes very narrow margins between the therapeutic and toxic doses, and plasma antibiotic levels may need to be measured (e.g. aminoglycosides) to reduce complications.

- Common complications are allergic responses, renal and hepatic failure, atypical infections in immunocompromised patients, difficulties in taking antibiotics by ingestion or injection, and the risk of antibiotics in pregnancy (theoretical teratogenicity of folate antagonists, such as trimethoprim; beta-lactams are the safest group in pregnancy and when breast feeding).

- Beta-lactams (penicillins and cephalosporins) may cause: allergic responses (there is a 10% overlap between the two groups); encephalopathy (particularly with intrathecal injection); drug fever; and bone marrow suppression. Second-generation cephalosporins include cefuroxime and third-generation cefotaxime, ceftazidime and ceftriaxone. Imipenem is a broad-spectrum beta-lactam.

- Aminoglycosides (gentamicin, tobramycin) and glycopeptides (vancomycin, teicoplanin) can both

produce ototoxicity and nephrotoxicity. Vancomycin
may potentiate aminoglycoside toxicity, while at high
infusion rates it can produce histamine release 'red man
syndrome'.

- Tetracycline, although having been replaced in many
cases by new antibiotics, is still a valuable treatment for
chlamydia. However, it should not be used in children,
or pregnant or breastfeeding women, as it can give rise
to brown staining of the teeth.

- Quinolones (ciprofloxacin) are central nervous
stimulants, and their action is potentiated by non-
steroidal anti-inflammatory drugs (NSAIDs);
macrolides (erythromycin) produce gastrointestinal
stimulation, and rarely ototoxicity and cardiac
arrhyhmias; sulphonamides (co-trimoxazole) may
produce a granulocytosis and renal failure; they are
contra-indicated in pregnancy; the last of this group is
metronidazole, which is a valuable treatment of gut
anaerobes, but can be hepatotoxic and is best avoided
in pregnancy.

- The wide choice of antibiotics, the potential side-effects
and the development of resistance have led to the
production of guidelines in most hospitals: these should
be observed, and advice taken from the microbiologist
and the physician in charge of infection control, in
difficult management decisions.

- Every effort should be made to culture the organism
before commencing antibiotic therapy. This includes
taking samples of blood (from more than one site),
urine, sputum, wounds, discharge, drains, and the tips
of all vascular cannulae that are removed.

Specific infections

- **Intra-abdominal** infection will not resolve without
initial abscess drainage. Organisms include enterococci,
coliforms and anaerobes. Combination antibiotics
are usually required, together with treatment of
yeast colonization. Second- or third-generation
cephalosporins, combined with metronidazole or a
broad-spectrum beta-lactam, such as imipenem, are
appropriate.

- Diarrhoea associated with *Clostridium difficile* is treated by an oral preparation, initially metronidazole, possibly through a nasogastric tube. If this is unsuccessful, vancomycin is used.
- In spite of routine **urinary** catheterization in the ICU, severe bacterial infection is uncommon, although candidiasis is increasingly encountered. In severe bacterial infection, the organism must be identified. The common treatment is with co-trimoxazole or a cephalosporin.
- **Respiratory** infections such as chronic bronchitis and uncomplicated community-acquired infection can be treated with amoxicillin on its own or combined with clavulanic acid (co-amoxiclav). Mixed infections are managed with second- or third-generation cephalosporins, while the mixed organisms of aspiration pneumonia should have metronidazole added to these regimens.
- **Ventilator-associated pneumonia (VAP)** encountered in an ICU, like many cannula infections, is commonly caused by a resistant organism, usually *Staphylococcus aureus* or *Pseudomonas aeruginosa*; MRSA is treated with high levels of intravenous vancomycin. Colonization of cannulae with this organism and yeast is an indication for removal of the cannula. *Pseudomonas aeruginosa* in these situations is best treated with a combination of antibiotics to avoid the development of further resistance. Examples are an aminoglycoside with a broad-spectrum penicillin, such as azlocillin or piperacillin.

CLINICAL CONSENT

- Patients have a fundamental legal and ethical right to determine their well being and a valid consenting process for invasive procedures, including surgery, is an absolute prerequisite. The surgeon performing the procedure is legally responsible for consent but may delegate this function to a colleague who is knowledgeable about the procedure.
- A patient may consent by gestures, orally or in writing. For the consent to be valid, the patient must be

competent, should be in receipt of the relevant information and must not be under duress.

- The consent process consists of information provision, discussion and decision making before signing the consent form; this may take place over one or more meetings, depending on the nature of the operation and the urgency of the procedure; the latter may limit the quantity of information given but should not affect its quality.
- An oral consent is legally valid, provided the patient was adequately counselled on the procedure. Conversely, a signed form may not be valid if the patient was not counselled or given the necessary time to make a valid judgement.

- When general or regional anaesthetic is required the anaesthetist should address the benefits and risks of the anaesthetic with the patient in the pre-assessment clinic or ward when seeking consent.

- The doctor obtaining consent for an operation should ensure that the patient is **competent**, fully **informed**, and voluntarily **agrees** to the procedure.
  - **Competence** is the ability to understand the nature, purpose and possible consequences of the procedure.
  - Patients with psychiatric or mental problems may have enough understanding to accept or reject an investigation or treatment, but information may have to be delivered during lucid intervals, and piecemeal or repeatedly.
  - If a patient complies with an investigation or treatment, even if they do not understand its implication, it may be undertaken, provided it is in the patient's best interest.

- The clinical need for the surgery should be discussed with the patient's carers and next-of-kin, who should be involved in the decision making.

- Compulsory treatment may be undertaken in a non-compliant patient under the Mental Health Act of 1983 and its 1998 Associated Code of Practice, but if the treatment is in any way controversial, the matter should be referred to the courts for approval.

- **Children** and minors require persons with 'parental responsibility' to give consent on their behalf; consent is required not only for surgical procedures but also for routine investigations.

- The law considers a child of 16 years of age to have adult rights. A younger child may consent, provided they have a clear understanding of all issues, but their decision can be overruled in the UK (except in Scotland).
- If the parent or guardian of a child under 16 years of age refuses a clinician's proposed management, the clinician can apply to the courts if they consider the management is in the best interest of the patient.
- Under the 1989 Children's Act, it is possible to obtain consent from the courts for a specific procedure without making the child a ward of court (e.g. giving a life-saving transfusion to the child of a Jehovah's Witness).

- Emergency life-saving surgery on a patient unable to give consent must not be withheld but should be proceeded with, following consultation with colleagues involved in the care and counselling of the next-of-kin.
  - In an emergency, in a mentally incompetent patient or an incompetent child, a clinician may have to proceed with the procedure but may also have to justify this decision later in a court of law.

- A patient has a right to know about all aspects of their disease and to be involved in all management decisions – it is the clinician's job to provide this **information** in a sensitive and comprehensive fashion.
  - Even if a patient does not want to know, they should still be made aware of the basic details of their disease and its management; withholding information because it could do serious harm is the exception, but in that case it should be fully recorded and will have to be justified if the decision is challenged.
  - The information should be given, and the consent obtained, by the person who is to undertake the procedure. There should be a witness present, usually a qualified nurse, and this information should be documented.
  - The patient should be told the reason for and the purpose of the operation, the benefits, effects, risks

and possible consequences, and the management of expected and unexpected operative findings.

- They should be told what they are likely to experience, what type of anaesthesia will be used, details of the postoperative monitoring, and about the management of pain and bodily functions.
- The amount of detail depends on the intelligence, knowledge and understanding of the patient. It is helpful to know their education level, occupation and cultural beliefs, and this may be obtained from other members of the team.

Consent for research

● Research usually takes the form of a clinical trial of drugs, surgery and/or radiotherapy and must have approval of the local research ethics committee. The patient is counselled by the clinician and the clinical trials nurse on all aspects of the trial and about their freedom to withdraw at any time. A written consent form must be signed.

Consent for organ donation

● The procedure is an opt-in system of signing a donor card and/or registering with the regional transplant support service.
● In the case of brainstem death, if the potential donor had not previously consented, agreement must be obtained from the next-of-kin.

Refusal or withdrawal of consent

● A competent adult is entitled to refuse treatment and this must be documented following counselling on the treatment proposed. Refusal of a surgical procedure should not affect the provision of other means of care to which consent is given.
● Consent may be given for a particular procedure but refused for a possible additional procedure (consent may be given for a colectomy but not for a colostomy,

if needed). If the surgeon considers it is unsafe to proceed under the patient's stipulated conditions, he/she is not obliged to operate but should permit the patient to obtain a second opinion.

- Withdrawal of consent is permitted at any time after it is given. If it happens during an operation (in a conscious and competent patient), the surgeon should stop the procedure, if it is safe to do so, and address the patient's concerns. If abandoning the operation at this point would endanger the patient's life, the surgeon is required to complete the procedure.

ANAESTHESIA

- Anaesthesia allows surgery to proceed in an unhurried, precise fashion, reducing operative mortality and morbidity.
- Anaesthesia is not a normal physiological state, nor a benign intervention. Although mortality has been reduced from 1:1200 (1960 statistics) to 1:100 000 (2002), anaesthesia still carries potentially life-threatening complications. One therefore needs to know the preparation for anaesthesia, the principles of its delivery and patient monitoring, its dangers and complications, and the contra-indications to proceeding with surgery under anaesthesia.

Principles of anaesthesia

- Anaesthesia involves:
  - Administration of drugs:
    (a) Hypnotics
    (b) Analgesics
    (c) Muscle relaxants.
  - Maintaining the airway and ventilation
  - Maintaining the circulatory volume and haemoglobin
  - Maintaining metabolic homeostasis – acid–base control through ventilation and maintaining renal perfusion, and monitoring and managing blood glucose
  - Temperature control.

Patient assessment

- Anaesthetists commonly measure the severity of patient co-morbidity, and assess the risk of anaesthesia according to the ASA scale:
    - ASA I. Healthy patient. The pathological process requiring surgery is localized, e.g. a fit young patient with an inguinal hernia.
    - ASA II. Mild to moderate systemic disease which may/may not be related to the pathological process requiring surgery, e.g. a patient on medication for hypertension.
    - ASA III. Severe systemic disease limiting activity, e.g. a patient with angina on walking 200 yards.
    - ASA IV. Severe systemic disease posing a constant threat to life, e.g. a patient with angina at rest.
    - ASA V. A moribund patient unlikely to survive 24 hours with or without surgery, e.g. an elderly patient with septic shock from perforated diverticular disease.
    - Suffix E is added to indicate emergency cases.

Premedication

- Modern anaesthetics have reduced the need for premedication but treatment with one or more of the traditional 12 'As' (anxiolysis, amnesia, analgesia, anti-sialagogue, anti-emetic, adjunct to anaesthesia, antivagal, antacid, antihistamine, antibiotic and antithrombotic) may still exist.
- **Anxiety** may not respond to reassurance and may require a benzodiazepine.
- **Analgesia** may be needed for existing pain. Opioids are sedative and suppress respiration. The NSAIDs inhibit the release of prostaglandins, prostacyclins and thromboxane, which sensitize pain receptors; but impairment of platelet function may affect haemostasis. Topical local anaesthetic cream to anaesthetize needle sites is valuable in children.
- **Anti-emetics** include ondansetron and metoclopramide.
- **Antacids** may be needed, especially in the third trimester of pregnancy, and **antibiotics** are needed to

prevent endocarditis in congenital and valvular heart disease, in the case of insertion of artificial valves, and before implantation of prostheses.

- **Antithrombotic** agents may be indicated (pages 15 and 584).
- Pre-existing diseases may require continuation of medication, such as in steroid cover in asthmatics, use of bronchodilators, in epilepsy and in cases of hypertension. Monoamine-oxidase inhibitors should be stopped 2–3 weeks pre-operatively because of their potential for interaction with certain anaesthetic drugs.
- Children with their parents, who fully understand what is going to happen, usually do not require any pre-medication, but many patients with needle phobia and with previous bad experiences may need sedation with midazolam, temazepam or ketamine. These produce calm relaxation, but rational verbal communication should still be possible; sedation should not be so deep as to interfere with reflex responses.

Maintenance of airway

- **Manual emergency control** is achieved by opening the mouth and clearing debris and false teeth, extending the neck and using the jaw thrust to pull the jaw forward by pressure behind the ramus of the mandible on each side.
- A **face-mask** must be in full contact; with an oropharyngeal airway in place, this is only possible if the patient is unconscious or after neuromuscular blockage.
- The **laryngeal mask airway (LMA)** is used an as alternative to endotracheal intubation in much general, dental and facial maxillary surgery, but it is not suitable for use in the prone position, or for longer and more complex surgery, where higher ventilatory pressures may be required and there is a risk of aspiration.
- The **endotracheal tube** can be sealed with a tracheal cuff, allowing positive pressure ventilation, and also protection of the airway from aspiration of gastric contents, while allowing transluminal suction to clear pus and other foreign material from the pulmonary tree. Usual sizes used are 9 mm for an adult male,

8 mm for an adult female. In patients under the age of 10 years a cuff is not required to seal the trachea, and neonatal sizes are from 2 mm diameter.

- An endotracheal tube can only be introduced in an unconscious patient, or with the use of neuromuscular blockade. In difficult airways it can be introduced over a fibreoptic scope or through blind, oral or nasal intubation.
- Double lumen tubes, used for thoracic and thoracoabdominal procedures, allow ventilation of one lung so that the other lung can be collapsed for access to the thoracic cavity.
- Emergency access to the airway can be obtained by inserting a needle through the cricothyroid membrane or proximal trachea, or by a **tracheostomy**.

Induction and maintenance of anaesthesia

- Anaesthesia involves maintaining a balance between hypnosis, analgesia and relaxation through continuous monitoring, and by supporting the function of vital organs.
- Suppression of consciousness can be likened to sleep with diminished sensory processing, motor hypotonia, disconjugate eye movements and ventilatory depression. However, with the drug-induced state there is no arousal on stimulation, and protective reflexes, particularly of the airway, are reduced or lost.
- Anaesthetic agents are delivered intravenously, by inhalation, or by both these routes.
- The aim of **induction** is to put an awake patient rapidly to sleep, while controlling the airway with an LMA or an endotracheal tube. This rapid effect is usually by intravenous anaesthetic within one arm-to-brain circuit while remembering the effects of apnoea, and a 10–20% fall in cardiac output, which can produce dangerous hypotension, particularly in hypo-volaemic patients. These effects may be partly blunted by fentanyl. Intravenous agents are thiopentone or, more commonly, propofol. Inhalation induction is more controlled, and may be preferable in children and in

patients with potential airway problems. Common inhalation agents are isoflurane and sevoflurane.

- **Analgesics** reduce the stimulatory effects of tissue damage on mechanoreceptors, thermoreceptors and chemoreceptors. This reduces the dose of anaesthetic required and improves cardiovascular stability.
- **Muscle relaxants** such as atracurium allow lower doses of inhalation anaesthetic to be given, improving safety, particularly in abdominal surgery. Relaxation can also be provided by local anaesthesia, and epidural or spinal anaesthesia.
- **Ventilation** maintains oxygenation and normo-carbia, avoiding increased intracranial pressure in neurosurgery.
- The **maintenance** of anaesthesia can be through intravenous agents, e.g. propofol, or, more commonly, by inhalation agents, e.g. combinations of isoflurane, nitrous oxide and oxygen.
- The response to inhalation agents is variable – maintenance is dependent on continuous monitoring and adjustment.
- Stages of anaesthesia resulting from the use of inhalation agents are:
    - From commencing anaesthesia until consciousness is lost: normal pupils, muscle tone and breathing
    - Excitation: dilated pupils, loss of blink reflex, breath-holding, coughing and struggling
    - Surgical anaesthesia: pupils constrict then gradually dilate, depression and eventually paralysis of breathing, loss of muscle tone and laryngeal reflexes
    - Apnoea, loss of reflex activity and fixed, dilated pupils – fatal if airway and ventilation are not supported.

Monitoring

- The **pulse oximeter** is attached to the earlobe or a finger, and its two photodetectors compare the wavelengths of oxygenated and deoxygenated haemoglobin in the superficial tissues to produce the SaO_2 measurement. It is unreliable in saturations of <70%, and can give false readings in carbon monoxide poisoning, severe anaemia, and with circulating dyes; there is a delayed response to sudden oxygen desaturation.

- Continuous **electrocardiograph (ECG)** monitoring gives heart rate and rhythm; and alterations of the trace can indicate changes in serum potassium and calcium, and myocardial ischaemia. Non-invasive blood pressure measurement is essential for basic monitoring. For more precise rapid and accurate measurements – as in major changes of fluid balance and the use of inotropes – an **arterial line** measurement is advised. In the critically ill patient, a **transoesophageal Doppler probe** may be used to monitor cardiac output.

- **Urine output** is measured by use of a catheter connected to a urometer, and **blood gases** provide important information on **oxygenation** and **acid–base balance**. When cerebral function measures are required, as in carotid endarterectomy, **electroencephalograph (EEG)**, cerebral blood flows through isotope clearance, and **transcranial Doppler** may be appropriate.

Dangers and complications of anaesthesia

- Awareness under anaesthesia is a cause of great distress to the patient. It occurs in a paralysed patient with inadequate anaesthesia; the patient is aware of conversation, surgical manipulation and pain.

- The airway is easily obstructed in the anaesthetized and recovering patient as the tongue falls backwards into the airway, particularly in the obese patient and if there are any abnormalities of the mandible or with neck extension. Turning onto the side and a chin lift or jaw thrust are used to open the upper airway.

- Anaesthesia paralyses autonomic as well as sensory and motor pathways, interfering with vegetative function and having a potentially profound effect on body physiology. Smooth and cardiac muscle function is affected, and glandular secretion together with airway, baroreceptor and chemoreceptor reflexes, and the central control of circulation, respiration and temperature.

- Contractility and cardiac output are reduced and bradycardia may be accompanied by arrhythmias. Peripheral vasodilatation includes the splanchnic bed, and loss of baroreceptor control can give rise to profound hypotension, especially in hypovolaemic patients. Renal blood flow, glomerular filtration rate and urine production are all reduced.
- Breathing is obtunded leading to hypoventilation, hypoxia and hypercarbia. Loss of upper airway tone, bronchodilatation and loss of gag reflex and airway control promote aspiration of oropharyngeal secretions. With loss of gastric reflexes, this can lead to regurgitation and aspiration of gastric contents. This is particularly seen in emergency anaesthesia, e.g. obstetric cases.
- The metabolic effects of hypoperfusion and hypo-ventilation are respiratory acidosis, hyperkalaemia, and slow clearance of anaesthetic and other drugs. Insulin production is reduced, with resultant hyperglycaemia, and some agents are hepatotoxic, leading to further metabolic disruption.
- In the central nervous system, cerebral blood flow is increased, intracranial pressure rises, cerebral meta-bolism is reduced, and at various phases there may be increased or decreased electrical activity.
- There is loss of temperature control and protective shivering; hypothermia is accentuated by vasodilatation, exposure of the body and thoracic and abdominal cavities to a cold theatre, cold appliances and cold gases and fluids.
- Hypothermia increases blood viscosity and sickling, interferes with coagulation, and shifts the oxygen–haemoglobin dissociation curve to the left. There is bradycardia, leading to arrhythmias and possible cardiac arrest. Neonates, children and the elderly are particularly susceptible to hypothermia.
- The unconscious patient is susceptible to pressure damage, particularly malnourished individuals. There is loss of protective withdrawal or postural changes, and these effects are accentuated by low perfusion, leading to pressure damage on heels, elbows and areas in contact with appliances, and with lithotomy and trolley poles. Superficial nerve injury may occur (page 759).

- Excessive traction strain and angulation can dislocate joints, fracture bone and pull on nerves, e.g. brachial plexus.
- Excess forces can damage the back, producing lumbar or cervical disc protrusion.
- Manipulation around the head can damage the cornea, where the blink reflex has been abolished, and the retina, together with crowns in teeth. Diathermy pads must be evenly applied, and contact with earthed metal appliances avoided, to prevent diathermy burns.
- Endotracheal intubation produces powerful sympathetic responses of tachycardia and hypertension, and powerful airway reflexes that can result in laryngeal spasm.
- The anaesthetist may have to cope with major haemorrhage, unscheduled splenectomy, myocardial infarction, cardiac arrhythmias and cardiac arrest.
- Other catastrophic events include acute hypersensitivity and anaphylaxis caused by anaesthetic agents (these may be difficult to diagnose under anaesthesia).
- Medico-legal problems include patient awareness under anaesthesia and surgery on the wrong patient, or undertaking the wrong operation.
- The commonest postoperative complications are nausea and vomiting, and until airway reflexes are fully recovered there is a danger of aspiration of oropharyngeal and regurgitated gastric secretions. Prolonged ventilation may be complicated by ventilator-acquired pneumonia, particularly with resistant organisms.
- Other postoperative complications, including venous thrombosis, are considered on page 54.
- **Local anaesthesia** produces sensory, autonomic and sometimes motor paralysis. Spinal and epidural anaesthesia causes hypotension, and may be complicated by a dural leak, postoperative headache, haematoma and, rarely, infection.
- Occasionally, local anaesthetics can produce an anaphylactic reaction. Overdose may cause bradycardia, reduced muscular contraction and hypotension. Treatment includes intravenous atropine, fluid and vasopressors. Cerebral toxicity includes numbness of

the tongue and mouth, light-headedness, visual disturbances, twitching, restlessness and epilepsy. The effect on the respiratory centre may produce hypoventilation, apnoea and coma.

- **Neuromuscular agents** may produce anaphylactoid reactions and bradycardia, arrhyhmias, myalgia, raised intracranial pressure, hyperkalaemia, and suxamethonium-related malignant hyperpyrexia in susceptible individuals (page 72).

Prevention of complications of anaesthesia

- **Positioning** and careful handling of the head, taping down eyelids, placing heel and head pads, and padding trolley and lithotomy poles, metal contacts and beneath tourniquets, should prevent nerve injuries, pressure sores and diathermy burns.
- False teeth should be removed prior to leaving the ward. Intubation must avoid crowns and loose teeth.
- Hypothermia is avoided by keeping the patient covered, and the use of warm-air blankets for long procedures. Theatre temperature and humidity are maintained at optimal levels to avoid heat loss. Large fluid and blood replacements, and cardiopulmonary bypass fluids, must be warmed to body temperature.
- The anaesthetist must be ready at all times to manage haemorrhage, and cardiac, respiratory and metabolic changes.

HAEMOSTASIS

Normal haemostasis

- Haemostasis (cessation of bleeding) after division of blood vessels in surgery or trauma results from the contraction of elastic arteries and spasm of smaller muscular arteries, and the formation of platelet plug and fibrin clot by normal coagulation mechanisms. *In vivo*, the extrinsic system is activated by release of

tissue factor from damaged tissues. This is supported
by intrinsic activation by thrombin.

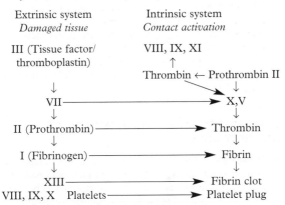

Extrinsic system
Damaged tissue

Intrinsic system
Contact activation

III (Tissue factor/
thromboplastin)

VIII, IX, XI
↑
Thrombin ← Prothrombin II
↓

VII ─────────────────→ X,V
↓

II (Prothrombin) ─────────→ Thrombin
↓

I (Fibrinogen) ──────────→ Fibrin
↓

XIII ──────────────→ Fibrin clot

VIII, IX, X Platelets ─────────→ Platelet plug

Measures of haemostasis and coagulation pathways

Test	Description	Measures	Normal value
Bleeding time	Time taken for cessation of bleeding from a superficial cut	Platelet function	4 min
APTT (activated partial thromboplastin time)	Time taken for blood to clot in a test tube when stimulated with kaolin	Intrinsic system (VIII, IX)	30–45 s
INR (international normalized ratio of prothrombin time)	Time taken for citrated plasma to clot in a test tube when stimulated with thromboplastin (III) and calcium (expressed as a ratio of a control time)	Extrinsic system (I, II, V, VII, X)	Ratio 1.0–1.3 (12–15 s)
Thrombin time	Time taken for plasma to clot when stimulated with thrombin	Fibrinogen deficiency	10–15 s
D-dimer	Monoclonal antibody test for fibrin fragments	*In-vivo* activation of the coagulation mechanisms	<0.3 mg/L

Disorders of haemostasis

Haemophilia A

Definitions

- Lifelong tendency to haemorrhage.
- Pathology: factor VIII deficiency.
- Aetiology: abnormal gene on X chromosome, sex-linked.
- Affects: males – all sons of haemophiliacs are not affected, all daughters of haemophiliacs are carriers, 50% of sons of carriers are haemophiliacs, and 50% of daughters of carriers are carriers.

Clinical features

- Painful spontaneous bleeding into joints and muscles.
- Deformity of bone and joint may develop in the long term.
- Less commonly: haematuria, epistaxis, gastrointestinal bleeding.
- Intracranial bleeding – may be fatal.

Investigations

- Genetic testing of chorionic villous sampling – antenatal diagnosis for children of carriers.
- INR: normal.
- APTT: prolonged.
- Factor VIII: <50 units/100 mL.

Treatment

- Intravenous freeze-dried factor VIII concentrate – for spontaneous bleeding or if surgery is planned.
- Genetic counselling.

Haemophilia B (Christmas disease)

- Factor IX deficiency results in a similar but less severe condition to haemophilia A.
- Diagnosis is confirmed by reduced factor IX level.
- Treatment is with intravenous freeze-dried factor IX concentrate.

Von Willebrand's disease

- Mild common bleeding disorder resulting from lack of von Willebrand's factor – a carrier for factor VIII, inherited in an autosomal dominant fashion.
- Usually presents with epistaxis or ecchymosis, but severe bleeding may occur after surgery.
- APTT is prolonged, factor VIII clotting activity is reduced and levels of von Willebrand's factor are reduced.
- Treatment is with desmopressin, or, in severe cases, von Willebrand's factor containing factor VIII concentrates.

Disseminated intravascular coagulation (see page 96)

Liver failure

- Liver failure results in reduced synthesis of vitamin K-dependent clotting factors (II, VII, IX, X) and fibrinogen, reduced clearance of plasminogen activator, and thrombocytopenia secondary to hypersplenism.
- Preparation of the jaundiced patient for surgery is described in the section on jaundice (page 16).

Renal failure

- Uraemia results in platelet dysfunction and thrombocytopenia, which may manifest as gastrointestinal haemorrhage or excessive operative bleeding.
- Treatment is by dialysis and platelet transfusion.

Anticoagulant therapy (see page 15)

BLOOD TRANSFUSION

- Blood is essential for life, carrying nutrients to, and removing waste from, the organs of the body, providing an inflammatory response to tissue injury, and containing the factors needed to maintain haemostasis.
- Prompt and appropriate management of blood disorders and blood loss is therefore essential to survival. When the onset of these problems is rapid, and they are severe, blood transfusion may be necessary, examples being

severe haemorrhage associated with trauma and major surgery, and some obstetric emergencies; blood products may be needed to control problems of coagulation.

- Blood, however, is not always available and transfusion is not without problems. It is important to understand the process of collection of blood, and the uses and complications of transfusion.

Collection, storage and distribution

- Donors are screened for anaemia, hepatitis B and C, and the human immunodeficiency virus (HIV), and donate 450 mL ± 50 mL.
- Blood is typed for ABO and rhesus factors, and in the UK, following anxiety concerning variant Creutzfeld-Jakob disease (vCJD), it is leukodepleted.
- Leukodepletion reduces the risk of febrile reaction, reduces the risk of developing antibodies to human leukocyte antigen (HLA), reduces the risk of contracting cytomegalovirus (CMV), vCJD, human T-cell leukaemia virus, and reduces the risk of immunomodulation effects of leukocytes.
- Filtering removes 99% of leukocytes, but also reduces red blood cells by 10%, and is accompanied by the loss of the beneficial effects of immunomodulation, e.g. in transplanted organs.
- The 320 mL ± 30 mL of resultant donation has a haematocrit of 0.5–0.7, and is preserved in optimal additive solution (SAG-M) and anticoagulant. It is stored at 2–6°C and has a 35 day shelf life. However, progressive loss of 2,3-diphosphoglycerate (2,3-DPG) gradually reduces the red blood cell oxygen-carrying capacity.
- **Platelet concentrates** are obtained by centrifugation of four donations or by plasmapheresis from a single donor; red cells are returned to the donor.
- FFP is obtained by snap freezing to preserve clotting factors. Rapid thawing produces cryoprecipitate; the technique is used to provide factor VIII and fibrinogen.
- **Predonated blood**, collected over the month before elective surgery, usually provides 2 units.

- The use of predonated blood is limited to operations with a well-defined moderate blood loss, such as hip replacement, and the guarantee of surgery before the expiry date of the donation. Although the technique avoids the problems of cross-infection and foreign antibodies, it is subject to the same problems of transfusing the wrong blood and bacterial contamination as with other forms of blood transfusion.
- Pre-operative **acute normovolaemic haemodilution** may be undertaken immediately before surgery, replacing the blood loss with crystalloid and using the collected blood as necessary during the operation.
- Peroperative **cell salvage** is collection of blood lost into a body cavity, filtering and washing it, and infusing it back into the patient as required.
- When **collecting and delivering** blood from the blood bank fridge, the details on each package must be compared with the documentation. On arrival in the ward or theatre, details of identification are confirmed with the patient, if this is possible, and with their wristband and notes.
- When **transfusing blood**, regular (usually quarter-hourly) observation of temperature, pulse and blood pressure are taken, and urine output is monitored for volume and any bloody discoloration during the course of the transfusion.

Indications for transfusion

- **Whole blood** is used in major haemorrhage such as in trauma and peptic ulcers, and for major surgery, such as cardiac and cancer surgery. In an emergency, O-negative blood is given, but most laboratories can provide cross-matched blood within 30 minutes.
- Blood may be required when tissue oxygenation is compromised, such as in the case of a reduced haemoglobin, and reduced carbon dioxide and arterial oxygen saturation. Haematocrits of <28% have an increased incidence of myocardial infarction. The level at which transfusion is considered is usually taken as 8 g of haemoglobin/dL, although the critical level of oxygen transport is not reached until the measure is

5 g of haemoglobin/dL. The latter is based on previously healthy individuals, and other factors such as age, smoking, pulmonary disease, hypertension and diabetes markedly influence management.

- Consideration is also given to transfusion of cellular components or plasma fractions. **Packed cells** are more appropriate in patients with existing or potential heart failure.
- Fresh frozen plasma may be required to reverse anticoagulation in liver disease and in disseminated intravascular coagulation (DIC), and the addition of 1 unit of FFP for every 9–10 units of whole blood transfused should be considered.
- **Platelet concentrates** are advisable in massive transfusion, and when the platelet count falls below 5×10^9/L, the partial thromboplastin time (PTT) is 3–5 seconds above the upper limit of the normal control, or fibrinogen falls below 0.8–1.0 g/L.
- **Fibrinogen** may be indicated in DIC (page 96).
- **Human albumin 4.5%** maintains circulating colloid osmotic pressure and, in leukodepleted collection, is safe from cross-infection. The results of its use in high-risk patients, however, have not been universally beneficial.
- Plasma substitutes [e.g. Gelofusine (B. Braun Medical Ltd, Chapeltown, Sheffield, UK), Haemaccel (Hoechst Marion Roussel Ltd, Uxbridge, Middx, UK)] are useful to restore circulating volume.
- When dealing with potential blood loss in a **Jehovah's Witness**, when it has been confirmed that blood transfusion is denied, their wishes must be honoured: the surgeon may wish to pass such a patient on to a colleague.
- Those involved with surgery in those refusing blood transfusion must keep peri-operative blood loss to a minimum and consider all other forms of treatment, such as haematinics for iron deficiency, folic acid, the use of erythropoietin, and antifibrinolytic drugs such as aprotinin.
- Although much is known of the structure and synthesis of haemoglobin, it has not yet been produced in a satisfactory form for human intravascular oxygen transport.

- Recombinant activated factor VII (rFVIIa) has shown promise when used in critically ill trauma patients. There was enhanced haemostasis at the site of injury, without systemic activation of coagulation.

Complications of transfusion

- Major blood transfusion is defined as replacement of the equivalent of the total blood volume within 24 hours.
- The effects of such a transfusion are to dilute leukocytes, platelets and coagulation factors. This, together with the infusion of citrate anticoagulant, increases the risks of bleeding and may progress to DIC and acute respiratory distress syndrome.
- Studies by the Serious Hazards of Transfusion Group in the UK have shown delivery of the wrong blood to be the commonest complication, and the need to ensure maximum checks, particularly at the point of delivery, cannot be overemphasized.

Immunological problems

- Incorrect incompatible blood produces an **acute haemolytic transfusion reaction**, presenting with fever, rigors and hypotension. Haemolysis produces haemoglobinaemia, haemoglobinuria, jaundice and blocking of glomeruli, producing oliguria and progressing to renal failure. There is loin pain and dyspnoea.
- Immune haemolysis is usually caused by ABO incompatibility; non-immune haemolysis is caused by bacterial contamination of blood.
- Hypersensitivity to donor plasma proteins (1% incidence of all transfusions) presents as urticaria and is treated with antihistamines.
- The transfusion must be stopped immediately in the case of all transfusion reactions. Blood should be taken and returned with the offending unit to the blood bank, an infusion of crystalloid should be commenced to overcome hypotension and mannitol given to promote urine flow. If renal failure occurs, haemodialysis is required and acute respiratory failure may require ventilation.

- **Delayed haemolytic transfusion response** can occur with recurrent transfusion, with the development of red cell antibodies.
- **Urticarial transfusion reaction** is related to plasma protein fractions and may be accompanied by itching. More serious responses, particularly with repeated transfusion of immunoglobulin A antibody, may result in an **anaphylactic transfusion reaction**, requiring urgent resuscitation.
- **Transfusion related acute lung injury** is related to HLA antibodies in donor plasma reacting to recipient leukocytes producing acute hypoxia and dyspnoea which may require ventilation. **Graft versus host** reaction to foreign HLA antibodies may also involve other organs.
- Reaction to **platelet antibodies** is not usually severe and is limited by the 10-day life of this component.
- Post-transfusion **purpura** is an unusual delayed complication. It is mediated by antiplatelet antibodies and a profound thrombocytopenia develops; treatment is by high-dose i.v. immunoglobulin.
- **Immunomodulatory effects** of transfusion are a global downregulation of the immune response in all transfused patients. These are the result of subtle effects of donor leukocytes, transfusion having been shown to be an independent risk factor in infection, with a higher incidence of recurrence of malignancy.
- Immunomodulation improves transplantation results in patients with prior transfusion. It may be associated with a higher incidence of cancer recurrence in those undergoing transfusion during cancer surgery.

Non-immune transfusion complications

- **Febrile non-haemolytic transfusion reaction**, as with major incompatibility, may present with hypotension. It is associated with bacterial contamination. The pyrogen response is to metabolic products of bacterial and viral contamination of donor blood.
- Major transfusion may lead to **cardiac failure**. The use of packed cells must be considered.
- **Hyperkalaemia** is commonly encountered, particularly in older stored blood, together with

hypocalcaemia, reduced 2,3-DPG and hypothermia, when large quantities of blood recently collected from a cold store are transfused.

- A large number of **infective agents** have been reported with blood transfusion, although these have been reduced with the practice of leukodepletion. They include hepatitis A, B and C; HIV I and II; parvovirus; CMV; malaria; babesiasis; brucellosis; trypanosomiasis and syphilis.

- **Iron overload** can give rise to haemosiderosis. Each unit contains 250 mg of iron, whereas the normal excretion is 1 mg/day. This is a particular problem in repeated transfusions, such as in patients with sickle-cell anaemia.

- **Local thrombophlebitis** is common at infusion sites, particularly when using small veins. A dedicated blood delivery line should be used and as wide-bore a needle as possible.

- A major factor in blood transfusion has been the increasing cost following the introduction of leuko-depletion and the use of cellular components from overseas, where the risk of vCJD is considered to be lower.

SURGICAL PROCEDURES

- For those following a surgical career, demonstration and supervision of surgical technique in the operating theatre is supplemented by skills courses, at both basic and advanced levels.

- The safety of patients and personnel is paramount; it requires shielding from radiation and lasers, and careful handling of heavy instruments and appliances, be these mechanical, electrical or optical. Anaesthetic gases are removed by scavenger systems and appropriate air flow through the theatre; this also controls the cleanliness, warmth and humidity of the air, ensuring that exposed operation sites on patients are not subjected to heat loss and dehydration.

- The identification of the patient is confirmed on their arrival in the operating theatre. This is by asking them (if they are awake) and from their identification wristband and their notes. The signed consent form, the operation and the marked site are confirmed, from the consent form, the notes and the patient. (Anaesthesia is considered on page 24.)

- Patients are positioned on an operating table to allow optimal access for the proposed procedure, whilst taking into account pressure areas where skin, nerves and other tissues could be damaged, avoiding metal contact that could produce an electrical burn when using diathermy.

- Antiseptic solutions, such as povidone iodine, spirit and chlorhexadine, are used to reduce pathogens over the operating site and operating drapes are used to exclude the non-prepared areas from the operating field.

- Sterile techniques are used to prevent contamination of the operation, but of equal importance is control of the spread of infection between patients and staff, particularly harmful organisms such as MRSA, hepatitis B and HIV. When such infections are known to be present, double-thickness protection is used by the operating team and for the drapes over the patient. Particular care is taken when handling sharp instruments and needles, and disposable material is double-bagged and incinerated.

- Students should attend operating sessions to learn appropriate dress and behaviour with regard to sterile areas, sterile operating fields, and sterile instruments and artefacts. They should assist at one or more operations to learn the techniques of scrubbing up and donning gown and gloves.

- Trainees must be able to safely handle and use surgical instruments, and be familiar with the names and categories of common instruments. They must be familiar with the key stages of common procedures, including: positioning and preparation; the use of tourniquets; relevant anatomy; instruments; incisions; haemostasis; sutures; prosthetic materials; wound closure; and drains.

- Operation notes and postoperative instructions must be complete, and student and trainee must be involved with the postoperative management of their patients.

POSTOPERATIVE CARE

- On completion of surgery, the patient is usually transported to a recovery area prior to return to the ward; seriously ill patients may be transferred directly to the ICU (page 88).
- The recovery area is adjacent to the operating theatre, and looked after by its staff. Here, time is allowed for the elimination of all effects of a general anaesthetic. This ensures that observations are stable, the airway, breathing and circulation are controlled, and consideration is given to pain management.
- On return to the ward the responsible clinician must be identified. He or she must be aware of the patient's history, what has been undertaken in the operating theatre, both routine and any untoward events, and there should be written as well as verbal instruction passed on concerning subsequent management.
- On arrival on the ward, all patients should have pulse, blood pressure, respiratory rate and temperature measured, and these and their state of alertness should be recorded. The patient's disease and the procedure undertaken determine monitoring, drugs and fluid balance, and subsequent management of the heart, chest, alimentary tract and the wound.

Pain and analgesia

- Pain is a major cause of morbidity after surgery and from its complications. It is a subjective experience and only perceived by the sufferer; there is great variation between subjects. It varies with the site, intensity, timing, quality and personal circumstances, including physiology, personality traits, psychosocial and cultural background, the patient's control of events and coping strategies, their fear, anxiety and previous experience, together with the attitude of the surgical team.
- Many patients are not able to indicate the severity of pain, but some idea is obtained from facial expression and posture, accompanied by tachycardia and raised blood pressure.

- A verbal rating of 'none', 'mild', 'moderate' or 'severe' is usually adequate. The use of a linear 10 cm scale, extending from none to the worst imaginable pain, and multidimensional scales, such as the Minnesota Multiphasic Personality Inventory, are usually only used in the measurement of chronic pain states.

Physiology

- Nociceptive fibres are widely distributed throughout the body, particularly in the skin and musculoskeletal system.
- Responses to pin-prick, incisions and temperature are carried in myelinated fast responding Aδ fibres. Multimodal receptors, responding to pressure, inflammatory mediators, including bradykinin and some heat responses, are carried in slower responding unmyelinated C fibres.
- Pain fibres pass centrally through the spinothalamic and spinoreticular tracts and, to a lesser extent, in the dorsal column; the level of awareness starts in the thalamus.
- Negative feedback is provided by a number of inhibitory neurotransmitters, including gamma-aminobutyric acid, endorphins, encephalins and 5-hydroxytryptamine.
- Positive feedback substances such as P and N-methyl-D aspartate, make pain outlast the stimulus and may be responsible for chronic pain states.

Analgesics

- Postoperative pain can be managed with a relatively small number of analgesics.
- **Paracetamol** (acetaminophen) 1 g qds (up to 4-hourly) is an effective oral, centrally acting antipyretic and analgesic drug for mild and moderate pain. It is cheap and safe. It is well absorbed from and not irritant to the stomach and reactions are rare. However, overdose (5–7 g) can produce fatal hepatic necrosis.
- **NSAIDs** are oral cyclo-oxygenase-1 (COX-1) inhibitors and are highly effective against moderate to severe inflammatory pain. However, inhibition of the actions of COX-1 also produce platelet and renal dysfunction, bronchoconstriction and loss of gastric

mucous protection. Non-steroidal anti-inflammatory drugs must therefore be used cautiously in young and brittle asthmatics, those with coagulopathies, active gastric ulceration and renal impairment (particularly in the elderly or for prolonged courses).

- Development of COX-2 inhibitors may reduce gastrointestinal and renal side-effects. Aspirin and other NSAIDs are contra-indicated in children (under 12 years of age) because of their association with the **renal** failure of Reye's syndrome.

- **Opioids** bind to the opioid receptors throughout the body, acting as agonists, particularly to μ (mediators of supraspinal analgesia, euphoria and dependency) and κ (mediators of sedation, nausea and spinal analgesia).

- **Opiates** are extracts of naturally occurring opium, but the term opioid also includes their synthetic equivalent. Morphine is the gold standard by which not only the opioids but other analgesics are assessed. It is most effective when given as an intravenous bolus of 1–3 mg in the adult, the dose being titrated against the response, with careful monitoring of respiratory and cardiac function.

- Codeine is methylated morphine. Although it has less respiratory depression, it is also a less potent analgesic than morphine. It has less central nervous system depression and is often the first-choice analgesic in intracranial neurosurgery. Other useful opioids are dihydrocodeine and oxycodone, together with tramadol, a weak opioid agonist.

- Complications of the opioid group include nausea, vomiting, constipation, dysphoria, dry mouth, meiosis, tachycardia, urinary retention and central nervous system depression.

- **Entonox** is a mixture of 50% oxygen and 50% nitrous oxide and is used as a fast-acting analgesic that does not accumulate, and can be self-administered by triggering through a close-fitting face mask. It is useful for short periods of analgesia, such as dressing changes and in labour.

- **Local anaesthetic agents** such as lidocaine (lignocaine) and the longer-acting amethocaine can be used.

Pain management

- Pain can be reduced or avoided with adequate pain relief. The team should be ready to treat the severe pain expected in abdominal and chest wounds, and must be appreciative of patient variation, analgesia being a basic human right, limited only by the ability to achieve it.
- Effective pain management, possibly under the guidance of a multidisciplinary acute pain team, improves postoperative mobilization, reduces respiratory complications and venous thrombosis, and alleviates anxiety, promoting normal sleep and early recovery.
- Treatment should commence pre-operatively, when pain is present, and towards the end of an operative procedure, using intravenous analgesia and regional blocks or infiltrating wound edges with long-acting local anaesthetic or by epidural techniques.
- Postoperative pain has two components: **background** pain is a constant aching pain, related to disease and the operative incision, and **breakthrough** pain is an acute exacerbation, related to movement, coughing, dressing changes and physiotherapy. The former is managed with long-acting drugs, while the latter may respond to short-acting medication.
- Nausea and vomiting may be treated with cyclizine 50 mg 6–8 hourly; to this may be added, or given as an alternative, ondansetron 4 mg qds.
- For mild to moderate postoperative analgesia in patients who can take oral preparations, NSAIDs with or without codeine derivatives are effective. Absorption is slow and therefore the route is for background rather than breakthrough pain. Suppositories have a similar effect but may be less acceptable to patients and staff.
- Severe pain is best treated with intravenous morphine. This can be accurately titrated against the response, and is suitable for background and breakthrough pain. The technique, however, requires an indwelling cannula and careful monitoring of side-effects.
- Patient-controlled analgesia (PCA) enables the patient to deliver small aliquots of analgesic through a pre-programmed syringe driver with a lock-out period to

prevent overdose. The drug is usually morphine, with 1–3 mg boluses and a lock-out period of 5 minutes.

- PCA is also applicable to subcutaneous and epidural analgesia. With the subcutaneous route absorption is more rapid than through the gut, and therefore the technique can be used for breakthrough as well as background pain. Absorption is less predictable if the peripheries are poorly perfused. A subcutaneous needle may be painful and cause bruising; it is less suitable in children and needle phobics.

- **Epidural analgesia** is very effective if the painful region can be targeted. This is particularly so with lower limb surgery, but it is also beneficial in abdominal procedures, promoting rapid mobilization, and reduced respiratory problems and deep venous thrombosis. It is an excellent means of achieving postoperative analgesia. The technique, however, requires expert anaesthetic and nursing care for the introduction and subsequent monitoring of the cannula and drug delivery. Lignocaine or morphine may be used.

- Postepidural headache can be severe and can persist for many weeks, implying continued leakage of cerebrospinal fluid through a dural defect. This may require sealing with a 'blood patch' (the introduction of 1 mL of the patient's blood into the epidural space). The technique may also produce hypotension, respiratory depression and urinary retention.

- Epidural haematoma and abscess formation, although rare, can produce severe pressure effects on the spinal cord, with paralysis, which may be permanent; the collection must be removed as an emergency.

- Other analgesic techniques include topical applications, such as a fentanyl patch, inhalation of entonox, and the traditional intramuscular injection, usually of 10–15 mg of morphine, although the latter may be painful and has a variable rate of absorption.

Fluid balance (see also page 55)

- Major surgery is usually accompanied by a period of fasting and fluid deprivation and, in patients with altered consciousness and those undergoing alimentary procedures, this period may be prolonged.

- Further fluid losses may be by aspiration through a nasogastric tube, diarrhoea and vomiting, an intestinal fistula, and sequestration of fluid in various body cavities and tissue spaces. Fluid input must match losses and urine output, and, when fluid balance is a critical part of management, timed measures of urine output are obtained by catheterization.

- Adult daily fluid requirement is 2.5–3.0 L (equivalent to 30 drops per minute of an intravenous infusion) and urinary output 60 mL/hour. Consideration must also be given to electrolyte and carbohydrate requirements and, if starvation is pronounced or likely to be prolonged, to parenteral nutrition.

- Sodium requirement is 170 mmol daily, but as a result of increased corticosteroid secretion related to operative injury, there is sodium retention for 1–2 days after surgery. Sodium requirements can be provided as normal saline (0.9 g/dL sodium chloride, equivalent to 154 mmol of sodium per litre).

- Potassium supplementation starts after 24 hours, if intravenous therapy is likely to last more than a few days. The daily requirement of 60 mmol is usually provided by using 1-litre bags of fluid supplemented with 20 mmol of potassium chloride. Higher concentrations must not be used as they may give rise to cardiac irregularities and arrest.

- 5% dextrose provides 50 mg/mL, and various combinations of 5% dextrose and dextrose/saline can be made up to satisfy the daily requirements for sodium and carbohydrate.

- Fluid intake should ensure at least 30 mL and preferably 60 mL of urine per hour in patients with normal renal function.

Gastrointestinal tract

- Nausea and vomiting are the commonest cause of delayed hospital discharge in day case surgery. This is usually related to the effect of the anaesthetic and other drugs and is commonest in gastrointestinal, ENT and gynaecological procedures.

- Paralytic ileus is usual after abdominal procedures and may occur after spinal surgery. The duration depends on the initial disease, particularly the degree of inflammation and the amount of gut dissection. It is accompanied by distension, nausea and vomiting, constipation and lack of flatus. Diagnosis is by a tympanitic silent abdomen and, on a plain abdominal radiograph, a dilated, air-filled gut.
- Treatment is nil by mouth, intravenous fluids, a nasogastric tube if nausea and vomiting are present, and as much mobility as possible. The latter is achieved by frequent changes of position in bed-bound subjects, and frequent rectal examination, to evacuate gas and to exclude any pelvic inflammatory cause of the problem.
- In the absence of any infection, gut motility usually returns after 1–2 days, but may be absent for many weeks in chronic sepsis.
- Postoperative drinking can commence once gut sounds are present and distension is minimal. Eating is encouraged when the appetite returns, the abdomen is soft and flatus is being passed; this occurs 2–3 days after small gut resection, and 4–5 days after large gut procedures.

Mobility

- Postoperative physiotherapy and early mobilization speed up the return of normal physiological function.
- The incidence of pressure sores, joint stiffness and muscle wasting is reduced, as are pulmonary problems, deep venous thrombosis and urinary retention.
- Pain control is essential to enable activity to take place.

Wound care

- Incisions are best made along the natural lines (Langer's lines) of cleavage where healing is under least tension. However, incisions also have to provide optimal exposure for the proposed operation and they can be in any direction.

- Good cosmetic healing is obtained by perfect apposition of the skin edges. This is possible in wounds produced by cutting instruments, such as a knife, but may not be so in trauma and dirty wounds.
- Wounds of less than 1 cm can be closed with stick-on 'butterfly' stitches [Steri-strips (3M Health Care Ltd, Loughborough, Leics, UK)] used to pull the edges together, provided the adjacent skin is dry and any tension does not pull them off. Clips and sutures are effective in larger wounds. The former are usually quicker to apply and remove, but sometimes do not control cutaneous bleeding.
- Clean wounds are covered by a dry dressing or a spray-on sealant. If there are no complications, they may be left alone until it is time to remove the clips or sutures. The tissue seal is watertight after 36 hours, and, if left undisturbed, allows showering and short baths, avoiding massage of the wound.
- Clips and sutures are removed once healing of the skin and subcutaneous tissues is sufficient to retain apposition during the anticipated subsequent activity. Subcuticular absorbable sutures do not require removal and provide a good cosmetic result.
- In wounds of the head and neck, where the blood supply is good and skin movement is minimal, clips and sutures can be removed after 3–5 days, checking apposition, the amount of swelling and any gaping of the wound edges. If in doubt, alternate clips or sutures can be removed and the remainder removed the following day.
- In wounds of 10–15 cm in length and where there is minimal tension, such as hernias and appendicectomy incisions, sutures can be removed after 1 week. For longer wounds, particularly of the chest and abdomen, that are subject to coughing and movement, clips and sutures should be left for 10–14 days.
- Drains may be intended for blood, lymph, inflammatory discharge or lavage fluid; these usually stop draining within 1–3 days. The drainage is measured and accounted for in fluid balance. The drain is removed once it has stopped draining or has minimal drainage.

- Suction drainage is used for rapid drainage of blood and/or lymph from closed spaces, e.g. chest or axilla.
- Chest drains have an underwater seal and are kept below the level of the patient. They drain air as well as blood, preventing a tension pneumothorax. They can be removed once they stop bubbling and fluid drainage has ceased. This is usually after 1–3 days.
- Drains in abscesses or placed alongside a gut anastomosis are left for 4–5 days. This allows healing, and the body's defences to combat infection and close down infected cavities. They can be removed once drainage ceases and clinical signs indicate that infection is controlled.

3

Postoperative complications

POSTOPERATIVE COMPLICATIONS

HAEMORRHAGE

- Primary haemorrhage is identified and controlled at operation but postoperative haemorrhage may be **concealed** in a body cavity, or in the depth of the wound or a limb, as well as **revealed** through a wound or drain.
- **Reactionary** haemorrhage occurs within a few hours of an operation when normovolaemia and normotension return and vasospasm relaxes; unseen, unsealed or inadequately tied vessels then bleed. Bleeding is accentuated by coagulopathy, from massive transfusion, and pre-operative and peroperative anticoagulation, possibly culminating in disseminated intravascular coagulation (page 96).
- Small vessels usually thrombose but may leave a residual haematoma, which can become secondarily infected and may require drainage when presenting with a mass or pyrexia.
- Massive haemorrhage produces hypovolaemia, fainting, anxiety, tachycardia, hypotension, hypoxia and reduction of urinary output. It requires fluid replacement, usually with blood, and catheterization to measure urine flow.
- Preoperative preparation includes resuscitation and treatment of coagulation defects with fresh frozen plasma, protamine sulphate, vitamin K, platelets, factor VII and fresh blood. Occasionally imaging may be required to identify the bleeding site but this must never delay essential surgery.
- **Secondary haemorrhage** occurs 5–15 days post-operatively and is usually the result of infective erosion of previously sealed vessels. If massive, it requires the treatment already outlined, but local control of haemorrhage through an infected base is more difficult, and may require proximal ligation of bleeding vessels.

- Remember that postoperative haemorrhage may be unrelated to the primary operation, examples being oesophageal varices, acute gastric erosions, colonic diverticula and ruptured abdominal aneurysms.

Water and electrolyte regulation

Definitions

- Extracellular water and electrolytes are controlled by ADH (or vasopressin) secreted by the posterior pituitary, which reduces renal diuresis and retains water.
- Osmoreceptors in the anterior hypothalamus regulate plasma osmolality (within 280–295 mmol/kg) by a feedback mechanism controlling ADH secretion.

DISTURBANCE OF FLUID AND ELECTROLYTE BALANCE

- Postoperative urine output should be at least 30 mL/hour and preferably 60 mL/hour.
- In order to maintain urine output, fluid loss must be compensated. This includes revealed and concealed haemorrhage, sequestrated losses (such as in paralysed gut, body cavity, ascites, pleural effusions), vomiting, diarrhoea, fistulae, vasodilatation (e.g. beta blockers increasing circulatory capacity), prolific sweating (e.g. fever), low intake (such as in upper alimentary disease) and peri-operative restriction. It is also common in burns, and may occur with renal loss and inappropriate diuretic therapy.
- Clinical features of hypovolaemia include thirst, a dry mouth and tongue, an inelastic skin, sunken eyes and the signs noted in the table below. There may also be muscle cramps and postural dizziness; impaired cerebral perfusion leads to confusion and eventual coma.

Clinical signs of hypovolaemia; 500 mL of fluid can be lost without any change

Features	Mild	Moderate	Severe
Hypovolaemia (mL)	1000	1500	2000+
Pulse rate (bpm)	110–120	121–140	140+
Systolic blood pressure (mmHg)	Orthostatic hypotension	<100	<80
Urine output (mL/hour)	20–30	<20	Nil
Peripheral perfusion	Cold	Cold and pale	Cold, clammy and cyanosed
Capillary refill	Normal	Delay	Marked delay
Cerebrovascular	None	Anxiety	Drowsy

- Investigations for non-haemorrhagic hypovolaemia (decreased extracellular volume) show the effects of haemoconcentration, with an increased haematocrit, a rise in plasma proteins, urea and creatinine, and an increase of urine osmolality.
- Symptoms are thirst, muscle cramps, nausea and postural dizziness.
- Treatment is by replacement of appropriate fluid, i.e. blood for haemorrhage, appropriate calories for daily requirement, intravenous nutrition for starvation, fluid replacement of losses and daily requirements, taking note of sodium, potassium, calcium and trace elements.
- The estimated volume of loss is added to a 3 L daily requirement. The table above provides an initial guide; pulse, blood pressure and urinary output indicate progress. A central venous pressure (CVP) line is essential and rapid infusion can be continued while levels of 0–5 mmHg are present. With repeated fluid challenges of 200 mL over 10-minute intervals, the level rises to 8–10 mmHg; this indicates that filling is optimal, warning that the rate must be slowed to maintenance levels.

Increased extracellular volume

- Peripheral oedema is caused by NaCl (sodium chloride) retention by the kidneys and an expansion of the extracellular volume by 2 L (15%) or more is clinically detectable. Precipitating factors are:

- Heart failure: fall in cardiac output releases antidiuretic hormone (ADH) and activates the renin–angiotensin mechanism, releasing aldosterone
- Protein malnutrition: results in hypoalbuminaemia and a fall in plasma oncotic pressure, leading to a shrinkage in circulatory volume, which, in turn, stimulates volume expansion and increases venous pressure, producing oedema
- Hepatic cirrhosis: marked peripheral vasodilatation and hypoalbuminaemia result in water and sodium retention and oedema formation
- Renal disease: a fall in glomerular filtration rate leads to sodium retention and oedema formation.
- Treatment is for the underlying cause of the oedema.
- Diuretic therapy may be used for any cause of systemic extracellular volume overload and stimulates the excretion of NaCl and water.

Hyponatraemia

- Sodium content in the extracellular compartment is regulated with the water content by chemoreceptors and volume receptors.
- Sodium deficiency may be the result of NaCl deficit or be a result of water excess.
- Hyponatraemia, with a decreased extracellular volume, is caused by loss of salt and water through the gut or the kidney; it is much more common than hypernatraemia.
- Overhydration can cause cardiac failure, and can also produce or accentuate renal and hepatic failure. Hyponatraemia can be produced by absorption of water from cystoscopic procedures, and is accentuated by subsequent encouragement to drink large volumes of fluid; polydipsia may be a psychological problem.
- The syndrome of inappropriate ADH secretion occurs after trauma (including surgery), malignancy (classically small cell pulmonary tumours), severe infection, drugs (such as cytotoxic agents and lithium), vasculitic disorders and sickle-cell disease.

- It may occur after the stress of surgery, Addison's disease, hypothyroidism and severe hypokalaemia.
- Symptoms include shortness of breath, pulmonary added sounds, ankle and sacral oedema, hepatomegaly, ascites and pleural effusions. Hyponatraemia is defined as a plasma level of <130 mmol/L, and confusion, followed by convulsions and coma, occurs in severe cases (plasma level <115 mmol/L).
- Treatment is of the underlying cause, increasing salt intake as needed.

Hypernatraemia

- Sodium retention as a result of an increase in aldosterone production is a temporary postoperative event but it may be accentuated by the infusion of normal or hypertonic saline.
- Other causes of hypernatraemia are primary hyperaldosteronism (Conn's syndrome), essential hypernatraemia, some rare renal conditions, and, in children, diarrhoea and salt poisoning, which may be difficult to differentiate. The condition may occur in diabetes insipidus (DI) and excessive water loss, as in an osmotic diuresis and nephrotoxicity (e.g. drug induced).
- Hypernatraemia is defined as a level of >160 mmol/L. Symptoms may involve the gastrointestinal tract, where vomiting and diarrhoea can accentuate the problem. There is thirst, nausea and vomiting; when severe it gives rise to convulsions and coma.
- Treatment is with hypotonic saline. (Be aware that 5% dextrose may produce water intoxication, with coma and convulsions; it is best avoided or delivered very slowly.)
- Pituitary DI, resulting from ADH deficiency, is treated with desmopressin (vasopressin analogue); this increases urine osmolality.
- Renal DI is usually the result of drug toxicity and is treated by withdrawal of the offending drug.

Hypokalaemia

- Serum $[K^+]$ is affected by:
  - Dietary intake (80–150 mmol/day)

- Uptake of K^+ (potassium ion) into cells (acidosis and α-adrenergic agents reduce, insulin and β-adrenergic agents stimulate uptake)
- Renal excretion (increased by alkalosis and aldosterone, decreased by acidosis)
- Gastrointestinal losses.

- Postoperative hypokalaemia may be produced by inadequate postoperative potassium supplementation or excess use of diuretics.
- Symptoms are lethargy and muscle weakness, paralytic ileus and ventricular dysfunction. Electrocardiograph (ECG) shows prolonged PR interval, T inversion and, classically, U waves.
- Treatment is with potassium chloride supplement, preferably via the oral route. Intravenous therapy must be closely monitored by ECG and biochemistry. Associated hypomagnesaemia must also be corrected.

Hyperkalaemia

- Hyperkalaemia occurs in renal failure, overdosage, transfusion of large volumes of old blood, tissue destruction (e.g. ischaemia, tumour breakdown, burns), leukaemia, malignant hyperthermia, primary aldosteronism, Cushing's syndrome, pyloric stenosis, with non-steroidal anti-inflammatory drugs (NSAIDs) and liquorice. It also occurs in renal drug toxicity, such as with angiotensin-converting enzyme (ACE) inhibitors and potassium-sparing diuretics.
- Patients are acidotic and hypoxic. Typical ECG changes are peaked T waves, a widened QRS complex and, eventually, asystole.
- Treatment is with intravenous calcium gluconate (10 mL of 10%) or intravenous sodium bicarbonate (1.26%), to correct associated acidosis, progressing, if necessary, to an insulin/glucose infusion (10 units in 50%), to increase transfer of potassium into the cells. Calcium exchange resins may also be tried but as potassium rises, usually as a result of progressive renal failure, dialysis may be required.

Low urine output

- Urine output is a valuable marker of postoperative fluid balance. Oliguria is defined as urine output of <35 mL/hour, and anuria is complete absence of urine output.
- Failure to pass urine may be related to the surroundings, with lack of privacy, postoperative pain, spinal surgery or epidural anaesthesia. This can be confirmed by percussion, palpation or ultrasound of the enlarged bladder. Flow may be helped by standing, seclusion and the sound of running taps.
- Accurate measurement requires urinary catheterization and this may also overcome postrenal problems of urethral, prostatic and bladder neck obstruction. Catheterization must be undertaken with full aseptic precautions and patency must be assured, if necessary by flushing with saline.
- Other postrenal causes of bladder and ureteric obstruction include tumours, surgical injury, ureteric ligation (particularly with operations around the cervix) and retroperitoneal fibrosis.
- Renal failure may be caused by renal disease, such as acute tubular necrosis, glomerular and interstitial nephritis, hepatorenal syndrome, diabetic nephropathy, hypoperfusion, toxicity from radiological contrast material, myoglobin and drugs (aminoglycosides, antibiotics, NSAIDs and ACE inhibitors).
- Prerenal causes include hypovolaemia, cardiac and septic shock, renal artery disease and aortic dissection.
- Clinical features of low urinary output reflect the cause. Hypovolaemia is managed with aliquots of 200–250 mL of fluid through a wide-bore needle, until the CVP rises and urine outflow increases.
- Renal failure may be accompanied by fluid retention with increased blood pressure, increased circulating volume, raised CVP, pulmonary added sounds, peripheral oedema, and rising potassium, blood urea and creatinine.
- Treatment is by fluid reduction, potassium reducing measures and, if necessary, haemofiltration or dialysis.
- Urinary tract infection is usually associated with catheterization, emphasizing that the use of catheters must be as limited as possible and aseptic insertion

techniques must be faultless. In spite of these precautions, low urine production, the presence of a foreign body and pre-existing urinary tract infection promote this complication.

- The usual treatment for urinary tract infection is encouraging urine flow with a high intake and prescribing mist potassium citrate, to produce alkaline urine. These methods may not be appropriate for the postoperative period, and a bladder washout may also be required.

DIABETES INSIPIDUS

Definitions

- DI results from ADH deficiency or insensitivity to its action and may be caused by hypothalamic/pituitary surgery, head injury, tumours (craniopharyngioma, glioma, metastatic deposits of some visceral cancers), infections (tuberculosis, meningitis), renal disease (renal tubular acidosis) and other rare diseases (sarcoidosis, histiocytosis)

Clinical features

- Polyuria, nocturia, compensatory polydipsia

Investigation

➤ High plasma (>295 mmol/kg) and low urine osmolality.
➤ Raised plasma sodium.
➤ High 24-hour urine volumes with failure of correction on fluid deprivation (water deprivation test).
➤ ADH administration results in urine concentration in pituitary disease but has no effect in renal disease.

Treatment

➤ Excision of hypothalamic tumour or intracranial space-occupying lesion.
➤ Medical therapy: desmopressin (vasopressin analogue) has a variable response and requires close monitoring.

ACID–BASE BALANCE

- Disturbances in acid–base balance result from altered excretion of carbon dioxide by the lungs, impaired excretion of hydrogen ions by the kidney, or from the production of lactic acid and other metabolic changes associated with critical illness.
- It is caused by acid generation, impaired acid excretion or bicarbonate loss in the gut or kidney.
- The anion gap = $([Na^+] + [K^+]) - ([HCO_3^-] + [Cl^-])$ is normally 10–18 mmol/L.
- Acidosis with a normal anion gap is the result of increased gut or renal HCO_3^- loss or decreased renal H^+ excretion; the HCO_3^- is then replaced by Cl^- to maintain electrical neutrality.
- Acidosis with a high anion gap is caused by unmeasured anions (lactate and organic acids or phosphates and sulphates in renal failure or salicylate poisoning).

Respiratory acidosis

- **Respiratory acidosis** occurs in type 2 (ventilatory) respiratory failure (abnormalities of mechanics and control of respiration, e.g. chest trauma, respiratory depression by opiates and anaesthesia), where Po_2 falls, Pco_2 rises and pH falls.
- Once respiratory acidosis has been established for a few hours, the kidney compensates by retaining bicarbonate – as a result the fall in pH may not indicate the severity of the acidosis, and bicarbonate and base excess (SBE) rise.
- Treatment is by correction of underlying causes, and supporting respiratory function with ventilation if necessary (page 90).
- Type 1 (hypoxaemic) respiratory failure [e.g. consolidation, pulmonary embolism (PE)] usually results in a fall in Po_2 and Pco_2, and is not initially associated with respiratory acidosis.

Respiratory alkalosis

- **Respiratory alkalosis** occurs in hyperventilation, where Po_2 rises, Pco_2 falls and pH rises.

- Acute cases occur in anxiety states, and can be managed by rebreathing into a bag.
- The state may also be observed in patients having mechanical ventilation, and can be corrected by adjustments of the ventilator settings.

Metabolic acidosis

- **Metabolic acidosis** is defined as a fall in pH resulting from anything other than respiratory causes. Po_2 is normal (unless the patient also has respiratory failure) and Pco_2 is normal, or low if there is respiratory compensation, and SBE is low (a large negative value).
- The arterial pH changes only slightly, but:
  - In metabolic acidosis there is a significant fall in $[HCO_3^-]$
  - In metabolic alkalosis there is a significant rise in $[HCO_3^-]$
  - In respiratory acidosis there is a significant rise in $Paco_2$
  - In respiratory alkalosis there is a significant fall in $Paco_2$.
- Metabolic acidosis occurs in sepsis and other states of critical illness (such as after cardiac arrest, major surgery or severe injury), with ischaemic bowel (page 568), in diabetic ketoacidosis.
- Clinical effects are hyperventilation and breathlessness.
- Treatment is by management of the underlying cause, good fluid balance management, and maintenance of renal and respiratory function. Bicarbonate containing Hartmann's solution may be used as resuscitation fluid in these patients (sodium bicarbonate 50 mL of 8.4% i.v.). Many patients require intensive care to facilitate tissue perfusion and oxygenation, with inotropes and mechanical ventilation; the latter also removes excess carbon dioxide. Diabetic ketoacidosis requires intravenous insulin.

Metabolic alkalosis

- **Metabolic alkalosis** is a rise in pH from non-respiratory causes. Po_2 and Pco_2 are usually normal and bicarbonate rises. It occurs in milk-alkali syndrome (excessive ingestion of milk and alkali in peptic ulcer disease) and with excessive vomiting in pyloric stenosis; in the latter, chloride ions are lost, resulting in hypochloraemic alkalosis.

- It may also occur with thiazide and frusemide diuretics, and in hypokalaemia.
- The clinical effects are apathy, confusion and drowsiness, with respiratory depression.
- Treatment is by abstaining from milk and alkali, rehydration with replacement of potassium and chloride, and management of the underlying condition.
- Also replenish Na^+, K^+ and Cl^- in the extracellular compartment to enhance renal excretion of HCO_3^-.

CARDIAC PROBLEMS

- Surgical patients are subject to changes in heart rate and rhythm, and reduced coronary perfusion; this may produce, or accentuate pre-existing, ischaemia.
- Tachycardia can reduce coronary perfusion and may be a result of hypovolaemia, hyperpyrexia, hyperthyroidism, anaemia, hypertension and ischaemic heart disease.
- Bradycardia (a heart rate of <60 bpm) is seen in hypothermia and hypothyroidism, but it may be caused by drugs (digitalis, beta blockers), and pre-existing ischaemia or heart block. General anaesthesia can convert partial to complete heart block.
- Peroperative cardiac **arrhythmias** are common and induced by many changes in body physiology. They are usually benign nodal or ventricular ectopics, but extreme physiological changes may give rise to potentially fatal ventricular arrhythmias.
- Causes of arrhythmias include general anaesthesia, vagal stimulation from laryngoscopy and endobronchial stimulation of the carina, pain, hypoxia, hypercarbia, electrolyte disturbances (particularly hypokalaemia and hyperkalaemia, and acidosis), hypovolaemia and hypervolaemia, hypotension and hypertension, hypothermia and hyperthermia, toxaemia, sepsis, and hypothyroidism and hyperthyroidism.

- Auricular fibrillation (AF) may be a result of mitral valve disease, ischaemic heart disease, thyrotoxicosis and hypertension, and may have been missed preoperatively. Fast AF may be difficult to diagnose clinically, but should be suspected when there is a sudden increase in heart rate. It may lead to cardiac failure and embolic complications.
- **Coronary perfusion** occurs in diastole and is reduced in tachycardia, hypotension, and reduced oxygen delivery due to anaemia, hypoxia, arrhythmias, drugs and abdominal distension. High epidural blocks (above C6) block cardiac responses to hypotension.
- Associated **myocardial infarction** may be silent. Atypical pain must be differentiated from oesophageal reflex, pleuritic pain and musculoskeletal pain. Although classically occurring on the third postoperative day, it may be during and immediately after surgery. Persistent hypo-perfusion produces irreversible damage to vital organs.
- Cardiac disease must be recognized and the cause diagnosed. ECG monitoring should be continuous perioperatively, particularly in the very young, the elderly, sick patients and all the conditions listed above.
- Patients are best treated in a cardiac or intensive care unit (ICU), where routine blood gases, electrolytes and 12-lead ECG monitoring are available. Treatment may involve management of the airway, breathing and circulation. Heart block, if recognized preoperatively, should be treated by pacing; uncontrolled fast fibrillation may require cardioversion.
- Myocardial infarction is treated with opioids and nitrate medication, supplementary oxygen, and beta blockers: the latter reduce myocardial demand for oxygen. Thrombolysis cannot usually be considered when anything more than minor surgery has been undertaken. Cardiogenic shock (pump failure) requires intensive monitoring and inotropic support in an ICU; mortality is still in the region of 90%.

RESPIRATORY PROBLEMS

- Postoperative pulmonary problems are common, particularly atelectasis and infection, but pneumothorax and PE must also be considered. Intubation, and other anaesthetic manipulations, traumatize the upper respiratory tract and the tracheobronchial tree, while general anaesthesia reduces ciliary movement.

- Dry gases produce desiccation, with viscid secretions and production of debris. This is accentuated by aspiration of oropharyngeal secretions and gastric acid, particularly in non-starved emergency surgery, such as caesarean section. Ventilation may not be uniform throughout the pulmonary tree and this promotes segmental collapse.
- Postoperative sedation, pain and diaphragmatic splinting by abdominal distension and bandaging reduce pulmonary expansion, and respiratory movement is also reduced in previous pulmonary disease, smokers, obesity, musculo-skeletal and cerebrovascular problem, and in the elderly and debilitated. These various factors may reduce vital capacity to 45% and function residual capacity to 20%.
- Hypoxia (defined as a Pao_2 of <12 kPa) may be caused by:
  - Lack of alveolar ventilation (airway obstruction, atelectasis, pneumothorax)
  - Deranged perfusion (pneumonia, oedema, acute respiratory distress syndrome)
  - Lack of alveolar perfusion (PE, shunting, pneumo-thorax, atelectasis).
- The airway is easily obstructed in the recovering patient, when sedation causes the tongue to fall backwards, particularly in the obese patient, and snorting and gasping noises are heard. The patient is turned on their side, and a chin lift, head tilt or jaw thrust is used to open the upper airway.

Atelectasis

- **Atelectasis** (alveolar and bronchopulmonary segmental collapse) may produce minimal, clinical or radiological signs; it should be suspected if there is a sharp rise in temperature or change in blood gases.
- Massive collapse produces dyspnoea, restlessness, tachypnoea (>20 breaths per minute), and is accompanied by lack of air entry, tracheal shift and a white-out on chest radiograph. Oxygen saturations

of <93% and central cyanosis are indications for urgent management (remember that >5 g/dL of unsaturated haemoglobin is required to produce central cyanosis and this may not be possible in severe anaemia).

- Treatment involves the use of nebulizers and supplementary oxygen, together with skilled physiotherapy and sometimes flexible bronchoscopy, to remove the occluding plug of inspissated debris.
- Antibiotics are only needed if there is secondary infection. Ventilation is required if infection progresses, or if there is diffuse collapse; it facilitates aspiration and this may also be helped by insertion of a minitracheostomy.

Pneumonitis and pneumonia

- **Pneumonitis and pneumonia** may be the result of aspiration or be secondary to atelectasis and pre-existing disease. Common causative organisms are *Haemophylus influenzae*, *Streptococcus pneumoniae* and Gram-negative anaerobes. Atypical organisms are encountered in immunosuppressed patients.
- Clinically there is pyrexia, tachypnoea, tachycardia, cough, purulent sputum (possibly blood stained), and increased respiratory effort, progressing to confusion and coma.
- There are widespread added sounds, reduced air entry and bronchial breathing, with diffuse changes on radiographs.
- Treatment is by physiotherapy and the appropriate antibiotic for the cultured or probable organism. Supplementary oxygen is required, but in chronic respiratory disease with retained carbon dioxide respiratory drive is dependent on hypoxia rather than hypercarbia; in these cases, when there is lack of improvement, deteriorating blood gases or a tiring patient, ventilation may be required, facilitating removal of secretions and pus, and adequate oxygenation.

Adult respiratory distress syndrome

- **Adult respiratory distress syndrome (ARDS)** is due to pulmonary capillary endothelial damage

allowing alveolar flooding, probably initiated by proinflammatory cytokines.
- It is characterized by progressive hypoxaemia, reduced lung compliance with normal left atrial pressure, and infiltrates on chest X-ray.
- It may result from severe sepsis, but may also be encountered postoperatively as a result of a transfusion reaction, massive blood transfusion or disseminated intravascular coagulation.

Pneumothorax

- **Pneumothorax** may be produced perioperatively by ventilatory hyperinflation and misplaced central lines.
- It is accompanied by dyspnoea, cyanosis and tachypnoea. On the affected side there are absent breath sounds, reduced chest expansion with a raised ribcage, hyper-resonance and, in a tension pneumothorax, tracheal shift.
- Chest radiograph shows absent pulmonary markings and lung collapse.
- Emergency treatment is by aspiration of air through the second intercostal space in the midclavicular line. For large and persistent defects, a drain is inserted in the fifth intercostal space in the midaxillary line and this is attached to an underwater seal drainage bottle beneath the patient's bed.

ALIMENTARY PROBLEMS

- Abdominal surgery is prone to septic complications related to the wide variety of organisms contained in the gut. Problems also include nausea and vomiting, haemorrhage, paralytic ileus, adhesions and intestinal obstruction.
- Management of most of these conditions involves nil by mouth, possibly with the insertion of a nasogastric tube, intravenous fluids with accurate fluid balance, airway, breathing and circulation resuscitation routines in acute cases, and parenteral nutrition in the chronic state.
- **Nausea and vomiting** are common after general anaesthetic and sedative drugs. They also may be

related to analgesics and antibiotics. They are more frequent in women with a past history of migraine and motion sickness, after gynaecological procedures, after long operations, and middle ear, squint and gastrointestinal operations. They may be indicative of obstruction and infection. Symptomatic management can be with metoclopramide or cyclizine.

- **Gastrointestinal haemorrhage** may be from oesophageal tears (Mallory–Weiss), varices, peptic ulceration or an ischaemic colon; it is accentuated by anticoagulants and NSAIDs. Diagnosis may require upper or lower alimentary endoscopy, and treatment with H_2 receptor antagonists, oesophageal banding and arteriographic embolization.

- **Paralytic ileus** is usual after gut surgery but usually resolves after 24 hours. It may be prolonged after retroperitoneal haemorrhage and operative procedures, spinal surgery and sepsis. The treatment is that of the cause, with nasogastric suction and intravenous fluids until the problem resolves. Acute gastric dilatation can be severe and the associated vomitus may produce airway and inhalation problems. Identification and nasogastric aspiration are essential.

- **Postoperative adhesions** are the commonest cause of intestinal obstruction and 1% of all laparotomies are for this complication. They also produce 15–20% of the causes of infertility, and generalized abdominal pelvic pain and dyspareunia. They are commoner with large bowel procedures and subsequent surgery takes longer, is subject to gut perforation complications and the need for intensive care.

- **Peritonism** may result from non-infective causes, such as blood, urine, bile, and pancreatic and gastric juices in the peritoneal cavity, but secondary infection is likely and the treatment is that of the cause, with peritoneal toilet. Air under the diaphragm is a diagnostic feature of peptic and other gut perforations, but, postoperatively, air persists under the diaphragm for at least 10 days and is therefore not a useful diagnostic sign.

- **Peritonitis** is usually secondary to bowel infection, such as appendicitis and diverticulitis, and to pelvic inflammatory disease. It may follow one of the disorders of the previous paragraph. Postoperative peritonitis may be a result of prior infection, but also result from gut contents, possibly through inadvertent perforation, as in dissection of dense adhesions, or leakage from a gut anastomosis.

- Symptoms of peritonitis include malaise, pain, pyrexia, tachycardia, distension and paralytic ileus. Localization of infection and abscess formation may lead to a palpable mass, or a pelvic or subphrenic abscess. A pelvic abscess can be palpated on rectal examination as a boggy, tender pelvic swelling, accompanied by tenesmus and watery diarrhoea.

- Subphrenic collections are more difficult to diagnose. There may be hiccups, shoulder tip pain, basal signs of pulmonary consolidation and an effusion, but ultrasound or computer tomographic imaging may be necessary for localization (pus somewhere, pus nowhere = pus under the diaphragm). Drainage of these abscesses may be possible by percutaneous techniques under ultrasound guidance, but may require surgical incision, debridement and insertion of a drain. Appropriate antibiotics are usually necessary.

- **Fistulae** connect loops of gut, the gut and another viscus (following discharge of an abscess from both sites), and the gut with the exterior; they are usually secondary to an inflammatory or neoplastic process. Cutaneous fistulae from high in the alimentary tract give rise to substantial fluid and electrolyte losses, requiring replacement. Digestive enzymes in the effluent can produce skin maceration, requiring barrier creams and closely applied stick-on bags to collect the discharge.

- Acute inflammatory fistulae usually heal spontaneously provided there is no distal obstruction. Chronic fistulae require extensive radiological investigation to determine the site and the cause of the problem, and to determine whether surgical intervention is needed or is likely to be successful in treating the condition.

NEUROLOGICAL PROBLEMS

- The aim of sedation and general anaesthesia is to reduce the level of consciousness, but these effects may be more than expected or may be prolonged postoperatively, particularly in the elderly, where confusion may be a feature of known or unsuspected dementia.

- Postoperative confusion is seen in the early postoperative period for up to 2–5 days, and is associated with prolonged hospital stay and convalescence. Causes are peri-operative hypotension and hypoxia, cardiovascular incidents, sepsis, and the side-effects of opiates, via intravenous or patient-controlled analgesia systems, other analgesics and withdrawal of habituated drugs.
- Altered consciousness is also seen with drugs, including analgesics, particularly opioids and benzodiazepines, excess local anaesthetic from regional, epidural or other sites, and central toxic effects of alcohol, recreational drugs, and hepatic and renal failure.
- Known or unknown cerebrovascular disease may cause peri-operative problems, including intracranial aneurysms, thromboembolic disorders and raised intracranial pressure, from trauma, tumours and epilepsy. Arterial disease may also be accentuated by hypertension, arrhythmias and coagulation defects.
- A number of clinical syndromes may produce an altered level of consciousness: these include hypoxia (producing cerebral ischaemia and preterminal coma), hypercarbia (levels of >9 kPa produce coma), hypotension (exacerbates cerebral ischaemia), hyponatraemia, hypernatraemia and hypothermia (coma occurring around 30°C).
- Some endocrine states may produce coma: these include hypoglycaemia and hyperglycaemia, hypothyroidism and addisonian crises.
- Other central nervous symptoms include **headache**. A mild headache frequently follows anaesthesia. A cerebrospinal fluid leak following lumbar puncture or drainage procedures usually subsides within 1–2 days of lying flat and rehydration, but may require epidural injection of a few millilitres of the patient's own blood (blood patch) and may persist for a number of weeks.
- Delirium tremens is an acute confusional state that may occur postoperatively in patients deprived of their regular alcohol consumption. It is monitored by serum potassium and managed by sedation and controlled reintroduction of alcohol.

- **Spinal and epidural blocks** may be complicated by needle damage, meningitis, haematoma and abscess formation, producing spinal cord compression, particularly in patients with coagulation problems. The effects must be recognized, documented, and pressure released urgently to reduce permanent damage.
- Certain positions on the operating table can produce **nerve palsies**, characteristically the ulnar nerve being compressed at the elbow and the common peroneal nerve around the neck of the fibula in a lithotomy position. Pre-existing nerve injuries must be fully documented.

FEVER

- Fever is defined as a temperature of >38.3°C and may be a result of infection at various sites, including the wound, the respiratory tract, the urinary tract, cannulae, the abdomen, and cutaneous lesions, such as ulcers (the term pyrexia also denotes a raised temperature).
- Infection typically occurs on the third postoperative day but may arise earlier if there is pre-existing disease. Children, the elderly, diabetics, immunocompromised patients and alcoholics are particularly susceptible.
- Fever also occurs in non-infectious conditions, including atelectasis, venous thrombosis, haematoma formation, transfusion reactions, myocardial infarction, some tumours (e.g. renal carcinoma), connective tissue disorders, drug reactions, and as falsified by malingerers. The latter can be achieved by exchanging thermometers and should be suspected with a sudden temperature rise without accompanying tachycardia or respiratory change. It can be excluded by carefully observing the patient and by taking the temperature using other techniques.
- Postoperative fever may be caused by coexistent disease, particularly malaria in the tropics, or in patients who have recently visited these areas.
- **Malignant hyperthermia** is an inherited disorder triggered by suxamethonium and producing a massive rise in metabolic rate. Temperature exceeds 40°C and is accompanied by rapid myolysis, hypoxia, raised potassium

levels and renal failure. The mortality is 70% but is reduced by management in an ICU, cooling by heavy fans, cold damp sheets, ice packs over axillae and large neck vessels, and, possibly, cardiopulmonary bypass.

- **Hypothermia** is encountered after exposure, cold water immersion and myxoedema. Thermoregulation is reduced under general anaesthesia and the body can cool to the temperature of the environment; this is accentuated by exposure, opening of body cavities, and delivery of cold blood and fluids. Patients with myxoedema, children and the elderly are particularly susceptible.

- Deliberate cooling, usually for cardiac surgery, is achieved by immersion of the anaesthetized patient in an ice cold bath or by cold fluid circulation through a cardiopulmonary bypass. Cardiac arrhythmias, including ventricular tachycardia, occur below 27°C and cardiac arrest at 20°C.

- Cooling in the operating theatre can be reduced by ensuring a warm environment (22–23°C), covering the anaesthetized patient, warming devices (warm water under mattresses and hot air surrounds), and warming blood and other intravenous fluids. The body's natural response to cold is shivering, which increases metabolic rate, but also produces hypoxia.

WOUND PROBLEMS

- Wound infections are one of the commonest complications of surgery.
- Wounds commonly ooze for a number of hours, particularly with coagulation problems, allowing entry of skin bacteria. Contained haematoma may also become infected by blood-borne organisms. Abdominal wounds are prone to infection, from contamination from existing peritonitis or from gut contents.
- The incision may have been made through infected lesions and wounds are classified into: clean (no contamination); clean to contaminated (minimal contamination); contaminated (significant contamination); and dirty (pre-existing bacterial infection in the operating field). This classification

determines the subsequent risk of infection, its severity and the likely organisms involved.

- Rational antibiotic prophylaxis is associated with reduced infection rates in all categories of wounds, but there is little indication in clean wounds and aseptic surgery.
- Wounds are best left undisturbed but should be inspected when infection occurs. This is suspected from malaise, pyrexia, and increasing rather than decreasing pain and tenderness. On examination, there is cellulitis, swelling and possibly discharge.
- After 3–5 days, suppuration may be present and pus is released by removal of one or more sutures or deeper exploration to remove infected haematomas or other abscesses. The discharge and pus are cultured and, if cellulitis and systemic effects persist, appropriate antibiotics are administered.
- **A burst abdomen** is a full-thickness dehiscence of part or all of the wound. The discharge is of a pink serosanguinous fluid, usually without infection or marked discomfort. The bowel is seen through the residual sutures or bursting through them.
  - The condition usually occurs on the 10th day, but discharge and diagnosis may be earlier. The aetiology is multifactorial: often a single continuous suture tears out of the musculofascial layer, this being promoted by distension and coughing. Poor healing may be the result of underlying disease, such as malignancy, anaemia, jaundice, pre-existing infection, malnutrition and immunosuppression.
  - Treatment is to cover the exposed bowel with saline-soaked packs and bandaging around the abdomen, while the patient is prepared for general anaesthetic (with a nasogastric tube and an intravenous infusion). The wound is repaired with deep, interrupted, full-thickness sutures and an antibiotic is prescribed if there are signs of infection.

CANNULA PROBLEMS

- Intravascular cannulae are essential for monitoring and treating severe disease, but they are not without

complications. Even wide-bore cannulae tend to
thrombose and all cannulae may develop painful
thrombophlebitis of a superficial vein, producing a red,
tender, palpable hard cord.

- Failed cannulae must be removed, and the cannula tip
  sent for culture. Cannulae frequently harbour infection
  and this should be suspected as the cause of an
  undiagnosed pyrexia; organisms may be obtained on
  blood culture.

- Attempts should be made to sterilize valuable lines with
  appropriate antibiotics, but if infection persists the line
  must be removed and, if necessary, repositioned.

VENOUS THROMBOEMBOLISM

Deep venous thrombosis

- The classic triad (Virchow's) in the aetiology of
  thrombosis is stasis, damage to the vessel wall and
  altered constituents of the blood. General anaesthesia
  and surgery interfere with all these factors. Stasis under
  general anaesthesia is prominent in the legs, with loss of
  tone and absence of contraction of the muscle pump.
  Endothelial wall damage is unavoidable at operation
  sites and this, together with the release of other
  inflammatory mediators, promotes both coagulation
  and clot lysis.

- Risk factors are elderly and obese patients, major
  abdominal/pelvic surgery, peri-operative immobility,
  intra-abdominal malignancy and previous deep venous
  thrombosis (DVT).

- DVT probably commences during an operation but
  symptoms usually appear after 7–10 days.

- Symptoms include pain, swelling of the calf and ankle,
  calf tenderness that may be accentuated by plantar
  flexion or dorsiflexion, and pyrexia.

- Propagation of thrombus may extend into the popliteal,
  femoral and iliac veins, producing oedema and the
  typical white leg (phlegmasia alba dolens, as seen
  postpartum). When the thrombosis extends throughout
  the venous system, the leg becomes blue from venous

stasis (phlegmasia caerulia dolens); this may progress to venous gangrene, which has an amputation rate of 50%.

- The condition may be bilateral and may extend into the inferior vena cava. Surprisingly, symptoms of all forms of DVT are minimal in at least 50% of cases. Other serious consequences are PE, and lower limb venous incompetence and its long-term sequelae.

- Diagnosis of DVT is suspected on clinical grounds and confirmed by duplex ultrasonography. Treatment includes prophylactic use of supportive compression stockings to reduce stasis under anaesthesia and when lying in bed, pneumatic compression devices during surgery, and prophylactic and therapeutic anticoagulation (page 15).

Pulmonary embolism

- PE produces breathlessness, chest pain and haemoptysis. These may be associated with fever, a plural rub and focal bronchial breathing. Chest radiographs usually show minimal signs, but there may be segmental consolidation, pleural thickening and a pleural effusion. A V/Q scan compares the distribution of an inhaled isotope with that of an intravenous injection of isotope: mismatch of the two scans indicates the perfusion defect. Computerized tomography (CT) is usually diagnostic.

- A massive PE is accompanied by sudden chest pain, cardiovascular collapse, and the vagal stimulation produces a desire to defecate. The outcome may be fatal. The ECG shows a tachycardia and the classic signs of right heart strain of an S wave in lead 1, and a Q wave and inverted T wave in lead 3 (S1Q3T3). Pulmonary angiography demonstrates the occlusion of a pulmonary artery or one of its major branches.

- Postoperative management of PE is difficult, as thromolysis of the embolism, the treatment of choice, could produce fatal haemorrhage. Embolectomy by an endovascular route or open surgery may be indicated in extreme situations.

- Standard treatment is anticoagulation with heparin followed by long-term warfarin treatment. Inferior vena caval filters may be of use for recurrent emboli or when anticoagulants produce adverse effects.

NUTRITION

Nutritional support

- 50% of surgical patients suffer protein energy malnutrition. Starvation may result from neoplasia, sepsis, pancreatitis and injury (trauma, surgery, burns), and energy requirements are increased in these processes. They are also accompanied by changes in metabolism. There is alteration of catecholamine and cortisol production, and resistance to insulin.
- Assessment of fluid loss can be difficult in vomiting, diarrhoea, enterocolitis, wound loss, loss through drains and fluid shift across damaged membranes. Assessment reveals loss of skin turgor and skin fold thickness, and weight loss. Markers include biological (albumin and total protein), immunological and increased lymphocytes.
- Nutritional support is required for:
  - Severely malnourished on admission
  - Moderately malnourished unable to eat adequately in the short term
  - Normally nourished undergoing surgery and not expected to eat for a week or more postoperatively, such as those with heavy sedation, intubation, dysphagia, extensive bowel surgery, paralytic ileus and conditions requiring additional calorie intake.
- The aim of nutritional therapy is to achieve a positive nitrogen balance and to provide adequate calories for energy requirements:
  - Nitrogen requirements = nitrogen loss (24-hour urinary urea in mmol $\times$ 0.028 + 2), generally = 3–6 g/day
  - Energy requirements = 50% as glucose polymers + 30% as fat
  - Electrolytes + vitamins + trace elements (added to feeds).

Starvation

- When exogenous energy sources are unavailable, the following endogenous stores are mobilized:

– Triglycerides (in adipose tissue) produce 30.06 kJ/g on oxidation
– Glycogen (in liver) produces 17.22 kJ/g on oxidation.
- They maintain glucose homeostasis, conserve body nitrogen and provide endogenous fuels to meet energy needs.
- The adaptation to fasting or starvation is initiated by a restriction in carbohydrate calories and not by total energy withdrawal.
- Therefore, providing lipid calories alone to meet energy needs does not prevent the normal adaptive response to fasting.
- The metabolic features of starvation are:
  – Decrease in metabolic rate
  – Decrease in glucose oxidation
  – Decrease in muscle protein breakdown
  – Increase in adipose tissue energy use.

Short-term starvation (postoperative 1–14 days)

- Adaptation in liver enzyme activity results in:
  – Fatty acid oxidation
  – Ketogenesis (as a result of increase in plasma glucagon to insulin concentrations)
  – Gluconeogenesis
  – Decreased urea production
  – Fall in protein synthesis and breakdown.
- These result in a fall in energy expenditure.
- Lipolysis and production of ketone bodies in the liver reaches a maximum within 3 days.
- Ketone bodies provide the main energy source for the brain (as they cross the blood–brain barrier) and greatly reduce glucose requirements and spare muscle protein breakdown.
- Reduction in liver glucose output decreases whole body glucose production by half.
- Gluconeogenic precursors are:
  – Glycerol from lipolysis
  – Alanine and glutamine from muscle protein catabolism (glucose–alanine cycle)
  – Lactate from glucose metabolism in glycolytic tissue (Cori cycle).

Re-feeding

Complications of re-feeding a semi-starved or cachetic patient are:

- Fluid overload: leads to fluid retention and congestive cardiac failure
- Mineral depletion: extracellular phosphorus concentration may fall to <1 mg/dL leading to muscle weakness, paraesthesiae, seizures, coma and cardiopulmonary failure
- Glucose intolerance: caused by inability of insulin to stimulate glucose uptake and oxidation
- Gastrointestinal dysfunction: as a result of protein loss from intestinal mucosa and pancreas
- Cardiac arrhythmias: occur during early phases of re-feeding.

Prevention of re-feeding complications during the first week:

- Evaluate fluid and electrolyte abnormalities
- Evaluate cardiovascular abnormalities.

Malabsorption

Definitions

Defined as failure to absorb essential dietary requirements in the small bowel; causes:

- Inadequate digestion: in post-gastrectomy, exocrine pancreatic insufficiency, cystic fibrosis and Zollinger–Ellison syndrome
- Inadequate absorptive surface: in short bowel syndrome, jejuno-ileal bypass, inflammatory bowel disease (Crohn's disease)
- Small bowel mucosal abnormalities: in coeliac disease, Whipple's disease, tropical sprue, amyloidosis and radiation enteritis
- Deficient bile salt pool: found in blind loop syndrome, Crohn's disease and small bowel fistulae
- Lymphatic obstruction: intestinal lymphangiectasis and malignant lymphoma.

Clinical features

- Crampy, abdominal pain
- Diarrhoea
- Abdominal distension
- Weight loss
- Anaemia
- Malabsorption is diagnosed during pre-operative assessment requiring nutritional work-up, soon after surgery or as a long-term consequence of surgery.

Treatment
➤ Surgical: in blind-loop syndrome, fistulae or Crohn's disease.
➤ Nutritional therapy.

Enteral nutrition

- Feeding may be by:
  - Mouth, if able to swallow and the feeds are palatable
  - Fine-bore nasogastric tube
  - Percutaneous endoscopic gastrostomy, when feeding is required for prolonged periods (after head injury or stroke)
  - Jejunostomy catheter, placed at laparotomy and brought out through the abdominal wall.
- Main prerequisite: a functional gastrointestinal tract.
- Advantages over parenteral nutrition:
  - Less complicated to administer; the diet content can be a normal feed that has been emulsified for tube feeding
  - Nutritional requirements are better known
  - Supplies gut-specific fuels, glutamine and short-chain fatty acids
  - Prevents atrophy of intestinal mucosa and the pancreas
  - Preserves intestinal mucosal and pancreatic secretory enzyme activity
  - Prevents cholelithiasis by stimulating gall bladder motility
  - Less expensive.

'Elemental' diets

Monomeric and oligomeric formulas:

* Indications: severely impaired digestive function (Crohn's disease, radiation enteritis, short bowel syndrome)
* Require minimal digestive function for absorption
* Are associated with bowel cramps and diarrhoea
* Are hyperosmolar and unpalatable.

Polymeric diets

Polymeric diets contain nitrogen in the form of whole proteins, carbohydrates as glucose polymers, and lipids as long-chain and medium-chain triglycerides. They are categorized into:

* Blenderized food formulas:
  - Poor palatability, require trans-nasal tube or percutaneous gastrostomy
  - Have a high fibre content (4–8 g/L) and are suitable for long-term enteral feeding.
* Milk-based formulas:
  - Palatable
  - Hyperosmolar
  - High protein content.
* Lactose-free formulas:
  - Most commonly used
  - Protein source: casein and soy
  - Carbohydrate source: corn syrup (glucose polymers) and starch (sucrose)
  - Fat source: corn and soy oil and medium-chain triglycerides
  - They are diets with a variable nutrient composition.

Tube feeding

* Trans-nasal tubes: placed so that the tip lies in the distal stomach or the duodenum.
* Gastrostomy or jejunostomy tubes: placed endoscopically or surgically, for long-term feeding.
* Continuous or intermittent controlled feeding with the aid of alarmed delivery pumps.
* Jejunostomy feeds are continuous; gastrostomy feeds may be given at 4- to 6-hourly intervals.

- Complications:
  - Mechanical: inadvertent intubation of the tracheobronchial tree in the unconscious patient
  - Nasopharyngeal irritation: lessened by small-calibre tubes (8 or 9 French gauge)
  - Tube blockage: requires intermittent irrigation
  - Metabolic: disturbances in fluid and electrolyte balance
  - Gastrointestinal symptoms: nausea, vomiting and abdominal pain – lessened by maintaining a semi-recumbent position and keeping the gastric residue to a minimum
  - Diarrhoea is associated with hypertonic feeds, antibiotic use and non-absorbable sorbitol (present in tube-administered medications).

PARENTERAL NUTRITION

- Parenteral feeding is needed for patients with heavy sedation, intubation, dysphagia, extensive bowel surgery, paralytic ileus and conditions requiring additional high calorie intake.
- It corrects specific nutritional deficiencies and prevents the adverse effects of malnutrition when the gastrointestinal tract cannot be effectively or safely used.

Peri-operative nutrition

In surgical patients who are malnourished, nutritional therapy may not affect clinical outcome unless the presence of malnutrition is an independent contributor to postoperative complications.

- Peri-operative central feeding should not be given routinely to surgical patients.
- Patients who are severely malnourished may benefit from pre-operative parenteral nutrition.
- Parenteral feeding is applicable to patients who cannot or are unlikely to tolerate oral or enteral feeding for 7 or more days.

Peripheral vein nutrition

- Indications:
  - Short-term use to cover postoperative period
  - As an interim measure when deciding on enteral or intravenous feeding.
- Composition: hypotonic dextrose with amino acids and low osmolar fat emulsions.
- Complications – superficial phlebitis; incidence reduced by:
  - Use of an in-line filter (0.45 or 0.22 μm)
  - Inclusion of an antiphlebitic mixture of heparin and hydrocortisone in the nutrient solution
  - Application of glyceryl trinitrate patches.

Central parenteral nutrition

- To administer total parenteral nutrition, a wide-bore dedicated subclavian or jugular line is required to infuse 2.5–3.0 L of fluid nutrient to the superior vena cava or right atrium.
- Central feeding lines may be:
  - A standard single lumen central line – a temporary measure, which must be changed every few days
  - A tunnelled silicone feeding line.
- Parenteral solutions supply all basic nutrient requirements (fluid, protein, carbohydrate, fat, macrominerals, trace minerals and vitamins):
  - Proteins: essential and non-essential amino acids to maintain nitrogen balance and replete lean-tissue mass in catabolic states (requirement: 0.8–1.5 g/kg per day)
  - Carbohydrate: in the form of dextrose has nitrogen-sparing effects; some tissues (red and white blood cells, bone marrow and renal medulla) require glucose as they are unable to oxidize fatty acids; other tissues (brain) prefer glucose as a fuel
  - Glucose stimulates insulin secretion, reduces muscle protein breakdown and inhibits hepatic glucose release; the amount of glucose oxidized is directly proportional to the amount administered; this should not exceed 7 mg/kg per min (11 760 kJ/day).

- Fat: infused as a 10% (4.62 kJ/mL) or 20% (8.4 kJ/mL) solution with an osmolality of 270–340 mmol/L
- Providing a proportion of infused calories as lipid reduces plasma insulin levels, sodium and water retention, carbon dioxide production and liver fat deposition
- A minimum of 5% of total calories as fat is necessary to prevent essential fatty acid deficiency
- Generally, 25–50% of daily caloric intake should be in the form of fat emulsions and the infusion rate should not exceed 2.94 kJ/kg per hour
- Electrolytes, vitamins and trace elements are administered concurrently.

- Large bags of high-energy lipid emulsion typically deliver for frail individuals 8–10 g of protein, 3.15 kJ of carbohydrate and 3.15 kJ of fat. Normal requirements are 10–16 g of protein, 8.4 kJ of carbohydrate and 4.2 kJ of fat. In sepsis, higher requirements within the 3 L are 16–20 g of protein, 9.24 kJ of carbohydrate and 5.04 kJ of fat. Minerals and vitamins are added as required just prior to carbohydrate transfusion.

Monitoring

- Baseline concentrations of glucose, electrolytes, creatinine, urea nitrogen, magnesium, phosphorus, calcium, triglycerides, amino transferases, alkaline phosphatase and bilirubin.
- Monitoring should be by blood sugar 4-hourly; electrolytes and creatinine daily; calcium phosphate and liver function tests every third day; and trace elements every 2 weeks.

Complications

- Mechanical: injuries during cannulation: pneumo-thorax, haemothorax, vascular injury, brachial plexus injury, thoracic duct injury, air embolism, deep vein thrombosis.
- Electrolyte disturbances: require daily monitoring and correction.

- Metabolic complications: usually caused by inappropriate nutrient administration or inadequate monitoring (e.g. hyperglycaemia requiring insulin).
- Metabolic bone disease may occur in long-term parenteral feeding.
- Infections: catheter-related sepsis is common and life-threatening.
- Presence of subcutaneous infection along the catheter tunnel or catheter tip (with positive blood cultures) requires catheter removal and repositioning. The risk of infection is reduced by the use of an in-line filter (0.45 or 0.22 μm).
- Parenteral antibiotic therapy is started immediately and modified following pathogen sensitivity results.
- Prevention is by attention to the catheter site and by not infusing other solutions or medications through the same port. The line should not be used for blood taking or for measurement of central venous pressure.
- Liver abnormalities: are the commonest of gastrointestinal complications of parenteral feeding. They are usually transient biochemical abnormalities and, rarely, histological abnormalities may be present. They are more common in infants.
- Biliary complications: occur in patients in prolonged (>4 weeks) infusional therapy (incidence: 5%) – acalculous cholecystitis, gall bladder sludge and cholelithiasis.

Home parenteral nutrition

- Indicated for gastrointestinal failure in:
  - Inflammatory bowel disease
  - Severe short bowel syndrome
  - Radiation enteritis
  - Malignant disease.
- Venous access is by subcutaneously tunnelled silastic catheter (attached to subcutaneous port), exiting low on the anterior chest wall.
- Infusion is controlled by volumetric pump fitted with air and occlusion alarms and in-line filter (0.22 μm). When not in use the catheter is primed with heparin solution.

- The infusional calorific distribution and requirements depend on what the patient is eating and absorbing and their level of physical activity.

Complications

- Micronutrient deficiencies
- Carbohydrate overfeeding
- Venous thrombosis
- Chronic liver disease
- Cholelithiasis
- Metabolic bone disease
- Catheter-related septicaemia (coagulase-negative staphylococci, *Staphylococcus aureus* and candida)
- Superior vena caval thrombosis – rare complication (preventable by heparinization of intravenous infusions or by warfarin therapy).

4

Systems management

MANAGEMENT OF SYSTEMIC DISEASE

Surgical patients, particularly the elderly, commonly have disease of more than one system that may require management before, during or after surgery. This section considers the management of systemic disease and critical illness, including intensive care.

Patients with any diseases are likely to require surgery at some time in their lives. In most cases this does not influence their surgical management. However, in some instances, particularly in cardiovascular disorders, specific treatment, possibly in an intensive care unit (ICU), may be needed in the peri-operative period and attention must always be given to coexistent drug therapy (page 12).

Sepsis is of particular importance to the surgeon because it may be the indication for surgery and is a serious postoperative complication.

Surgery, like other disciplines, is also concerned with end-of-life issues, in the management of palliative care and of the dying patient.

INTENSIVE CARE UNIT

- The ICU provides intensive monitoring and support with the most advanced therapeutic measures available within an institution, under the direction of an intensive care specialist, with involvement of all specialist medical and surgical teams as required. It is an expensive facility and must have strict entry and discharge criteria.
- Nursing in the ICU is provided on a one-to-one basis, allowing continuous monitoring and individual attention to the patient's skin, pressure areas, mouth care, lines, catheters, wounds, drains, stomas and other clinical measures, medication, dialysis, and ventilation and circulatory support.
- Other ICU staff may include: physiotherapists, pharmacists, dieticians, nutrition specialists and physicists.
- The ICU environment is controlled to reduce heat and fluid losses from unconscious and exposed patients,

the staff wearing theatre garb. Airflow promotes good infection control, and aseptic techniques must be meticulous for all invasive procedures in an environment that often houses immunocompromised patients, and where resistant organisms must be contained.

- Intensive care management is appropriate for:
  - Multiple organ failure
  - Immediately postoperative patients where there is a continued need for ventilatory or circulatory support
  - Respiratory failure requiring intubation and mechanical ventilation
  - Circulatory failure in circumstances where this cannot be managed by a coronary care or high dependency unit (HDU)
  - Where abnormal manipulation of cardiorespiratory physiology may improve outcome, e.g. serious head injury
  - Where there is a high risk of requiring a sudden escalation in support.
- The failure of individual organs is considered under postoperative care (page 54).

Assessment of the critically ill patient

- General principles: history, examination and investigation. History, usually obtained from other clinicians and relatives, identifies the primary and coexistent disease, e.g. asthma, myocardial ischaemia and endocrine abnormalities.
- Severity: vital signs – pulse, blood pressure including postural falls, temperature, respiratory rate; CVP monitoring; features of dehydration, weight changes and urine output; blood gases; full blood count; urea, electrolytes and liver function tests; and coagulation status.

Systems support

- An ICU provides critical support for the body systems, both individually and collectively, the latter being a key factor in the management of severe trauma, generalized sepsis, shock and multiple organ dysfunction syndrome.

- A prime feature of intensive care is maintaining access to relevant parts of the body by: catheterization, intubation, endoscopy, laparoscopy and thoracoscopy. Vascular access is a key to blood sampling, fluid delivery, monitoring, dialysis and mechanical assistance to the circulation.

Respiratory system

- **Management of the respiratory system** is a major role as ventilation is not usually available in high dependency or coronary care units.
- **Hypoxia** is an early feature of a number of systemic diseases, such as shock and sepsis, as well as direct lung trauma and primary lung disease.
- Hypoxia produces endothelial and alveolar wall disruption, increasing capillary permeability and oedema, and progressing to acute lung injury. In a ventilated patient PaO_2 in kPa should be only 10 less than the inspired O_2 concentration (FIO_2); in acute lung injury PaO_2 is less than or equal to 47.5 kPa (200 mmHg) for $FIO_2 > 60\%$; in more severe cases, ARDS, PaO_2 is ≤ 40 kPa. Arterial oxygen saturation can be continuously monitored by a pulse oximeter, which is an effective and non-invasive painless device attached to the finger or ear. It can be influenced by altered peripheral perfusion and should be supplemented by blood gas estimations. It provides an early warning monitor.
- Admission to ICU may be because of airway obstruction, such as difficult intubation and facial trauma. The first priority is to secure an airway, usually by endotracheal intubation, but if necessary by tracheotomy.
- Introduction of an endotracheal tube requires paralysis but the patient may then breathe spontaneously.
- Indications for **ventilation** are inadequate gas exchange, dyspnoea or a tiring patient.
- Augmentation of breathing may be by non-invasive as well as invasive measures, such as continuous positive airway pressure through a tight-fitting face or nasal mask, or inspiratory pressure support through a triggered machine such as the Bird ventilator.
- Invasive positive pressure ventilation may be by a prescribed volume (e.g. 6–10 mL/kg at a rate of 12–20 breaths per minute), as in a volume-controlled

ventilator, or by a set pressure. Other adjustments are related to end-expiratory pressure and the timing of inspiration/expiration, usually 1:2. In extreme circumstances extracorporeal transmembrane oxygenation may be delivered.

Cardiovascular system

- **Cardiovascular** management involves much sophisticated measurement, but commences with simple measurement of pulse and blood pressure. Tachycardia is an early cardiovascular response to sepsis, shock and many surgical problems, while postural hypotension, followed by progressive hypotension, is a sign of reducing cardiac output.
- Intensive care may be required for severe primary heart disease, such as ischaemia, valvular dysfunction and dysrhythmias, and when secondary causes place excessive demand on cardiac output, both groups progressing to pump failure.
- **Twelve-lead electrocardiograph** identifies rate, rhythm, conduction abnormalities, atrial and ventricular dysrhythmias and areas of ischaemia. Echocardiography identifies cardiac anatomy, regional wall motion abnormalities, left ventricular dysfunction, valvular function and intracavity thrombus. Thallium scans can assess myocardial perfusion, while the use of isotopes in multi-gated acquisition scans of the beating heart identify hypokinetic, akinetic and dyskinetic areas, and measure the left ventricular ejection fraction.
- **Coronary angiography** provides information on heart chambers, valves, great and coronary vessels, and measures pressures and gradients, cardiac output and facilitates calculation of vascular resistance. Access also allows endomyocardial biopsy and evaluation of intracardiac electrical activity.
- **Arterial lines** provide accurate measurement of blood pressure and arterial samples for blood gas analysis.
- **Central venous pressure (CVP)** monitors right atrial pressure and provides a useful marker for fluid replacement. Severe fluid losses are replaced through a

wide-bore needle until the CVP starts to rise.
Thereafter aliquots of 200–250 mL are infused, a
3 mmHg rise after an aliquot indicating that optimal
filling is being reached. Urine output should be
>0.5 mL/kg per hour. Fluid replacement is then
continued at the daily requirement.

- A pulmonary wedge pressure is obtained through a line
floated through the right side of the heart, through the
pulmonary artery and wedged into an arterial tributary;
it provides an indication of pressure in the left side of
the heart. A mixed venous oxygen saturation is
obtained, and this should be approximately 70–75%.

- Direct and indirect measures of the left and right sides
of the heart help to determine whether they are
working effectively in tandem.

- Cardiac dysrhythmias may be sensitive to appropriate
medication, cardioversion or cardiac pacing. Ventricular
fibrillation and cardiac arrest may require defibrillation.

- If poor cardiac output continues after adequate refilling
of the circulation, and urine output remains low,
inotropes may be required. Pulmonary ventilation
reduces the work of breathing and also cardiac load,
and may be of value in these instances.

- A failing heart may be amenable to support by intra-
aortic balloon counterpulsation or, when they are
available, ventricular assist devices and
cardiopulmonary bypass, the ultimate management
being cardiac transplantation.

- **Renal failure** in the presence of adequate perfusion
requires diagnosis and immediate fluid restriction,
control of potassium being by carbohydrate and insulin
infusion, progressing to venovenous filtration or
haemodialysis.

Fluids and acid–base balance

- **Fluid balance** is an essential component of intensive
care management and, in chronic illness and starvation,
the need for parenteral nutrition. Fluid loss may be
through haemorrhage, vomiting and diarrhoea,
nasogastric tubes, drains, fistulae, stoma and sweating,
and (more difficult to measure) sequestration into the

gut, body cavities, movement into the third space and losses caused by leaking membranes. Metabolism is altered in the critically ill patient by release of catecholamines and cortisol, and an increased energy requirement of up to 30%.

- **Acid–base balance** (page 62) is monitored by regular arterial blood gas measurements, and maintained by optimizing respiratory and renal function, and treating sepsis and other causes of critical illness. Bicarbonate containing Hartmann's solution may be used as a resuscitation fluid in these patients.
- Severe **metabolic acidosis** following cardiac arrest, and in other critical illness, may be corrected urgently by administration of 50–100 mmol of 8.4% sodium bicarbonate solution i.v. (1 mL contains 1 mmol).

Alimentary system

- **Starvation** may be related to the lack of food during the peri-operative period, but also with associated conditions, such as personal neglect (as in dementia), diarrhoea, vomiting, dysphagia, chronic sepsis and neoplasia. Clinical presentation is of weight loss, general wasting, loose clothing and reduced skin fold thickness. Blood tests may show reduction of albumin, prealbumin, transferrin and lymphocyte count, but these are non-specific and are not an accurate guide to replacement needs.
- Normal **enteral feeding** (page 80) is the best treatment, using a balanced diet. This is possible if gut motility is not disturbed. Tube feeding may be delivered through a nasogastric or nasojejunal tube or percu-taneously to the stomach [percutaneous endoscopic gastrostomy (PEG)] or jejunum. A balanced diet with added vitamins and electrolytes may be commenced and delivered through the tube.
- Parenteral feeding may be required when the bowel is non-functioning: indications include a protracted postoperative course, short bowel syndrome and gastrointestinal fistulae.

- A wide venous line is required, preferably a tunnelled subclavian or internal jugular line. Total **parenteral nutrition** contains a balance of protein, carbohydrate and lipid, together with water, electrolytes and vitamins. Protein is usually provided with the balance of 40% essential and 60% non-essential amino acids. Carbohydrate as glucose (16.8 kJ/g) and lipid emulsion (37.8 kJ/g) is currently provided in a single bag for 24-hour use, reducing the need for repeated changes and potential infection. Total parenteral nutrition is managed by a multidisciplinary team, including doctors, nurses, pharmacists and dieticians. Good glycaemic control is essential.

Sepsis

- **Fever** >38.3 C is very common in the critically ill, but may arise from infective and non-infective causes.
- **Sepsis** (page 114) is present in 70–80% of patients entering an ICU. It is often the result of Gram-negative infection, but is also encountered in multiple organ failure, hypovolaemic shock, severe trauma, particularly when accompanied by marked tissue damage such as in burns, fat embolism, crush injury, liver and immunological disease, obstetric causes (abruptio placentae, amniotic fluid embolus and pre-eclampsia) and malignancy.
- **Natural immunity** is reduced in critical illness, probably linked to poor nutrition and abnormal renal, metabolic and endocrine function. Natural barriers are breached by endotracheal tubes and vascular lines, while mucosal barriers are broken by trauma and ischaemia. Alongside these changes, secretions accumulate in recumbent sedated and anaesthetized patients, allowing overgrowth of bacteria, and promoting and sustaining sepsis.
- **Acquired immunodeficiency** may be divided into neutropenia, T-cell deficiency, broad-spectrum immunodeficiency (haematological, malignant, chemotherapy and post-transplant), hypogamma-globulinaemia, splenectomy and complement deficiencies.

- **Neutropenia** is caused by viral and severe bacterial infections, and by drug reactions. It is classified as mild, with total counts of $1.0–1.8 \times 10^9$/L, moderate $0.5–1.0 \times 10^9$/L and severe 5×10^9/L, and results in impaired killing of bacteria and fungi. The signs of infection may be minimal; while Gram-positive organisms are the commonest infection, Gram-negative infection, particularly *Pseudomonas* bacteraemia, is lethal in 50% of patients within 24 hours. In severe neutropenia, therefore, if the infective agent has not been identified, broad-spectrum antibiotics, possibly meropenem with an aminoglycoside, should be instituted, together with metronidazole if there is gut involvement.
- If this regimen is unsatisfactory, additional vancomycin or teicoplanin are included, to cover Gram-positive organisms and amphotericin B, for treatment of fungal infection.
- The commonest cause of **T-cell deficiency** is infection with the human immunodeficiency virus, but immunosuppressive treatment must also be considered. Infections are often caused by atypical bacteria, but also include viral, fungal and parasitic agents. Viral infections include herpes simplex, herpes zoster, cytomegalovirus, hepatitis B, Epstein–Barr and papilloma viruses. The number of antiviral agents is increasing, but toxic effects, such as renal impairment, must be monitored. Ganciclovir is the first-line treatment for cytomegalovirus.
- Common fungi are *Histoplasma capsulatum* and *Cryptococcus*, while parasitic infections include *Pneumocystis* (treated by high-dose co-trimoxazole); toxoplasmosis (treated with pyrimethamine/sulfadiazine); and cryptosporidiosis, presenting with unresolved diarrhoea; the latter, being usually resistant to medication, is treated symptomatically.
- **Hypogammaglobulinaemia** frequently presents with recurrent respiratory and gastrointestinal infections. Complement deficiency is usually associated with systemic lupus erythematosus. Splenectomy carries a 1% annual risk of serious sepsis, common organisms being *Streptococcus pneumoniae*, *Haemophilus influenzae* and *Escherichia coli*.

Coagulation

- **Disseminated intravascular coagulation (DIC)**
  is accompanied by release of thrombin, producing
  deposition of fibrin in the microvasculature, and also
  increased plasmin, leading to fibrinolysis and
  spontaneous haemorrhage into the gut or other organs,
  or at any trauma site, such as an operative incision or
  cannula insertion.
- Diagnosis is initially clinical, based on the presence of
  organ dysfunction and haemorrhage, and usually non-
  specific changes of coagulation factors and platelets,
  a reduction of fibrinogen levels, and an increase in
  prothrombin time, activated partial thromboplastin
  time (APTT) and fibrin degradation products. D-dimer
  antigen is raised, indicating the presence of thrombin
  and plasmin.
- Treatment of DIC is that of the underlying cause, the high
  mortality usually being related to the aetiological factor.
  In view of the conflicting problems of haemorrhage and
  coagulation, a delicate balance has to be maintained
  between transfusion of platelets, fresh frozen plasma
  and cryoprecipitate, to maintain fibrinogen levels, while
  considering use of heparin to reduce microthrombosis;
  the involvement of a haematologist is essential.
- Other coagulation defects encountered in the ICU
  include iatrogenic platelet dysfunction, following
  massive transfusion, aspirin and sequestration of
  platelets in major surgery, particularly cardiac. There
  may also be platelet dysfunction in renal failure, while
  liver disease can interfere with the production of factors
  II, VIII, IX and X.

Shock

- Shock is a clinical state resulting from inability of the
  body to maintain tissue perfusion, which is characterized
  by tachycardia, hypotension, pallor, cool and clammy
  skin, impaired conscious level and, eventually, coma. It is
  commonly encountered in the critically ill. Causes of
  shock: **cardiogenic** – pump failure (e.g. after myocardial
  infarction); **hypovolaemic** – low vascular volume (after
  haemorrhage and dehydration); **septic** – there may be a

warm periphery and pyrexia initially, with increased cardiac output and peripheral vasodilatation; and **anaphylactic** – peripheral vasodilatation.

- Shock is accompanied by multiple organ damage. The brain suffers, with clouding of consciousness, progressing to lethargy, disorientation and delirium. In the lungs, capillary oedema promotes hypoxia and peripheral ischaemia. There is progressive renal and liver failure, with accumulation of lactic acid and a falling pH. The terminal event is usually the release of endotoxins from an ischaemic gut. There may be associated DIC. The mortality increases from 50% with a single organ to 80% with three or more organs involved.

Nervous system

- A cardinal role for the ICU is the management of the unconscious patient. Many patients are anaesthetized to facilitate ventilatory support but failure of most systems, as well as primary intracranial pathology, can have marked cerebral consequences.
- Cardiac arrest produces unconsciousness within seconds and permanent brain damage within minutes. The effect of failure of other systems, while not so immediate, can be equally devastating. These include hypertension, hypotension, hypoxia, hyperpyrexia, hypothermia, extremes of metabolic acidosis and alkalosis, renal and hepatic failure, sepsis, hyperglycaemia and hypoglycaemia, hypersecretion and hyposecretion of the pituitary, adrenal and thyroid glands, and altered metabolism of drugs, including alcohol.
- Coma from intracranial pathology usually results from the haemorrhage, thrombosis and embolism of cerebrovascular disease, but raised intracranial pressure and neuronal damage may also be caused by infection, neoplasia and trauma.
- Generalized convulsive status epilepticus (GCSE) is a specific problem presenting to the ICU. It may be secondary to the conditions mentioned above, the first manifestation of epilepsy, or occur in a known epileptic who has not taken their drugs, or who has intercurrent disease.

- Phase one in the progression of GCSE is a marked increase in metabolic activity, producing tachycardia, hypertension and hypoglycaemia. After 30 minutes compensatory mechanisms begin to fail.
- In phase two GCSE there is failure of autoregulation, oxygen requirement exceeds supply, and there is a resultant rise in intracranial pressure and electromechanical dissociation; seizures become minimal and there is progressive neuronal damage.
- Emergency management is by endotracheal intubation and ventilation to secure the airway, preventing gastric aspiration and providing adequate oxygenation.
- Subsequently it is essential to make a diagnosis. History is obtained from attendant clinicians, relatives and associates. Examination may reveal a stroke or associated disease, and specific tests may include blood culture, lumbar puncture and cerebral imaging.
- Drug management progresses through benzodiazepines (lorazepam) to hydantoins (phenytoin and fosphenytoin) to phenobarbitone. If this regimen is unsuccessful, general anaesthesia is maintained with electroencephalograph monitoring, while an appropriate drug regimen is established.
- Rapid initial control of GCSE is essential because mortality at 30 minutes is 3.7% but rises after an hour to 35%. Most cases occur in known epileptics who have missed out on their drug therapy and have a good prognosis. The overall mortality of 25% is largely the result of coexistent disease.
- 70–80% of patients with severe sepsis or multiple organ failure develop some form of neuropathy or myopathy. The precise mechanism of these conditions is unknown, although there is a relationship to steroids and neuromuscular blocking agents, at least in patients with acute asthma. The cellular changes may be related to inflammatory mediators disrupting the microcirculation. Subsequent hypoxic neuronal damage can expose them to the toxic effects of neuromuscular drugs. Histological findings include primary axonal degeneration of peripheral motor and sensory fibres, and scattered atrophic muscle fibres, with a variable degree of necrosis.

- When these signs are observed during the recovery phase, it is still important to exclude causes of spinal cord compression, such as trauma, neoplasia and infection, as well as myasthenia gravis, muscular dystrophies and Guillain–Barré syndrome.
- There may be electromyogram evidence of denervation, but investigations are usually non-specific. Management is directed at the underlying critical illness, with prolonged physiotherapy and rehabilitation for the involved muscles. Recovery is related to the severity of the problem. Milder forms recover completely within a few weeks, but the remainder take several months and recovery may be poor in cases of necrotizing myopathy.

Follow-up

- Many ICUs provide an outreach programme to follow up sick patients transferred to the HDU (where the patient–nurse ratio is 2:1 and ventilation is not usually available) and to acute wards. They may also advise on the need for admission to ICU, and on measures for preserving organ function, such as drugs, fluids and nutritional support.

HIGH DEPENDENCY UNIT

- High level of nursing and monitoring, but 2:1, rather than the 1:1 nurse/patient ratio of an ICU, and fully backed up by all hospital specialist teams.
- Admission to the HDU is usually upon failure of one rather than multiple systems, and patients do not usually require mechanical ventilation.
- Strict control of infection and its management is necessary.
- The HDU is valuable for preoperative optimization of seriously ill (physiologically compromised) patients, particularly emergency admissions.
- Postoperative care requiring intense monitoring of one or more systems is provided.
- For patients who may need treatment in, or have just been discharged from, the ICU. Most patients requiring

an HDU level of preoperative care will need admission to ICU postoperatively.

BRAINSTEM DEATH

- The critical condition of all ICU patients means that staff are frequently managing end-of-life events, making decisions on withdrawing and withholding treatment. Brainstem death makes such decisions possible, as no recovery has ever been recorded following properly conducted brainstem death testing. When such a patient is retained on a ventilator for religious or family reasons, asystole occurs within a few days.
- 10–15% of deaths in UK ICUs are brainstem deaths occurring after trauma, intracranial haemorrhage and drowning. Recovery from cardiac arrest usually results in a persistent vegetative state rather than brainstem death and presents a difficult problem of long-term management.
- The UK code of management of brainstem death is in three stages: preconditions; exclusions; and clinical testing.
- **Preconditions** are that the patient is in an unresponsive coma and that their condition is a result of irreversible brain damage of known aetiology.
- All the following reversible causes must be **excluded**:
  - Drugs such as narcotics, hypnotics, tranquillizers and muscle relaxants
  - Hypothermia – the core temperature must be above 35°C
  - Circulatory, including a recent circulatory arrest
  - Metabolic, such as hyponatraemia and hypo-glycaemia
  - Endocrine, such as a hypothyroid state.
- **Clinical state** and **clinical tests** are performed by at least two doctors (one a consultant, the other with at least 5 years' post-registration experience), who are unconnected with the family or any proposed organ donation. The tests are repeated twice by both doctors independently or together – the time interval not being specified.

- There should be no response in any of the following brainstem reflexes:
  - No pupillary response to light
  - No corneal reflex
  - No vestibulo-ocular reflex (20 mL of ice-cold water is injected into each external auditory meatus in turn over a 1 minute period. A normal response is deviation of the eyes towards the stimulus)
  - No motor response to central stimulation (absence of facial movement to pressure over the supraorbital notch on each side)
  - No gag reflex to stimulation of the fauces
  - No cough reflex to bronchial stimulation
  - No spontaneous breathing. This test is carried out by removing the patient from the ventilator without risking further ischaemic damage and it involves blood gas analysis. The patient is pre-oxygenated with 100% oxygen for 10 minutes and the partial pressure of carbon dioxide in arterial blood allowed to rise to 5 kPa or above. The patient is then disconnected from the ventilator, oxygen at a rate of 6–10 mL being insufflated into the trachea through a catheter to maintain adequate oxygenation. The Pa_{CO_2} is allowed to rise to over 6.65 kPa for the lack of spontaneous respiratory effort to be confirmed.
- The legal time of death is that of the completion of the first set of brainstem tests, and death is certified after completion of the second set of tests, regardless of when active support is withdrawn. The patient is reconnected to the ventilator after completion of the first set of tests, but only after the second set if organ donation is being considered; the testing clinicians must not be involved with these decisions. Further tests are undertaken if pre-existing respiratory disease invalidates apnoea testing on account of the high resting Pa_{CO_2}, or when facial trauma or other disease prevents all the criteria of brainstem testing. Also, additional testing is required for neonates and young children.
- Additional tests include cerebral angiography, radio-nucleotide scanning and transcranial Doppler ultrasono-graphy to confirm the absence of the anterior and posterior cerebral circulation, there being a minimum

mean arterial blood pressure of 80 mmHg. Electro-encephalography using auditory and sensory evoked responses is available as an additional test in children.

- Brainstem death indicates irreversible brain damage, but other organs are often functioning normally or have the potential for full recovery; they are therefore ideally suited for use in transplantation (page 592). Some cultures do not permit the use of organs for these purposes, but in the UK there is generally the desire to donate organs, many individuals having written a living will to this effect. When this is not so, permission is required from the next of kin. Although they may be supportive, the timing of this request is very difficult when the decision is being made to stop ventilatory support. It is therefore essential that the team involved in the certification of death is not involved in the request or any other aspects of organ donation.

OBESITY

- Obesity is the result of energy intake exceeding needs; a small daily excess can lead to a large accumulation of fat over a period of years.
- Obese patients are termed overweight where there is a 10% increase above normal, and morbidly obese when there is a 20% increase. The latter is accompanied by a 25% increase in mortality risk.
- Morbid obesity is defined as 45 kg above the ideal weight for height, age and sex, or a body mass index of more than 45.
- The cause of obesity is ill defined; genetic and environmental factors are probably both involved. The *ob* gene is expressed in brown and white adipose tissue; mutations of this gene are associated with the high plasma levels of leptin found in obesity.
- Smoking is an important co-factor in mortality, but although obesity is common on stopping smoking, it is not a contraindication to stopping, as the risk associated with smoking 20 cigarettes per day is equivalent to 20 kg.

- Obese patients have increased plasma lipoprotein cholesterol fractions, triglycerides, uric acid, and fasting and postprandial glucose, predisposing to ischaemic heart disease, cerebrovascular disease, hypertension and non-insulin-dependent diabetes.
- The mechanical load decreases exercise tolerance and increases osteoarthritic changes, back pain, proneness to accidents and reduction in chest wall compliance, reducing vital capacity and giving rise to dyspnoea.
- These patients are prone to postoperative complications partly as a result of cardiorespiratory problems but also because of variable response to a distribution of drugs through their systems and increased incidence of deep vein thrombosis.
- They are subject to hiatus hernia, gallstones, chole-cystitis, infertility and neoplasms of the gallbladder, large bowel, prostate, ovary, uterus and breast.
- Obesity is assessed by comparison with tables of ideal weight for height from which the body mass index (weight in kg/m^2 in height) is calculated.
- Obesity in teenagers is accompanied by an increase in the number of fat cells, but in later life there is an increased amount of fat in each cell, rather than an increased cell number.
- Management of obesity is primarily medical, with diet control, reduction in caloric intake, long-term change in eating habits and modification of lifestyle, with support from a team of psychiatrists, physicians and nutritional experts.
- Patient motivation and education are directed towards the principles of energy intake and expenditure, and the health benefits of weight control.
- Exercise regimens are essential, as weight reduction is difficult to achieve without exercise.
- Drug therapy is useful in the short term and as an adjunct to a dietary regimen (fenfluramine – 'slimming pill').
- Surgery should only be considered in well motivated, well informed and low risk patients, supported by a full team with surgical expertise and lifelong follow-up (page 433).
- Measures include wiring of jaws, which permits liquid feeds only and is a temporary measure.

- A gastric balloon is positioned endoscopically; it is of limited value (may cause bowel obstruction).
- Gastric plication or vertical banded gastroplasty reduce the size of the stomach; they can be effective in the well motivated patient.

THE ELDERLY PATIENT

- Old age is not a disease and the marked variation in individuals means that the physiological rather than the chronological age of each patient and their individual systems must be identified.
- The ageing process is one of continuous cellular loss and gradual failure of physiological function, producing a wide spectrum of pathological changes. In the cardiovascular system, loss of pacemaker cells can give rise to arrhythmia, and loss of muscle compliance reduces stroke volume, cardiac volume and cardiac reserve. The replacement of elastin with collagen fibres, and progressive atherosclerosis, reduces coronary blood flow, and increases peripheral resistance and blood pressure, producing postural hypotension.
- In the respiratory system, loss of compliance of the chest wall, kyphosis and reduction of respiratory reflexes is accompanied by parenchymal cell loss and reduction of elastic recoil, widening of the airways increasing dead space and reducing vital capacity.
- Bone and marrow reduction can produce anaemia, pancytopenia and reduction of the immune response.
- Reduction of glomeruli and their vascularity reduces filtration rate, and the ability to deal with altered alkaline and acidic load. Prostatic enlargement may contribute to renal failure.
- In the alimentary tract, gut motility is reduced, with consequent constipation; and with loss of appetite and teeth, there may be malnutrition.
- Muscle size and bulk decrease, and skin becomes more fragile and bruises easily.
- In the musculoskeletal system, rheumatoid arthritic changes are common and may themselves be an

indication for surgery. They produce pain, limited movement accompanied by weakness of ligaments and joints, and potential for subluxation and peroperative damage.

- Osteoporosis produces kyphosis, bowing of the long bones and flexion deformities, and limited respiratory excursion.
- In the central nervous system, dementia increases markedly over the age of 80 years, although reversible causes such as hypoxia, infection, drugs, hypoperfusion, hypothyroid, and visual and hearing loss, must always be excluded. Atherosclerotic changes in carotid and vertebrobasilar territories may produce stroke and add to parenchymal changes. Central control of temperature, appetite and thirst may be diminished, peripheral nerve conduction reduced, such as in pain perception, and autonomic degeneration may reduce cardiovascular and other reflex responses.
- These various factors must therefore be taken into account when assessing an elderly patient for surgery. Findings must be fully documented and discussed with the patient and their relatives. Their preoperative condition must be optimized, and in high-risk patients an alternative to surgery must be considered. Postoperative monitoring must be comprehensive, any postoperative complications being rapidly treated, possibly in an ICU.

PALLIATIVE CARE

- Palliative care is the total care of patients, and their families, when they are beyond curative treatment or when they are suffering from a terminal illness.
- Advanced cancer, acquired immune deficiency syndrome (AIDS) and progressive neurological disease form the spectrum of illnesses requiring palliative care.
- Palliative care forms a partnership between the carers and the patient and family members, and aims to achieve the highest possible quality of life for the patient and the family.

- Treatment is of physical symptoms, sustains nutrition, and supports the patient's psychological, social and spiritual needs.
- Palliative care is administered by a multidisciplinary team consisting of a palliative care physician, Macmillan and community nurses, physical and complementary therapists, social workers, volunteers (including family members) and priests; specialist services (surgical, oncological, microbiological and immunological input) are available on request.

Breaking bad news

- Unpleasant or unwelcome clinical information must be given to the patient (and to the family) with counselling to minimize the distress and anxiety that it will cause.
- Clinical realities are communicated at a pace acceptable to the patient and the family with the required support that will relieve anxiety, enhance hope and promote confidence in the palliative care team.
- The quantity of information given is based on how the patient regards the illness at the time and the strategies used by the patient in coping with the information.
- The various uncertainties associated with the care of terminal illness are addressed through a relationship built up by the care team with the patient and the relatives based on trust, mutual respect and transparency.

Emotional support

- Terminally ill patients and some family members experience significant psychological problems that may conflict with care plans; denial is used as a coping strategy to avoid the anxiety that is associated with the diagnosis. Professional counselling is necessary when denial interferes with acceptance of treatment.
- Anxiety, anger and depression are normal emotions associated with terminal illness; once recognized, these are treated by counselling and with anxiolytic and

antidepressant drugs, which enable the patient to improve their emotional quality of life, retain self-assurance and self-respect, and to prepare for the future.

Symptom management

Cancer pain

- Pain is caused by nerve stimulation or nerve dysfunction; analgesic therapy is commenced along the three-step analgesic ladder:
  - Mild pain is treated with non-opioids (aspirin 600 mg or paracetamol 1 g 6-hourly)
  - Moderate pain is treated with weak opioids (codeine 60 mg or buprenorphine 200–400 µg 6- to 8-hourly, sublingually)
  - Severe pain is treated with strong opioids (dextro-moramide 5–20 mg orally; pethidine 50–100 mg i.m.; morphine or diamorphine 5–10 mg i.m. 4- to 6-hourly).
- 'Breakthrough pain' not controlled by regular dosage is addressed by the addition of a quick-release form of morphine for rapid onset to be given as often as necessary, or fentanyl 200 µg lozenge (one or two doses per pain episode) or as adhesive patches releasing 25 or 50 µg hour for 72 hours; these additional measures are assessed over 3 days and the regular dosage upgraded (a laxative and an anti-emetic are usually needed with morphine).
- Visceral pain originating from the abdomen or pelvis is often poorly localized and may be referred to other sites, and adequate pain relief may not be sustained with drugs as the disease progresses. Destruction of nerve tissue with alcohol or phenol by image-guided needle administration to nerve roots and plexuses provides long-term palliation (coeliac plexus block, subarachnoid neurolysis or chemical cordotomy). Spinal catheter administration of diamorphine into epidural or subdural spaces provides a patient-controlled delivery system to alleviate diffuse somatic and visceral pain and associated symptoms.
- 'Incident pain' is due to spinal, bone or joint malignancy and is brought on by physical activity;

control may be achieved by optimizing opioid dose regimens or by spinal administration.
- Rehabilitation is through physical and occupational therapies and modifying levels of activity with appropriate lifestyle changes.
- Surgical stabilization of spinal, bone or joint lesions gives lasting relief and must be considered in patients with a life-expectancy of a few months or longer.
- Morphine-resistant pain is usually the result of muscle spasm associated with neuropathic or bone pain and is treated by non-drug methods involving transcutaneous electrical nerve stimulation (TENS), acupuncture, physiotherapy and occupational therapy.

Respiratory symptoms

- Breathlessness, cough and haemoptysis are managed by a combination of reducing awareness and fear by counselling and emotional support, with oxygen therapy and air humidification and a strong opioid and a benzodiazepine.

Gastrointestinal symptoms

- Nausea and vomiting are distressing and are frequently opioid or chemotherapy induced; they may also be a result of:
  - Functional gastric stasis, which responds to prokinetic agents (metoclopramide or domperidone)
  - Renal failure, which may respond to haloperidol or methotrimeprazine
  - Raised intracranial pressure or vestibular disturbance, which respond to cyclizine
  - Constipation that is caused by opioid therapy or neurological lesions is treated with dietary modifications and laxatives (bulk formers and peristalsis stimulants)
  - Diarrhoea is a frequent symptom in AIDS but is less common in malignant disease and may be caused by laxative overuse; non-specific anti-diarrhoeal agents (loperamide or codeine) may be tried.
- Additional therapies include:
  - Cholestyramine for post-irradiation diarrhoea
  - H_2 receptor blockade for Zollinger–Ellison syndrome

- Pancreatin for steatorrhoea
- Cyproheptadine for carcinoid syndrome.
- **Bowel obstruction** in advanced cancer is caused by extrinsic tumour compression, intraluminal or adhesion obstruction, post-irradiation fibrosis or motility disorders caused by tumour infiltration.
- Partial obstruction may progress to complete obstruction during the course of the disease.
- Intravenous diamorphine, hyoscine, haloperidol, cyclizine and methotrimeprazine may be used individually or in combination to alleviate the accompanying nausea and colic.
- Surgical decompression is required for gastric outlet obstruction (gastro-enterostomy), high small bowel obstruction (entero-enteral bypass) or colonic obstruction (ileostomy or colostomy). Radiologically and endoscopically placed stents are gaining popularity. Entero-cutaneous fistulae are a frequent surgical complication.

Cachexia and malnutrition

- The majority of patients with advanced cancer or AIDS develop cachexia before death and it is common in those with solid tumours.
- Cachexia is caused by tumour products causing lipolysis and proteolysis and by cytokines produced as a response to the tumour. Significant, progressive weight loss may be a sequela to anti-cancer therapy.
- Intensive nutritional therapy (enteral or parenteral nutrition) has limited effect on complications of anti-cancer treatment and has no effect on survival; however, the provision of high-calorie, small and pleasant meals, and involving the patient and family in choosing and preparing the menu, improves appetite, gives a sense of well-being and builds confidence.

Mood changes

- Psychological reactions to incurable diseases include anxiety, fear, anger, sadness and depression, which are resolved over time by the patient and the family with professional counselling. In a minority of cases, these mood changes remain unresolved and progress to psychiatric illness that requires specific evaluation and management.

- Confusion is found in elderly patients with impaired memory, hearing or sight, and presents as forgetfulness, disorientation, changes in mood or behaviour, and is caused by delirium (reversible) or dementia (irreversible).
- Screening instruments such as the hospital anxiety and depression scale, and mood disorder and mental status schedule for cognitive impairment, assist in the recognition of these states.

THE DYING PATIENT

- The direction and culture of medical practice is towards curing disease and preserving life. When this is not possible it may be looked on as failure.
- Nevertheless, surgeons, like other clinicians, have the responsibility to ensure that patients die with dignity, and in a setting of their choice.
- This is not always possible when death may be precipitate and occasionally unexpected; there are few biochemical or haematological markers that can reliably predict the time of death.
- Where there is hope for prolongation of quality life, it is desirable to treat anaemia, infection and arrhythmias; however, this must not perpetuate false hopes of survival.
- There may be reluctance from the clinician to expect that death is inevitable when the diagnosis is unknown, when patients and relatives are unaware of the serious-ness of the situation, or from the fear of shortening life or withholding treatment, or when cultural, spiritual or medico-legal aspects are unresolved.
- When death is anticipated, time must be given for full discussion with the patient and relatives and to answer questions. The surgical team must speak with one voice, avoiding any conflicting messages. There must be confidence for everyone that everything that could have been done has been done, with full knowledge and

professionalism. The patient's general practitioner
should be informed and contact numbers must be
available for relatives, priest and all others involved.

Hospital versus home care

- Terminally ill patients must be consulted on where they
  wish to be cared for when planning their management;
  most patients wish to die at home but less than a
  quarter manage to do so.
- Patients may become frightened or insecure or lose
  confidence with home care support and seek terminal
  care in a hospital or hospice, where there is the
  infrastructure for the provision of various support
  services.
- Terminal care at home requires home assessment and
  upgrading of home facilities and the organization of
  primary care teams that may include family members.

Religious and cultural support

- Religion and cultural background offer comfort and
  strength to the terminally ill patient and solace to the
  relatives. Their needs are variable, depending on the
  individual religious and cultural affiliations, and their
  availability.
- People with religious values are dependent on external
  sources for spiritual strength, and access to priests and
  articles of worship must be made available. Those who
  profess not to hold religious values may object to such
  material or counselling, as may a small minority who
  derive spiritual solace and strength from within
  themselves.

Death and bereavement

- The diagnosis of dying is an important clinical skill.
  The patient becomes bed-bound by progressive
  weakness, food is neglected and fluids are taken
  eventually only in sips, with an inability to take drugs
  orally. The patient drifts into a semi-coma.

- When death is inevitable, all investigations, monitoring and non-essential medication should stop. This usually also includes intravenous therapy.
- Symptomatic control is essential and includes management of nausea and vomiting, pain, dyspnoea and agitation. Oral drugs are converted to subcutaneous, possibly using a syringe driver. Mouth care and gentle cleanliness may include catheterization. Psychological support may be required if there is any element of distress.
- The grief of relatives of a patient dying of a terminal illness affects their emotional, physical and social well-being. Clinical staff, particularly palliative care teams, can provide support and bereavement counselling to relatives, who should feel that they and the patient have experienced a good death.
- Relatives cope with grief by the dual process of 'loss-orientated' behaviour (confronting grief) and by 'restoration-orientated' behaviour (avoiding grief).
- Grief counselling supports and guides the relatives through these processes towards a good outcome, with restoration of their emotional and physical well-being.

5

Management of surgical disease

SEPSIS

- Injury to the body produces an inflammatory response, which has local features (pain, heat, redness, swelling and loss of function) and systemic features.
- **Systemic inflammatory response syndrome (SIRS)** is defined as two or more of the following:
  - Temperature $>38°C$ or $<36°C$
  - Heart rate >90 bpm
  - Respiratory rate >22 breaths per minute or $Paco_2$ <4.2 kPa (32 mmHg)
  - White blood cell count >12, $<4 \times 10^9/L$ or $>10\%$ of immature forms.
- **Sepsis** is SIRS resulting from infection.
- The **immune system** defends the body against infection, and mediates the inflammatory response.

Innate immunity

Innate immunity is the body's first line of defence. It is immediately available but non-specific, and has no memory, i.e. it always responds in the same way to the same pathogen. It comprises:

- **Physical and chemical barriers:** skin, tears, saliva and gastric acid
- **Cellular defences:** macrophages, mast cells, neutrophils, basophils, eosinophils, monocytes and natural killer (NK) cells
  - **Macrophages** release: platelet activating factor (PAF); prostaglandins and leukotrienes – causing vasodilatation, chemotaxis of neutrophils and eosinophils; nitric oxide and free oxygen radicals that are antimicrobial; and cytokines.
  - **Cytokines** released into the circulation include: tumour necrosis factor alpha, interleukins – particularly interleukin-1 (IL-1) and 6, and interferons. In the brain they produce fever, somnolence and anorexia; in the bone marrow they stimulate production of leukocytes; and in the liver the production of acute phase proteins, including C-reactive protein (CRP), fibrinogen and complement.

- **Neutrophils** and **monocytes** phagocytose pathogens, then kill them intracellularly. Monocytes also produce further tissue macrophages. The granules released from **basophils** and **eosinophils** are toxic to extracellular pathogens.
- **Mast** cells release histamine, heparin, degradation enzymes, prostaglandins and leukotrienes.
- **NK cells** are large granular lymphocytes that provide first-line defence against intracellular pathogens, particularly viruses. Abnormal cells not expressing normal human leukocyte antigen markers are vulnerable to NK cell attack.

- **Humoral responses** involve: the complement system, the coagulation pathway and the contact system. These are activated directly by pathogen wall components or indirectly by cellular released mediators:
  - **Complement proteins:** bind to antibodies; are inflammatory mediators; activate mast cells and platelets; are chemotactic to neutrophils, monocytes, eosinophils and basophils; and also promote microbial cell lysis.
  - The **coagulation pathway** is activated by fibrin and Hageman factor; fibrinolysis is also increased. Activation of the **contact system** releases bradykinin, causing vasodilatation, smooth muscle contraction and pain.
  - **Acute phase proteins** bind and inactivate micro-organisms **(opsonization)**.

Specific immunity

- Specific immunity takes about 4 days to develop after first exposure to the pathogen. It is specific and has memory, which results in an immediate response on subsequent exposure – the basis of vaccination.
- Bone marrow precursors migrate and differentiate into thymic (T)-lymphocytes, and B-lymphocytes of the fetal liver and adult bone marrow. Most are produced in fetal life, but also originate from stem cells in adults. They both recognize antigenic receptors on antigen-producing cells.

- **T-lymphocytes** have antigen receptors (TcR) that recognize degraded antigen fragments associated with self molecules of the major histocompatibility complex (MHC) – located on chromosome 6 in a human. They are of two types: CD4 or CD8.
- CD4 cells recognize extracellular antigens deposited by liposomal pathways, associated with class II MHC. They become T-helper (Th) cells by bonding with dendritic cells containing antigen. **Dendritic cells** have receptors for PAMPs, and have strong phagocytic properties to ingest antigen. They travel in the lymphatic system to lymph nodes, and in the bloodstream to the spleen – to bind with CD4 cells.
- CD8 cells recognize intracellular antigen degraded in proteolytic structures termed proteosomes, and associated with class I MHCs. With the help of Th cells, they divide and differentiate into CD8 target cells (Tc) that are capable of killing cells with the same antigen.
- **B-lymphocytes** have antibody molecules on their surface which fold to match antigen-binding fragments (Fab) on pathogens. On reaching lymph nodes or the spleen they differentiate and proliferate into plasma cells (memory B-cells). These long-lived cells rapidly produce high affinity antibody when the same pathogen is encountered.
- Delayed hypersensitivity is a further response to intracellular pathogens, where large numbers of activated macrophages release cytokines and other mediators. It may result in tissue damage in chronic infection, e.g. tuberculosis and leprosy.

Systemic inflammatory response

- Pro-inflammatory cytokines affect the endothelial cells of the microcirculation, causing vasodilatation and increased permeability, activate coagulation mechanisms, and cause platelet and neutrophil activation.
- **Septic shock** is the clinical state of shock where sepsis is the underlying cause. Vasodilatation causes hypotension, tachycardia and increased cardiac output.

Severe SIRS is mediated by tumour necrosis factor (TNF)-alpha, IL-1 and PAF, which produce fever and anorexia, progressing to confusion and coma.

- **Multiple organ dysfunction syndrome (MODS)** results from increased tissue oxygen requirements and microthrombosis. Features include: increased respiratory rate (an early sign of sepsis); changes in blood gases, renal and liver function tests (LFTs); raised white blood cell count and deranged clotting mechanisms (partial thromboplastin time, activated partial thromboplastin time, fibrin). Inflammatory markers such as IL-1, IL-6, CRP, procalcitonin and von Willebrand's factor are raised.

Management of sepsis

- Identify the source of the infection: culture wounds, discharge, urine, blood, and faeces; replace and culture intravascular lines; take chest radiograph for pneumonia or effusions; ultrasonography or computerized tomography (CT) for chest and abdominal cavities to look for abscesses/collections.
- Initial management of septic shock is the ABC of resuscitation, ensuring adequate airway and breathing, if necessary in an intensive care unit (ICU), and maintaining the circulation.
- Abscesses in wounds, beneath the skin or in a body cavity, must be drained surgically or under radiological guidance.
- Appropriate antibiotics are given according to specific culture and sensitivity findings, or, if the organism is not known, based on the presumed origin of the infection after consultation with a microbiologist.
- Circulatory support aims to achieve central venous pressure of 8–12 mmHg, mean arterial pressure of 65–90 mmHg, and urine output of >0.5 mL/kg per hour. This may require: intravenous fluid, inotropes and vasopressins, such as noradrenaline and dobutamine. In acute cases adrenaline may be required to provide both alpha and beta sympathomimetic activity (dopamine, while improving renal blood flow, may cause bowel ischaemia and is not advised).

- Oxygen is administered using a Venturi mask, which delivers a specific concentration of oxygen, or a reservoir bag, to achieve peripheral capillary O_2 saturation >90%, or central venous oxygen saturation of >70%. Severe cases are managed by intubation and ventilation, but a protective lung strategy is used: tidal volume is limited to 6–8 mL/kg, mean airway pressures of <36 cm H_2O, relatively high positive end-expiratory pressure (PEEP) (5–15 cm H_2O), a limited fraction of oxygen in inspired air (up to 0.6).
- Continuous venovenous haemofiltration may be required for renal failure, using high volume flows (30 mL/kg per minute). Filtration prior to renal failure has not proved effective in removing inflammatory mediators.
- Blood sugar should be maintained at 4.4–6.1 mmol/L using insulin, and steroid may be given (300 mg hydrocortisone/24 hour) to prevent adrenal insufficiency. Activated protein C may reduce 28-day mortality by 6.1%.
- Patients with MODS are best managed in an ICU. Mortality for these patients is 45%.

HIV AND AIDS

- Acquired immunodeficiency syndrome (AIDS) was first recognized 1981 in the USA.

Aetiology

- Human immunodeficiency virus-1 (HIV-1, a retrovirus) identified in 1983, nine subtypes or clades.
- Subtype B is the predominant clade in USA and Europe.

Epidemiology

- WHO/UNAIDS estimate 40 million people infected worldwide; 28 million in sub-Saharan Africa.
- UK 2001 total of 41 200 infected. Risk categories: 15 100 homosexual/bisexual, 11 200 heterosexual, 4200 undetermined.
- 71% of new UK infections in persons from Africa or who had sexual intercourse while there.

Pathogenesis and natural history

- Transmission is by the following means:
  - Sexual – vaginal and rectal sexual intercourse
  - Materno-fetal/vertical
  - Parenteral – intravenous drug use
  - Blood/blood products
  - Percutaneous and mucocutaneous exposure
  - Xenotransplantation.
- HIV-1 – lymphotrophic and neurotrophic virus. Short half-life of approximately 2 days with high replicative capacity in lymphoid tissue and peripheral CD4+ lymphocytes.
- High turnover of CD4+ lymphocytes (up to 2×10^9/day).
- Direct viral cell killing, apoptosis or other immune mechanisms lead to progressive depletion of CD4+ lymphocyte populations with suppression of cell-mediated immunity.

Investigation

- HIV antibody tests; enzyme-linked immunosorbent assay, immunofluorescent assay, Western blot.
- P24 antigen, culture of plasma and/or peripheral blood mononuclear cells, qualitative polymerase chain reaction.
- Quantitative measures of plasma viral load – RNA/DNA amplification techniques; reverse transcriptase polymerase chain reaction, nucleic acid sequence based amplification, branched-chain DNA assay.

CLINICAL MANIFESTATIONS/ CLASSIFICATION

CDC classification (1992)

- Category A – acute HIV infection, asymptomatic, persistent generalized lymphadenopathy.
- Category B – mildly symptomatic HIV disease.
- Category C – AIDS surveillance defining diseases.

From acquisition of HIV infection, the medium time to symptomatic HIV disease/AIDS is approximately 8–10 years in untreated individuals.

Acute HIV infection

Transiently symptomatic illness in 40–80% of cases, associated with high levels of viraemia. Symptoms: pharyngitis, fever, maculopapular rash, lymphadenopathy. There is HIV antibody seroconversion within 3–12 weeks.

Symptomatic HIV disease (not AIDS)

Constitutional symptoms appear after 1 month: oropharyngeal candidiasis, oral hairy leukoplakia, seborrhoeic dermatitis, molluscum contagiosum, recurrent oral/peri-anal/vulval/penile herpes simplex (HSV) infection, thrombocytopenia. Peripheral generalized lymphadenopathy (>2 cm diameter, bilaterally symmetrical, smooth, rubbery, mobile, non-tender) common.

SYMPTOMATIC HIV DISEASE/AIDS

Major opportunistic infections/ clinical syndromes

Respiratory disease

Pneumonia

- *Pneumocystis carinii* pneumonia (PCP).
  - Aetiological agent: fungus *P. carinii*, 85–90% of patients have CD4+ lymphocyte count <200/mm^3. Interstitial pneumonitis.
  - Symptoms: dry cough, fever, dyspnoea.
  - Signs: often minimal, tachypnoea, crackles.
  - Investigations: oximetry, arterial blood gases (resting and exercise), chest X-ray, bronchoscopy, detection of *P. carinii* with Giemsa stain, toluidine blue-O, fluorescent antibody techniques in bronchoalveolar lavage (BAL) fluid in 95%.

- Treatment: i.v./p.o. co-trimoxazole or i.v. pentamidine. Corticosteroids if hypoxic (Po_2 <70 mmHg).
- Complications: pneumothorax, respiratory failure.

- Pulmonary tuberculosis (TB). Leading cause of death worldwide in persons infected with HIV.
  - Aetiological agent: *Mycobacterium tuberculosis*. It results from reactivation of latent infection or primary infection. Clinical presentation varies with stage of HIV disease; incidence of extrapulmonary disease more common with CD4 count <100/mm^3.
  - Symptoms: cough, fever, dyspnoea, weight loss, night sweats.
  - Signs: consolidation, pleural effusion, extrapulmonary signs, lymphadenopathy, hepatomegaly, splenomegaly.
  - Investigations: purified protein derivative (PPD), chest X-ray (mediastinal adenopathy, coarse interstitial or localized infiltrates, disseminated or miliary pattern, pleural effusion), sputum examination and culture for acid- and alcohol-fast bacilli (AAFB), bronchoscopy/BAL, mycobacterial blood cultures.
  - Treatment: standard antituberculous therapy, rifampicin, isoniazid, pyrazinamide and ethambutol (RIPE) for 2 months; rifampicin and isoniazid for 4 months. Consider directly observed therapy, twice/thrice weekly treatment regimens.

- Bacterial pneumonia.
  - Aetiological agents: *Streptococcus pneumoniae* and *Haemophilus influenzae* common, *Staphylococcus aureus* (intravenous drug users), *Pseudomonas aeruginosa*, other Gram-negative organisms. These occur at all levels of CD4+ counts.
  - Symptoms: clinical presentation is typically with fever, chills, cough, pleuritic chest pain and dyspnoea.
  - Investigations: chest X-ray shows segmental or lobar consolidation, pleural effusion, cavities (*S. aureus*, *P. aeruginosa*). Gram stain and culture of sputum. Positive blood cultures are common with pneumococcal pneumonia.

– Treatment: there is a prompt response to appropriate antibiotic therapy, macrolides, extended spectrum cephalosporin.

Neoplastic disorders

- Kaposi's sarcoma (KS). Associated with human herpes virus 8 (HHV-8). Usually cutaneous and/or mucosal KS.
  - Symptoms: cough, bronchospasm, dyspnoea.
  - Investigations: chest X-ray shows coarse, poorly defined nodular densities throughout lung fields. Pleural effusions are common. Hilar adenopathy is uncommon. High resolution CT scan, bronchoscopy ± transbronchial biopsy.
  - Treatment: highly active antiretroviral therapy (HAART), systemic chemotherapy.
- Lymphoma. Usually non-Hodgkin's B-cell type. Extranodal involvement is usual in advanced HIV disease.
  - Symptoms: thoracic manifestations include pleural effusion, hilar/mediastinal lymphadenopathy, reticular nodular infiltrates, and alveolar consolidation. Primary effusion lymphoma is associated with HHV-8.
  - Investigations: chest X-ray, CT scan, bronchoscopy, mediastinoscopy.
  - Treatment: systemic chemotherapy.

Bowel manifestation in AIDS

- Chronic enteritis and neoplastic lesions of the bowel are associated with intussusception in HIV infection and include infective enteritis, lymphoid hyperplasia, Kaposi's sarcoma and non-Hodgkin's lymphoma of the bowel:
  - Diagnosed by contrast-enhanced abdominal ultrasound and CT scans
  - Treated by surgical reduction of intussusception and resection of bowel containing causative lesion.

Central nervous system disease

Meningitis

- Cryptococcal meningo-encephalitis is the most common manifestation of disseminated cryptococcosis in patients with CD4+ counts <100/mm^3.
  - Aetiological agent: *Cryptococcus neoformans* encapsulated yeast.
  - Clinical presentation may be non-specific.
  - Symptoms and signs: headache, fever, confusion, nausea and vomiting, meningism, cranial nerve abnormalities.
  - Investigations: diagnosis confirmed by lumbar puncture and cerebrospinal fluid (CSF) examination – raised opening pressure in >60%, pleocytosis variable, positive India ink stain, positive cryptococcal antigen in 90%.
  - Treatment: amphotericin B ± 5-fluorouracil, fluconazole.
- TB meningitis.
  - Symptoms: headache, fever, confusion, cranial nerve abnormalities.
  - Investigations: contrast CT scan may show basal meningeal enhancement, CSF examination (raised CSF protein, pleocytosis, decreased glucose, AAFB stain and culture).
  - Treatment: rifampicin, isoniazid, pyrizinamide, ethambutol ± corticosteroids.
- Bacterial meningitis (*S. pneumoniae, H. Influenzae, Neisseria meningitidis, Listeria monocytogenes*) is uncommon.

Focal brain disorders

- Cerebral toxoplasmosis is the commonest cause of focal mass lesions in patients with advanced HIV disease and a CD4+ count <200/mm^3.
  - Aetiology: caused by reactivation of latent infection by protozoa *Toxoplasma gondii*. 95% of patients have positive anti-toxoplasma immunoglobulin G (IgG).
  - Symptoms and signs: headache, confusion, fever, seizures, focal neurological symptoms and signs depending on location of lesion(s) in the central nervous system (CNS).

- Investigations: contrast CT and magnetic resonance imaging (MRI) demonstrate multiple bilateral ring enhancing lesions/abscesses in 80–90% of cases, often with mass effect/oedema. Brain biopsy of lesion is indicated to establish diagnosis if not responding to standard therapy after 2 weeks.
- Treatment: sulfadiazine or clindamycin and pyrimethamine.

Other causes of brain abscess and focal lesions: tuberculous, pyogenic, nocardia and cryptococcosis

- Primary CNS lymphoma.
  - Aetiology: Epstein–Barr virus associated B-cell lymphoma in patients with advanced HIV disease, CD4 count <100/mm³.
  - Symptoms and signs: variable – altered mental state, seizures, focal neurological deficits.
  - Investigations: CT/MRI, solitary, weakly enhancing lesion with mass effect, typically in periventricular region. Biopsy required for definitive diagnosis.
  - Treatment: responds to chemotherapy; radiation therapy gives poor results with a mean survival rate of 2–5 months.
- Progressive multifocal leukoencephalopathy.
  - Aetiology: demyelinating condition, CD4 count usually <100 mm³. Caused by jC virus (papovavirus).
  - Symptoms: presents with focal neurological deficits, altered mental status, seizures. Typically causes subcortical white matter lesions with no mass effect on MRI (high intensity signal on T_2-weighted images).
  - Treatment: no specific treatment but antiretroviral therapy to reverse HIV immunosuppression may induce remission.

Ophthalmologic disease

Cytomegalovirus retinitis

- Typically associated with CD4+ count <50 mm³.
- Symptoms: may be asymptomatic, floaters, decreased visual acuity and progressive blindness.

- Investigation: ophthalmological diagnosis of necrotizing retinitis with perivascular exudates and haemorrhages.
- Treatment: systemic intravenous ganciclovir, foscarnet orcidofovir, oral valganciclovir, intravitreal fomivirsen.

Other ophthalmological conditions

- Other ophthalmological conditions include micro-angiopathic retinopathy with cotton wool spots, varicella zoster retinitis, toxoplasma chorioretinitis, herpes zoster ophthalmicus, syphilis uveitis in HIV.

Gastrointestinal disease

Oropharynx

- Oral candidiasis is the commonest intra-oral lesion in HIV-infected individuals.
  - Aetiology: caused predominantly by *Candida albicans*. Clinically: pseudomembranous, erythematous, hyperplastic, or angular cheilitis.
  - Symptoms: pseudomembranous candidiasis presents as white lesions/plaques on buccal mucosa, floor of mouth, palate, tongue, which may be painful.
  - Treatment: topical antifungals, nystatin or clotrimazole. Systemic treatment with azoles, fluconazole or itraconazole is more effective. Parenteral amphotericin B may be required for azole-resistant candidiasis.
- Oral hairy leukoplakia. Epstein–Barr virus-associated white lesions, typically on lateral borders of tongue. Cannot be scraped off. Usually asymptomatic and requires no treatment.
- HSV infection. Lesions often multiple and recurrent. May be extensive.
  - Treatment with aciclovir, valaciclovir or famciclovir.
- KS. Most common intra-oral neoplasm in AIDS patients.
  - Symptoms and signs: painless, flat or raised dark red or purple lesions on hard and soft palate. Oral lesions often associated with visceral lesions. Painful if ulcerated.
  - Treatment: local radiotherapy or systemic chemotherapy.
- Warts (human papilloma virus – HPV). Clinical presentation, asymptomatic, multiple flat papules or exophytic papillomas or condylomata.

- Recurrent aphthous ulceration. Intensely painful ulcers on labial and buccal mucosa, tongue and palate. Minor, major and herpetiform variants occur. Major aphthous ulcers usually require topical steroids.
  - Investigation: exclude HSV infection prior to steroid treatment.
  - Treatment: in refractory cases systemic treatment with corticosteroids and/or thalidomide may be required.

Salivary glands

- Benign, bilateral enlargement, CD8+ cell infiltration. Painless but associated with xerostomia. May respond to antiretroviral therapy.

Oesophagus

- Oesophageal candidiasis.
  - Aetiology: *Candida albicans* is the commonest cause. It occurs in individuals with CD4+ counts <100/mm^3. The majority will also have oral thrush.
  - Symptoms and signs: commonly presents with dysphagia, odynophagia, heartburn.
  - Investigations: barium swallow shows 'moth-eaten' diffuse mucosal irregularity. Oesophagoscopy with oesophageal brushings or biopsy gives the definitive diagnosis.
  - Treatment: fluconazole or itraconazole; amphotericin B if azole resistant.
- CMV and HSV ulceration affects middle to lower third of oesophagus. Indistinguishable endoscopically.
  - Treatment: ganciclovir/foscarnet for CMV; aciclovir for HSV.
- KS, lymphoma and squamous cell carcinoma uncommon.

Stomach

- Disorders cause symptoms of nausea, vomiting, early satiety, haematemesis, melaena. Endoscopy and biopsy usually required to establish diagnosis(es).

- CMV infection causes ulceration similar to that of the oesophagus.
  - Treatment: ganciclovir or foscarnet.
- KS. 40% have concomitant cutaneous or nodal KS.
  - Symptoms: often asymptomatic, occasionally may cause haematemesis.
  - Treatment: systemic chemotherapy.
- Non-Hodgkin's lymphoma. May cause obstructed outlet syndrome, haematemesis or melaena.
  - Treatment: systemic chemotherapy.

Pancreatitis

- Idiopathic, alcohol, hyperlipidaemia, HIV drug-related (didanosine, pentamidine, zalcitabine), CMV.

Enteritis and colitis/diarrhoea

- Infective diarrhoea is common in HIV-infected individuals.
  - Aetiology: common pathogens of small intestine include cryptosporidia, microsporidia, giardia, *Mycobacterium avium* complex (MAC). Common pathogens of large intestine include *Salmonella* sp., *Campylobacter* sp., *Shigella*, *Clostridium difficile*, MAC, *Entamoeba histolytica*. CMV colitis occurs with CD4+ count <100 mm^3.
  - Symptoms and signs: small bowel diarrhoea manifest by large volume, watery stools, dehydration and electrolyte disturbance, and large bowel diarrhoea by frequent small-volume stools with mucus, pus and blood. If severe, patient may present with toxic megacolon.
  - Investigations: send stools for microscopy for AAFBs, ova, cysts and parasites, and culture. Upper and lower endoscopy with biopsies is often essential to establish diagnosis.

Anal/peri-anal disorders

- Increased incidence warts (HPV), HSV ulceration and candidal infection.
  - Treatment: standard HPV treatments such as cryotherapy, and topical acid/podophyllin/

podophyllotoxin application may fail and surgical excision of lesions may be required.

- Increased incidence of fissures and trauma with anal receptive sexual intercourse. Fistulae, bacterial abscesses occur. Increased incidence of HPV-related squamous cell carcinoma in HIV-infected homosexual men.

Hepatic and hepatobiliary disease

Hepatitis

- High rates of co-infection with hepatitis A, B and C viruses (HAV, HBV, HCV). Exclude in the presence of abnormal LFTs $\pm$ jaundice.
- HIV immunosuppression may accelerate progression to chronic hepatitis B and C liver disease and chronic hepatitis increasing cause of mortality in HIV-infected individuals.
- Treatment of hepatitis B and C in HIV-infected individuals is evolving, with 3TC, adefovir, and tenofovir available for HBV and interferon-alpha plus ribavirin available for HBC.

Viral infections

- Other viral infections in HIV-infected individuals include CMV, HSV and adenovirus.

Drug-associated dysfunction/toxicity

- Drug-induced hepatitis is common with many of the drugs used in HIV treatment. Eosinophils in peripheral blood or liver biopsy may help diagnosis. If LFTs >5× normal, this usually requires dose reduction or discontinuation. Antiretroviral drugs are also associated with hepatic steatosis.

Acalculous cholecystitis

- Presents with severe right upper quadrant colicky pain, nausea, vomiting, pyrexia. Thickened gallbladder wall with no gallstones on ultrasound study.
- Indistinguishable from symptomatic gallstone disease.
- Technetium-hepatic iminodiacetic acid (HIDA) scan may confirm diagnosis. Associated most commonly with CMV, *Cryptosporidia* or *Campylobacter*.

Sclerosing cholangitis

- Clinical and cholangiographic picture analogous to that seen with primary idiopathic sclerosing cholangitis.
- Ultrasound demonstrates dilatation and thickening of bile duct walls.
- Endoscopic retrograde cholangiopancreatography shows beading of bile ducts $\pm$ oedematous swollen ampulla with papillary stenosis.
- Most commonly associated pathogens include cryptosporidia, CMV, microsporidia and MAC.

Neoplastic liver disease

- KS, usually as part of disseminated disease, non-Hodgkin's lymphoma, hepatocellular carcinoma.

Haematological disease

- Anaemia (HIV, mycobacterial infection, CMV, drugs, malignancies), leukopenia, neutropenia (HIV and drug related), and thrombocytopenia (immune mediated).
- Neoplastic disorders – non-Hodgkin's lymphoma, Hodgkin's disease.

Dermatological and musculoskeletal disease

- Xeroderma, seborrheic dermatitis, viral infections (molluscum contagiosum, common warts, HSV, shingles), other infections (staphylococcal, mycobacteria, fungi, bacillary angiomatosis), scabies, eosinophilic folliculitis – pruritic papular eruption.
- Neoplastic skin disorders – KS, basal cell carcinoma, squamous cell carcinoma.
- Myositis/myopathy (HIV, drug related – azidothymidine zidovudine/AZT), pyomyositis (*S. aureus*).

ANTIRETROVIRAL THERAPY

- AZT, first antiretroviral agent licensed in 1987. 1996 saw introduction of HAART with 70% decline in HIV-related mortality and morbidity.
- HAART usually comprises two nucleoside reverse-transcriptase inhibitors (e.g. AZT, 3TC) + non-nucleoside

- reverse transcriptase inhibitor (e.g. efavirenz) or protease inhibitor (PI, ritonavir/lopinavir).
- Indications for treatment include symptomatic disease/ AIDS, CD4+ count <350/mm^3, depending on symptoms, rate of decline of CD4 count and viral load. Aim of treatment is to improve symptoms, suppress virological replication and induce immune recovery.
- The initiation of antiretroviral therapy may result in immune reconstitution syndromes – acute flare or exacerbation of underlying infection as a result of renewed immune responsiveness.
- Appropriate therapy guided by history of antiretroviral prior exposure, use of viral resistance assays, therapeutic drug monitoring, drug toxicities and concomitant clinical disorders.
- The British HIV Association (BHIVA) publishes guidelines for the treatment of HIV-infected adults with antiretroviral therapy.

TROPICAL AND SUBTROPICAL DISEASES

CANCERS OF THE TROPICS

Tropical regions show a high incidence of certain solid tumours that are uncommon in temperate and industrialized countries.

Oropharyngeal cancer

Definitions

- Squamous cell carcinoma of the oral cavity and pharynx is associated with the cultural habit of chewing and retaining betel quid in the mouth and/or smoking locally made cheroots (chutta and bidi).

Clinical features

- Presents as a red or white plaque that may bleed to touch, which progresses to ulceration with spread to the cervical nodes.

Investigation
➤ Diagnosis is by mucosal or core nodal biopsy.

Treatment
➤ Early lesions are excised with block dissection of the cervical nodes. Advanced tumours may respond to primary radiotherapy and/or systemic or infusional chemotherapy (bleomycin, vincristine and methotrexate).

Nasopharyngeal cancer

Definitions
● Poorly differentiated (non-keratinizing) squamous cell carcinoma of the nasal passages is associated with the Epstein–Barr virus infection, foods containing dimethylnitrosamine and inhalation of wood smoke (used to keep the thatch of dwellings free from rodents).

Clinical features
● Presents with enlarged cervical lymph nodes, nasal obstruction, epistaxis or deafness or cranial nerve palsy (from invasion of skull base).

Investigation
➤ Diagnosis is by mucosal or nodal biopsy.

Treatment
➤ Primary radiotherapy with adjuvant chemotherapy (nitrogen mustard).

Primary upper small intestinal lymphoma (PUSIL) (Mediterranean lymphoma)

Definitions
● Tumour of the proximal small bowel in children.
● Endemic in subtropical and Mediterranean regions.

- Associated with cell-mediated immune deficiency from malnutrition and chronic diarrhoeal disease.

Clinical features
- Insidious onset of abdominal symptoms, diarrhoea and weight loss.

Investigation
➤ Diagnosed by small intestinal mucosal biopsy.

Treatment
➤ Poor prognosis in established disease.
➤ Chemotherapy is palliative.

Burkitt's lymphoma

Definitions
- A tumour of children, associated with the mosquito-borne Epstein–Barr virus and the reovirus type 3, and recurrent malarial infection.
- A non-Hodgkin's lymphoma arising from B-lymphocytes. Endemic in the rainforest belt of equatorial Africa and New Guinea.

Clinical features
- A multi-focal tumour involving facial bones, abdominal and retroperitoneal organs, long bones and, rarely, the brain.
- Jaw tumours are the commonest and extend into the gums, the orbit or the nasopharynx.

Investigation
➤ Core needle biopsy confirms the diagnosis ('starry sky' appearance on histology).
➤ Radiology: absence of dentine lamina dura of tooth sockets and osteolytic changes.
➤ Laparoscopic staging to assess visceral involvement.

Treatment

➤ Primary chemotherapy with cyclophosphamide, vincristine, methotrexate and/or cytosine arabinoside.
➤ Surgical debulking of abdominal lesions following chemotherapy hastens remission.
➤ Good early remission with chemotherapy with an excellent prognosis for solitary extra-abdominal lesions (87% survival at 10 years); poorer survival with multiple or abdominal lesions (25–50% at 10 years).

Kaposi's sarcoma (KS)

Definitions

● A tumour involving skin, with frequent visceral and bone involvement with sporadic, endemic and epidemic forms.
● Associated with the cytomegalic virus antigen, histocompatibility antigen (HLA-DR5) and the AIDS syndrome with T-lymphocyte deficiency.

Clinical features

● The sporadic (classic) form presents with multiple small nodules and plaques and generally runs a benign course with occasional visceral involvement.
● The epidemic form in sub-Saharan Africans and in the AIDS syndrome is progressive, with oropharyngeal and visceral lesions with cachexia, debility, skin hyperpigmentation and nodal metastases.
● Also seen in the immunosuppressed transplant recipient.

Investigation

➤ Low CD4 cell count ($<300/\mu L$) or low CD4:CD8 cell ratios carry a poor prognosis.

Treatment
➤ Sporadic form responds well to oral alkylating agents or to radiotherapy.
➤ Endemic form responds to primary chemotherapy (actinomycin D, vincristine and imidazole carboximide).
➤ Lesions, when confined to a limb, producing disabling deformity may necessitate amputation.
➤ Surgical debulking following downstaging with chemotherapy is indicated for large tumours.

INFECTIONS OF THE TROPICS

Tropical ulcer

Definitions
● Found in the feet and lower legs of farm workers, caused by barefoot walking, trivial trauma, rodent/insect bites associated with chronic malnutrition.
● Causative agents: fusiform bacilli and Vincent's organism.

Clinical features
● Acute ulcer: tender inflammatory swelling with blistering and serosanguinous discharge and necrosis of the overlying skin, resulting in a painful ulcer with raised, rolled edges; slough covering the floor exudes foul-smelling pus.
● Chronic ulcer: when unhealed over a period of 1–3 months becomes relatively pain-free and odourless with little discharge; the base is fibrotic and there may be underlying bony changes.

Investigation
➤ Wound swabs and smears for culture/sensitivity and microscopy.

Treatment

➤ Broad-spectrum penicillin (ampicillin 0.5–1.0 g 6-hourly, amoxicillin or co-amoxiclav 250–500 mg tds for 2–4 weeks).
➤ Wound toilet and moist dressings.
➤ Surgical debridement and skin grafting for ulcers >2.5 cm.

Complications

- Long-standing ulcers show pseudo-epitheliomatous hyperplasia with surface irregularity mimicking neoplasia
- Squamous carcinomatous change may occur in non-healing ulcers, necessitating below-knee amputation and block dissection of the inguinal nodes.

Buruli ulcer

Definitions

- A chronic ulcerating skin lesion found over the trunk and limbs in farm workers, caused by *Mycobacterium ulcerans* infection.

Clinical features

- Starts as a subcutaneous nodule that enlarges in size, becomes fixed to overlying tissues and ulcerates.
- It is painless with irregular undermined skin edges and a pale, necrotic slough covering the floor.

Treatment

➤ Small pre-ulcerative lesions may be excised under a local anaesthetic; established ulcers require wide excision and skin grafting, with broad-spectrum antibiotic therapy.
➤ Bacille Calmette–Guérin (BCG) vaccine confers partial immunity in children.

Veld sore

Definitions

- Diphtherial skin infection (*Corynebacterium diphtheriae mitis*) producing ulceration.

Clinical features

- Painful vesicle that ulcerates.
- Ulcer becomes chronic, punched-out and circular with a greyish scaly base and undermined edges.
- Concomitant systemic illness with fauceal infection.

Treatment

➤ Diphtheria antitoxin 20 000 units s.c. or i.m. given near the sores, with the sores dressed with antitoxin.
➤ Penicillin 600 mg daily or erythromycin 250 mg tds for 5 days.

Cancrum oris (Noma)

Definitions

- An infective gangrene of the face or gum caused by *Fusobacterium* (*F. fusiforme*), Vincent's organisms (*Borrelia vincenti*).
- Affects malnourished children under 9 years of age who may have oral sepsis or an undercurrent febrile illness.

Clinical features

- Early features are a sore mouth and swollen gums with fetor and salivation, progressing to ulceration of the gum with loosening of teeth.
- Infection spreads to involve the cheek, which is red and brawny and ulcerates (sequestration of the underlying bone is a late complication).
- Healing results in contracture of the cheek with trismus.

Investigation

➤ A mixture of organisms are usually isolated from the oral mucosa.

Treatment

➤ Broad-spectrum antibiotic and antimalarial therapy with blood transfusion (to correct anaemia).
➤ Tube feeding of vitamin-enriched high protein–calorie diet and iron therapy.
➤ Elective surgery following healing, with excision of scar tissue and reconstruction of the cheek by pedicled skin flap.

Yaws and pinta (endemic treponematoses)

Definitions

● A non-venereal infection caused by the spirochaetes *Treponema pertenue* (yaws) and *T. carateum* (pinta).
● Acquired in childhood and associated with overcrowding, poor hygiene and poverty.

Clinical features

● An itchy papule marks the entry site in an exposed part of the body, which may occasionally ulcerate with minimal constitutional disturbance and painless regional lymphadenopathy.
● Primary lesion heals after 3–6 months, with secondary cutaneous or mucosal lesions manifesting later as necrotic gummatous skin and bony lesions resulting in scarring and deformities.
● Nasal and pharyngeal involvement leads to tissue destruction and secondary infection.

Investigation

➤ Diagnosis is essentially clinical and epidemiological (dark field microscopy of exudates or serology cannot distinguish from syphilis).
➤ X-ray examination demonstrates late bony lesions.

Treatment

> ➤ Benzylpenicillin 600 mg i.m. single dose for children
> aged <6 years, 1.2 g for children aged 6–15 years and
> 2.4 g for adults (in cases of penicillin allergy, erythromycin
> or tetracycline 500 mg qds orally is given for 15 days).

Genital ulcers

	Syphilis	Chancroid	Herpes	LGV*	Granuloma inguinale
Infective agent (sexual contact)	*Treponema pallidum*	*Haemophilus ducreyi*	*Herpes simplex*	*Chlamydia trachomatis*	*Calymmato-bacterium granulomatis*
Genitals, perineum, upper thigh	Papule leading to ulcer	Papule/pustule leading to ulcer (multiple)	Grouped vesicles	Vesicle/papule leading to shallow ulcer	Papules leading to granulo-matous ulcer
Symptoms/ signs	Painless not tender	Painful tender	Painful tender	Painless	Painless
Inguinal nodes	Not tender discrete	Tender matted	Tender discrete	Tender firm	Not involved
Complica-tions	Spontaneous healing	Slow healing relapses	Healing with recurrences	Sinus/fistulae urethral/rectal strictures	Lymphatic obstruction scarring
Treatment	Procaine penicillin/ tetracycline	Trimethoprim/ erythromycin	Oral and topical aciclovir	Tetracycline/ erythromycin	Trimethoprim/ tetracycline

*Lymphogranuloma venereum

Typhoid

Definitions

- Typhoid (enteric fever) is caused by endotoxin
  produced by the typhoid bacillus, with a worldwide
  prevalence in conditions of poor sanitation and poverty.

- Transmission is through contaminated drinking water and by the faeco-oral route.
- The bacillus multiplies in the Peyer's patches of the ileum and in the mesenteric lymph nodes and may thence spread to the liver or spleen. The infected Peyer's patches may undergo necrosis and ulceration, resulting in haemorrhage or perforation.
- Bacilli are excreted in stools, urine or bile, with the gallbladder serving as a reservoir and a source of re-infection and converting the patient into a carrier.

Clinical features

- Fever, headache, high temperature, slow pulse and bradycardia and abdominal cramps with diarrhoea.
- Bleeding from an ulcer presents with melaena (haemorrhage is uncommon).
- Ulcer perforation may occur in the third week of onset of symptoms, with sudden deterioration and signs of peritonitis.

Investigation

➤ Moderate leukocytosis of $5–6 \times 10^9$/L; a rise of $>15 \times 10^8$/L indicates abdominal sepsis.
➤ Blood and occasionally stool cultures are positive for typhoid bacillus.
➤ Widal test is positive (rise in O antibody titre) in established disease.
➤ Abdominal X-ray may show mucosal oedema/ulceration in distal small bowel.
➤ Free intraperitoneal air on X-ray, with a leukocytosis of $>15 \times 10^9$/L indicates perforation.

Treatment

➤ Chloramphenicol 50 mg/kg i.v. in divided doses daily with amoxycillin 0.25–0.50 g 8-hourly or co-trimoxazole 1 g 12-hourly or tetracycline 250–500 mg 6-hourly for 12 days.

➔

> ➤ Intravenous fluid and electrolyte replacement therapy and bowel rest.
> ➤ Mucosal bleeding requires blood transfusion (rarely surgical resection of the ulcer-bearing segment for control of haemorrhage).
> ➤ Perforation with peritonitis is treated by emergency laparotomy, oversewing of perforation and lavage; perforations may be multiple and loculated abscesses require drainage.
> ➤ Three negative stool cultures are necessary before discharging the recovering patient.

Complications

- Management of the typhoid carrier:
  - Elective cholecystectomy for reservoir of infection in the gallbladder
  - For residual infection in the liver, in addition to the cholecystectomy the common bile duct is drained with a T-tube and the patient placed on oral chloramphenicol and tetracycline for 12 days until three successive bile cultures are negative, followed by negative stool cultures.

Leprosy

Definitions

- A minimally infective bacillary disease with a worldwide incidence but endemic in Africa, the Far and Middle East and South America.
- *Mycobacterium leprae* in the lepromatous form spreads through the upper respiratory tract and occasionally the skin.
- A vigorous host cellular response results in tuberculoid lesions; a poor host response results in the bacilli multiplying in the skin, subcutaneous tissue or bone, producing lepromatous lesions.
- Bacilli invade peripheral nerves producing a polyneuritis, which is the main cause of the deformities and disabilities of this disease.

Clinical features

- Early skin lesions are hypopigmented or depigmented, with anaesthetic patches and tingling or numbness in the extremities.
- In tuberculoid and borderline leprosy, nerves are affected early with nerve thickening, pain, sensory loss or motor paralysis (neuropathic lesions).
- In lepromatous disease, bacillary infiltration of the facial skin, muscle and bone produces the characteristic 'leonine facies' and 'saddle-nose'.

Investigation

➤ Test for positive smears from skin snips from lepromatous lesions.

Treatment

➤ Lepromatous patients are nursed in isolation until nose and throat swabs are free of bacilli; tuberculoid patients are not infectious.
➤ Restore general health with nutritional and emotional support and counselling and occupational therapy.
➤ Three drug regimen of dapsone 100 mg daily (1–2 mg/kg), rifampicin 600 mg once monthly and clofazimine 300 mg once monthly for at least 2 years; ethionamide or prothionamide is used in the presence of dapsone resistance.
➤ Acute neuritis, a reaction to drug therapy is treated immediately with prednisolone 40–60 mg orally daily.
➤ Most hand deformities respond to massage, wax baths, electrical muscle stimulation (faradism) and splinting.
➤ Foot drop may require tendon transfer surgery and severe joint deformities and muscle palsies are corrected by capsulotomies, tendon transfers and arthrodeses.
➤ Postoperative physiotherapy and occupational therapy and fitting of custom-made appliances assist functional recovery.
➤ Cosmetic surgery for facial, nasal and auricular deformities facilitates emotional recovery and social rehabilitation.

Tuberculosis

Definitions

- A bacillary disease of poverty and social deprivation of worldwide distribution, but endemic in Asia, Africa and Latin America with a prevalence of 100–500 per 100 000 population (mainly in young adults).
- The human form (pulmonary TB) is spread by droplet transmission (sputum of patients with pulmonary disease).
- The bovine form (much less common) is acquired through the consumption of unpasteurized milk or dairy products.
- Bone and joint TB involves the vertebrae (Pott's disease), large joints and occasionally long bones through blood spread.

Clinical features

- Insidious onset with nocturnal fever, productive cough, cervical lymphadenopathy, anaemia, weight loss or amenorrhoea.
- Abdominal discomfort, pain, distension or diarrhoea (in bovine disease); mucosal ulceration of the small bowel or hypertrophic scarring may lead to perforation or subacute obstruction with a high incidence of peritoneal seeding.
- Haematogenous spread from the bowel may present with a non-tender hepatomegaly with caseating lesions.

Investigation

- ➤ Tuberculin (Mantoux/Heaf) skin test is strongly positive.
- ➤ Hypochromic, normocytic anaemia, raised erythrocyte sedimentation rate and a leukocytosis.
- ➤ Chest X-ray shows an active or a healed primary lung focus or pleural involvement (empyema).
- ➤ Abdominal X-ray: calcification in mesenteric nodes, liver or spleen; barium enema: characteristic mucosal lesions in the ileo-caecal region.
- ➤ Image-guided core needle biopsy of enlarged regional or mesenteric nodes may show caseation, and an ascitic tap, acid-fast bacilli.

Treatment

➤ Oral therapy for 6 months with isoniazid and rifampicin (3–6 tablets daily of the combined preparation) with an initial 2-month course of pyrazinamide and ethambutol or streptomycin; the initial phase is designed to reduce the bacterial population rapidly and to prevent the emergence of drug-resistant strains.

➤ Relapse or recurrence necessitates the full regimen to be recommended under strict supervision.

➤ Surgery is reserved for complications of lung suppuration, bowel obstruction, fistulation or abscess formation.

➤ Vertebral and joint disease requires debridement and stabilization.

Pyomyositis

Definitions

● A pyogenic infection of the skeletal muscle by *Staphylococcus aureus* leading to abscess formation.

● It has a sporadic worldwide incidence but is prevalent in tropical Africa and New Guinea.

● Predisposing factors are chronic ill health, anaemia, vitamin C deficiency and malnutrition, immune-deficiency syndromes, immunosuppression and muscle trauma.

● It affects any voluntary muscle, but occurs mainly in the trunk or root of limbs.

Clinical features

● Pyrexia and malaise with painful swelling and tenderness over the affected muscle with developing signs of abscess formation (distinguish from guinea worm abscesses in endemic areas, which are intermuscular and usually produce an anterior tibial compartment syndrome in the leg).

Investigation

➤ *Staphylococcus aureus* is isolated from blood cultures in the invasive phase or from abscess aspirate.

Treatment

➤ Systemic broad-spectrum antibiotic therapy in the early inflammatory phase.
➤ Small abscesses may respond to aspiration.
➤ Large abscesses are surgically drained, curetted and packed, or primarily closed under antibiotic cover.

Actinomycosis

Definitions

● Opportunistic infection by a branching Gram-positive anaerobic bacillus (*Actinomyces israeli*), associated with malnutrition or chronic ill health, sporadic incidence in the Americas, Africa, Middle and Far East.
● Rare infection of subcutaneous, oral and visceral tissue with a tendency to spread through the bloodstream.
● 50% of infections involve the abdomen as sequelae to surgical operations.

Clinical features

● A discharging sinus, which may contain characteristic yellow 'sulphur' granules.
● May present as a liver or lung abscess with constitutional symptoms.

Investigation

➤ Aspirate from abscess or discharge from the sinus may contain Gram-positive bacilli.

Treatment

➤ Sensitive to a wide range of antibiotics (penicillin, sulphonamide, erythromycin, tetracycline and chloramphenicol) in high and prolonged dosages; clindamycin is preferred when bone is involved.
➤ Surgical drainage of a chest or abdominal abscess as an adjunct to antibiotic therapy.

SUPERFICIAL MYCOSES

Mycetoma

Definitions

- Caused by saprophytic fungi maduromycetes and actinomycetes gaining entry through skin breaches, usually in the foot or leg.
- Sporadic incidence in North Africa, India and South America.
- It is a chronic, slow-growing inflammatory swelling of the subcutaneous fat and overlying skin characterized by micro-abscesses containing coloured fungal particles, which are discharged through multiple cutaneous sinuses.

Clinical features

- Painless long-standing swelling of the leg or dorsum of foot with multiple discharging sinuses.
- Constitutional symptoms are generally absent.

Investigation

➤ X-ray changes: peri-osteal new bone formation with underlying patchy para-osteal erosion; honeycombing of the medulla with cystic cavities; diffuse bony thickening with increase in bone density and loss of definition.
➤ Host antibody titres specific to the fungus are raised and are diagnostic.

Treatment

➤ Actinomycetoma responds to dapsone 1–2 mg/kg orally or rifampicin 0.6–1.2 g orally daily combined with streptomycin 15 mg/kg i.m. daily for 2–4 weeks (resistant infections may respond to ciprofloxacin, imipenem, sodium fusidate and sulphonamide). Maduromycetoma responds to ketoconazole 200–400 mg daily for 2–3 weeks.

➔

> Surgical excision removes all infected tissue, sparing tendons, nerves and vessels (avoiding spillage of granules into the wound). Amputation is reserved for loss of function or extensive bony involvement.

Paranasal aspergillus granuloma

- Caused by *Aspergillus flavus* and presents with proptosis or maxillary swelling.
- It is painless and slowly progressive.
- Treatment is by conservative surgery and adjuvant radiotherapy.

Phycomycoses

- Infections of the nasal cavity by phycomycetes, which extends into the paranasal sinuses and the subcutaneous tissue of the mid-face.
- Diagnosed by plain radiology and tissue biopsy.
- Responds to amphotericin-b and ketoconazole. Surgical excision is reserved for established lesions.

Rhinoscleroma

Definitions

- A chronic, slowly progressive painless inflammatory growth in the nose and upper respiratory passages caused by a Gram-negative bacillus, *Klebsiella rhinoscleromatis*.

Clinical features

- Gross deformity of the nose with destruction of nasal passages and spread of infection to cervical lymph nodes.

Investigation

> Identification of characteristic foam cells in tissue smears.

Treatment

> Excision of lesion with reconstruction of the nose, maxilla and/or upper lip. Early stage lesions respond to streptomycin 1 g i.m. daily for a month.

Rhinosporidiosis

- An infection of the nasal mucosa by a yeast-like organism, *Rhinosporidium seeberi*.
- Friable, polypoid or pedunculated lesions on the nose and face.
- Lesions are excised and mucocutaneous defects reconstructed.

Chromoblastomycosis

- A chronic skin infection caused by pigmented fungi.
- Warty, verrucose lesions which slowly enlarge and may cause deformities of the extremities.
- Early stage lesions respond to itraconazole 100–400 mg daily orally, and late stage lesions to itraconazole combined with flucytosine 150 mg/kg daily.
- Surgical excision is reserved for advanced lesions.

Phaeohyphomycosis

- A skin infection of pigmented fungi that presents as large fibrous cysts containing the fungi.
- Lesions are best excised.

Lobomycosis

- A rare fungal infection of subcutaneous tissue producing plaques and keloid-like scars.
- Treatment is by excision.

PROTOZOA

Malaria

Definitions

- Surgical disease in the tropics is often treated in patients suffering from or debilitated by recurrent malarial infection.
- Malaria is endemic in most parts of Africa, the Middle-East, Asia, Central and South America.

- There are four types of *Plasmodium* species transmitted by a variety of mosquitoes.
- Red cells are invaded and haemolysed by the parasite, with resultant anaemia and organ-specific complications dependent on parasite virulence and load.

Clinical features

- Intermittent or recurrent fever with chills and rigors.
- Tender hepatosplenomegaly.

Investigation

➤ Thick blood film (Leishman, Giemsa or Field stained) demonstrates the parasite; thin film measures parasitic count per field (disease intensity).

Treatment

➤ Chloroquine (orally or i.m.) 25 mg/kg body weight over 3 days; amodiaquine 1.4–2.4 g over 2–4 days, or prima-quine 7.5–15.0 mg daily for an adult, and 0.25 mg/kg for a child for 15 days (in chloroquine resistance).

Complications

- Blackwater fever causes rapid haemolysis and, with accompanying dehydration, may lead to renal tubular necrosis and failure.
- Cerebral malaria may lead to coma and is treated by quinine 600 mg i.v. 8-hourly over 7 days.

Visceral leishmaniasis (kala-azar)

Definitions

- Caused by protozoal parasite *Leishmania*, transmitted by the sandfly bite.
- The infection may be cutaneous, mucocutaneous or involve the internal organs and the reticulo-endothelial system (visceral leishmaniasis).
- It is endemic in parts of Europe, Africa, the Middle East, Asia, South and Central America.

Clinical features

- Undulating fever of characteristic pattern (double rise in 14 hours).
- Anaemia as a result of haemorrhagic episodes.
- Ulcerating lesions of the face, nose or mouth.
- Rapid splenomegaly with hepatomegaly and regional lymphadenopathy.

Investigation

➤ Blood films may show the parasite as Leishman–Donovan bodies.
➤ Aspirate from the spleen (or involved lymph nodes, liver and bone marrow) is the best means of parasite isolation.

Treatment

➤ Sodium stibogluconate and meglumine antimonate 20 mg 5b(v)/kg IV or 1 M for 20–30 days.
➤ Splenectomy may be indicated for a huge splenomegaly or in cases resistant to drug therapy; post-splenectomy pneumococcal vaccination, penicillin and antimalarial prophylaxis is required for debilitated patients.
➤ Skin lesions may be treated with diathermy, cryo-surgery or curettage.

Amoebiasis

Definitions

- An endemic protozoan infection of worldwide distribution by *Entamoeba histolytica*, transmitted by the faeco-oral route as a result of poor hygiene and sanitation (water-borne transmission is unusual).
- Causes ulceration of the colonic mucosa resulting in bleeding, granuloma and stricture formation or perforation.
- May invade the peri-anal skin, liver, lung or brain.

Clinical features

- Presentation is similar to that of typhoid enteritis, with mucoid, blood-streaked diarrhoea and colicky abdominal pain, which becomes generalized when the colon becomes oedematous or friable, with the risk of perforation of a mucosal ulcer and peritonitis.

- Severe colitis in children is a fulminating, necrotizing inflammation producing ileus, peritonitis and toxic shock, with a fatal outcome.
- A palpable, tender, mobile mass in the abdomen is an inflammatory mass (amoeboma) or an abscess causing bowel obstruction or fistulation to the abdominal wall or to an adjoining bowel loop.
- Amoebic skin ulceration around abdominal stomas and the perineum is the result of surgical procedures performed oblivious to the underlying infection.
- Amoebic liver abscess presents with low-grade fever, malaise, anaemia and right upper abdominal pain or tender hepatomegaly.

Investigation

➤ Fresh stool smears reveal motile, haemophagous trophozoites and cysts.
➤ Colonoscopy may reveal mucosal ulcers or the presence of trophozoites in mucosal scrapings or biopsy.
➤ Gastrografin enema may demonstrate a granuloma, stricture or an intussusception.

Treatment

➤ Oral metronidazole 1.4 g or tinidazole 2 g daily for 3 days cures uncomplicated colitis.
➤ In fulminating illness commence fluid and electrolyte therapy with colloid or blood transfusion and i.v. metronidazole 500–800 mg 8-hourly for 5 days.
➤ Progressive abdominal distension, signs of developing peritonitis or haemorrhage requires surgical exploration and resection of the involved colon and drainage of peritoneal collections.
➤ Liver abscesses are aspirated under image guidance under cover of metronidazole 400 mg 8-hourly i.v. over 5–10 days.
➤ Repeated aspiration may be required for residual collections.

➔

➤ A right pleural effusion may precede abscess rupture into the pleural cavity; chest drainage is then required.
➤ Asymptomatic carriers are treated with diloxanide furoate 500 mg 8-hourly orally for 10 days.

FLUKES (TREMATODES)

Schistosomiasis (bilharziasis)

Definitions

● An infestation of the urinary tract and/or bowel by the trematodes *Schistosoma haematobium*, *S. mansoni*, *S. intercalatum* and *S. japonicum*, prevalent in Africa, the Middle East, South America, the Caribbean and the Far East.
● These parasites are found in freshwater snails and infect humans when they bathe in infected ponds and rivers.
● They enter the body through skin penetration, mature in the liver and settle in the bladder or bowel mucosa, where they produce ova, initiating a chronic inflammatory response with fibrosis.
● Parasite-induced squamous metaplasia is linked to a high incidence of squamous carcinoma of the bladder (*S. haematobium*) and colon (*S. japonicum*) in endemic areas.

Clinical features

● Urinary tract: dysuria, frequency and terminal haematuria; ureteric fibrosis leads to signs of obstructive uropathy on the affected side; bladder fibrosis results in a contracted bladder; infection of the seminal vesicles may result in secondary infertility; renal involvement is rare.
● Bowel: usually asymptomatic; a heavy worm load produces abdominal pain, loose motions containing blood and mucus; advanced lesions may produce bowel strictures with signs of subacute bowel obstruction.

- Hepatomegaly with portal and periportal fibrosis resulting in portal hypertension and splenomegaly.
- Inflammatory polyps of the rectosigmoid produced by chronic infestation may cause tenesmus and bloody diarrhoea (they are not premalignant).
- Lung, brain or spinal cord involvement is rare and may present with dyspnoea, seizures or nerve root compression.

Investigation

➤ Urine or stool microscopy and bladder or rectal mucosal biopsy demonstrate parasitic ova.
➤ X-ray abdominal and pelvis show calcified lesions in the ureter and/or bladder.
➤ Intravenous urography may show ureteric strictures causing obstructive uropathy.
➤ Cystoscopic appearance of 'sandy patches' in the mucosa is diagnostic.

Treatment

➤ Early infestation responds well to praziquantel 40–60 mg/kg in divided doses orally for 1 day.
➤ Ureteric stenosis may respond to dilatation or require reconstruction of the stenosed segment or resection and re-implantation.
➤ Contracted (small volume) bladder is enlarged by incorporating a segment of bowel or stomach (ileocystoplasty or gastrocystoplasty).

Liver flukes

Definitions

- *Clonorchis sinensis* and *Fasciola hepatica* are flukes, found in fresh waterways, that infect humans consuming contaminated watercress and fish, respectively, with sporadic epidemics in Europe, the Far East and Australia.
- The larvae migrate from the gut to the intrahepatic ducts through the ampulla of Vater, where they mature into adult flukes.

- Infection is associated with an increased risk of cholangiocarcinoma.

Clinical features

- Early features: urticaria, upper abdominal pain and diarrhoea with hepatomegaly, malaise and anaemia.
- Late features: cholecystitis, ascending cholangitis with obstructive jaundice from duct calculi or fibrosis and/or pancreatitis.

Investigation

➤ Tests for eosinophilia.
➤ Egg and fluke counts in faecal smears.

Treatment

➤ *Clonorchis sinensis*: oral praziquantel 40–120 mg/kg for 1–2 days.
➤ *Fasciola hepatica*: oral bithonol 30–50 mg/kg in divided daily doses for up to 15 days.
➤ Gallstones or biliary strictures caused by dead worms and eggs may require cholecystectomy with biliary drainage.
➤ Acute pancreatitis is treated by standard methods (see pancreas page 476).

Lung fluke

Definitions

- Lung fluke infection (*Paragonimus westermani*, *P. africanus* and related species) is contracted by eating infected freshwater shellfish or raw wild boar meat (intermediary hosts).
- The flukes migrate to the lung, where they induce an inflammatory reaction and form granulomas.
- Endemic in the Far East, Africa and the Americas.

Clinical features

- Recurrent cough productive of rust-coloured sputum containing the eggs of the parasite.

- May progress to recurrent episodes of broncho-pneumonia, with lung fibrosis and abscess formation.
- Neurological signs from a space-occupying lesion as a result of egg deposition in the brain is a rare complication of the disease.

Investigation
➤ Chest X-ray shows changes similar to pulmonary tuberculosis, with foci of calcification or cavitation.
➤ Smears of sputum and stool may demonstrate parasitic ova.

Treatment
➤ Oral praziquantel 25 mg/kg daily for 2 days or niclofolan a single dose of 2 mg/kg is effective in eradicating the disease.
➤ Pulmonary abscess responds to aspiration.

ROUND WORMS (NEMATODES)

Gut round worms

Hookworm

Definitions
- Caused by *Ancylostoma duodenale* and *Necator americanus*, hookworm is the commonest cause of anaemia and hypoproteinaemia in the tropics and the subtropics and an important cause of co-morbidity in the surgical patient.
- Worm larvae penetrate the skin from soil contaminated by human faeces containing ova; larvae then migrate to the lung and thence to the small intestine, where they mature and lay eggs.

Clinical features
- 'Ground itch' at the site of larval entry with an irritating vesicular rash.
- Fever and a dry cough with wheeze and dyspnoea may follow.

Investigation
➤ Stool smears show parasitic ova.
➤ Peripheral blood smear: hypochromic, microcytic anaemia and eosinophilia.

Treatment
➤ Single oral dose of albendazole 400 mg or levamisole 150 mg is curative; re-infection is, however, common.

Cutaneous larva migrans (creeping eruption)

Definitions
● Caused by larvae of non-human form of hookworm that are unable to complete their normal life cycle in the human host and remain burrowed under the skin, producing an intense and persisting itch.
● Endemic in most tropical and subtropical countries.

Clinical features
● Red, itchy papule at site of entry and larval tracts in hands, feet and abdomen in established disease.

Treatment
➤ Oral thiabendazole 25 mg/kg twice daily for 5 days.

Strongyloidiasis

Definitions
● Larvae of the nematode worm *Strongyloides stercoralis* penetrate the skin when it is in contact with soil contaminated by faeces. They migrate through the lungs and mature in the small bowel mucosa to adult worms and lay eggs, which are excreted.
● Endemic in most tropical and subtropical countries.

Clinical features

- Itchy skin rash with petechial haemorrhage at entry site and creeping eruptions caused by larval migration in the skin.
- Mucoid diarrhoea with malabsorption of fat and fat-soluble vitamins and a protein-losing enteropathy.
- Granulomas (rarely abscesses) may form in lung or bowel.

Investigation

➤ Leukocytosis and eosinophilia.
➤ Stool microscopy and cultures for ova and larvae.

Treatment

➤ Oral thiabendazole 25 mg/kg twice daily for 2–5 days or ivermectin 200 µg/kg daily for 2 days for chronic infection.
➤ Excision of bowel or lung granuloma or drainage of abscess.

Oesophagostomiasis (helminthoma)

Definitions

- The nematode *Oesophagostomum* (a natural parasite of monkeys) is transmitted to humans through faecal contamination of food.
- It penetrates bowel (ileocaecal) mucosa and produces inflammatory and later granulomatous lesions in the bowel wall.
- Sterile abscesses and adhesions may involve adjacent bowel loops and/or the abdominal wall.

Clinical features

- Abdominal pain of short duration localized to the right lower quadrant.
- Tender abdomen and a mass may be palpable.
- Acute appendicitis may be simulated in the acute phase of the disease.

Investigation
➤ Normal blood count with no eosinophilia.
➤ Contrast imaging of bowel may demonstrate a filling defect in the wall; must be distinguished from a tumour by colonoscopic biopsy.

Treatment
➤ Responds to oral tiabendazole 25 mg/kg 12-hourly for 3 days or ivermectin 200 μg/kg daily for 2 days.
➤ Surgery is required for bowel obstruction or drainage of abscesses.

Ascariasis

Definitions
● A nematode infection (*Ascaris lumbricoides*) endemic in the tropics and subtropics, with children of 3–9 years of age having the highest rate of infection.
● Infection is through the faeco-oral route.
● The eggs develop into larvae, which migrate through the cardiorespiratory system before settling in the lumen of the small bowel, where the adult worms lay eggs that are carried in the faeces and contaminate the soil.

Clinical features
● The majority of infected individuals have few or no symptoms.
● With increasing worm load nutritional disturbances are observed in children, resulting in growth retardation.
● Larval granulomas may form in the liver and, rarely, in other organs.
● Presents as acute or acute-on-chronic bowel obstruction.
● An ill-defined mass corresponding to the worm bolus may be palpable.
● Small bowel obstruction is caused by a worm bolus, or a bowel loop heavily loaded with worms may twist, strangulate or perforate.

- Strangulation may also be produced by a volvulus or intussusception of the worm-loaded loop, resulting in peritonitis.

Investigation

➤ Diagnosis is by stool ova counts with blood eosinophilia and a raised IgE antibody titre, and occasionally by the passage of adult worms.

➤ Abdominal X-ray may show features of bowel obstruction and may occasionally reveal a worm bolus.

➤ Small bowel opacification with barium may show worms in the lumen as cylindrical filling defects.

Treatment

➤ Subacute bowel obstruction resolves on bowel rest and cautious commencement of oral anti-helminthic therapy (levamisole 120–150 mg as a single dose, piperazine 4 g as a single dose or mebendazole 100 mg twice daily for 3 days).

➤ Dead or dying worms resulting from drug treatment may convert a partial into a complete obstruction, which is relieved surgically by milking the worm bolus down the bowel or by its removal through an enterotomy.

➤ When bowel viability is compromised, resection becomes imperative.

➤ Invasion of the bile and pancreatic ducts by worms from the duodenum may result in cholangitis, extrahepatic cholestasis or acute pancreatitis.

Tissue round worms

Filariasis; elephantiasis; and onchocerciasis: river blindness

Definitions

- Threadlike worms (*Wuchereria bancrofti*, *Brugia malayi et timori*, loa loa and *Onchocerca volvulus*) infect the human host in their larval forms through the bite of the mosquito, *Chrysops*, and the *Simulium* fly.

- Found throughout the tropical regions of Asia, Africa, China, the Pacific and the Americas.
- The larvae mature into adult worms in the lymphatic system or subcutaneous tissue, producing recurrent inflammation and fibrosis, with lymphatic obstruction in the limbs and scrotum with skin thickening and induration.

Clinical features

- Early features in wuchereria infection are recurrent febrile episodes and lymphangitis, with limb swelling and peripheral lymphadenitis involving the inguinal, axillary, cervical or epitrochlear nodes; occlusion of mesenteric lymphatics results in lymph escaping as chylous ascites, chylothorax, chylous diarrhoea or chyluria.
- Chronic phase:
  - Wuchereria infection produces brawny oedema and skin changes (elephantiasis)
  - Onchocercal infection produces skin nodules with patchy depigmentation and loose skin folds (leopard skin and hanging groin) and, more significantly, corneal opacities and blindness (river blindness).
- Loa loa produces smooth subcutaneous swellings of the limbs (calabar swelling) and may cause acute arthritis with effusion, meningo-encephalitis or choroidoretinitis.

Investigation

➤ Microfilaria are demonstrated in nocturnal blood smears (*Wuchereria* spp) and in skin snips (*Onchocerca* spp).
➤ Mazzotti test: a test dose of oral diethylcarbamazine produces intense itching and a skin rash in onchocerciasis.
➤ A serological immunochromatographic test (ICT) is highly sensitive and specific for bancroftian filariasis.
➤ Lymphangiography of a swollen limb demonstrates extreme dilatation and tortuosity of the affected lymphatics.

Treatment

➤ Oral diethylcarbamazine 150–200 mg tds for 2–3 weeks clears both microfilaria and adult worms from the circulation but is ineffective in closed cavities (hydrocoeles).

➤ Single oral dose of ivermectin 50–200 µg/kg is effective in onchocerciasis but eye infection may require i.v. suramin.

➤ Excision of onchocercal nodules and skin folds reduces worm load and disease progression and achieves cosmesis.

➤ Leg swelling is treated by physical measures and avoiding dependency.

➤ Surgical:
  - Excision of subcutaneous tissue and abnormal skin with skin grafting in the leg
  - Hydroceles and scrotal swellings are excised with redundant scrotal tissue.

Dracunculiasis (Guinea worm infection)

Definitions

● Filarial infection (*Dracunculus medinensis*), found in parts of Latin America, Africa, the Middle East and India, is transmitted in drinking water containing water-fleas infected with worm larvae.

● The larvae migrate from the gut in blood or lymph to the subcutaneous tissue, where the worms mature and release the larvae through a skin blister when in contact with water.

Clinical features

● Presents as a subcutaneous blister or a discharging ulcer, usually in the leg but may occur in the hip girdle, groin or scrotum or on the back, with preceding pyrexia, malaise, giddiness or urticaria.

● Occasionally the worm may be visible or palpable beneath the skin.

● Secondary infection of a blister or ulcer may result in a pyogenic abscess or tetanus.

Treatment

➤ Tiabendazole 25 mg/kg 12-hourly orally for 3 days is
  effective in controlling the infection (eradication is
  difficult as re-infection is common).

TAPEWORMS (CESTODES)

Hydatid disease (cystic echinococcosis)

Definitions

- *Echinococcus granulosus* and *E. multilocularis* are
  small tapeworms that infect humans through food
  contaminated by infected canine or rodent faeces.
- Endemic in sheep, camel, buffalo and deer farming
  regions of Australia, New Zealand, the Middle East,
  Africa, China, Russia and South America. Sporadic
  episodes occur in North America and Europe.
- The larvae penetrate the bowel wall and reach
  the liver or lungs and slowly mature into hydatid
  cysts.

Clinical features

- Non-specific abdominal or chest symptoms with
  malaise and tiredness.
- Hepatomegaly resulting from cyst formation (rarely
  jaundice or portal hypertension).
- Brain cysts may present as space-occupying lesions
  (lung cysts are quiescent).
- Anaphylactic shock may be produced by the rupture
  of large cysts.

Investigation

➤ Eosinophilia with lymphocytosis in peripheral blood
  smear.
➤ Characteristic cystic calcification in lung and liver on
  imaging.

Treatment

➤ Surgical excision of hydatid cysts in the liver or lung (following aspiration and sterilization with 1% cetrimide solution); bone cysts (rare) may require amputation.

➤ Albendazole therapy 10–50 mg/kg daily for 30 days controls and eradicates widespread disease; used in conjunction with surgery to reduce risk of recurrence.

➤ Liver resection or liver transplantation for advanced multilocular disease.

Bladderworm

Definitions

● A tapeworm infection (*Coenurus cerebralis*) of the brain transmitted by eating raw fruit and vegetables contaminated by infected animal faeces. Ingested eggs hatch into larvae in the gut and migrate to the brain, where they form cysts.

● Sporadic incidence in Africa and the Americas.

Clinical features

● Cysts in the brain produce raised intracranial pressure with focal neurological signs, confusion, epilepsy or paralysis.

Treatment

➤ Praziquantel in large doses (200–500 mg/kg) may be effective in controlling the disease.

➤ Craniotomy and cyst removal may prevent deterioration of cerebral function.

Bowel tapeworms

Definitions

● Tapeworms that infect the bowel are pork (*Taenia solium*), beef (*Taenia saginata*), fish and dwarf tapeworms, which are endemic in pork, beef and fish farming regions worldwide.

- Infection is acquired through consumption of contaminated, poorly cooked meat or fish.

Clinical features

- Usually asymptomatic within the bowel; rarely, a large, dead tapeworm may cause bowel obstruction.
- Weight loss, passage of segments.

Treatment
➤ Praziquantel 10 mg/kg as a single oral dose or miclosamide 2 g to be chewed over an hour.

Complications

- Cysticercosis is caused by the larval form of *Taenia solium*, which spreads via the bloodstream and causes significant morbidity.
- Brain involvement causes epilepsy and cerebral ataxia; treated with praziquantel and corticosteroids under neurological supervision.

Sparganosis

Definitions

- Larval infection by the tapeworm *Spirometra*, affecting muscle, bowel, mesentery, kidney, heart and brain; endemic in South-East Asia and Africa.
- Transmitted by drinking contaminated water containing the larvae or from eating raw snakes or by using raw frogs as poultice (both of which have eaten aquatic creatures infected with the larvae).

Clinical features

- Painful, migratory subcutaneous swellings in the chest, breast and legs, which may ulcerate, discharging the worm (sparganum).
- Worms proliferate by budding and may spread rapidly, producing haemoptysis, hepatosplenomegaly, lymph-oedema or cerebral disease. Eye involvement causes conjunctivitis and peri-orbital oedema.

> **Treatment**
> ➤ An invariably lethal disease with no effective treatment
> (praziquantel has failed.)

Myiasis (fly maggots of tumbu and bot flies in living tissue)

Definitions

- The larvae that hatch from the eggs of these flies penetrate the skin (from contaminated clothing) and mature into adults.
- Domestic animals and rodents are the definitive hosts.

Clinical features

- Itchy, painful rash at site of entry; later a small papule forms, containing a developing larva and serous fluid.

> **Treatment**
> ➤ Larvae may be squeezed or teased out.
> ➤ Occasionally requires surgical excision.

POISONING BY ANIMALS

Snake bites

Definitions

- Poisonous snakes are:
  - Elapidae (cobras, kraits and mambas): venom has a generalized neurotoxic/myotoxic effect
  - Viperidae (adders and vipers): venom has a local cytotoxic effect with tissue swelling and necrosis; it produces shock from bleeding owing to increased vascular permeability and renal failure
  - Hydrophiidae (sea snakes): venom is similar to that of the Elapidae, producing anticoagulation and muscle necrosis; also causes convulsions or respiratory paralysis

- Colubridae or back-fanged snakes (the boomslang):
  venom has a haemolytic effect that may cause renal
  failure
- Atractaspididae (the asps) produce autonomic
  symptoms and fever, with blistering and necrosis of
  bite site.
- There is no reliable means of distinguishing one species
  from another except by appearance and scale patterns.

Clinical features

- Severe pain and swelling of the bite site with blistering
  progressing to skin necrosis and thrombosis of
  superficial vessels.
- Systemic envenoming is indicated by:
  - Extensive swelling or bruising of bite site
  - Cardiac or haematological abnormalities.
- Systemic effects are:
  - Bilateral ptosis, conjunctival oedema or external
    ophthalmoplegia
  - Inability to open mouth, protrude tongue or swallow
  - Bleeding from gums or gastrointestinal bleeding
  - Glossopharyngeal nerve palsy, muscle pain, weakness
    and limb stiffness, or impaired consciousness
  - Respiratory distress as a result of pulmonary oedema
  - Hypotension resulting from splanchnic vasodilatation
  - Myocardial toxicity.

Investigation

➤ ECG abnormalities.
➤ Coagulopathy.
➤ Myoglobinuria.

Treatment

➤ Observe patient closely and give analgesia for local
  pain.
➤ Withhold treatment in the absence of local or
  systemic signs of poisoning when 2 or more hours
  have elapsed after the bite (the snake may be
  harmless!).

➔

➤ Calm and reassure patient; maintain verbal communication; monitor vital signs and level of consciousness.

➤ Do not suck, incise or cauterize the bite site or apply a tourniquet; apply dry dressing and firmly apply crepe bandage and immobilize affected part in a splint to prevent the spread of toxin in superficial tissues.

➤ Before antivenom is given a test dose of 1:100 dilution of the antivenom in normal saline is given intra-dermally (20–50 mL of specific antivenom in 1:3 dilution is given i.v. over 1–2 hours and may be repeated in the absence of an adequate response; an anaphylactic reaction may be counteracted by i.m. administration of 0.5 mL of 1:1000 adrenaline).

➤ Ventilatory support for neurotoxicity and respiratory failure.

➤ Blood/colloid transfusion is indicated for hypovolaemic shock (secondary to a bleeding diathesis or haemolysis).

➤ Antitetanus and antibiotic prophylaxis.

➤ Delayed debridement of non-viable skin and muscle, decompress compartment syndrome caused by muscle swelling.

➤ Renal failure (as a result of haemolytic crisis or muscle necrosis) is treated with optimal fluid and electrolyte replacement and by monitoring hourly urinary output (dialysis is rarely required).

Spider bites and scorpion stings

Definitions

- Venomous spiders are distributed worldwide and produce local tissue damage (the brown recluse spider), neurotoxicity or cardiac toxicity (the black widow, hourglass, button, red-black and banana spiders) causing respiratory failure.
- Scorpions with fatal stings, particularly in children, have a wide tropical distribution in North Africa, the Middle East, the Americas, the Caribbean and Asia.

Clinical features

- Bites and stings are painful with local inflammation and may progress to necrosis and ulceration of the site.
- Systemic effects are fever, rigors, drowsiness, jaundice and coma.
- Acute pancreatitis as a result of exocrine stimulation with sphincter spasm (black scorpion sting).
- Haemolytic crisis and jaundice (black widow spider bite).

Treatment

➤ Wound toilet and splinting of involved part.
➤ Delayed debridement of bite site rarely needed.
➤ Systemic poisoning is treated with specific antivenom and urinary output monitored with fluid and diuretic therapy as indicated.

Fish stings

Definitions

- Caused by sting rays, weaver fish, scorpion fish, stone fish and the Portuguese- man-of-war.
- The venoms consist of vasoactive agents and enzymes and produce local pain, necrosis and cardiac, muscle and neurological toxicity.

Clinical features

- Nausea, vomiting (caused by autonomic nervous stimulation)
- Cardiac arrhythmias
- Respiratory distress
- Convulsions.

Treatment

➤ Immerse stung limb in warm water and remove spine, fish membrane and foreign material from wound.
➤ Give parenteral analgesia and tetanus toxoid and antibiotic prophylaxis for large wounds.

➔

> ➤ Maintain adequate airway and prepare for cardio-pulmonary resuscitation for respiratory failure or vasopressor therapy for hypotension.
> ➤ Antivenom is available for scorpion fish sting.

Jellyfish, sea anemone, sea urchin, star fish, octopus and cone shell

Definitions

- Similar properties to fish venom and produce severe pain, inflammation or urticaria.
- Depresses respiration and produces muscle paralysis leading to respiratory failure and death (the box jelly fish, the blue-ringed octopus and the cone shell).

Treatment

> ➤ Remove venomous tentacles or spines stuck to the skin and bathe the area with commercial vinegar or baking soda in water (deeply embedded spines require surgical removal).
> ➤ Cardiopulmonary resuscitation with mechanical ventilation is required if the patient becomes cyanosed or comatose.

AINHUM

- Progressive fibrous constriction at the base of the fifth toe resulting in spontaneous auto-amputation of the toe.
- Probable racial predisposition afflicting those of African descent.

ANAEMIAS

Definitions

Anaemia is defined as a decrease in the level of haemoglobin in the blood below the reference level for age and sex and results in a decreased oxygen-carrying capacity of the blood. There are three types:

- Normocytic normochromic (normal MCV):
  - Acute blood loss
  - Anaemia of chronic disease
  - Infection
  - Collagen disease
  - Malignancy
  - Endocrine disease.
- Hypochromic microcytic (low mean cell volume, MCV):
  - Iron deficiency
  - Thalassaemia
  - Anaemia of chronic disease
  - Sideroblastic anaemia.
- Macrocytic (high MCV):
  - Impaired DNA synthesis as a result of vitamin B_{12} and folate deficiency (found in liver disease and chronic alcoholism)
  - Abnormalities of DNA synthesis (found in sideroblastic anaemia, erythroleukaemia and chemotherapy)
  - Post gastrectomy.

Clinical features

Clinical symptoms depend on severity and rapidity of onset:

- Lassitude, malaise, easy fatiguability and muscle weakness
- Headache, faintness and breathlessness
- Palpitations, angina of effort, tachycardia, systolic murmur and heart failure
- Pallor, papilloedema and retinal bleed (rare)
- Intermittent claudication.

Investigation

➤ Haemoglobin below 13 g/dL for men and 12 g/dL for non-pregnant women.
➤ MCV is measured electronically but may be calculated from the packed cell volume (PCV) and red cell count (RCC) [MCV = PCV/RCC ×1000 fL] (normal range 82–96 fL in adults and 70 fL up to 2 years of age).

➜

➤ Mean cell haemoglobin (MCH), MCH = Hb/RCC pg (normal range 27–33 pg), is raised in macrocytosis and lowered in all states with a low MCV.

➤ Mean cell haemoglobin concentration (MCHC), MCHC = Hb/PCV% (normal range 31.7–34.1%), is raised in spherocytosis and decreased in iron deficiency and anaemia of chronic disease. It is normal in the thalassaemias and haemoglobinopathies (and is used to distinguish these from iron deficiency).

➤ Peripheral blood film identifies red cell morphology (as normocytic, microcytic or macrocytic, and normo-chromic or hypochromic).

➤ Bone marrow smears: increased cellularity is found in iron deficiency, haemolysis and hypersplenism and megaloblastic anaemias; also in marrow infiltration (leukaemias, lymphomas and metastatic carcinomas); hypocellular marrow is characteristic of aplastic anaemia (iron stain: iron in red cell fragments (siderotic granules) excludes iron deficiency; iron stores are generally increased in pernicious anaemia, thalassaemia, sickle-cell disease, siderotic anaemias and haemosiderosis). The normal iron store in adults is 5 g (found in haemoglobin 2–3 g and the reticulo-endothelial system 0.5–1.5 g).

➤ Serum iron-binding capacity and soluble transferring receptor assay.

➤ Anaemia resulting from suspected blood loss into the gastrointestinal tract or urogenital system requires appropriate stool/urine analysis and imaging.

NORMOCYTIC AND MICROCYTIC ANAEMIAS

Normocytic anaemia

Definitions

Causes:

- Blood loss
- Chronic disease

- Blood diseases: aplastic and haemolytic anaemias
- Endocrine diseases: pituitary, thyroid and adrenal cortical hypofunction.

Iron deficiency

Definitions

Insufficient iron for haem synthesis as a result of depleted iron stores. Causes:

- Occult blood loss from gut or uterus
- Poor dietary intake
- Increased demands in growth and pregnancy
- Decreased absorption (post gastrectomy).

Clinical features

- Brittle nails and hair; koilonychia
- Glossitis and papillary atrophy
- Angular stomatitis
- Dysphagia (Plummer–Vinson syndrome).

Investigation

➤ Blood film: microcytic hypochromic red cells, target cells, poikilocytosis (variations in shape) and elliptocytosis ('pencil' cells).
➤ Low serum iron.
➤ Raised total iron binding capacity is found in inflammations/infections (normal range 15–250 mg/L).

Treatment

➤ Treat underlying cause of iron deficiency (chronic blood loss, malabsorption).
➤ Replenish iron stores by oral iron therapy: ferrous sulphate 200 mg bd or tds for 4–6 months (ferrous gluconate or fumarate may be substituted in cases of poor tolerance).
➤ Parenteral iron is given to replenish iron stores rapidly in the presence of continuing blood loss (usually from the gastrointestinal tract).

MACROCYTIC ANAEMIAS

Definitions

- A proportion of red cells are enlarged (MCV >98 fL): oval macrocytosis is seen in megaloblastic anaemias and round macrocytosis in liver disease, hypothyroidism and alcoholism.
- Differentiated into megaloblastic and non-megaloblastic anaemias.

Megaloblastic anaemias

Vitamin B$_{12}$ deficiency and pernicious anaemia

Definitions

- Failure of intrinsic factor production resulting from gastric mucosal atrophy or vitamin B$_{12}$ malabsorption or postgastrectomy.
- An autoimmune disease producing antibodies to parietal cell and intrinsic factor, and may predispose to gastric carcinoma.

Clinical features

- Pigmentation, anorexia, weight loss and diarrhoea.
- Angular stomatitis and atrophic glossitis.
- Insidious neurological changes: paraesthesiae, loss of proprioception and ataxia leading to progressive polyneuropathy and paraplegia.

Investigation

➤ Blood film: macrocytes and hypersegmented polymorphs; raised MCV.
➤ Bone marrow film: megaloblastic erythropoiesis.
➤ Reduced serum vitamin B$_{12}$ (normal range 160–925 µg/L).
➤ B$_{12}$ absorption test (Schilling test): oral administration of 1 µg of labelled cyanocobalamin followed by a flushing dose of 1000 µg i.m. of non-radioactive B$_{12}$;

➜

a 24-hour urine collection estimates the percentage of the oral dose excreted, indicating level of absorption. The test is repeated with addition of intrinsic factor orally; in pernicious anaemia B_{12} malabsorption is corrected by intrinsic factor.

➤ Therapeutic trial: 1 μg of vitamin B_{12} i.m. daily for 7 days with a rise in haemoglobin of 1 g/dL suggests deficiency.

➤ Deoxyuridine suppression test: determines nature and severity of B_{12} deficiency.

Treatment
➤ Hydroxocobalamin 1000 μg i.m. injections on alternate days for six doses followed by 1000 μg 3-monthly as maintenance.

Folate deficiency
Definitions
Causes:

● Dietary deficiency or malabsorption (coeliac disease and tropical sprue), or increased utilization (pregnancy and lactation) and in chronic haemolytic anaemias
● Antifolate drugs (antimalarials, trimethoprim) deplete borderline folate stores
● Haemodialysis or peritoneal dialysis.

Clinical features
● Insidious onset of anaemia with absent neurological complications (unlike B_{12} deficiency).

Investigation
➤ Red cell folate content (normal range 160–640 μg/L).
➤ Therapeutic trial: 100 μg of oral folic acid daily for 7 days with a rise in haemoglobin level by 1 g/L suggests deficiency.
➤ Deoxyuridine suppression test: determines severity and nature of folate deficiency.

Treatment

> 5 mg folic acid orally daily.

Complications

Macrocytosis without megaloblastic changes. Causes:

- Physiological: in newborn and pregnancy
- Liver disease and alcoholism
- Hypothyroidism
- Aplastic and sideroblastic anaemia
- Chemotherapy (azathioprine).

Sideroblastic anaemia

Definitions

- Inherited.
- Acquired: myeloproliferative or myelodysplastic disorder; drug or alcohol induced; lead poisoning.

Anaemias of chronic disease (secondary anaemias)

Definitions

- Impaired bone marrow response to the anaemia associated with decreased erythropoietin production and red cell survival. Causes:
  - Chronic infections (infective endocarditis, tuberculosis, osteomyelitis and fungal infections)
  - Chronic inflammatory disease (rheumatoid arthritis, systemic lupus erythematosus, polymyalgia rheumatica, inflammatory bowel disease)
  - Carcinomas and lymphomas.

Investigation

> Haemoglobin rarely falls below 8 g/dL.
> MCV is usually between 70 and 85 fL (lower in children).
> Neutrophilia with raised erythrocyte sedimentation rate and platelet count.

→

➤ Blood film: increased rouleaux formation.
➤ Low serum iron and total iron-binding capacity.
➤ Normal or raised serum ferritin (as a result of inflammatory process).

Treatment

➤ Oral iron therapy; treat underlying disease.

Aplastic anaemia

Definitions

- Marrow failure resulting in a pancytopenia because of stem cell population reduction.
- Predisposes to myeloblastic leukaemia (resulting from emergence of abnormal stem cell clones).

Causes are:

- Congenital (Fanconi's syndrome)
- Chemical agents (benzene)
- Ionizing radiation
- Infections (viral)
- Paroxysmal nocturnal haemoglobinuria.

Clinical features

- Anaemia with superadded infections.
- Ecchymoses, bleeding gums and epistaxis.

Investigation

➤ Peripheral film: pancytopenia with absence of reticulocytes.
➤ Marrow smear: hypocellular.

Treatment

➤ Red cell and platelet (leukocyte depleted) transfusion.
➤ Antibiotic therapy to combat infection.
➤ Bone marrow transplant for severe anaemia (<45 years of age).
➤ Immunosuppression with anti-lymphocyte globulin and ciclosporin may initiate remission.

Complications

- Failure of one stem cell line may produce a pure red cell aplasia, which is associated with a thymoma (30% incidence); thymectomy may induce remission.

HAEMOLYTIC ANAEMIAS

Definitions

- Caused by increased destruction of red cells in the circulation or in the reticulo-endothelial system (spleen) thereby shortening normal red cell lifespan of 100–120 days.
- Anaemia results when the marrow's capacity for red cell production is exceeded.

Investigation

➤ Increased red cell destruction (jaundice, hyperbilirubinaemia, raised urobilinogen in urine, reduced plasma haptoglobin and raised serum lactic dehydrogenase).
➤ Increased red cell production (reticulocytosis, marrow erythroid hyperplasia).
➤ Measurement of red cell survival by ^{51}Cr tagging.

INHERITED HAEMOLYTIC ANAEMIAS

Hereditary spherocytosis

Definitions

- Common autosomal dominant anaemia in Europeans (incidence 1:5000).
- Caused by red cell membrane defects.

Clinical features

- Usually jaundiced at birth.
- May present later with anaemia, splenomegaly and leg ulcers.

Investigation
➤ Blood film: spherocytes and reticulocytes.
➤ Haemolysis (raised bilirubin and urinary urobilinogen).
➤ Increased red cell fragility (swelling and lysis in hypotonic solution).
➤ Coombs' test negative (distinguishes from autoimmune haemolytic anaemias).

Treatment
➤ Splenectomy is curative; postponed until after childhood to reduce infection risk.

Complications
● Hereditary elliptocytosis is a similar but much milder condition, with only a minority of patients developing anaemia.

Sickle-cell disease

Definitions
● Sickle-cell anaemia is caused by inherited haemoglobin SS (homozygous) and AS (heterozygous) genotypes and is found in people of African, southern Mediterranean and Caribbean descent. The disease manifests only in the SS genotype, the AS, sickle-cell trait, being asymptomatic carriers.
● Low oxygen tension in the peripheral blood produces sickling of red cells, resulting in a haemolytic anaemia.
● Haemolysed cells are vaso-occlusive, causing infarcts in the spleen, liver and long bones, producing the sequestration syndrome and marrow failure.

Clinical features
● Anaemia, joint, bone or abdominal pain and generalized peripheral lymphadenopathy.
● Tender hepatomegaly and/or splenomegaly with tenderness over bone infarcts.

- Haemolytic jaundice.
- Haematuria following a severe crisis as a result of renal papillary necrosis.
- Long-term manifestations: susceptibility to infections, chronic leg ulcers and growth disorders in children, aseptic bone necrosis, pigmented gallstones, chronic renal disease and blindness.

Investigation

➤ Screening sickle test: pre-operative haemoglobin S (HBS) detection in at-risk ethnic groups.
➤ Blood film: shows sickling during crises.
➤ Bone radiology: avascular necrosis with partial collapse of the femoral head or severe joint deformity.

Treatment

➤ Haemoglobin SS patients for elective or emergency surgery may require exchange transfusion. There should be optimal tissue oxygenation during anaesthetic induction, operative and postoperative periods.
➤ Avoid unpressurized air travel, cold and dehydration.
➤ Treatment of sickle cell crisis
  - Oxygen
  - Hydration i.v.
  - Opiate analgesia
  - Treat infection
  - Hydroxyurea may resolve frequency of crises.
➤ Bone marrow transplant in severe cases.

Complications

- Osteomyelitis (usually *Salmonella* infection): the affected limb is swollen, tender and warm; appropriate systemic antibiotic therapy when started early leads to resolution.
- Abscess formation requires debridement of necrotic bone and drainage.
- Pathological fracture or vertebral collapse result from infarcts and may produce cord or nerve root compression; treat by immobilization (may require surgical splinting).
- Cerebral infarcts are rare.

Sickle-cell trait

- Asymptomatic condition where 50% of the haemo-globin is HBS. Sickling may still occur under extreme conditions, e.g. anoxia, critical illness.
- Avoid precipitating factors; maintain oxygenation and hydration during anaesthesia.

Glucose-6-phosphate dehydrogenase deficiency

Definitions

- A common cause of non-spherocytic haemolytic anaemia in Africa, the Middle East and the Mediterranean region.
- Glucose-6-phosphate dehydrogenase (G-6-PD) deficiency predisposes to haemolysis, as it is the rate-limiting enzyme of the pentose–phosphate shunt that produces reduced nicotinamide adenine dinucleotide phosphate (NADP) (which protects the red cell from the oxidative stress of anaerobic glycolysis).
- Sex-linked transmission affecting males, infants and children.
- Haemolysis is precipitated by drugs (sulfonamides, chloramphenicol, sulfasalazine, nalidixic acid and antimalarials); foods (broad beans – 'favism' – and food additives); infections (typhoid, malaria and viral hepatitis).

Clinical features

- Severe anaemia accompanied by jaundice in the presence of a precipitating factor.

Investigation

➤ Blood film: reticulocytes with irregular (bite) cells, blister cells and Heinz bodies.
➤ Raised serum bilirubin and lactate dehydrogenase enzyme.
➤ Screening test: cresyl blue dye decoloration in the presence of G-6-PD activity.
➤ Enzyme assay of G-6-PD activity.

Treatment
➤ Immediate discontinuation of the agent precipitating haemolysis.
➤ Treat infections vigorously with appropriate antibiotics (malaria must be treated with antimalarials not implicated in haemolysis, such as chloroquine and primaquine).
➤ Blood transfusion for severe haemolytic episodes.

Pyruvate kinase deficiency

Definitions
● Inherited, autosomal recessive transmission.
● Defect in red cell metabolism with reduced adenosine triphosphate synthesis, producing 'rigid' red cells.

Clinical features
● Presents in childhood with anaemia of variable severity.

Investigation
➤ Blood film: distorted (prickle) cells and reticulocytes.
➤ Low pyruvate kinase activity (by enzyme assay).

Treatment
➤ Blood transfusions.
➤ Splenectomy may improve prognosis.

Thalassaemias (Mediterranean anaemia)

Definitions
● An inherited haemolytic disease of southern Mediterranean and north African communities resulting in reduced synthesis of the globin chains (beta-chain in beta-thalassaemia and alpha-chain in alpha-thalassaemia).

- Only dominant (homozygous) disease (thalassaemia major) manifests as an anaemia in early childhood, requiring lifelong blood transfusions leading to iron overload (the latter is associated with growth retardation, multiple endocrine deficiencies, pancreatic insufficiency and diabetes mellitus).

Clinical features

- Anaemia and failure to thrive, with gross splenomegaly.
- Haemorrhagic tendency and pathological fractures.

Investigation

➤ Peripheral blood film: gross hypochromia, nucleated red cells and numerous target cells.

Treatment

➤ Parental counselling.
➤ 6–8 weekly transfusions with red cell concentrates.
➤ Folic acid supplementation.
➤ Desferrioxamine infusions (chelating agent) to prevent iron overload.

BLOOD TRANSFUSION IN THE TREATMENT OF SEVERE ANAEMIA

- Blood transfusion is a highly effective but temporary therapy for anaemia.
- Indications: acute haemolysis (G-6-PD deficiency), acute sequestration crises (sickle-cell), aplastic crisis and in cases of late pregnancy or haemorrhage aggravating an underlying anaemia.
- Risks: hypersensitivity reactions and transmission of infection (viral hepatitis, AIDS and malaria).
- Exchange transfusion: when an equal volume of the patient's blood is replaced by transfused blood, used in treating neonatal jaundice, severe anaemia in late pregnancy, sickle-cell crises and cerebral malaria (with a high parasitaemia).

ANAEMIAS IN THE TROPICS

- Anaemia is an important cause of co-morbidity in the tropics for patients undergoing surgery. They require pre-operative assessment and treatment of chronic infections, nutritional work-up in protein–calorie malnutrition, and peri-operative supportive measures for patients with sickle-cell anaemia, G-6-PD deficiency and thalassaemias.
- Secondary anaemias are also caused by chronic parasitic infections, malaria, visceral leishmaniasis, trypanosomiasis, tuberculosis, schistosomiasis and hookworm.

ONCOLOGY

Cancers

Cancers are tissues that escape the controlling mechanisms of cell proliferation and cell death. They show the following features:

- Abnormalities in cell proliferation
- Abnormalities in cell differentiation
- Abnormalities in intercellular and stromal relationships.

Most cancers are monoclonal (caused by a single gene mutation) and arise from a single cell line. These mutations may be inherited or acquired.

Carcinogenesis

Carcinogenesis is the conversion of normal cells into tumour cells and is a multistage sequence of events (initiation → promotion → tumour formation).

- DNA damage or alteration in the genome results in an oncogene that initiates transformation into a tumour cell.
- In tumour cells normal cell proliferation is unchecked by apoptosis (programmed 'physiological' cell death)

and leads to 'perpetual' survival of increasing cell numbers, resulting in tumour formation.
- Tumour growth results from the loss of normal intercellular adhesion (by downregulation of E-cadherins), degradation of the surrounding stroma (by metalloproteinases) and by the initiation of angiogenesis (growth of tumour blood vessels and lymphatics).
- Escape from immunological surveillance by inactivation of major histocompatibility antigens and cadherins.
- Invasion of surrounding structures is assisted by motility factors (integrins) and matrix metalloproteinases (degrade stromal matrix).

Cancer genes

The genesis of cancer involves the input of cancer genes that bring about sequential changes, transforming normal cells into cancer cells; the following have been studied:

- Cell multiplication is stimulated by proto-oncogenes and inhibited by anti-oncogenes
- Proto-oncogenes are activated into oncogenes by carcinogens
- Anti-oncogenes (tumour-suppressor genes) inhibit excessive cell proliferation by binding to gene mutations and repairing damaged DNA
- Mutator genes repair DNA damage during replication and that caused by carcinogens
- Ced genes control apoptosis; overexpression of some of these genes inhibits apoptosis and promotes carcinogenesis
- Telomerase enzyme prevents the normal shortening of chromosomal ends (telomeres) during cell division that leads to natural cell death and permits continued cell division found in tumour growth.

All cancers appear to involve multiple sequential genetic alterations involving oncogenes, tumour-suppressor genes, mutator genes and apoptosis genes.

Carcinogens

A carcinogen is any environmental factor that increases the risk of cancer development.

- Chemical carcinogenesis: a multistep process involving an initiation–promotion sequence; a chemical initiator (carcinogen) produces gene damage and mutation and promoters induce tumour growth in tissue sustaining gene damage.
- Radiation carcinogenesis: radiant energy (ultraviolet light and ionizing radiations) produces genetic damage and mutations by inducing the formation of oxygen-free radicals.
- Infective agents as carcinogens: some DNA and RNA viruses and bacteria (*Helicobacter pylori*).

Spread of cancer

Metastases are islands of cancer cells found distant from the primary tumour with no direct continuity; metastases spread by:

- Lymphatics: tumour cells grow into lymphatics, embolize and invade adjacent tissue or enter regional lymph nodes where they may be destroyed, remain dormant or multiply
- Blood vessels: tumour cells invade capillaries and venules, are conveyed in the bloodstream to distant sites, where they migrate out of the vessels by proteolysis
- Transcoelomic: tumour spread occurs in a visceral cavity from one structure to another by detachment and migration of tumour cells (Krukenberg's tumours).

Clinical features

Cancers may present as:

- A mass lesion or an ulcer
- An obstructing lesion in a hollow viscus

- Pressure symptoms or pain from invasion of adjacent structures
- Pain resulting from tumour infarction
- Haemorrhage from invasion of large vessels.

Paraneoplastic syndromes are constitutional disturbances unrelated to the local effects of the tumour or metastases; effects may manifest as:

- Endocrine: ectopic hormone secretion as a result of malignant transformation
- Metabolic: found in all tumours (mechanism not understood)
- Haematological: anaemia (all tumours), erythrocytosis (liver and renal carcinoma), red cell aplasia (thymoma) and disseminated intravascular coagulation (mucinous carcinomas)
- Neurological: effect of tumour autoantibodies (peripheral neuropathy, cerebellar degeneration, carcinomatous myelopathy)
- Musculoskeletal: polyarthritis (breast carcinoma), systemic lupus erythematosus-like syndrome (lymphoma) and dermatomyositis (lung carcinoma).

Investigation

Tumour assessment:

➤ TNM staging describes the size of primary tumour (T) or depth of invasion, extent of regional nodal disease (N) and presence of metastases (M)
➤ Imaging: plain radiology, ultrasound, CT and MRI scans assess the primary tumour and radioisotope body scans the presence of metastases
➤ Grading: indicates aggressive potential and is based on the degree of cellular differentiation, nuclear pleo-morphism and mitotic activity
➤ Tumour markers: chemicals secreted by tumours into the circulation, titres of which may indicate extent and/or spread.

Treatment

➤ Treatment (primary and adjuvant therapies) is based on:
  – The natural history of the disease
  – Type, grade and stage of the tumour
  – Age and frailty of the patient
  – Results of clinical trials
  – Whether the treatment is curative or palliative.
➤ Primary tumour is treated by surgery, radiotherapy, chemotherapy, hormonal therapy or any combination of these:
  – **Surgery:** complete excision with/without excision of regional lymph nodes; palliative excision (debulking) of large/extensive lesions. Surgery is determined by the tumour type, grade, stage and tumour biology and the anatomical site. Surgical reconstruction following tumour excision may be required for functional or cosmetic reasons
  – **Radiotherapy:** used as primary treatment of radiosensitive tumours (seminoma, localized Hodgkin's disease), when tumours are inoperable (brainstem lesions), or when preferred to surgery for a better functional or cosmetic result (laryngeal cancer, basal cell cancer of the face). Pre-operative radiotherapy is used to downstage a tumour, enabling complete excision. Postoperative radiotherapy is used to sterilize the surgical field to reduce the incidence of local recurrence. May be used as an adjuvant to chemotherapy in acute leukaemias
  – **Chemotherapy:** usually used in the adjuvant setting following surgery; cytotoxic agents may be used in combination with each drug, acting on a different phase of the cell cycle and ensuring that their toxicities do not overlap
  – **Endocrine therapy:** drugs are used to antagonize the action of hormones that sustain tumour growth (tamoxifen or aromatase inhibitors in breast carcinoma and gonadorelin analogues or anti-androgen (diethylstilboestrol) in prostatic carcinoma

➔

- **Immunotherapy:** Bacille Calmette–Guérin vaccine and some cytokines modulate the immune response, producing tumour remission (interferons and interleukin-2 in melanoma and renal carcinoma)
- **Combined treatments:** surgery and radiotherapy are needed to treat locally advanced tumours where the two modalities have complementary roles in achieving local control of the disease, with preservation of structure and function; chemotherapy combined with surgery is required when there is a high probability of micrometastatic disease requiring systemic treatments, with effective local control.
- Metastatic malignancy in regional lymph nodes.
- All the above modalities are used to treat clinically involved nodes in the regional drainage sites and those at high risk of harbouring metastases. Surgically removed nodes provide information to stage the primary tumour.

Chemotherapy

Cytotoxic agents act by interfering with DNA synthesis and may be used in combination, acting at different phases of the cell cycle (thereby ensuring their toxicities do not overlap). They are grouped as follows:

- Alkylating agents (cyclophosphamide, nitrogen mustards, platinum)
- Antimetabolites (methotrexate, 5-fluorouracil, purine analogues)
- Intercalating agents (anthracyclines)
- Spindle poisons (vinca alkaloids, taxanes)
- Miscellaneous agents (procarbazine, hydroxycarbide).

Optimal drug dose and dose intensity (drug dose per unit time) are necessary to achieve a cure; drugs are given as pulsed or intermittent therapy which allows large doses to be given with rest periods for normal tissue recovery, or as continuous infusions with doses adjusted to permit normal tissue recovery during treatment.

Radiotherapy

- Ionizing radiation or energy from ionized particles causes DNA damage, thereby producing tumour regression.
- Ionizing radiation consists of gamma rays (produced by the decay of radioactive isotopes, radionuclides) and X-rays, the penetration of which is dependent on the voltage.
- Electron beams decay with depth and are used to treat superficial lesions.
- Treatment planning: the total dose, fractionation and treatment duration are calculated on the characteristics of the radiation beam, tumour volume and location.
- Shielding of normal anatomy during treatment is by radiation field mapping, dose adjustment, angulation of beam and protecting adjacent structures with shields.
- Radiation protection of patients and personnel is based on radiation safety guidelines.

SKIN

- Surgeons, like all clinicians, see many cutaneous lesions either as the presenting complaint or as an incidental finding.
- A confident diagnosis facilitates a clear explanation to the patient and appropriate management, be this surgical, referral to another department or a conservative approach.
- The skin may be an indicator of underlying systemic disease.

Colour

- Pallor: anaemia, hypoalbuminaemia, uraemia.
- Yellow: uraemia, jaundice, mepacrine.
- Blue: chloroquine, mercurial products, methaemoglobin and cyanosis.
- Pigmentation: pregnancy (melasma gravidarum), Addison's disease, haemochromatosis, Wilson's disease, ectopic adrenocorticotropic hormone (ACTH), Cushing's disease, Nelson's syndrome, pellagra, acanthosis nigricans and sunburn.

- Gold: arsenic and cytotoxic drugs.
- Pigmented spots: café au lait of neurofibromatosis and Peutz–Jeghers syndrome.
- Orange: carotenaemia.
- Purple: polycythaemia and purpura from any cause.
- Depigmentation: albinism, vitiligo, pernicious anaemia, Addison's disease, autoimmune disorders, scleroderma, syphilis, leprosy and tuberculosis.

Nails

- Colour changes mirror those in the previous section.
- Half-and-half nails with proximal white and distal brown colouring of renal failure.
- Red moon bases of congestive cardiac failure.
- Brown: smoking and fungal infection.
- Clubbing: chronic respiratory disorder, cyanotic, cardiac, inflammatory bowel disease and cirrhosis.
- Koilonychia: spoon deformity of iron deficiency.
- Beau's lines: transverse mark showing delayed growth, often associated with severe illness.
- Splinter haemorrhages: bacterial endocarditis and vasculitis.
- Deformity of psoriatic involvement.
- Onycholysis: premature separation from nail plate as a result of trauma, infection, thyroid disease.
- Onychogryphosis: curved horny thickening of the nail as a result of trauma; also pits, ridges and white markings.
- Ingrowing toenails (page 738), infected nails, paronychia (page 195).
- Subungual lesions: haematoma, glomus tumours, exostoses and malignant melanomas.

Associated diseases

- Rheumatoid: nodules.
- Osteoarthritis: Heberden's nodes.
- Gout: tophi.
- Hyperlipidaemia: xanthelasma. Crohn's disease, sarcoid and amyloid infiltration.
- Collagen diseases: vasculitic.

Cutaneous manifestations of malignancy

- Acanthosis nigricans: gut.
- Ichthyosis and keratosis: gut.
- Ectopic ATCH syndromes: bronchus and gut.
- Dermatomyositis: gut.
- Erythema gyratum repens: bronchus and gut.
- (Superficial) thrombophlebitis migrans: pancreas and stomach (Trousseau's sign).
- Peutz–Jeghers pigmentation: testes and ovaries.
- Multiple basal cell carcinomas: medulloblastoma (Gorlin's syndrome).
- Cysts and osteomata: colon (Gardiner's syndrome).
- Sebaceous tumours: gastrointestinal (Torr, Muir).

Pruritus

- Itching is a feature of many skin diseases, including dermatitis, urticaria and psoriasis, and may indicate infestation by mites, lice and fleas.
- Itching is common in pregnancy, obstructive jaundice, liver and renal failure, blood dyscrasia, malignancy, iron deficiency, diabetes, hypothyroidism, as a side-effect of certain drugs and in psychiatric conditions.
- Treatment is of the cause; calamine lotion to soothe symptoms.

Dermatitis

- Dermatitis is the commonest skin disorder. The term is often used interchangeably with eczema, although the latter is best retained for the endogenous form of the disease.
- Skin changes are initially inflammation, producing redness and oedema and the marked irritation and subsequent scratching, causing excoriation, weeping and secondary bacterial infection.
- Dermatitis is commonest in hands, as a result of exposure such as prolonged dehydration or fluid immersion, abrasion (e.g. fibreglass), and acid, alkalis, aldehydes, solvents, acrylics and resins.

- Dermatitis may also be caused by soaps, cosmetics, latex and base metals of jewellery.
- **Allergic responses** are mediated through the release of immunoglobulin E, complement mast cells and prostaglandin inhibitors. Allergens include pollen, house-dust mites, food stuffs (such as cow's milk), nuts, additives, spices and shellfish, and are reported with most drugs, particularly beta-lactams.
- The clinical effects of allergy are fever and urticaria.
- **Acute anaphylaxis**, occasionally related to the above allergens as well as insect bites and stings, can give rise to bronchospasm, laryngospasm and hypotension, producing dyspnoea, hypoxia, cyanosis, nausea, vomiting and diarrhoea. Emergency treatment is intramuscular adrenaline, oxygen and intravenous fluids, followed by chlorphenitamine and steroids. Once identified, sufferers must carry 1:1000 adrenaline, possibly in the form of a self-injection pen.

Psoriasis affects 2% of the population, particularly young adults, producing silvery-grey sharply defined scaly plaques, marked over the extensor surfaces of elbows, knees and involving the nails.

Skin, its appendages and subcutaneous tissues are subject to many **congenital**, **traumatic**, **inflammatory**, **neoplastic** and **degenerative lesions**.

- Many of these lesions require surgical management for cosmetic reasons, and the diagnosis or eradication of malignancy.

Congenital lesions

- Congenital skin lesions include dermoid cyst, along the line of fusion of primitive skin folds (external angular dermoids of the lateral end of the eyebrow), and sinuses and fistulae (pilonidal and branchial). Arteriovenous malformations are considered on page 590.

Trauma

- **Wounds** commonly require surgical management, such as debridement, closure and revision; while burns also require skilled fluid management.

- **Scars** may become **hypertrophic** or **keloid,** where they extend into the surrounding tissues, the latter being common in young black Africans.
- Scars should be left to mature for at least 6 months, by which time hypertrophic scars usually regress and become paler. Keloid is difficult to manage as it tends to recur, but may respond to repeated injections of triamcinolone or steroid patches.
- Prolonged pressure may produce **callosities,** particularly with coexistent neuropathy (page 773).
- **Pressure ulcers** may occur in bed-bound debilitated patients; contributory factors are poor nutritional status, anaemia, skin changes of ageing and low body mass index.
- Pressure ulcers are graded as:
  - Skin erythema and oedema, with or without induration (grade 1)
  - A blister or abrasion (grade 2)
  - Full-thickness skin loss (grade 3)
  - Skin loss with underlying tissue destruction (grade 4).
- Ulcers are debrided, using regular dressings to remove slough and protect the surrounding skin, and correcting anaemia and nutrition.
- Once slough is removed and the base covered with fresh granulation, skin grows in from the edges; grade 3 and 4 ulcers usually require skin grafting or myocutaneous flap transposition.
- Prevention is by meticulous nursing care, pressure areas being washed and gently massaged, together with 2-hourly turning. For high risk patients, special mattresses should be used, these being filled with air or water to provide uniform support over dependent areas.

Infection

- Infection commonly breaches cutaneous barriers through minor abrasions, such as insect bites, and may be secondary to extension from deep-seated infections, as in sinuses and fistulae. It may complicate surgical wounds or be transmitted via the bloodstream.

- It commonly follows an underlying dermatological disease, such as dermatitis or psoriasis.
- Infection is severe in patients with diminished natural resistance, such as in diabetes, increased steroid production or administration and immunodeficiency.
- General measures of treatment of cutaneous infection include:
  - Antibiotic management of cellulitis when this is not resolving spontaneously with the appropriate antibiotic (where possible, confirmed with sensitivities)
  - Additional drainage of abscesses, debridement of residual abscess cavities, slough, recurrent glandular infected tissue and foreign material
  - Skin grafting of large residual areas, either at the time of excision through normal tissue, or once a clean granulating base is available.
- The initial tissue response to infection is cellulitis; this may be accompanied by malaise and fever, and regional lymph node enlargement.
- Streptococcal cutaneous infection is accompanied by marked erythema and oedema (erysipelas). Staphylococcal infection is more localized, producing **boils** (furuncle), which are small abscesses in hair follicles.
- **Carbuncles** result from infection of a number of hair follicles and the spread of the infection to the subcutaneous tissue, with areas of necrosis and sinus formation.
- **Acne** is an infection of sebaceous glands and is common after puberty, when the number and activity of the glands increases under hormonal control.
- **Rashes** may be flat, macular or raised, papillary or plaques (when greater than 1 cm), may produce fluid-filled vesicles, may break down when scratched (excoriation) and may discharge (weeping eczema). They may be the cutaneous manifestation of a systemic disease, with fever and toxic effects, e.g. viral infections (mumps, measles, chicken pox). These may be contagious.

Cutaneous vasculitis

- Aetiology: bacterial infection (streptococcal, gonococcal, tuberculosis, leprosy), hepatitis B,

lymphoma, drugs (sulphonamides, thiazides, captopril), tartrazine, and autoimmune disorders (SLE, PAN, scleroderma).
- Associations: vasculitis of brain, heart, lung, gut.
- Appears as areas of palpable purpura.
- Investigations: skin biopsy and histology, and investigation of underlying conditions.
- Treatment: of underlying and associated conditions, usually steroids and immunosuppressants.

Hydradenitis suppurativa

Definitions

- A chronic suppurative, fibrosing lesion of the skin, originating in the sweat glands.
- Particularly found in the axilla, groin and perineum, it may penetrate the subcutaneous tissues, providing a number of discharging sinuses.
- Seen in the third and fourth decades of life with a male:female ratio of 1:3.
- Probable causation: disruption of sweat glands as a result of duct obstruction by keratin plugs with superimposed infection.
- Associated factors:
  - Hyperhidrosis
  - Trauma from repeated shaving
  - Use of chemical depilators.

Clinical features

- Multiple abscess formation in thickened, indurated skin.

Treatment
➤ Debride and lay open abscesses and sinus tracts with systemic antibiotic therapy (metronidazole and erythromycin).
➤ For non-healing areas, excision and split skin grafting is required.

Pilonidal abscess and sinus

Definitions

- Infection of the pre-sacral fascia and skin caused by exfoliating hairs penetrating the skin in the natal cleft, producing a discharging sinus or an abscess.
- Affects mainly young adults (male:female ratio 4:1).
- Occasionally found in the finger webs (hairdressers), umbilicus and toe webs.

Clinical features

- Swelling and pain in the natal cleft associated with a discharge.
- Inflammation and abscess formation or single or multiple discharging sinuses.

Treatment
- ➤ Early lesions respond to shaving and warm salt baths.
- ➤ Abscesses are drained, curetted and de-roofed to heal over a period of 2–3 months.
- ➤ Established sinus tracts (demarcated with methylene blue dye) are excised down to sacral fascia; primary skin closure under systemic antibiotic cover if not under tension; if not possible, releasing incisions or healing by secondary intention.

Other infections

- **Hand infections** may be around the nail bed (paronychia), around the tip of the finger (apical abscess), along the finger (whitlow, pulp abscesses), or secondary to penetration of the deep palmar or web spaces. Infection of tendon sheaths can result in tendon destruction, marked fibrosis and long-term immobility.
- All hand infections should be treated with appropriate antibiotics, adequate release of any purulent collections, and rest and elevation of the limb. In a mobile patient this involves the use of a sling, retaining the hand elevated to the opposite shoulder.

- Spreading subcutaneous infection and devascularized tissue produce widespread necrosis and gangrene in necrotizing fasciitis. Meleney's gangrene and Fournier's gangrene (scrotal gangrene) are often collectively termed synergistic gangrene. A mixture of organisms is involved, commonly Bacteroides, coliforms, anaerobic streptococci and staphylococci, accompanied by gas production and toxic myositis. Urgent excision and debridement of the affected areas, and broad-spectrum antibiotics, are needed in this life-threatening situation.

- *Clostridium perfringens* may be commensal in the alimentary tract. This Gram-positive spore-bearing rod produces a lethal myotoxin in acutely ischaemic muscle and following septic abortions, with gas production (gas gangrene). It has the sickly sweet smell of decaying apples. Local cellulitis is dark red but not very marked. Systemic effects are lethal unless the affected area is excised, often requiring limb amputation.

- **Tetanus** infection is uncommon in the UK thanks to childhood immunization with 0.5 mL of tetanus toxoid, this being repeated at 6 weeks, 6 months and 5-year intervals to retain immunity. The Gram-negative spore-bearing rod is present in animal faeces, and dirty wounds are therefore at high risk of contamination. The organism multiplies in dead and ischaemic tissue. The incubation period is usually 10–14 days and its powerful neuro-exotoxin produces lassitude, irritability and dysphagia, progressing to spasm of facial muscles (trismus, producing a characteristic, painful smile – risus sardonicus), rigidity of lockjaw, and generalized tonic–clonic spasms and convulsions. Treatment for spasms is with muscular relaxation and ventilation, debridement of the wound, which is not necessarily extensive, and treatment with penicillin, human and antitetanus immunoglobulin and commencement of tetanus toxoid immunization.

- A number of cutaneous infections are encountered in the **tropics**, particularly tuberculosis (lupus vulgaris), syphilis, yaws, leishmaniasis, paracoccidiomycosis, glanders and mycetoma (page 145).

- Although the majority of cutaneous infections are bacterial in origin, a variety of other organisms are involved.
- **Warts** (verrucae) are produced by the pox virus, and they have a hard central core with a roughened surface, common in children over knuckles and nail folds. Plantar warts are painful as they are driven inwards by the pressure of weight bearing. Although warts usually resolve spontaneously, they can be difficult to eradicate, as evidenced by the number of methods available; these include the application of podophyllin, freezing, salicylic acid, and curettage under local anaesthetic.
- **Herpes simplex** virus I produces painful lesions of the lips, and II of the genitalia, although neither is limited to these sites. The incidence is increased in immunocompromised patients. The cutaneous application of alcohol or spirit on the appearance of the discomfort alleviates the subsequent eruption; this may also be helped by an antiviral cream such as aciclovir.
- **Herpes zoster** is of importance to the surgeon as pain can precede the vesicular eruption along the dermatome of the involved peripheral nerve. It is therefore an important differential diagnosis when this is across the chest or abdomen.
- **Candida** is the most common fungal infection encountered. It is a human commensal with a worldwide distribution. Cutaneous infection is in moist areas, such as axillae and submammary, where it produces intertrigo (thrush – whitish moist rash causing discomfort and discharge). It may also produce paronychia, balanitis and vaginitis. Treatment is by improved local hygiene and local antifungal agents, such as nystatin, and oral therapy in severe and persistent cases.
- **Tinea**, the ringworm fungus, occurs as areas of scaling and hair loss, tinea capitis occurring on the scalp, tinea pedis (athlete's foot) around the webs and soles of the feet, causing scaling, maceration and sometimes blistering. It also occurs on the palms and medial thigh. Tinea unguium produces discoloration, subungual hyperkeratosis and fragmentation of the nail bed. Tinea corporis may produce the characteristic rings

on the body and an infection of the groin. Treatment is with local antifungal creams and, if necessary, griseofulvin.

- **Scabies** is produced by a burrowing mite attacking the webs of the fingers, wrists, elbows, breasts and genitalia causing irritation, excoriation, with a papular eruption and often secondary infection. Gamma benzine hexachloride must be applied to all parts of the body except the face and retained for 24 hours. Repeated application may be required and all clothing and linen must be laundered and, if possible, the animal source identified and, where possible, removed.

- **Head lice** (*Pediculosis capitis*) are common among schoolchildren and are highly contagious. Application of malathion 0.5% left overnight and removed with malathion shampoo, should be repeated 7 days later, but most effective control is probably achieved by repeated brushing and use of nit combs. Pediculosis pubis is a common infestation when large populations are congregated with poor hygiene facilities, such as in emergency refugee camps, and lice are an important vector in the spread of epidemic typhus.

Benign skin lesions

- **Pyogenic granuloma.** This bright red proliferating nodule is probably an acquired haemangioma, although a history of trauma is not always obtained. It usually resolves spontaneously, but if it persists, contact bleeding or secondary infection are a problem. It may be excised.

- **Telangiectasia.** Fine vessels, usually up to 1 mm in length; 5–10 are found on 5% of the population and they occur in various sizes and shapes; spider naevi have a central arteriole, and mostly consist of capillary and venous malformations. They may be multiple, as in hereditary telangiectasia, and occur in ageing. They may be under hormonal influence, as in raised steroids, liver disease and pregnancy. They occur in association with venous hypertension. Treatment, if required, can be with a laser or by injection with sclerosant, using a fine dermal needle and magnifying glass.

- **Glomus tumours** are subcutaneous arteriovenous abnormalities, found around the nail fold, subungual position and elsewhere over the body. They may be sensitive to touch and pressure, but sometimes extreme pain is associated with temperature change. Symptomatic lesions are excised. Subungual lesions can be identified by transillumination. They require the removal of the nail and lifting the tumour out from the nail bed.

- **Campbell de Morgan spots.** These are bright red capillary lesions of 2–3 mm in length that blanch on compression. The are asymptomatic but increase in number in old age.

- Reduction of the blood supply to an area (**ischaemia**) may result in tissue death (**necrosis**). The dead tissue may be incorporated into an organ (**infarct**), or through invading anaerobic organisms may undergo putrefaction (gangrene). The organisms may be saprophytic, producing superficial **dry gangrene**, e.g. a black, mummified ischaemic toe. Parasitic organisms produce **wet gangrene**, as in the invasion of acutely ischaemic muscle, and produce toxins and gas. **Gas gangrene** is classically caused by *Clostridium perfringens*, but can also be produced by anaerobic staphylococci and streptococci; spreading subcutaneous gangrene (page 538) may also be accompanied by gas production.

Benign skin tumours

- There are a large number of cutaneous tumours; most are small and can be managed conservatively, but excision is recommended if they are unsightly, if there is uncertainty about their benign nature, if they are painful, or interfering with vision or hearing. They can usually be excised under local anaesthetic.

- **Fibrous histiocytoma** is a firm, dermal red-brown nodule of 3–5 mm, usually found on the lower limb and asymptomatic.

- **Squamous cell papilloma** are pedunculated skin tags which are pink, soft and painless, but may catch and bleed. It is usually possible to tie them around the base.

- **Keratoacanthoma (molluscum sebaceum).** This lesion grows rapidly for 3–4 weeks and drops off after 2–12 months. It is usually painless; its main problems are the differential diagnosis from carcinoma and the residual scarring that may occur. It has a hard central core and an irregular raised surface. It is usually less than a centimetre but may be more than double this size.
- Turban tumour (hidradenoma) is a tumour of sweat glands of the scalp which may grow to a large size (hence its name).

Pigmented naevi

- **Intradermal naevi** are the commonest skin lesions and represent the Mongolian spot of children and the blue naevus of the adult. They are generally reddish-brown, may appear rapidly and may be flat or raised, with or without hair. They, like other naevi, derive from neural crest cells. Like juvenile naevi, they have no malignant potential.
- **Junctional naevi** occur at the epidermodermal junction and rarely may undergo malignant change.
- **Compound naevi** occur when melanocytes migrate into the dermis, the epithelial element usually becoming less prominent.
- **Arteriovenous (AV) malformations** (page 590).
- A number of other benign tumours develop of sebaceous sweat glands and hair follicles. They are small nodules without malignant potential.

Pre-malignant lesions

- **Bowen's disease** is a pigmented, red-brown, well-defined, scaly-crusted plaque. It is an intra-epidermal carcinoma in situ. When it occurs on the glans penis it is termed **erythroplasia of Queyrat**.
- **Solar keratosis** is scaling and crusting usually over exposed areas of the body. It may fissure and bleed, particularly when scratched. It carries a 10–15% incidence of malignant change. A related pigmented scleroderma pigmentosum carries similar potential.

- Marjolin's ulcer is malignant change in a chronic inflammatory ulcer.

Malignant cutaneous lesions

- **Basal cell carcinoma** usually arises on the face between the eyebrow and mouth as a pearly-pink smooth raised circumferential lesion, which gradually enlarges with central ulceration. Early excision is needed as the lesion continues to invade surrounding superficial structures, hence its name of rodent ulcer, but it rarely metastasizes.
- **Squamous cell carcinoma** is the commonest cutaneous malignancy, frequently arising from pre-existing skin changes. It has an irregular outline with early ulceration, which, once established, has a raised everted edge. It may enlarge rapidly and also metastasize early to lymph nodes and occasionally through the bloodstream. An enlarging crusting ulcerated lesion must be biopsied early and treated by wide excision with any involved lymph nodes, or by radiotherapy early in its development.
- **Malignant melanoma** presents as lentigo maligna (Hutchinson's freckle), superficial spreading melanoma and nodular melanoma forms. Early suspicion must be raised when pre-existing moles or freckles change their appearance. Typically itching, colour change, increasing size, ulceration, bleeding and halo pigmentation should raise suspicion. Satellite nodules, enlarged local lymph nodes and distant spread are bad prognostic features, and 5-year survival falls from 80% to 30% once these features are present.
  - Prognosis is related to depth of spread: when less than 1.5 mm there is a 90% 5-year survival, but when >4 mm this falls to 50% (Breslow's depth).
  - An incision biopsy may be required; a wide excision, including nodes, should be undertaken as early as possible.
- **Kaposi's sarcoma (KS)** is a purplish irregular lesion which gradually increases in size. It does not itch and is not usually painful, but may ulcerate. They were very uncommon except in mid-European Jews and

Africans, until the emergence of acquired immunodeficiency syndrome and other immunodeficient
syndromes (page 118). Local nodules may be excised
but the lesions respond to radiotherapy and
chemotherapy.

- Other malignancies encountered include carcinomas of
  sebaceous glands, lymphomatous infiltration (mycosis
  fungoides) and metastatic spread.

Benign subcutaneous tumours

- **Lipomas** are soft, single or multiple smooth or
  bosselated lesions that may fluctuate and
  transilluminate. They are usually asymptomatic but
  occasionally can be painful (Dercum's disease).
- **Neurofibroma** are common (pure neuromas and
  fibromas not so), usually with isolated occurrence;
  tethered to nerve sheath, therefore move from side to
  side but not longitudinally. Asymptomatic unless
  pressed (tingling) or in a confined space (root
  compression); no malignant potential.
- **Neurofibromatosis** (von Recklinghausen's disease):
  - **Type I:** cutaneous, congenital autosomal
    dominant with variable degree of expression; lesion
    vary from small skin tags to being a number of
    centimetres in diameter. Usually asymptomatic
    unless in confined space. Associations – café-
    au-lait spots (more than six is diagnostic), 5%
    neurofibrosarcomas, phaeochromocytomas, gliomas,
    meningiomas and 10% mental retardation.
  - **Type II:** central, bilateral acoustic and spinal
    neuromas, also autosomal dominant, present with
    hearing problems and nerve root compression.
  - **Plexiform neurofibromatosis:** congenital
    subcutaneous pigmented overgrowth of a region
    of the body; may be large and disfiguring,
    particularly if on the face.
- **AV malformations** (page 590).
- **Subcutaneous malignant lesions** include
  rhabdomyosarcomas, neurofibrosarcomas and
  angiosarcomas. Lymphangiosarcomas are occasionally
  encountered in long-standing lymphoedema.

● These various lesions are excised if they cause pain, disfigurement, or undergo malignant change.

Degenerative lesions

● **Seborrhoeic keratosis** (basal cell papilloma, senile wart). These flat well demarcated pigmented plaques are common in the elderly. They have a greasy rough surface and can be scraped off without bleeding. They can be disfiguring and are important in the differential diagnosis of basal cell carcinoma.

● **Ganglia** are smooth hemispherical firm cysts. They are weakly fluctuant and are usually filled with clear jelly which transilluminates; they are an outpouching of synovium from tendon sheaths or joints. They are commonly found over the dorsum of the hand and foot.
  – The ganglia can be ruptured by pressure, or traditionally by striking with the family bible, but they usually recur, and if they are causing discomfort or inconvenience, they should be excised intact.

● **Sebaceous cysts.** These lesions are found in the hair-bearing areas of the body, particularly the scalp, face and scrotum. They are hemispherical and always fixed to the skin, the punctum being found by gentle squeezing of the skin across its surface. These are usually mobile over the underlying subcutaneous tissues and may be fluctuant but not usually transilluminable, as the content is inspissated and sometimes foul smelling, degenerative epithelial tissue. It may give rise to a foreign body inflammatory response or the cyst may become secondarily infected, with surrounding inflammation.

● They occasionally ulcerate and may resemble a malignant ulcer (Cock's peculiar tumour).

● A sebacious horn is formed by the gradual build-up of secretion into a hard, conical skin protuberance.

● Because of recurrent infection, discharge, discomfort and inconvenience, the lesions of sebaceous cysts are usually excised with an overlying ellipse of skin, including the punctum. An infected cyst may require drainage of the abscess, with excision when the infection has subsided.

- **Other degenerative lesions** include arterial ischaemia (page 552) and neuropathy (page 773).

LUMPS, ULCERS, SINUSES AND FISTULAE

- The differential diagnosis of observable and/or palpable lesions can usually be made on clinical grounds using the features listed in the table below.

Features to consider in the description of lumps and ulcers

Feature	Definition
Pathogenesis	Tissue of origin: single/multiple
	Classification: congenital, trauma, inflammatory, neoplastic, degenerative
	Incidence: age; sex; familial; ethnic; occupational; environment
Symptoms	Time of appearance: progress; disappearance
	Precipitating, exacerbating and/or relieving factors
	Course of symptoms: pain; discharge
	Systemic effects: social history
Signs*	Site: anatomy; depth; relations
	External: colour; temperature; tenderness; shape; size; surface; edge; mobility
	(Edge: sloping; punched out; undercut; raised; everted)
	Internal: consistency; fluctuation; transillumination; compression; reducibility; cough impulse; thrill; pulsation; resonance; bruit
	(Base: slough; granulation; deep tissues; fixation; discharge)
	Surroundings: induration; spread; fixation; penetration; perforation; lymphangitis; nodes; veins; arteries; nerves; muscle; bone; joints

*Substitute 'edge' and 'base' for 'external' and 'internal' to describe ulcers.

- The tissue of origin is of primary importance, followed by consideration of the **five** components of the **surgical**

sieve: congenital, traumatic, inflammatory, neoplastic and degenerative (further pathological features of metabolic, hormonal, poisons, chemicals, idiopathic, psychiatric are less important in this context).

- A consideration with congenital lesions is whether they are an extension of normality, such as a prominent muscle belly, an unusually long xiphisternum or a deformed finger.
- Key points in the history are, **how long** the lesion has been present, is it **changing** in size, and is it **painful**.
- The tissue of origin may not be immediately obvious, such as the differential diagnosis of a lymph node over the carotid bifurcation, which could be a carotid body tumour; the differentiation of inflammatory and neoplastic lesions may also be difficult.
- Lumps may be **tender**, and tender areas may be caused by local trauma or tears of muscle or tendon fibres. Active and passive movements of the latter produce pain and in these cases a useful diagnostic test is the injection of a local anaesthetic.
- Lumps and areas of tenderness may also be made more or less prominent by contraction of the underlying or overlying muscle, such as the sternocleidomastoid or abdominal wall.
- When the diagnosis of a lump is in doubt on clinical grounds, **imaging** usually defines the site of origin and a probable diagnosis. This may be confirmed by fine-needle **cytology**, core needle histology, or by incision or excision biopsy of the lesion.
- **Excision biopsy** should ensure clear margins and, if this is likely to produce deformity or need skin grafting, a small incision biopsy is examined histologically so that subsequent surgery can be appropriately planned.
- **Biopsy of ulcers** should be taken from the active edge rather than the base, which is likely to be reported as non-specific inflammatory tissue.
- The term **tumour** literally refers to a swelling, such as an inflammatory mass. However, it has become synonymous with a **neoplasm**, which may be benign, or primary or secondary malignancy.

- **Cysts** are fluid-filled lesions that demonstrate fluctuation and transillumination, although the degree depends on their depth and the tension and consistency of their content.
- True cysts are lined by epithelium and may be congenital (e.g. branchial, dermoid) or acquired. The latter occur in exocrine (e.g. sebaceous, epididymal) or endocrine (e.g. thyroid, ovarian) glands, or extensions from an epithelial surface (e.g. implantation, dermoids, ganglia or bursae).
- False cysts are usually secondary to inflammatory changes (e.g. an abscess cavity, pseuodopancreatic cyst) or degeneration within a neoplasm. Invading parasites may be in their cystic phase (e.g. hydatid, cysticercosis).
- An **ulcer** is a discontinuity of an epithelium and may be caused by traumatic, inflammatory and malignant lesions. Degenerative changes of the blood supply, venous drainage and nerve supply to an area also produce epithelial loss.
- The various ulcers have characteristic edges (see table, page 204) indicating their progression or healing phases, while the base provides an indication of the depth of penetration.
- A **sinus** is a blind tract opening onto an epithelial surface and a **fistula** is a communication between two epithelial surfaces.
- In congenital sinuses and fistulae, the tract is usually lined by epithelial tissue (e.g. umbilical, branchial) and when excised, all this epithelial tissue must be removed to avoid recurrence.
- Acquired sinuses and fistulae are usually lined by granulation tissue. Persistence of these tracts may be the result of inadequate drainage (abscess), distal obstruction (gut fistulae), chronic inflammation (Crohn's disease), chronic infection (tuberculosis, syphilis), dead tissue (gangrenous core, bony sequestrum), the presence of a foreign body (infected prosthesis) or malignant disease.
- Eradication of acquired sinuses and fistulae is directed at these causes. Management of high gut fistulae includes replacement of the large fluid losses.

HEAD

CRANIAL NERVES (number of each pair usually given in roman numerals as below)

I. Olfactory nerve palsy

Definitions
- Rarely occurs in cribriform plate fracture.

Clinical features
- Loss of sense of smell.

Investigation
➤ Investigation of anterior cranial fossa basilar skull fracture (page 219).

Treatment
➤ Treatment of anterior cranial fossa basilar skull fracture.

II. Optic nerve palsy and interruption of the optic pathway

Definitions
- Optic nerve:
  - Retro-ocular tumour (page 257)
  - Multiple sclerosis
  - Temporal arteritis (page 564) – ischaemia from ophthalmic artery occlusion.
- Optic chiasm:
  - Pituitary adenoma (page 225)
  - Meningioma (page 224).
- Optic tract:
  - Craniopharyngioma.
- Optic radiation – via parietal and temporal lobes:
  - Malignant cerebral tumours (page 223)
  - Intracranial haemorrhage (page 224).

- Visual cortex:
  - Vertebrobasilar stroke (page 549)
  - Intracranial haemorrhage (page 222).

Clinical features

- Optic nerve:
  - Central or complete visual field loss on the affected side(s).
- Optic chiasm:
  - Bitemporal hemianopia – bilateral, lateral visual field loss.
- Optic tract:
  - Homonymous hemianopia – loss of the medial visual field on the side of the lesion, and the lateral visual field on the unaffected side.
- Optic radiation – parietal lobe:
  - Lower homonymous quadrantanopia – loss of the medial lower quadrant of the visual field on the side of the lesion, and the lateral lower quadrant of the visual field on the unaffected side.
- Optic radiation – temporal lobe:
  - Upper homonymous quadrantanopia – loss of the medial upper quadrant of the visual field on the side of the lesion, and the lateral upper quadrant of the visual field on the unaffected side.
- Visual cortex – unilateral:
  - Homonymous hemianopia, but with sparing of central fields – loss of the medial visual field on the side of the lesion, and the lateral visual field on the unaffected side.
- Visual cortex – extensive, bilateral:
  - Blindness
  - Pupillary reflexes are preserved.

Investigation

➤ Head computerized tomography (CT)/magnetic resonance imaging (MRI).
➤ Investigation of underlying conditions.

Treatment

➤ Treatment of underlying conditions.

III. Oculomotor nerve and nucleus palsy

Definitions

- Paralysis of extrinsic ocular muscles except superior oblique (IV) and lateral rectus (VI).
- Aetiology:
  - Brainstem stroke
  - Brainstem tumour
  - Intracavernous internal carotid artery aneurysm
  - Ipsilateral acute compressing intracranial haematoma (page 226)
  - Coning (page 230) – bilateral oculomotor palsy
  - Exophthalmic ophthalmoplegia (page 309)
  - Iatrogenic – ocular surgery.

Clinical features

- Divergent squint – failure of upward, downward and inward movement of the ipsilateral eye.
- Pupillary dilatation – ipsilateral.
- Ptosis – ipsilateral.

Investigation

➤ Head CT/MRI.
➤ Investigation of underlying conditions.

Treatment

➤ Treatment of underlying condition.
➤ Corrective surgery may be possible for strabismus (page 264) in non-acute cases.

IV. Trochlear nerve and nucleus palsy

Definitions

- Paralysis of superior oblique ocular muscle.
- Rarely occurs in isolation.
- Aetiology:
  - Brainstem stroke
  - Brainstem tumour

– Intracavernous internal carotid artery aneurysm
– Exophthalmic ophthalmoplegia (page 309)
– Iatrogenic – ocular surgery.

Clinical features

- Diplopia when walking downstairs – when the affected eye looks downwards and medially.

Investigation

➤ Head CT/MRI.
➤ Investigation of underlying conditions.

Treatment

➤ Treatment of underlying condition.

V. Trigeminal nerve and nuclear palsy

Definitions

- Paralysis of muscles of mastication and facial sensory loss.
- Aetiology:
  - Medullary and pontine stroke
  - Medullary and pontine tumour
  - Compression by acoustic neuroma (page 244)
  - Syringomyelia
  - Gradenigio's syndrome (page 241)
  - Causes of neuropathy (page 773).

Clinical features

- Deviation of the jaw.
- Loss of ipsilateral masseter strength – palpated when the teeth are clenched.
- Jaw jerk exaggerated – only for a bilateral lesion above the nuclei.
- Wasting of ipsilateral temporalis, masseter and pterygoids – lower motor neuron palsy.
- Sensory loss over ipsilateral forehead, ophthalmic, maxillary and mandibular regions.
- Sensory loss of ipsilateral cornea – absent blinking on touching the cornea with cotton wool.

- Loss of taste from anterior two-thirds of tongue –
  lesion affecting the mandibular division.

Investigation
➤ Head CT/MRI.
➤ Investigation of underlying condition.

Treatment
➤ Treatment of underlying condition.

- Trigeminal neuralgia (page 234).
- Ophthalmic and trigeminal herpes (page 235).

VI. Abducent nerve and nucleus palsy

Definitions
- Paralysis of lateral rectus muscle.
- Aetiology:
  - Brainstem stroke
  - Brainstem tumour
  - Intracavernous internal carotid artery aneurysm
  - Coning (page 230) in raised intracranial pressure –
    bilateral lateral rectus
  - Exophthalmic ophthalmoplegia (page 309)
  - Iatrogenic – ocular surgery.

Clinical features
- Convergent squint – failure of outward movement of
  the ipsilateral eye.

Investigation
➤ Head CT/MRI.
➤ Investigation of underlying conditions.

Treatment
➤ Treatment of underlying condition.
➤ Corrective surgery may be possible for strabismus
  (page 264) in non-acute cases.

VII. Facial nerve palsy

Definitions

Upper motor neuron:

- Contralateral paralysis of lower face – the upper face is bilaterally innervated
- Aetiology: stroke.

Lower motor neuron – Bell's palsy (page 235):

- Ipsilateral paralysis of the face
- Aetiology:
  - Demyelination
  - Degeneration
  - Compression by cerebellopontine angle tumour
  - Causes of neuropathy
  - Petrous temporal osteomyelitis from middle ear infection (page 241)
  - Herpes zoster infection of the geniculate ganglion – Ramsay Hunt syndrome (page 244)
  - Iatrogenic – during parotid surgery.

Clinical features

Upper motor neuron – contralateral:

- Drooping mouth angle
- Inability to puff-out the cheek.

Lower motor neuron – ipsilateral:

- Loss of frowning and facial creases
- Drooping lower eyelid
- Loss of eyebrow raising
- Loss of ability to fully close the eye – eye rolls upwards on attempting this
- Loss of ability to 'screw-up' the eyes
- Drooping mouth angle
- Loss of ability to 'puff-out' the cheek or whistle.

Investigation

➤ Head and facial CT/MRI.
➤ Investigation of underlying condition.

Treatment

➤ Treatment of underlying condition.
➤ Residual weakness:
  - Reconstructive surgery – a sling of temporalis fascia raises the edge of the mouth
  - Hypoglossal nerve transposition to facial nerve.

VIII. Vestibulocochlear nerve and nucleus palsy

Definitions

● Aetiology:
  - Acoustic neuroma (page 244)
  - Cerebellopontine angle tumours
  - Cerebellar abscess
  - Menière's disease (page 245)
  - Ramsay Hunt syndrome (page 244)
  - Glomus jugulare (page 246).

Clinical features

● Sensorineural deafness.
● Reduction of both air and bone conduction hearing on tuning fork tests.
● Tinnitus – 'ringing in the ear'.
● Vertigo – a sense of rotational movement, vomiting and inability to remain upright.
● Nystagmus – uncontrollable horizontal pendular movements of the eye, fast phase away from the side of the lesion.

Investigation

➤ Head CT/MRI.
➤ Audiometry.

Treatment

➤ Treatment of underlying condition.

IX. Glossopharyngeal nerve palsy

Definitions

- Occurs in bulbar and pseudobulbar palsy.

Clinical features

- Loss of taste from posterior one-third of tongue.
- Loss of gag reflex – danger of aspiration.

Investigation

➤ Investigation of bulbar and pseudobulbar palsy.

Treatment

➤ Treatment of causes of bulbar and pseudobulbar palsy (see below).

X. Vagus nerve palsy

Definitions

- Occurs in bulbar and pseudobulbar palsy.

Clinical features

- Uvula deviates away from affected side.

Investigation

➤ Investigation of causes of bulbar and pseudobulbar palsy (see below).

Treatment

➤ Treatment of bulbar and pseudobulbar palsy.

XI. Accessory nerve palsy

Definitions

- Motor function to sternomastoid and trapezius.
- Aetiology:
  - Occurs in bulbar and pseudobulbar palsy
  - Iatrogenic – posterior triangle neck surgery.

Clinical features

- Weakness of turning the head away from the affected side.
- Loss of shrugging ipsilateral shoulder.

Investigation

➤ Investigation of bulbar and pseudobulbar palsy.

Treatment

➤ Treatment of causes of bulbar and pseudobulbar palsy (see below).

XII. Hypoglossal nerve palsy

Definitions

- Motor function to the tongue.
- Aetiology:
  - Occurs in bulbar and pseudobulbar palsy
  - Iatrogenic – carotid surgery.

Clinical features

- Tongue deviates to affected side.
- Wasting of the tongue – lower motor neuron lesion.
- Fasciculation of the tongue – lower motor neuron lesion.

Investigation

➤ Investigation of bulbar and pseudobulbar palsy.

Treatment

➤ Treatment of causes of bulbar and pseudobulbar palsy (see below).

Bulbar and pseudobulbar palsy

Definitions

Bulbar palsy:

- Lower motor neuron paralysis of IX–XII cranial nerves
- Aetiology: X linked motor neuropathy – Kennedy syndrome, Guillain–Barré syndrome.

Pseudobulbar palsy:

- Bilateral upper motor neuron paralysis IX–XII cranial nerves
- Aetiology: motor neuron disease, multiple sclerosis, cerebrovascular disease (bulbar stroke).

Clinical features

Bulbar palsy:

- Kennedy syndrome – lower motor neuron weakness spreading proximally:
  - Lower limbs
  - Upper limbs
  - Face.
- IX–XII paralysis with:
  - Dysphagia
  - Dysarthria
  - Loss of gag reflex
  - Fasciculation of tongue and lower face.

Pseudobulbar palsy:

- Bilateral IX–XII paralysis with:
  - Dysarthria
  - Exaggerated jaw jerk
  - Gag reflex is preserved
  - Tongue is not wasted.

Investigation

➤ Genetic analysis – X-linked motor neuropathy.
➤ Central motor conduction time:
  - Raised threshold in motor neuron disease
  - Significantly prolonged in multiple sclerosis
  - Indicates degree of recovery at 6 months after stroke.
➤ Cerebrospinal fluid (CSF) immunoglobulins – multiple sclerosis.
➤ CT/MRI.
  - Demyelination in multiple sclerosis
  - Exclude intracranial tumours
  - Cerebral infarction shows as low density on CT after 2 days.

Treatment

General:

➤ Speech therapy
➤ Computer-assisted communication
➤ Physiotherapy
➤ Gastrostomy feeding
➤ Electric wheelchair
➤ Baclofen 5 mg tds orally, increasing to up to 100 mg daily; diazepam 5 mg tds orally – reduce spasticity in motor neuron disease.

Multiple sclerosis:

➤ Interferon beta as per product instructions – reduces duration and severity of relapse
➤ Prednisolone 20 mg i.v. daily for up to 2 weeks, reducing to 5 mg orally daily – reduces duration and severity of relapse
➤ Oxybutynin (anticholinergic) 5 mg tds orally – improves urinary urgency
➤ Intermittent self-catheterization – relieves impaired bladder emptying
➤ Laxatives – constipation
➤ Papaverine 30 mg/phentolamine 0.5 mg self-injection of the penile corpora – for impotence
➤ Propranolol (beta blockers) 40 mg tds – tremor.

Prognosis:

➤ Many die of aspiration pneumonia within 5 years.
➤ X-linked bulbar palsy – slower progression.

SCALP

- Meningocele/meningo-encephalocele (page 740).
- Sebaceous cysts (page 203).
- Lipomas (page 202).
- Turban tumours (page 200).
- Plexiform neurofibromas (page 202).
- Basal cell carcinomas (page 201).
- Squamous cell carcinomas (page 201).

Cirsoid aneurysms

Definitions

- Arteriovenous fistula on the forehead and scalp.
- Aetiology: post-traumatic.

Clinical features

- Pulsatile swellings over the forehead and scalp.

Investigation

➤ Duplex ultrasound.
➤ Angiography – rarely required.

Treatment

➤ Excision – if ligated the fistula reforms from minor tributaries.

Temporal arteritis (page 564)

SKULL

Microcephaly

Definitions

- Congenitally small cranium and brain.
- Aetiology: intrauterine infection, consanguinity, a feature of congenital syndromes, and a rare autosomal recessive condition.

Clinical features

- Head circumference >3 standard deviations below the mean.
- Features of associated congenital syndromes.
- Mental and physical retardation.

Investigation

➤ Serology for causes of intrauterine infection.
➤ Investigation of associated congenital syndromes.
➤ Head CT.

Treatment

➤ Genetic counselling for consanguinity and inherited syndromes.
➤ Management of mental and physical disabilities.

Anencephaly

- Fatal absence of cranium and hemispheres.
- Antenatal diagnosis – raised serum alpha fetoprotein at beginning of second trimester; confirmed by ultrasound.

Skull tumours

- Metastatic deposits, fibrous dysplasia and eosinophilic granulomas appear as lytic lesions on skull X-ray.
- Multiple myeloma may produce a pepperpot skull with multiple lytic lesions.
- Biopsy and histology may be required for an unidentified mass arising from the skull.
- Some metastatic deposits may be treated with radiotherapy.

Paget's disease (page 633)

Skull fractures

Definitions

- Linear fractures of skull vault or base – moderate trauma.
- Basilar fractures – severe trauma.
- Depressed fractures – severe focal trauma (hammer blow).

Clinical features

- Overlying bruising and swelling.
- Associated intracranial injury (page 226).

- Basilar fractures of the anterior fossa may result in:
  - Bilateral peri-orbital bruising (Panda sign)
  - CSF rhinorrhoea
  - Aerocele.
- Middle fossa fracture may result in CSF otorrhoea.

Investigation

➤ Skull X-ray if:
  - Loss of consciousness or amnesia
  - Clinically suspected fracture
  - CSF otorrhoea/rhinorrhoea
  - Neurological signs/fits.
➤ Head CT if:
  - Skull fracture with confusion, impaired consciousness, focal neurogical signs, fits
  - Persistent confusion or impaired consciousness after resuscitation
  - Deterioration of conscious level
  - Depressed skull fracture
  - Penetrating injury
  - CSF otorrhoea/rhinorrhoea
  - Difficulty in assessment.

Treatment

➤ Admission for observation:
  - Confusion, impaired consciousness
  - Skull fracture
  - Neurological symptoms
  - Difficulty in assessment
  - Social circumstance/other medical conditions.
➤ Prophylactic amoxycillin 500 mg tds for 10 days – basilar, depressed and compound linear fractures.
➤ Treatment of associated intracranial injury (page 226).
➤ Surgical repair of anterior fossa floor – persisting rhinorrhoea.

Depressed fractures

- Surgical exploration and elevation or debridement, closure of the dura and overlying tissues.

INTRACRANIAL CONDITIONS

Hydrocephalus

Definitions

- Increased CSF volume.

Obstructive hydrocephalus – impaired flow of CSF:

- Stenosis of the aqueduct of Sylvius
- Fourth ventricle lesion: Chiari type II and Dandy–Walker malformations.

Communicating hydrocephalus – impaired CSF reabsorption:

- Subarachnoid haemorrhage – premature infant
- Pneumococcal or tuberculous meningitis
- Leukaemic infiltration.

Clinical features

Infant:

- Enlargement of the head
- Mental and physical retardation
- Features of associated underlying condition.

Adult:

- Features of associated underlying condition
- Raised intracranial pressure (page 229):
  - Tense fontanelles
  - Headache – worse in the morning or on stooping
  - Vomiting
  - Confusion
  - Drowsiness – deterioration of conscious level
  - Coning (page 230) – may eventually occur.

Investigation

Infant:

➤ Ultrasound via the fontanelles.

➔

Adult:

➤ Skull X-ray:
  - Pathological calcification
  - Asymmetry
  - Neoplasm
  - Enlarged posterior fossa – Dandy–Walker syndrome
  - Enlarged anterior fossa – Chiari type II
    malformation.
➤ CT/MRI.
➤ Contrast ventriculography.

Treatment

Adult and progressive infant hydrocephalus:

➤ Surgical removal of obstructing lesion
➤ Drainage procedures:
  - Intracranial
  - Extracranial to right atrium, peritoneum or lumbar
    spinal cord.

Infant hydrocephalus without progression:

➤ Observation.

Intraventricular haemorrhage

- Premature infants
- Identified and followed by ultrasound
- Usually settles within 1–2 weeks – treatment is only
  required if hydrocephalus develops.

Intracranial abscess

Definitions

- Chronic space-occupying lesions.
- Spread of infection from:
  - Chronic otitis media
  - Frontal sinusitis
  - Lung abscess
  - Bronchiectasis
  - Miliary tuberculosis.

Clinical features

- Raised intracranial pressure.
- Sepsis.

Investigation

➤ CT: halo appearance from contrast uptake by surrounding hyperaemic tissue.

Treatment

➤ Cefotaxime 1 g bd to 4 g tds i.v..
➤ Aspiration via burrhole under local anaesthesia – repeated.
➤ Enucleation may be required.

Prognosis:

- 10% mortality
- Epilepsy is common.

Malignant intracranial tumours

Definitions

Primary:

- Glioblastoma
  - Commonest primary brain tumour
  - Affects adults
  - Occur in cerebral hemispheres.
- Astrocytoma:
  - Affect young adults
  - Occur in cerebral hemispheres and spinal cord.
- Medulloblastoma:
  - Affect young children
  - Occur in the cerebellum.

Metastatic:

- Secondary deposits, typically from: breast, bronchus, melanoma.

Clinical features

- Raised intracranial pressure (page 229).
- Hydrocephalus – posterior fossa tumours, particularly in children.

- Epilepsy.
- Behavioural change.
- Focal neurological signs according to location.
- Sensorineural deafness and tinnitus – acoustic neuroma.

Investigation

➤ CT/MRI – with and without contrast:
  – Calcification
  – 'Ring' contrast enhancement.
➤ Biopsy and frozen section histology at time of surgery.
➤ Investigations for primary tumour in metastatic cases.

Treatment

Primary:

➤ Surgical debulking and biopsy – most tumours
➤ Extensive surgical resection – possible for some astrocytomas
➤ Radiotherapy – good response for astrocytoma, poor response for other types
➤ Chemotherapy – improves survival for childhood tumours.

Metastatic:

➤ Radiotherapy, chemotherapy or hormonal therapy – depending on primary tumour
➤ Surgical resection sometimes possible for small solitary metastases.

Meningioma

- Slow-growing tumours arising from arachnoid cells.
- Occur mainly on the dura of the falx cerebri and base of the skull.
- Affects: adults, females > males; growth exacerbated by pregnancy.
- Treatment: neurosurgical resection is often curative – recurrence may occur with some invasive types.

Schwannoma and acoustic neuroma

- Benign Schwann cell tumours.
- Associated: neurofibromatosis.
- Occur on the dorsal spinal roots or VIII nerve – acoustic neuromas.
- Treatment: neurosurgical resection is curative.

Pituitary adenomas

Definitions

- Benign anterior pituitary tumours.
- May be non-functioning or produce anterior pituitary hormones.
- Associated: multiple endocrine neoplasia type 1 – parathyroid hyperplasia, pancreatic gastrinoma and pituitary adenoma.
- Abnormalities of antidiuretic hormone (ADH) (page 61).

Clinical features

- Bitemporal hemianopia.
- Endocrine disturbances:
  - Acromegaly or gigantism – growth hormone
  - Nipple discharge and amenorrhoea – prolactin
  - Cushing's syndrome – adrenocorticotropic hormone (ACTH).
  - Diabetes insipidus – lack of ADH production (page 61).

Investigation

➤ Serum assays of growth hormone, prolactin and ACTH.
➤ Skull X-ray – double-floor appearance to sella turcica.
➤ CT/MRI.
➤ Cavernous sinus venography – demonstrates extension into the sinus.

Treatment

➤ Surgical resection – trans-sphenoidal or transcranial.

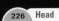

HEAD INJURY

Glasgow Coma Scale

- Conscious level is assessed by the Glasgow Coma Scale (GCS) (see table).
- Scale ranges from 15 = normal, down to 3; coma is defined as a GCS of 8 or less.

Response	Details	Score
Eye opening	Spontaneous	4
	Speech	3
	Pain	2
	None	1
Verbal response	Orientated	5
	Confused	4
	Inappropriate words	3
	Incomprehensible sounds	2
	None	1
Best motor response	Obeys commands	6
	Localizes pain	5
	Withdrawal from pain	4
	Flexion to pain	3
	Extension to pain	2
	None	1

Skull fractures (page 219)

Intracranial haematoma

Definitions

Acute subdural haematoma:

- Severe head trauma
- Associated: laceration to the surface of the brain.

Acute extradural (epidural) haematoma:

- Relatively mild trauma to the side of the head
- Middle meningeal artery bleeding
- Temporal bone fracture.

Chronic subdural haematoma:

- Relatively minor trauma in:
  - Elderly
  - Alcoholics
  - Clotting disorders.
- Small collection of blood gradually enlarges by osmosis.

Clinical features

Acute subdural haematoma:

- Immediate or rapidly developing coma.

Acute extradural haematoma:

- Consciousness is regained
- Gradual deterioration to coma over several hours.

Chronic subdural haematoma:

- Subtle symptoms develop over days or weeks
- Behavioural change
- Memory loss
- Symptoms and signs of raised intracranial pressure.

Investigation

➤ CT without contrast/MRI:
- Subdural haematoma:
  - Concavo-convex (crescentic) area over the surface of a cerebral hemisphere
  - Higher density than brain if <2 weeks' duration
  - Lower density than brain >4 weeks' duration
  - Cerebral oedema.
- Acute extradural haematoma:
  - Biconvex (fusiform) high density area adjacent to the vault.

Treatment

Acute subdural haematoma:

➤ Evacuation through a burrhole
➤ Craniotomy to deal with underlying cause
➤ Prognosis depends on associated brain injury.

➤

Acute extradural haematoma:

➤ Drainage through a burrhole.

Chronic subdural haematoma:

➤ Drainage through burrholes.

Infants:

➤ Aspiration via the anterior fontanelle
➤ Occasionally shunts are placed.

Diffuse axonal injury

- Microscopic damage to axonal tracts containing myelinated sensory and motor fibres following major head trauma.
- Symptoms range from concussion to coma.
- Treatment is by rehabilitation.
- Prognosis:
  - Ranges from complete recovery to vegetative state
  - The longer the duration of coma the greater the permanent deficit.

Subarachnoid haemorrhage

Definitions

- Haemorrhage into the subarachnoid space.
- Aetiology:
  - Rupture of a berry aneurysm of the anterior, middle or posterior cerebral, or internal carotid arteries
  - Haemorrhage from arteriovenous malformation.
- Associations: hypertension, polycystic kidney, Marfan's syndrome, Ehlers–Danlos syndrome, pseudoxanthoma elasticum.
- Affects: men <40 years of age, and women >50 years of age.

Clinical features

- Sudden severe occipital headache.
- Focal neurological deficit may be present.

- Coma.
- Deterioration to death, or gradual recovery.

Investigation

➤ CT without contrast/MRI:
  - High density blood in CSF pathways <48 hours after haemorrhage
  - Hydrocephalus may develop >2 weeks after haemorrhage.
➤ Lumbar puncture – bloodstained CSF or xanthochromia >12 hours after haemorrhage.
➤ Four vessel cerebral angiography – identifies causal lesion.

Treatment

➤ Atenolol 50–100 mg daily orally – for control of blood pressure.
➤ Neurosurgery for patients who have regained consciousness:
  - Obliteration of the aneurysm with a clip
  - Carotid artery ligation – for large aneurysms, but may cause stroke.

Prognosis:

  - 25% die within 24 hours
  - A further 25% die within 1 month from further haemorrhage.

Raised intracranial pressure

- Aetiology:
  - Severe head injury
  - Intracranial haematoma (page 226)
  - Intracranial tumour (page 223)
  - Hydrocephalus (page 221).
- Features: headache – worse in the morning or on stooping; vomiting; diplopia; papilloedema; depressed consciousness and eventually coma.

- Coning occurs when pressure forces the brain through the tentorium or foramen magnum:
  - Ipsilateral, dilated, unreactive pupil
  - Medullary compression: bradycardia, rising blood pressure, slow, irregular respiration.
- A pressure monitoring 'bolt' may be screwed through the cranium to monitor intracranial pressure.
- Investigation and treatment is that of the underlying conditions.

Brain death (page 100)

Vegetative state

Definitions

- A state where the cerebral cortex is not functioning but the brainstem survives.
- Aetiology:
  - Anoxic brain injury – prolonged resuscitation in shock (page 96)
  - Severe head injury
  - Subarachnoid haemorrhage.

Clinical features

- Coma.
- Spontaneous respiration is possible.

Investigation

➤ Clinical diagnosis.
➤ CT/MRI – underlying cause.

Treatment

➤ Prognosis: some recovery within 3 months if from diffuse axonal injury.

FACE AND JAWS

Sinusitis

Definitions

- Infection of paranasal sinuses.
- Aetiology:
  - Acute infection: pneumococcus, streptococcus, staphylococcus, *Haemophilus influenzae*, *Klebsiella pneumoniae*
  - Chronic infection: tuberculosis, syphilis, fungal infection.
- Associated: obstructed sinus drainage, e.g. nasal polyp.

Clinical features

- Nasal obstruction and rhinorrhoea.
- Pain in cheek or upper teeth – maxillary sinusitis.
- Headache – frontal sinusitis.

Investigation

➤ X-ray – opacification or fluid level in the sinus.
➤ Microbiology swab.
➤ Antroscopy – identifies cause of osteal obstruction.

Treatment

➤ Amoxicillin 500 mg tds orally for 3–10 days
➤ Ephedrine 0.5% nasal drops qds
➤ Persisting cases:
  - Lavage of sinuses
  - Mucosal resection
  - Removal of obstructing lesions
  - Antrostomy.

Complications

- Chronic sinusitis
- Pott's puffy tumour – osteomyelitis of the skull
- Orbital cellulitis (page 256)
- Intracranial infection (page 222).

Carcinoma of the paranasal sinuses

Definitions

- Aetiology: cigarette smoking, chronic inhalation of wood smoke.

Clinical features

- Cervical lymphadenopathy.
- Epistaxis.
- Local invasion.

Investigation

➤ Biopsy and histology.
➤ CT – shows local extent.
➤ Chest X-ray/CT – identifies lung metastases.

Treatment

➤ Radiotherapy.
➤ Neck dissection for involved nodes.
➤ Prognosis:
  – Poor.

Maxillary fractures

Definitions

- Le Fort I:
  – Low-facial impact
  – Separated fragment comprises: palate, maxillary alveolar processes and lower two-thirds of pterygoid plates.
- Le Fort II:
  – Mid-facial impact
  – Separated fragment is pyramidal in shape.
- Le Fort III:
  – Superior impact
  – Whole face separates from the skull.

Clinical features

- Severe facial swelling and bruising.
- Mobility of fracture segment.

Investigation

➤ X-rays.
➤ CT.

Treatment

➤ Open reduction and intermaxillary fixation.
➤ Le Fort II and III may require antrostomy, packing and bone-grafting.

Mandibular fractures

Definitions

● Significant trauma – multiple fractures.
● Common combinations:
  – Condyle and opposite region of body
  – Condyle and opposite angle
  – Bilateral subcondylar (parade ground fracture).

Clinical features

● Pain and swelling.
● Difficulty speaking or eating.
● Visible or palpable discontinuity of the alveolar margin and teeth.

Investigation

➤ X-rays – lateral, oblique and panoramic.

Treatment

➤ Children:
  – Intermaxillary fixation for 10–14 days
  – Remodelling corrects residual deformity over 3 years.
➤ Adults:
  – Open reduction and intermaxillary mandibular fixation for 4–6 weeks
  – Union assessed by releasing fixation and biting on a tongue depressor – pain indicates that further fixation is required.

Alveolar fractures of the mandible and maxilla

- Separation of a fragment of the alveolar margin with the associated teeth.
- Mobility of a number of teeth with the alveolar fragment.
- Treatment: repositioning, and holding with circum-dental wires for 6 weeks.

Trigeminal neuralgia

Definitions

- Unexplained condition causing relapsing paroxysms of trigeminal pain.
- Aetiology: unknown.

Clinical features

- Intense pain over distribution of trigeminal nerve for up to 1 minute.
- Usually unilateral, but may subsequently occur contralaterally.
- One or more nerve divisions may be affected.
- Recurs in bouts after weeks or months.

Investigation

➤ Exclusion of other pathology, such as compression of nerve by tumour.

Treatment

➤ Carbamazepine 100 mg bd orally.
➤ Severe cases:
  – Thermocoagulation of ganglion
  – Section of sensory root by posterior fossa microsurgery.
➤ Prognosis:
  – Remission for months or years
  – Older patients have shorter periods of remission.

Herpes zoster (shingles)

Definitions

- Shingles – painful cutaneous eruptions in the distribution of a dermatome.
- Aetiology: reactivation of varicella zoster virus infection in a dorsal root ganglion.
- Typically affects the trigeminal ganglion.
- Associated: previous chicken-pox.

Clinical features

- Severe unilateral shooting pains over selective divisions of the nerve.
- Characteristic vesicular rash follows.
- Skin eruption dries and heals over 2 weeks.

Investigation

➤ Characteristic clinical appearance.
➤ Virus isolated from vesicular fluid.

Treatment

➤ Skin care – avoid secondary infection.
➤ Analgesics.
➤ Aciclovir 800 mg five times daily orally for 7 days – may reduce post-herpetic neuralgia.
➤ Prognosis:
   – Incomplete recovery over months.

Complications

- Ramsay Hunt syndrome: facial paralysis, sensorineural deafness and vertigo.

Bell's palsy

Definitions

- Term used to describe unilateral lower motor neuron facial paralysis from disease of the nerve within the facial canal.

- Aetiology:
  - Demyelination – most cases
  - Degeneration of the nerve.

Clinical features

- Unilateral lower motor neuron facial palsy.

Investigation

➤ Investigation of:
  - Multiple sclerosis
  - Middle-ear disease
  - Generalized disorders causing neuropathy: diabetes, Lyme disease (borreliosis), sarcoidosis and Guillain–Barré.
➤ Electrodiagnostic studies – distinguish demyelination from degeneration.

Treatment

➤ Most recover spontaneously:
  - Demyelination: complete recovery over a few weeks
  - Degeneration: incomplete recovery over several months.
➤ Residual weakness:
  - Reconstructive surgery – a sling of temporalis fascia raises the edge of the mouth
  - Hypoglossal nerve transposition to facial nerve.

EAR

Outer ear

Congenital abnormalities

Definitions

- Microtia – small deformed pinna.
- Anotia – absent pinna.
- Associated:
  - Atresia of the external meatus

– Corresponding degree of abnormality of the middle and inner ear
– Congenital syndromes.

Treatment
➤ Surgical exploration and creation of a meatus.
➤ Hearing aid.
➤ Treat before 2 years of age to allow normal speech development.
➤ Surgery in bilateral cases one side at a time – it may worsen hearing loss.

Accessory auricles
● These can be excised.

Pre-auricular cysts and sinuses
● These can be excised if they become infected.

Bat ears
● These can be surgically corrected after 6 years of age.

Otitis externa

Definitions
● Inflammation of the external auditory canal.
● Pathology: staphylococcal, streptococcal infection, fungal infection, herpes zoster (page 244), contact dermatitis, seborrhoeic dermatitis.
● Fungal infection complicates:
  – Immunosuppression
  – Antibiotic therapy
  – Bacterial infection.

Clinical features
● Staphylococcal infection:
  – A boil in the ear canal.
● Streptococcal infection:
  – Spreading cellulitis.
● Fungal infection:
  – Discharge of musty hyphal material – resembles wet newspaper.

Treatment

Staphylococcal infection:

➤ Discharges spontaneously
➤ Local warmth and ear drops.

Streptococcal infection:

➤ Amoxicillin 500 mg tds orally.

Fungal infection:

➤ Remove hyphal material
➤ Clotrimazole 1% ear drops tds

Herpes zoster:

➤ Spontaneous resolution.

Contact dermatitis:

➤ Avoid cause, e.g. nickel spectacle frames.

Seborrhoeic dermatitis:

➤ Cetrimide topically.

Otitis externa malignans

Definitions

- Destructive infection of the external auditory canal and pinna.
- Pathology: pseudomonal infection.
- Associations: diabetic, immunocompromised.
- Affects: the elderly.

Clinical features

- Local and systemic sepsis.
- Cranial nerve palsy VII, IX–XII.
- Gradenigo's syndrome (page 241).

Treatment

➤ Ceftazidime 1 g tds i.v. in combination with other broad-spectrum antibiotics.
➤ Drainage of subperiosteal pus.

➜

> ➤ Debridement of necrotic bone.
> ➤ Prognosis:
>   – Recurrent infection occurs – review for 6 months
>   – May be fatal.

Complications

- Osteomyelitis of temporal bone.
- Intracranial infection.

Exostosis of the external auditory canal

- Commonest benign tumour of the external ear.
- Bilateral bony projections into the canal.
- May impair hearing.
- Removed with a burr.

Ceruminomas

- Benign ceruminous gland tumour.
- Firm masses under the skin of the outer meatus.
- Can be excised.
- Recurrence and malignant change may occur.

Squamous cell carcinoma (page 201)

- Occurs at the meatus or auricle.

Basal cell carcinoma (page 201)

- They may be pre-auricular or post-auricular.

Cauliflower ear

- Post-traumatic deformity of the pinna.
- Haematoma deep to the perichondrium compromises the blood supply of the cartilage, leading to scarring.
- Haematoma may be aspirated with a wide-bore needle.
- Sometimes requires drainage incision along the margin of the helix.

Impacted wax

- Removed by syringing with water after softening with olive oil.

The middle ear

Otosclerosis

Definitions

- Spongy bone formation in the region of the stapes footplate.
- Aetiology: autosomal dominant inheritance.
- Associations: pregnancy, osteogenesis imperfecta.
- Affects: young adults.

Clinical features

- Combined conductive and sensorineural deafness.

Investigation

➤ Pure-tone audiometry:
  - Similar reductions in air and bone conduction
  - Most pronounced at 2 kHz.
➤ X-rays – lucent and sclerotic changes.

Treatment

➤ Sodium fluoride can promote recalcification over a 2-year period.
➤ Hearing aids.
➤ Stapedectomy and reconstruction of the ossicular chain.
➤ Risk of perilymph fistula following surgery: avoid violent nose blowing, flying and strenuous exercise.

Acute suppurative otitis media

Definitions

- Acute infection of the middle ear.
- Aetiology: follows respiratory infection.
- Pathology: *Streptococcus pneumoniae* or *Haemophilus influenzae*.
- Affects: children.

Clinical features

- Earache.
- Systemic sepsis.
- Red bulging drum on otoscopy.
- Conductive deafness.

Investigation

➤ Bacteriology swabs.
➤ X-rays of mastoid – exclude mastoiditis.
➤ Immunoglobulin electrophoresis – hypogammaglobulinaemia is a cause of recurrent infection.

Treatment

➤ Analgesia.
➤ Amoxicillin 250 mg tds orally <10 years of age, 500 mg tds orally >10 years of age.
➤ Ephedrine 0.5% nasal decongestant drops qds
➤ Surgical drainage by incising the drum (myringotomy) – persisting infection.

Acute mastoiditis

Definitions

- Acute infection of the mastoid air sinuses.
- Aetiology: complication of untreated otitis media.

Clinical features

- Inflammation, pain and tenderness over the mastoid region.
- Cranial nerve palsies sometimes occur.
- Gradenigo's triad:
  - Headache
  - Trigeminal pain
  - Lateral rectus palsy.

Investigation

➤ Mastoid X-rays – demonstrate breakdown of air cells.

Treatment

➤ Ampicillin 500 mg qds i.v.
➤ Surgical drainage by mastoidectomy.
➤ Nerve palsies resolve with treatment of the underlying condition.

Chronic serous otitis media (glue ear)

Definitions

- Chronic inflammation of the middle ear – viscous secretions prevent normal ossicular function.
- Aetiology: poor drainage of middle ear via eustachian tubes.
- Associations: adenoidal hypertrophy.
- Affects: infants and small children.

Clinical features

- Fluctuant hearing loss.
- Delayed language development.
- Recurrent ear infection.
- Identified on routine screening.

Investigation

➤ Examination with an operating microscope.
➤ Pure-tone audiometry – determines severity of hearing loss.
➤ Tympanometry – a screening test, detecting negative middle ear pressure.

Treatment

➤ Myringotomy and insertion of a grommet.
➤ Adenoidectomy – improves eustachian drainage.
➤ Prognosis:
  - Grommet extrudes within a year, repeated insertion sometimes needed.

Chronic suppurative otitis media

Definitions

- Tubotympanic disease:
  - Repeated infection of the middle ear
  - Aetiology: perforation of the tympanic membrane, cleft palate.
- Attico-antral disease:
  - Cholesteatoma – locally destructive epidermoid cyst arising from the tympanic membrane.

Clinical features

- Smelly discharge from the ear.
- Conductive hearing loss.

Investigation

➤ Ear swabs for aerobic and anaerobic culture.
➤ Audiograms assess hearing loss.
➤ Mastoid X-rays – exclude mastoiditis.

Treatment

➤ Amoxicillin 250 mg tds orally <10 years of age, 500 mg tds orally >10 years of age.
➤ Cleaning of debris and discharge from the ear canal.
➤ Surgical excision of cholesteatoma.
➤ Surgical reconstruction of the drum – 2 years later.
➤ Radical mastoidectomy – sometimes necessary.

Complications

- Cranial nerve palsies.
- Subperiosteal abscesses over the mastoid.
- Intracranial infection:
  - Meningitis
  - Brain abscesses
  - Thrombophlebitis of the sigmoid sinus.
- Tympanosclerosis – scarring of the tympanic membrane.
- Adhesive otitis – fusion of the ossicles.

Traumatic rupture of the tympanic membrane

- Small perforations heal spontaneously; large perforations and perforations from hot metal fragments (welding injuries) do not.
- Examination under an operating microscope and eversion of the edges of the perforation encourage healing.
- Surgical repair with a graft of skin, vein, temporalis fascia or banked tympanic membrane homograft at 3–6 months.

The inner ear and vestibulocochlear nerve

Herpes zoster oticus and Ramsay Hunt syndrome

- Herpes/varicella zoster infection of the vestibular or genicular ganglia produces intense pain in the ear, followed within a few days by a vesicular rash on the external ear or face.
- Ramsay Hunt syndrome – the combination of sensorineural deafness, vertigo and facial paralysis.
- Treatment: pain relief and aciclovir 800 mg five times daily orally for 7 days.
- Prognosis: facial nerve function recovers in 60%; pain may persist.

Acoustic neuroma

Definitions

- Benign tumour of the acoustic nerve.
- Bilateral cases occur in type II neurofibromatosis.

Clinical features

- Sensorineural deafness.
- Tinnitus.
- Vertigo.

Investigation

➤ Audiometry – shows sensorineural deafness.
➤ Computerized tomography/magnetic resonance imaging – confirms diagnosis and distinguishes from temporal bone meningioma.

Treatment

➤ Neurosurgical resection.

Menière's disease

Definitions

- An unexplained condition causing intermittent vertigo and hearing loss.
- Pathology: possibly intermittent endolymphatic duct obstruction.
- Aetiology: unknown, possibly viral infection.
- Usually unilateral.
- Affects: mainly adult women.

Clinical features

- Intermittent attacks of vertigo, sensorineural hearing loss and tinnitus.

Investigation

➤ Pure-tone audiometry – on repeated visits shows the fluctuant hearing loss.
➤ Caloric tests – abnormal in three-quarters of cases.

Treatment

➤ Prochlorperazine 5 mg tds orally.
➤ Cinnarizine 30 mg tds orally.
➤ Surgery: ablation of the labyrinth, drainage of the saccus endolymphaticus, insertion of a grommet into the tympanic membrane, cervical sympathectomy, or vestibular nerve section.
➤ Prognosis:
  – 60% of cases resolve spontaneously.

Glomus jugulare

Definitions

- Neuroendocrine tumour of jugular bulb.
- Pathology: paraganglionoma.
- Affects: mainly women, around 50 years of age.

Clinical features

- Pulsatile tinnitus.
- Sensorineural deafness.
- Otoscopy – red mass behind the tympanic membrane (setting sun sign).

Investigation

- ➤ Operating microscope examination confirms diagnosis.
- ➤ Audiography – sensorineural hearing loss.
- ➤ Computerized tomography shows enlargement of the jugular bulb and erosion of the hypotympanum.
- ➤ 24-hour urinary vanillylmandelic acid (VMA) identifies endocrine function in some tumours.

Treatment

- ➤ Observation – auditory symptoms alone.
- ➤ Radiotherapy – cranial nerve involvement.
- ➤ Surgical resection following pre-operative embolization – sometimes possible.

Noise-induced hearing loss

- Audiograms: early loss at 4 kHz, followed by high and then low frequency.
- Treatment: hearing aids.

Barotrauma

- Sudden pressure changes in flying or diving rupture inner ear membranes, producing endolymph fistula, sensorineural deafness, tinnitus and vertigo.
- The fistula test: induces nystagmus and vertigo by raising and lowering the external ear pressure by a pumping action on the tragus.

- Treatment:
  - Bed rest with the head raised – allows healing within 10 days.
  - Surgical closure of the fistula.

Presbyacusis

- Age-related hearing loss causing difficulty in understanding speech – hearing aids offer some improvement.

ORBIT

Peri-orbital disease

Dermoid cysts

- Congenital subcutaneous cystic swellings – usually over the external angular process of the frontal bone – treatment is by excision.

Herpes zoster ophthalmicus (shingles)

Definitions

- Herpes/varicella zoster infection of the trigeminal ganglion.

Clinical features

- Painful vesicular rash in territory of ophthalmic division of trigeminal nerve.
- Gradually subsides over weeks.
- Post-herpetic neuralgia persists for months.

Treatment

➤ Aciclovir 800 mg 5 times a day for 7 days – reduces vesicles and pain if started early.
➤ Aciclovir 3% eye ointment 5 times a day until 3 days after healing.
➤ No treatment is effective for post-herpetic neuralgia.

The eyelids

Ptosis

Definitions

- Drooping of the eyelid.
- Aetiology:
  - Congenital
  - Third-nerve palsy
  - Horner's syndrome
  - Age-related weakness
  - Following cataract surgery
  - Conjunctival scarring post infection
  - Myasthenia
  - Blepharophimosis.

Clinical features

- Investigation of possible underlying condition.

Treatment

- ➤ Surgical correction – excision of ellipse of upper lid or plastic reconstruction.
- ➤ Conservative – for postoperative cases.
- ➤ Treatment of myasthenia.

Blepharitis

- Inflammation of the eyelid margins.
- Acute: allergic reactions.
- Chronic: staphylococcal infection – treated with fusidic acid 1% eyedrops bd.

Trachoma

Definitions

- Chronic conjunctival infection, leading to scarring.
- It occurs worldwide – leading cause of preventable blindness.
- Aetiology: results from infection by *Chlamydia trachomatis* – transmitted by the common fly.
- Affects: children of the developing world.

Clinical features

- Chronic inflammation of the conjunctiva.
- Entropion – inturning of the lid margin.
- Trichiasis – inturning of eyelashes.
- Corneal abrasion.
- Herbert's pits – depressions around the iris caused by scarring.

Investigation

➤ Clinical diagnosis.

Treatment

Active disease:

➤ Improved hygiene
➤ Tetracycline 500 mg qds orally for 21 days.

Mass treatment campaigns:

➤ Tetracycline 1% eye ointment bd, 5 days a month for 6 months.

Late stages:

➤ Surgical correction of entropion and trichiasis
➤ Removal of scar tissue and keratoplasty for corneal scarring.

Styes

- Red discharging swellings of the eyelid margin from staphylococcal infection of a hair follicle.
- Treatment: most resolve spontaneously; antibiotics for associated cellulitis.

Meibomian cysts (chalazion)

- Translucent swellings at the eyelid margin – treated by surgical drainage from inside the lid.
- Treatment: topical 0.5% erythromycin or bacitracin ointment 500 units/g with hot compresses. Incision and curettage may be required.

Entropion

- Inturning of the eyelid.
- Aetiology: idiopathic in the elderly, secondary to scarring from foreign body or trachoma.
- Treatment: protective contact lens, removal of eyelashes, surgical correction.

Ectropion

- Eversion of the eyelid.
- Aetiology: idiopathic in the elderly, secondary to scarring or facial palsy.
- Treatment: surgical correction.

The lacrimal apparatus

Acute dacryocystitis

- Infection of the lacrimal sac.
- Treatment: broad-spectrum antibiotics, surgical drainage if unresolved.

Chronic dacryocystitis

- Watering of the eyes from nasolacrimal duct obstruction in the elderly.
- Treatment: surgical drainage into the nose.

Congenital nasolacrimal duct obstruction

- Sticky eyes in the infant – relieved by massage of the sac and probing the duct.

Lacrimal gland tumours

- Hard irregular swellings, enlarging over several months.
- Treatment: pleomorphic adenomas – surgically excised, malignant tumours – radical resection or radiotherapy.

The eye

Conjunctivitis

Definitions

- Inflammatory condition of the conjunctiva.

- Aetiology:
  - Allergic
  - Irritants
  - Adenovirus
  - Gonococcus
  - Chlamydia.

Clinical features

- Red, inflamed conjunctiva.
- Usually bilateral.
- Allergic cases have associated hay fever, asthma or eczema.
- Adenoviral cases are contagious.
- Adult gonococcal and chlamydial cases – associated with venereal disease.
- Neonatal gonococcal and chlamydial cases – infected birth canal:
  - Gonococcal cases present within 3 days
  - Chlamydial cases present within 2 weeks.

Investigation

➤ Microbiology of swab – gonococcal cases.
➤ Serological tests for chlamydia antibodies.

Treatment

➤ Allergic – spontaneous recovery.
➤ Irritants – irrigation, betamethasone 0.1% eyedrops 2-hourly short term, artificial tears, vitamin C minimizes scarring; surgical removal of scar tissue.
➤ Adenovirus – spontaneous recovery over 2 weeks.
➤ Gonococcus:
  - Adult – ciprofloxacin 0.3% eyedrops every 15 minutes for 6 hours as an in-patient, gradually decreasing frequency of application over 21 days
  - Neonate – amoxicillin 100 mg/kg daily in divided doses until resolution.
  - Adult – doxycycline 100 mg bd for 14 days
  - Neonate – tetracycline 1% eye ointment bd until resolution.

Pterygium

- An ingrowth of conjunctiva onto the cornea – occurs in hot dusty countries – treatment is by surgical removal.

Iritis

Definitions

- Inflammatory conditions of the iris
- Associations: sarcoidosis, seronegative arthritis, tuberculosis, syphilis, leprosy, cytomegalovirus infection in acquired immunodeficiency syndrome (AIDS).

Clinical features

- Unilateral red eye.
- Pain.
- Photophobia.
- Blurred vision.
- Reduced acuity.
- Pupillary constriction.
- Keratic precipitates.

Investigation

- ➤ Investigation of associated systemic condition.
- ➤ Lumbar puncture in syphilitic cases – identifies neurosyphilis.

Treatment

- ➤ Treatment of associated systemic condition.
- ➤ Betamethasone 0.5% eyedrops 2-hourly initially – seronegative arthritis.
- ➤ Prednisolone up to 1 g intravenously per day short term in acute condition, then 7.5 mg orally per day maintenance dose – Behçet's syndrome and sarcoid.
- ➤ Ganciclovir 5 mg/kg bd intravenously for 21 days – cytomegalovirus iritis in AIDS.
- ➤ Benzylpenicillin 1.2 g qds intravenously for up to 4 weeks – syphilitic cases.
- ➤ Isoniazid 300 mg daily for 6 months – tuberculous cases.
- ➤ Surgical removal of scarred lens – lepromatous iritis, which does not respond to treatment.

Keratitis

Definitions

- Inflammation of the cornea.
- Aetiology: bacterial infection secondary to trauma from contact lenses or a foreign body.

Clinical features

- Localized corneal opacity.
- Staphylococci and streptococci – yellow, oval, suppurating opacity.
- Pseudomonas – thick ground-glass exudate in an irregular ulcer.
- Enterobacter – grey-white exudate in a shallow ulcer with ring-shaped corneal infiltrates from endotoxins.

Investigation

➤ Microbiology of corneal scrapings.

Treatment

➤ Ciprofloxacin 0.3% eyedrops every 15 minutes for 6 hours, gradually reducing to 4-hourly over 14 days, continuing for 21 days.

Dendritic ulcer

- Herpes simplex causes a characteristic multi-fronded ulcer – demonstrated with fluorescein/rose Bengal staining.
- Treatment: aciclovir eye ointment 3% five times daily.

Scleritis

- Association: rheumatoid arthritis and collagen disorders.
- Investigation and treatment are those of the systemic conditions.

Congenital glaucoma

Definitions

- Congenital condition where raised intra-ocular pressure causes blindness.

- Pathology: impaired drainage of the anterior chamber – occluded angle of anterior chamber; rising intra-ocular pressure damages the optic nerve.
- Aetiology: abnormal mesodermal tissue at angle of anterior chamber.
- Affects: infants >2 months of age.
- Usually bilateral.

Clinical features

- Buphthalmos – huge enlargement of the eyes.
- Photophobia.
- Corneal clouding.
- Excessive lacrimation.

Investigation

➤ Examination under anaesthesia.
➤ Ophthalmoscopy.
➤ Measurement of intra-ocular pressure by tonometry.
➤ Gonioscopy.
➤ Measurement of horizontal and vertical corneal diameter.

Treatment

➤ Surgery to establish a communication between the anterior chamber and Schlemm's canal.

Acute (closed-angle) glaucoma

Definitions

- Acute condition where sudden rise in intra-ocular pressure may cause blindness.
- Pathology: acutely impaired drainage of the anterior chamber – obstruction at the periphery of the iris.
- Aetiology: narrow anterior chamber angle.
- Affects: patients aged >40 years with peak incidence at 60–70 years of age.
- Usually affects one eye at a time.

Clinical features

- Coloured rings around light sources days or weeks beforehand.
- Visual loss over several hours.
- Severe orbital pain.
- Red and watery eye.
- Pupil is oval, dilated and poorly reactive to light.

Investigation

➤ Measurement of intra-ocular pressure by tonometry – raised at 60–70 mmHg.
➤ Goniometry (slit lamp) to assess risk for unaffected eye – narrow anterior chamber angle.

Treatment

➤ Emergency – immediate treatment:
  - Pilocarpine 2% eyedrops every 5 minutes – relieve the acute episode
  - Acetazolamide 500 mg i.v.
  - Surgical peripheral iridectomy – if unrelieved within a few hours.
➤ Prevention of further episodes, and protection of unaffected eye:
  - Pilocarpine 1% eyedrops to the unaffected eye
  - Bilateral laser iridotomy.

Chronic simple (open-angle) glaucoma

Definitions

- Chronic condition where a gradual rise in intra-ocular pressure causes field loss and eventually blindness.
- Pathology: chronically impaired drainage of the anterior chamber – obstruction in the trabecular network.
- Aetiology: unknown.
- Usually bilateral.

Clinical features

- Gradual visual field loss.
- Eventual blindness.

Investigation

➤ Ophthalmoscopy – cupping of optic disc, central retinal vessels displaced toward the nose.
➤ Perimetry – visual field defects: arcuate scotoma, enlarged blind spot, nasal step defect.
➤ Measurement of intra-ocular pressure by tonometry – raised at 30–45 mmHg.

Treatment

➤ Timolol 0.25% eyedrops bd
➤ Metipranolol 0.1% eyedrops bd, or adrenaline 1% eyedrops bd, or pilocarpine 0.5% eyedrops bd if no response.
➤ Laser trabeculoplasty – for resistant cases.

Congenital proptosis

● Associations: Apert's syndrome and Crouzon's syndrome.
● Surgical frontal and facial bone advancements reduce intracranial pressure, allowing more normal visual and mental development.

Orbital cellulitis

Definitions

● Infection of peri-orbital tissues.
● Aetiology: spread of infection from frontal and ethmoidal sinuses.

Clinical features

● Peri-orbital swelling and inflammation.
● General features of sepsis.

Investigation

➤ Blood and nasal swab cultures.
➤ CT/MRI – sinus infection, orbital or intracranial abscesses, cavernous sinus thrombosis.

Treatment

➤ Hospitalization.
➤ 4-hourly optic nerve function: pupil reaction, acuity, colour vision.
➤ Intravenous antibiotics:
  – Age <5 years: ampicillin 100 mg/kg daily in divided doses
  – Age >5 years: cefuroxime 750 mg and metronidazole 500 mg tds
➤ Surgical drainage of the orbit and sinuses – unresponsive cases.

Complications

- Complicated by frontal lobe abscesses and cavernous sinus thrombosis.

Fungal orbital cellulitis

- Occurs as mucormycosis in the immunocompromised, and as spread of aspergillosis from the nose in hot humid countries.
- Microscopy shows irregular hyphal branching in mucormycosis, dichotomous branching in aspergillosis.
- Treatment: amphotericin B 250 µg/kg increasing to 1 mg/kg intravenously daily if tolerated. Aspergillosis requires debridement of necrotic tissue.

Cavernous sinus thrombosis

- Presents like orbital cellulitis but progresses to high fever, vomiting and prostration, engorgement of facial and retinal veins, decreased acuity, decreased pupillary response to light and afferent defect, and proptosis.
- Rapid infusion contrast CT demonstrates a filling defect in the cavernous sinus.
- Treatment is benzylpenicillin 1.2 g tds and flucloxacillin 1 g qds intravenously, and possibly full heparinization.

Retro-ocular tumours

Capillary haemangioma

- Usually only cosmetic but rarely retro-ocular causing proptosis.

- Grows during the first year of life, then spontaneously involutes.
- If no improvement or threat of visual impairment steroid injections, surgical resection or radiotherapy may be required.

Cavernous haemangioma

- Produces unilateral proptosis in middle life or during pregnancy; treatment is surgical excision.

Optic nerve glioma

- A cause of unilateral visual loss in children.
- CT/MRI shows a fusiform enlargement of the optic nerve.
- Can be kept under observation; but progressive visual loss or high growth rate are indications for surgery, radiotherapy for intracranial extension.

Optic nerve meningioma

- A cause of unilateral visual loss in the middle-aged.
- CT/MRI show tubular thickening and CT shows calcification of the optic nerve.
- Can be kept under observation; but progressive visual loss or high growth rate on CT/MRI are indications for surgery.

Rhabdomyosarcoma

- A cause of proptosis in childhood.
- CT/MRI of chest and abdomen assess metastatic spread; biopsy confirms diagnosis.
- Treatment is with radiotherapy or chemotherapy; with orbital exenteration for recurrent or resistant cases.

Tumours of the fundus

Melanoma of the choroid plexus

Definitions

- Malignant melanoma may occur in the optic fundus.

- Aetiology: primary tumour of choroid, or metastasis from melanoma elsewhere.
- Affects: those in the 50–70 years age range.

Clinical features

- Visual field changes.
- Incidental finding on funduscopy.

Investigation

➤ Fluorescein angiography – large vessels within a small tumour are diagnostic of melanoma.
➤ Ultrasound/colour duplex – demonstrates tumour size.
➤ CT – demonstrates local extension.
➤ Intra-ocular biopsy – confirms diagnosis.

Treatment

➤ Enucleation of the globe.
➤ Localized radiotherapy by implanted plaques.
➤ 75% 5-year survival.

Options:

➤ Photocoagulation and localized resections – small tumour.
➤ Exenteration – extensive tumour.
➤ Chemotherapy – metastatic tumour.

Retinoblastoma

Definitions

- Primary malignant tumour of the retina.
- Aetiology: hereditary and sporadic cases.
- Affects: infants up to 2 years of age.
- Hereditary cases may be bilateral.

Clinical features

- White appearance to the pupil is noted by the parents (cat's eye).
- Raised white area on funduscopy.
- Untreated cases: strabismus, proptosis and fungation.

Treatment

Options:

➤ Enucleation with a long portion of optic nerve.
➤ Radiotherapy.
➤ Photocoagulation or cryotherapy – for small tumours.
➤ Chemotherapy – recurrence and metastases.

Prognosis:

➤ Survival is 85%.

Carotid–cavernous fistula

Definitions

● Aetiology: an aneurysm of the intracranial carotid artery ruptures into the cavernous sinus; basilar skull fracture.

Clinical features

● Rapid onset.
● Throbbing orbital pain.
● Buzzing noise in the head.
● Blurred vision.
● Pulsating proptosis – obliterated by compressing the ipsilateral carotid artery.

Investigation

➤ MRI/CT of the brain and intracranial circulation.
➤ Cerebral angiography.

Treatment

➤ The fistula may close spontaneously by thrombosis.
➤ Surgery – for visual impairment or problems resulting from proptosis.

Thyrotoxicosis (page 308)

Eye injury

Corneal abrasions

- Visualized with fluorescein staining – resolve spontaneously – chloramphenicol 1% eye ointment tds prevents infection.

Foreign bodies

Definitions

- Low velocity bodies impact in the cornea, e.g. from hammer and chisel.
- High velocity bodies can penetrate the globe, e.g. in metal grinding.

Clinical features

Corneal body:

- Red eye
- Visible body.

Intra-ocular body:

- Red eye
- Reduced acuity
- Hypopyon – pus in the anterior chamber
- Uveitis.

Late features:

- Cataract formation
- Retinal damage from metal toxicity.

Investigation

Corneal body:

➤ Abrasion or visible foreign body on fluorescein staining.

Intra-ocular body:

➤ X-rays with radio-opaque contact lens – localization.

Treatment

Corneal body:

➤ Remove under local anaesthetic with the tip of a needle.

Intra-ocular body:

➤ Remove within 24 hours to avoid complications.

Magnetic fragments:

➤ Anterior chamber – can be drawn out with an electromagnetic probe
➤ Posterior chamber – surgical exposure is required first.

Non-magnetic fragments:

➤ Surgical exposure and removal.

Hyphaema

Definitions

● Bleeding into the anterior chamber.
● Aetiology: moderate blunt injury.

Clinical features

● A fluid level of blood in the anterior chamber when sitting or standing.

Treatment

➤ Bed rest – prevents secondary haemorrhage.
➤ Atropine drops – restrict movement of the iris.
➤ Prednisolone drops – prevent uveitis.

Traumatic retinal detachment

● Sudden loss of vision some days after injury – requires urgent surgical intervention.

Globe disruption

● Shuttlecock injury.
● Surgical exploration and repair.

Cataracts

- Opacities of the lens.
- Aetiology: congenital, age, iritis, keratitis, radiation, injury.
- Treatment: surgical extraction and either placement of a synthetic lens or the use of glasses.

Refractive errors

Definitions

Hypermetropia (long sight):

- Light is focused beyond the retina
- Aetiology: short globe or weakly refractive lens or cornea.

Myopia (short sight):

- Light is focused in front of the retina
- Aetiology: long globe or strongly refractive lens or cornea.

Astigmatism:

- Aetiology: cornea has uneven curvature.

Clinical features

Hypermetropia:

- Initially it is possible to compensate by accommodation
- Difficulty with close vision (reading) over the age of 30.

Myopia:

- Recognized in childhood by routine eyesight tests
- Susceptible to retinal detachment, macular degeneration and primary glaucoma.

Astigmatism:

- Focal differences in different meridians through the eye.

Investigation

➤ Snellen chart – assesses distance vision.
➤ Jaeger charts – assess near vision.

➜

➤ Retinoscopy – determines lens power required to correct a refractive error.
➤ Electronic optometry – determines far and near points and refractive error.

Treatment

Glasses:

➤ Myopia:
  – Concave lenses.
➤ Hypermetropia:
  – Convex lenses reading glasses.
➤ Astigmatism:
  – Cylindrical lenses.

Contact lenses:

➤ Better at correcting large refractive errors.
➤ Hard lenses:
  – Less risk of infection or allergy
  – Cannot be worn continuously because the cornea becomes hypoxic.
➤ Soft lenses:
  – More prone to infection and allergy
  – Can be worn for long periods – gas permeable
  – Unable to correct astigmatism.

Refractive surgery:

➤ Surgical or laser incisions in the cornea flatten the lens – for myopia.

Strabismus

Definitions

● Loss of normal conformity of eye movements.

Non-paralytic strabismus:

● Failure of development of binocular reflexes
● Aetiology: may be secondary to a refractive error in one eye
● Usually develops between 1 and 3 years of age.

Paralytic strabismus:

- Extra-ocular muscle paralysis
- Aetiology:
  - Congenital: birth trauma
  - Acquired: head or orbital injury, meningo-encephalitis, multiple sclerosis, intracranial neoplasms, myasthenia gravis and thyrotoxicosis.

Clinical features

Non-paralytic strabismus:

- Angle of deviation of affected eye remains constant in all directions
- Convergent squint is most common
- The image from the affected eye may become suppressed (amblyopia).

Paralytic strabismus:

- Congenital cases usually have convergent squint (lateral rectus palsy).

Investigation

➤ Exclude disease of the eye.
➤ Assess refractive error.
➤ Investigate suspected underlying conditions.

Treatment

Non-paralytic strabismus:

➤ Glasses
➤ Occlusion – covering the unaffected eye stimulates development
➤ Orthoptics – visual exercises
➤ Surgery: repositioning, lengthening, shortening and denervation (injecting botulinum toxin) of muscles.

Paralytic strabismus:

➤ Prismatic glasses correct diplopia, but surgical correction is required.

Nystagmus

Definitions

- Rhythmic involuntary eye movements.

Horizontal nystagmus:

- Aetiology:
  - Disease of the semicircular canals, vestibulocochlear nerve, or vestibular nuclei
  - Cerebellopontine angle tumours
  - Idiopathic.

Vertical nystagmus:

- Aetiology: fourth ventricle lesions and tonsillar herniation through the foramen magnum.

Clinical features

- Jerking involuntary eye movement in one direction, with gradual return to the initial position.
- Induced by the patient fixing their gaze on the examiner's finger, particularly at the extremes of the horizontal range of eye movement.
- Horizontal nystagmus – movements in the horizontal plane:
  - Fast phase away from the side of the lesion – vestibular lesion
  - Fast phase towards the side of the lesion – cerebellar lesion.
- Vertical nystagmus – movements in the vertical plane.

Investigation

➤ Head CT/MRI.

Treatment

➤ Treatment of underlying condition.

Pupillary response abnormalities

- Acute compressing intracranial haematoma (page 226) – dilated ipsilateral pupil.

- Bilateral frontal intracranial haematoma pre-coning – normal pupils but failure of upward gaze.
- Coning (page 230) – bilateral pupillary dilatation.
- Ocular globe injury – dilated unreactive pupil.
- Optic nerve injury or disease – dilated pupil, unreactive to direct light but reactive to light in the contralateral eye.
- Optic tract disease – no effect on pupillary size but gives absent pupillary reflexes bilaterally to stimulation of the eye on the opposite side to the lesion.
- Oculomotor nerve injury – dilated pupil, unreactive to light stimulation of either eye, with a divergent paralytic squint.
- Argyll Robertson pupil – a feature of neurosyphilis; the pupil is small, irregular and unreactive to light, but reacts on convergence.
- Holmes–Adie pupil – a feature of myotonia; shows no normal reactions to light or convergence, but may slowly dilate in a darkened room.
- Investigation: CT/MRI to exclude intracranial tumours; MRI identifies demyelination; serological tests for syphilis; and investigations for multiple sclerosis (page 664).
- Treatment of the underlying conditions.

Horner's syndrome

Definitions

- Characteristic features resulting from loss of sympathetic nerve supply to the face.
- Pathology: damage to the cervical sympathetic chain.
- Aetiology: idiopathic, post-cervical or upper thoracic sympathectomy, trauma, brainstem vascular or demyelinating disease, carotid artery dissection, aneurysms of the aortic arch, cervical malignancy (lymph nodes, thyroid, skull base), chemodectoma and Pancoast tumours.

Clinical features

- Ipsilateral:
  - Meiosis – pupillary constriction
  - Ptosis
  - Vasodilatation and anhidrosis of the ipsilateral face.

Investigation

➤ Instil:
   – 4% cocaine into both eyes – the normal pupil dilates, the affected side does not
   – 1% hydroxyamphetamine – in preganglionic lesions both pupils dilate; in postganglionic lesions the pupil on the affected side does not.
➤ Investigation of underlying condition.

Treatment

➤ Treatment of underlying condition.

Field loss and blindness

Central retinal artery occlusion

Definitions

● Aetiology: embolism from carotid atheroma or from the heart.

Clinical features

● Sudden loss of vision in one eye.
● Light can be perceived.
● Decreased light reflex.
● Ophthalmoscopy: a pale fundus, with a bright macula – 'cherry-red spot'.

Investigation

➤ Carotid duplex – identifies atheromatous plaques.
➤ Echocardiography – identifies atrial thrombus or valve vegetations.

Treatment

Measures to restore vision:

➤ Lying flat
➤ Firm ocular massage for 15 minutes

→

➤ Acetazolamide 500 mg i.v. – to lower ocular pressure
➤ Inhaled 5% carbon dioxide to produce vasodilatation.

Prognosis:

➤ Success is unlikely.

Measures to reduce further embolism:

➤ Aspirin – carotid disease
➤ Anticoagulation – cardiac thrombus
➤ Removal of embolic source: carotid endarterectomy
  and atrial thrombectomy.

Amaurosis fugax

- Transient visual loss lasting for minutes or hours results
  from smaller emboli that do not cause complete
  occlusion.
- Treatment of embolic source (as above).

Retinal detachment

Definitions

- Aetiology: spontaneous, or may be precipitated by
  minor head trauma.
- Associated: myopia.
- Affects: most common in those >50 years old.

Clinical features

- Flashes of light – may occur days beforehand.
- Sudden blindness – dark shadow descends across the
  visual field.
- Funduscopy – detached portion of the retina appears
  grey.

Treatment

➤ Photocoagulation – early equatorial or posterior
  detachment.
➤ Cryotherapy – early peripheral detachment.
➤ Surgery: drainage of subretinal fluid, vitreous injection
  and microsurgical repair.

Macular degeneration

Definitions

- Common cause of blindness in Western countries.

Clinical features

- Gradual age-related deterioration of vision over years.
- Funduscopy: speckled pigmentation of the macular region.

Investigation

➤ Fluorescein angiography – increased fluorescence in some areas.

Treatment

➤ Laser photocoagulation – may reduce the risk of visual loss.

Orbital fractures

Definitions

- Depressed fractures of the zygomatic arch – from a direct blow.
- Fracture separations.
- Orbital blow-out fractures – blunt globe trauma (squash ball).

Clinical features

- Epistaxis – extension into maxillary sinus.
- Black eye.
- Subconjunctival haemorrhage – orbital floor injury.
- Flattening of the contour of the cheek.
- Anaesthesia in the infra-orbital nerve distribution – extension to the infra-orbital foramen.

Blow-out fracture:

- Diplopia – muscle entrapment
- Enophthalmos and strabismus.

Investigation

➤ X-rays.

Blow-out fracture:

➤ X-rays – opacity of maxillary sinus in orbital floor fracture
➤ Hess test (plotting eye movements on a chart) – restriction in the vertical plane
➤ CT – extent of fracture.

Treatment

➤ Osteotomy and repositioning or interposition of orbital floor plate – for diplopia, interference with mandibular function and infra-orbital anaesthesia.

Blow-out fracture:

➤ Antibiotic prophylaxis
➤ Avoid nose blowing
➤ Surgery and release of muscle entrapments – for diplopia or enophthalmos.

MOUTH

Additional teeth

● May be prone to infection and hence may require extraction.

Absent teeth

● Failure of eruption of a secondary tooth results from lack of space, abnormal position or dentigerous cysts; they can be identified by X-ray – extraction and re-implantation is possible.

Congenital syphilis

● Congenital syphilis may result in small tapered Hutchinson's incisors, and dome-shaped first upper Moon's molars.

Odontomes

- Hamartomas of dental tissue resulting in enamel pearls on a tooth or large round masses beneath the gums – larger masses are prone to infection, requiring excision.

Caries

Definitions

- Damage to teeth from bacteria and food debris.
- Pathology: bacteria penetrate the dentine, resulting in cavitation, then pulpitis, death of the pulp and dental abscess.
- Aetiology: *Streptococcus mutans* and bacterial plaque – food debris and sugar.

Clinical features

- Sticky fissure – a sharp probe sticks on the crown of the tooth – an early sign.
- Chalky appearance of softened enamel.
- Visible dental cavitation.
- Pulpitis causes toothache and sensitivity to heat or cold.
- Dental abscess causes pain and fever, which is relieved when the bone is penetrated, forming a periodontal cyst – the abscess may discharge externally forming a sinus.

Investigation

➤ Orthopantomogram X-ray – may demonstrate cavitation, periodontal cysts and abscesses.

Treatment

➤ Preventive: tooth brushing, avoiding refined sugar, and regular dental inspection.
➤ Clearing and filling of areas of cavitation.
➤ Drainage of pulpitis or dental abscess via the crown of the tooth, packing and amoxil 500 mg tds orally until sepsis subsides; with later root filling or crown.
➤ Apicectomy for recurrent root infection.
➤ Dental extraction for severe caries and acute abscess.

Vincent's angina

- Rapidly spreading ulceration from the gingival margins associated with *Borrelia vincenti*, *Spirochaeta denticola* and *Bacteroides melaninogenicus* infection, poor oral hygiene, smoking and general debilitation.
- Treatment: metronidazole 200 mg tds orally for 3 days; oral hygiene – chlorhexidine 0.2% mouthwash, hydrogen peroxide 6% mouthwash; improve general health.

Chronic gingivitis

- Gradual recession of the alveolar margins secondary to bacterial plaque can result in loss of teeth in old age – good oral hygiene, use of dental sticks and coating of exposed areas is useful.
- Chronic gingivitis also occurs in: acute leukaemias, uraemia, pregnancy and scurvy.

Dentigerous cysts

- Cystic swellings surrounding the crown of a tooth, preventing eruption; identified on X-ray when investigating failure of eruption of a secondary tooth – excised when extracting and re-implanting the tooth.

Dental impaction

- Failure of eruption of a secondary tooth because of lack of space results in absence of the tooth, aching and trismus in a young adult.
- Wisdom teeth – the third upper molars – are most often impacted; they are prone to infection and osteo-myelitis of the mandible may develop.
- Orthopantomogram identifies.
- Treatment: extraction.

Cold sores

- Herpes simplex infection transmitted by mucosal contact (kissing) results in painful vesicular lesions of the lips, which ulcerate – healing occurs over a 2-week period with periodic recurrences.

- Treatment: chlorhexidine 0.2% mouthwash avoids painful toothbrushing; aciclovir 200 mg five times daily orally for 5 days.

Oral candidiasis

- *Candida albicans* infection of the mouth appears as raised white patches, and occurs with antibiotic therapy and in immunocompromised patients.
- Treatment: amphotericin 10 mg lozenges qds for 10 days.

Syphilis

- Primary syphilis may appear as a chancre – a painless ulcer on the lips; and in secondary syphilis snail-track ulcers occur in the mouth.
- Treatment: doxycycline 200 mg bd orally for 14 days.

Cancrum oris

- Rapidly spreading gangrene of the mouth results from infection by Vincent's organisms – *Borrelia vincenti*, *Spirochaeta denticola* and *Bacteroides melaninogenicus* – and occurs in the severely debilitated and malnourished; associated with vitamin B deficiency.
- Treatment: metronidazole 500 mg tds i.v., hydrogen peroxide 6% mouthwash; surgical debridement; improve nutrition; later facial reconstruction – but many cases may be fatal.
- Oral manifestations of systemic disease: acquired immunodeficiency syndrome (page 118), Behçet's syndrome.

Aphthous ulcers

- Recurring multiple painful ulcers of unknown origin occur mainly in young women, but also associated with inflammatory bowel disease (page 435), Behçet's syndrome and coeliac disease.

- Treatment: hydrocortisone 2.5 mg lozenges qds, local anaesthetic lozenges, and caramellose sodium protective paste.

Osteomas

- Raised bony areas occurring in the midline of the palate, torus palatinus, and on the lingual aspect of the mandible, torus mandibularis.
- Treatment: excision may be required to allow denture fitting.

Leukoplakia and erythroplakia

- Premalignant raised white or red areas of oral mucosa, confirmed by biopsy and histology – 3% undergo malignant change within 5 years.
- Treatment: observation and avoidance of smoking.

Carcinoma of the mouth

Definitions

- Squamous carcinoma.
- Affects mainly elderly males; more common in the Far East.
- Aetiology: pipe, cigarette and chutta smoking; chewing tobacco, and betel nuts.

Clinical features

- Chronic bleeding oral ulcer with everted edges.
- Local invasion may cause: fixation, mandibular anaesthesia, otalgia, tongue wasting.
- Cervical node metastases.

Investigation

➤ Biopsy under anaesthesia and histology.
➤ CT/MRI assess local invasion.

Treatment

➤ Radiotherapy – for small tumours located where resection would interfere with function, and for fixed tumours.
➤ Radical resection and partial mandibulectomy with reconstruction using a 'Chinese' free vascularized radial forearm flap – for carcinoma of the floor of the mouth. Radiotherapy may cause bone necrosis.
➤ Neck dissection – cervical node metastases.
➤ Prognosis: up to 60% 5 years survival.

TONGUE

● **Glossitis:** occurs as a manifestation of systemic disease: pernicious anaemia, pellagra, agranulocytosis; and in oral candidiasis (page 274).
● **Wasting and weakness of the tongue:** occur in hypoglossal nerve palsy and bulbar palsy (page 215).

Carcinoma of the tongue

Definitions

● Squamous carcinoma.
● Affects mainly elderly males.
● Aetiology: pipe and cigarette smoking; chewing tobacco, alcohol.

Clinical features

● Painful ulcer or painless lump – usually on the lateral border.
● Referred otalgia – local invasion.
● Deviation of the tongue to the affected side – local invasion.
● Cervical node metastases – typically the jugulo-omohyoid node.

Investigation

➤ Biopsy under anaesthesia and histology.
➤ CT/MRI assess local invasion.

Treatment

➤ Partial glossectomy with skin grafting for small tumours, or pectoralis flap reconstruction for larger tumours.
➤ V resection – tumours of the tip of the tongue.
➤ Radiotherapy – large ulcerating and fixed tumours.
➤ Neck dissection – cervical node metastases.

PALATE

Cleft lip and palate

● Congenital failure of mesenchymal fusion affecting 1/800 births.
● Cleft lip:
  – Varying degrees of division of the upper lip extending from the vermillion border; mainly cosmetic rather than functional
  – Treatment: surgical repair after at least 10 weeks of age.
● Cleft palate:
  – Varying degrees of division of the palate from the uvula forwards; mainly functional – feeding difficulties, risk of aspiration, problems with speech development
  – Treatment: prosthesis for feeding; surgical reconstruction after 6–12 months.

Syphilitic gumma

● May result in a hole in the palate – treatment is that of the systemic disease and surgical reconstruction.

NOSE

Dermoid cysts

● Congenital cysts may occur on the bridge of the nose – treatment is excision.

Atresia of posterior apertures

- Occurs in 1/8000 births. Unilateral atresia causes chronic nasal discharge, bilateral atresia may result in neonatal death or cause feeding asphyxia.
- Investigation: listening in each nostril with a stethoscope tube, or attempting to pass a catheter into the nostrils.
- Treatment: surgical correction; urgent airway management, tracheostomy and tube feeding may be required in bilateral cases.

Acute rhinitis (coryza/common cold)

- Rhinovirus – picornavirus infection causing rhinorrhoea, sneezing, nasal obstruction and malaise.
- Treatment: rest, paracetamol up to 1 g qds, ephedrine 0.5% nasal drops relieve symptoms; but condition is self-limiting.

Simple chronic rhinitis

- Rhinorrhoea and nasal obstruction secondary to dusty environment or sinusitis.
- Treatment: avoid dust – use face-mask; betamethasone 0.1% nasal drops 3-hourly.

Wegener's granulomatosis

Definitions

- Necrotizing granulomatous vasculitic autoimmune condition of the respiratory tract, kidneys and skin.
- Affects mainly middle-aged males.

Clinical features

- Sinusitis and nose-bleeding.
- Breathlessness, pleurisy and haemoptysis.
- Flitting arthritis.
- Splinter haemorrhages.
- Punched-out skin lesions.
- Progressive renal failure – death within 1 year if left untreated.

Investigation

➤ Positive antineutrophil cytoplasmic antibody – supportive.
➤ Chest X-ray/chest CT may show cavitation.
➤ Multiple nasal biopsies may show granulomatous arteritis.
➤ Urinalysis may show red cells, casts, proteinuria.
➤ Renal biopsy may demonstrate renal involvement.

Treatment

➤ Cyclophosphamide 1–3 mg/kg and prednisolone 60 mg daily orally until remission is achieved.
➤ Renal transplantation may eventually be required.

Stewart's midline granuloma

● Rare T-cell lymphoma causing granulomatous inflammation and destruction of the mid-face.
● Affects mainly middle-aged females, presenting with chronic rhinitis and slow destruction of the mid-face, causing saddle-nose deformity and septal perforation, eventually resulting in death.
● Treatment: radiotherapy and debridement; reconstructive surgery or facial prosthesis.

Syphilitic gumma of the nose

● Occurs in congenital syphilis, with features of tertiary syphilis by 2 years of age – and tertiary syphilis – destructive granulomatous syphilitic gumma in late, untreated disease.
● Purulent nasal discharge, septal perforation and saddle-nose deformity.
● Facial X-rays show bony destruction, *Treponema pallidum* may be identified on dark-ground microscopy of nasal exudates. Serological tests confirm this but tests also remain positive after treatment.
● Treatment: cleanse nose with alkaline solution and remove sequestrum; benzylpenicillin 1.2 g qds for adults, and up to 300 mg/kg for children i.v. daily for up to 3 weeks.

Yaws (page 137)

- A tropical condition similar to syphilis, now believed to result from *Treponema pertenue* infection.
- Treatment: improve hygiene and nutrition; as for syphilis.

Tuberculosis (page 142)

- Mucosal infection causes unilateral chronic rhinitis; destructive tuberculoma causes septal perforation – mycobacteria may be identified or cultured from nasal discharge, biopsy may show caseating granulomas. Other investigation of systemic condition (page 142).
- Treatment: as systemic condition.

Leprosy (page 140)

- Lepromatous involvement of the nasal mucosa may cause bloodstained nasal discharge, nasal obstruction, and septal perforation.
- *Mycobacterium leprae* may be isolated from nasal discharge.
- Treatment: rifampicin 600 mg once a month orally, dapsone 100 mg daily orally and clofazimine 300 mg once a month orally for 2 years. Cleanse nose with alkaline solution.

Rhinoscleroma (page 146)

- Chronic rhinitis from *Klebsiella rhinoscleromatis* infection – occurs in poor rural areas of the Pacific Asian coast, Middle and Far East, Papua New Guinea, and Central and South America.
- Large, soft, inflammatory masses develop from the nasal mucosa and may protrude from the nostrils, causing nasal obstruction.
- Treatment: clofazimine 100 mg bd orally for 3 months; debulking operations may be required to relieve nasal obstruction.

Rhinosporidiosis (page 147)

- Bleeding raspberry-like nasal polyps presumed to result from fungal infection – sporangia can be identified, but no specific organism has been cultured. The condition occurs in India, Africa and South America.
- Treatment: diathermy excision.

Leishmaniasis (page 148)

- Protozoal skin and mucosal infection transmitted from other mammals to humans by sandfly bites; occurs in South America, Africa and Mediterranean regions.
- Painless facial ulceration takes months to heal, with subsequent scarring.
- Microscopy of ulcer smears: Leishman–Donovan bodies; oval cells with an eccentric nucleus.
- Treatment: where scarring is not important lesions can be left to heal spontaneously, otherwise sodium stibogluconate 20 mg/kg daily i.v. for at least 20 days.

Allergic rhinitis

- Sneezing, rhinorrhoea, nasal obstruction and conjunctivitis occurring as an allergic response to pollens, dust mites or other allergens.
- Onset in childhood with asthma and eczema – skin-prick tests identify allergens.
- Prophylaxis: avoid allergens; sodium chromoglycate 2–4% nasal spray qds.
- Treatment: azelastine 140 μg nasal spray bd or cetirizine 10 mg daily orally, and beclometasone 50 μg nasal spray qds.

Vasomotor rhinitis

- A similar condition to allergic rhinitis, but of unknown cause, with no identifiable allergen and no atopic association. Associated with nasal polyposis.
- Treatment: as for allergic rhinitis. If unresponsive, surgical division of nerve of pterygoid canal may be required for severe rhinorrhoea, and surgical reduction

of turbinates/resection of polyps for persisting nasal obstruction.

Rhinophyma

- Swelling of the tip of the nose from hyperplasia and fibrosis of sebaceous glands. Associated with acne rosacea.
- Treatment: dermabrasion – excess tissue is shaved off – re-epithelialization occurs from sebaceous glands but split skin grafts are sometimes required.

Capillary haemangiomas (page 590)

Nasal polyps

- Most arise in anterior ethmoidal air cells, growing into the nares causing: anosmia, speech defects, snoring, rhinorrhoea or bleeding.
- Multiple polyps occur with allergic and vasomotor rhinitis; polyps also occur with rhinosporidiosis and as malignant polyps.
- X-rays: expansion of ethmoidal sinus, opacity of maxillary sinus.
- Treatment: treatment of allergic and vasomotor rhinitis; transnasal polypectomy for persisting nasal obstruction.

Nasal fractures

- Type 1 (Chevallet): distal nasal bone and vertical septal fracture – requires manipulation under anaesthesia and nasal packing for up to 3 days.
- Type 2: C-shaped fracture of perpendicular plate of ethmoid and quadrilateral cartilage from lateral trauma – requires open reduction and packing.
- Type 3: perpendicular plate of ethmoid rotates backwards, septum collapses and nose turns upwards – from severe trauma – requires open reduction, packing and support with wires.
- Fractures >2 weeks old – require osteotomy to allow manipulation.

- Many fractures need not be manipulated if there is a high likelihood of further trauma, e.g. in boxers.
- Septal haematoma: bilateral red swellings of the septum may require surgical drainage and repair of subsequent septal defects.

Nasal foreign body

- Unilateral purulent nasal discharge in a child may result from an inserted foreign body.
- Treatment: remove item with forceps or sneeze out while occluding other nostril; if unsuccessful, push object back into pharynx and remove via the mouth.

Epistaxis (nosebleed)

- Usually arises from Little's area – anterior inferior septum.
- Spontaneous bleeding is exacerbated by hypertension, dry air and low atmospheric pressure, but bleeding may also result from trauma, inflammatory conditions, infection, neoplasia and conditions causing raised venous pressure or coagulopathy.
- Investigation: rhinoscopy and investigation of any suspected underlying condition.
- Treatment: pressing the ala onto the septum with a cold swab on the affected side. In case of continued bleeding, pack for 24 hours. Sometimes post-nasal packing under anaesthesia or cautery is required; rarely ligation of internal maxillary and anterior ethmoidal arteries for uncontrollable bleeding.

Snoring

- Results from partial obstruction of upper airway during sleep; rhinoscopy may demonstrate small nasopharynx, adenoidal hypertrophy, polyp or septal deviation. Some patients may wish to have resection of polyps, or surgical correction of septal deviation.

Sleep apnoea

- Occlusion of the airway during sleep causing cessation of airflow for >10 seconds; commoner in obesity, it causes snoring and lethargy – falling asleep at work.

- CT may show tongue–posterior pharyngeal wall distance <10 mm. Endoscopy or oxygen saturation monitoring during sleep are required to confirm diagnosis.
- Treatment: weight loss; use of continuous positive airway pressure apparatus at night; resection of polyps or other cause of obstruction; widening of the airway by resection of tonsils and soft palate.

PHARYNX

Bifid uvula

- Double uvula may be associated with a minor degree of cleft palate; if resection of adenoids is required, nasal speech will result – modified adenoidectomy should be performed.

Acute pharyngitis

- Occurs with rhinitis or laryngitis.

Vincent's angina

- Ulcerative infection by Vincent's organisms: *Borrelia vincenti* and *Bacillus fusiformis*, spreading from tonsils, causing high fever and a grey slough over the pharynx.
- Treatment: benzylpenicillin 1.2 g qds and metronidazole 500 mg tds i.v. until resolution.

Diphtheria

- *Clostridium diphtheriae* infection causes high fever and a characteristic grey-white membrane over the tonsils and palate, which bleeds on separation and obstructs the airway.
- Affects mainly children 2–5 years of age – spread by airborne droplets. It is associated with poor living conditions. It has been eliminated from the developed world by vaccination programmes.

- Treatment: observation and protection of the airway, antitoxin 10 000–30 000 units i.m. in suspected cases, and benzylpenicillin 25 mg/kg qds i.v. until resolution.
- Emergency tracheostomy or cricothyroidotomy may be needed for acute upper airway obstruction in severe cases.

Acute tonsillitis

- Group A haemolytic streptococcal infection causes sore throat, difficulty in swallowing, earache and cervical lymphadenopathy – swabs confirm microbiology.
- Treatment: penicillin V 500 mg qds for 10 days; children <5 years 125 mg, 5- to 12-year-olds 250 mg, and aspirin gargles.
- Complications: scarlet fever, rheumatic fever, peritonsillar abscess, otitis media, chronic tonsillitis.

Scarlet fever

- Group A haemolytic streptococcal throat infection can produce a toxin causing scarlet fever.
- Sore throat is followed after 2 days by an erythematous rash over the face, punctate erythema over the trunk and high fever. After 4 days the skin starts to peel. The condition usually settles over 1 week, but rheumatic fever (page 381) or glomerulonephritis may develop after 2 weeks.
- Treatment: benzylpenicillin 1.2 g qds i.v.; infants 300 mg, children aged 1–9 years 600 mg; converting to penicillin V once severe sepsis subsides.

Peritonsillar abscess (quinsy)

- An abscess between the tonsil and its bed causes high pyrexia, severe throat pain, and displacement of the tonsil medially and backwards so that it is obscured by the soft palate.
- Treatment: surgical drainage without anaesthesia using sinus forceps; children – drain face down when recovering from general anaesthesia; tonsillectomy 6 weeks later.

Chronic tonsillitis

- Repeated attacks of acute tonsillitis result in scarring and accumulation of calcified chronically infected material – tonsoliths.
- Persisting symptoms, chronic cough and sleep apnoea may result.
- Treatment: tonsillectomy; if unfit for surgery, long-term penicillin V. Lift out tonsoliths with probe.

Tuberculous tonsillitis

- Tuberculous tonsillar infection is the origin of tuberculous lymphadenitis (page 301).
- Treatment: tonsillectomy and treatment of the systemic condition.

Adenoidal hypertrophy

- Develops in childhood causing mouth breathing, toneless voice, and a pinched appearance to nostrils – identified by rhinoscopy and sometimes examination under anaesthesia.
- Treatment: breathing exercises; adenoidectomy only for severe symptoms.
- Complications of adenoidectomy: sepsis, otitis media, persistence of nasal speech.

Retropharyngeal abscess

- Suppuration of retropharyngeal nodes may result in accumulation of pus between buccopharyngeal and prevertebral fascia.
- Causes toxaemia, and breathing and feeding difficulties in an infant; X-ray shows swelling in the prevertebral region.
- Treatment: as in peritonsillar abscess.

Nasopharyngeal carcinoma (page 131)

- Occurs mainly in South-East Asia, and is associated with Epstein–Barr virus infection. It presents with epistaxis or cervical node metastases, and diagnosis is confirmed by endoscopy and biopsy.

- Treatment: radiotherapy.

Oropharyngeal and tonsillar carcinoma

Definitions

- Aetiology: smoking – particularly pipe or cigar, and heavy alcohol consumption.
- Affects mainly elderly males.

Clinical features

- Oropharyngeal carcinoma – sore throat, dysphagia, blood in saliva.
- Tonsillar carcinoma – Trotter's triad: conductive deafness, otalgia, unilateral elevation and fixity of the soft palate.
- Horner's syndrome (page 267).
- Cervical node metastases may be the only presenting feature.

Investigation

➤ Endoscopy and biopsy under anaesthesia.
➤ CT and chest X-ray: to demonstrate metastases.

Treatment

➤ Radiotherapy – for localized tumours; combined with neck dissection for involved lymph nodes.
➤ Surgical resection for tonsillar carcinoma. Commando operation: combined neck dissection, mandibulectomy and resection of tonsil, part of the palate and tongue base – for tonsillar carcinoma with cervical lymph node metastases.
➤ Symptomatic treatment for advanced cases.

Post-cricoid carcinoma

- Associations: Patterson–Kelly–Brown syndrome – post-cricoid web and iron-deficiency anaemia affecting

young women; and irradiation >20 years earlier for thyrotoxicosis.
- Presents with dysphagia.
- Treatment: radiotherapy for small tumours; pharyngolaryngectomy and radical neck dissection for larger tumours and involved cervical nodes.

Lymphoma

- Smooth enlargements of the pharyngeal tissues; diagnosis by incision biopsy under anaesthesia and histology and immunohistochemistry.
- Treatment: radiotherapy and chemotherapy: single agent, if low grade; combination, if high grade.

Adenocarcinoma of minor salivary glands

- Smooth enlargements of the pharyngeal tissues; diagnosis by incision biopsy under anaesthesia and histology.
- Treatment: wide excision with radiotherapy for palliation or recurrence.

Pharyngocoele

- An anterior pharyngeal pouch arising from the piriform fossa can develop from repeatedly raised intrapharyngeal pressure in glass blowers and trumpet players.
- A swelling appears just anterior to the sternomastoid on performing a Valsalva manoeuvre; confirmed by barium swallow or ultrasound with Valsalva manoeuvre.
- Treatment: surgical excision via neck incision.

Pharyngeal pouch

- A Zenker's diverticulum is a posterior herniation through Killian's dehiscence (between the thyropharyngeal and cricopharyngeal parts of the inferior constrictor muscle), occurring mainly in elderly men. Patients present with dysphagia, regurgitation of

food and sometimes aspiration; diagnosis is confirmed
by barium swallow with continuous screening.

- Treatment: dilatation of the cricopharyngeal sphincter
with bougies; endoscopic diathermy division of the wall
between the pouch and the oesophagus – Dohlman's
operation; or surgical excision via neck incision.

LARYNX

Laryngeal web

- Complete congenital occlusion of the larynx results in
stillbirth; partial occlusion causes stridor soon after
birth.
- Treatment: emergency tracheostomy and endoscopic
division of the web.

Laryngomalacia

- Congenital abnormal shape to the laryngeal inlet; rarely
problematic, it may cause respiratory distress.
- Treatment: tracheostomy and division of aryepiglottic
folds.

Laryngitis

Acute laryngitis

- Viral infection, alcohol and smoking inflame the larynx
causing hoarseness, sore throat, cough, malaise and
fever.
- Treatment: rest, avoid cause.

Laryngotracheobronchitis (croup)

- Parainfluenza virus, respiratory syncytial virus, and
rhinovirus infection in 1- to 2-year-olds causes stridor.
- Treatment: avoid sedation, moist air environment;
severe cases are admitted for observation.

Acute epiglottitis

- *Haemophilus influenzae* infection in 2- to 3-year-olds
causes stridor, high fever, painful swallowing, and

drooling; life-threatening airway obstruction may
be precipitated by instrument examination of the
throat.
- Treatment: admit for observation, moist air environment, cefotaxime 50–100 mg/kg bd i.v.
- Emergency tracheostomy or cricothyroidotomy may be
  needed for acute upper airway obstruction in severe
  cases.

Chronic laryngitis

- Cigarette smoke, alcohol, fumes, dusts produce chronic
  inflammation of the larynx, causing hoarseness and
  cough.
- Treatment: rest the voice, avoid causes.

Miscellaneous conditions

- Chronic inflammation of the nose, pharynx and larynx
  with similar presentations include: diphtheria,
  tuberculosis, syphilis, leprosy and mycotic infection.

Carcinoma of the larynx

Definitions

- Squamous carcinoma.
- Affects males aged 40–60 years.
- Aetiology: smoking (cigarette, cigar and pipe).

Clinical features

- Glottic (vocal cord) – hoarseness.
- Subglottic – presents late with stridor and respiratory
  obstruction.
- Supraglottic – presents late with cervical node
  metastases.

Investigation

➤ Direct laryngoscopy under general anaesthesia.
➤ Biopsy: histology.
➤ CT: local invasion and nodes.
➤ Chest X-ray: metastases.

Treatment
- ➤ Radiotherapy – for small tumours, preserves speech.
- ➤ Microsurgery – for small tumours in young patients, avoids radiation.
- ➤ Supraglottic laryngectomy – for small supraglottic tumours, preserves speech.
- ➤ Excision of vocal cord – for small mobile vocal cord tumours.
- ➤ Total laryngectomy and end tracheostomy – larger tumours.
- ➤ For advanced disease, laryngectomy reduces pain and risk of fungation. Radiotherapy may relieve obstructive symptoms if not resectable.

Leukoplakia
- Premalignant changes occur as raised white patches on the cords – biopsy and histology confirm the diagnosis.
- Treatment: observe, avoid smoking and alcohol.

Benign neoplasms
Papillomas, fibromas, chordomas, angiomas are excised endoscopically or via lateral laryngotomy.

Singer's nodes
- Repeated voice strain may result in bilateral grey nodules halfway along the vocal cords, causing hoarseness and loss of voice – identified on laryngoscopy.
- Treatment: rest voice – most resolve over weeks. Voice training prevents further problems.

Laryngocoele
- Repeated forced expiration by trumpet players and glass blowers can result in enlargement of air sac remnants of the laryngeal ventricle, between the true and false vocal cords.
- Typically affects those >50 years of age. The sac can protrude into the neck on coughing or blowing – external

laryngocoele, or be confined to the vallecula – internal laryngocoele.

- X-ray with Valsalva manoeuvre shows an air-filled sac.
- Treatment: an internal laryngocoele can be surgically marsupialized. An external laryngocoele can be surgically excised via the neck.

Angioneurotic oedema

- Sudden dyspnoea and stridor from laryngeal oedema in response to drug or food allergy.
- Treatment: give oxygen and maintain airway; adrenaline 500 μg i.m., chlorpheniramine 20 mg i.v., hydrocortisone 100 mg i.v.

Laryngeal trauma

- Blunt trauma or strangulation causes hoarseness, dyspnoea and dysphagia.
- Treatment: observe for 24 hours – if airway obstruction develops, intubate and explore surgically.
- High velocity blunt trauma and penetrating trauma cause haemorrhage and asphyxia – but severe disruption may create a natural surgical airway.
- Treatment: intubate, surgically explore and debride, with later reconstructive surgery or surgery for subsequent stenosis.

Thermal and chemical burns

- Cause airway obstruction from oedema.
- Treatment: observe for 24 hours – if airway obstruction develops, intubate, tracheostomy; later surgery may be needed for subsequent stenosis.

Laryngeal paralysis

- Laryngeal paralysis results from recurrent or superior laryngeal nerve palsy, myasthenia gravis, and, rarely, conditions of the central nervous system.
- Varying degrees of loss of power of speech, hoarseness and loss of speech; airway obstruction and risk of aspiration in bilateral adductor paralysis.

- Laryngoscopy identifies the pattern of cord paralysis. CT may identify tumour causing nerve palsy; other investigation of suspected underlying neurological conditions.
- Treatment: unilateral abductor paralysis requires only speech therapy; unilateral adductor paralysis requires Teflon injection and speech therapy; bilateral adductor paralysis requires tracheostomy, tube feeding; permanent paralysis may require laryngectomy and permanent tracheostomy.

SALIVARY GLANDS

Salivary gland swelling

Infection	
Acute	Viral (mumps)
	Bacterial parotitis
Recurrent	Obstruction, calculus, stricture
Chronic	TB, actinomycosis
Autoimmune	Sicca syndrome, Sjögren's syndrome
Calculus (sialolithiasis)	
Cysts	
Chronic inflammatory	Sarcoid
Drugs	Phenylbutazone
Allergy	Iodine
Neoplasia	
Benign	Pleomorphic adenoma
	Warthin's
Malignant	Adenocystic carcinoma
	Mucoepidermoid carcinoma
Systemic disease	Alcoholic cirrhosis
	Diabetes mellitus
	Pancreatitis
	Acromegaly
	Malnutrition

Mumps

- Contagious mumps virus infection causes epidemics in non-immunized children aged 4–12 years.

- After an incubation period of 3 weeks, malaise, fever, bilateral parotid swelling and arthralgia develop.
- Complications: orchitis, meningoencephalitis, pancreatitis, thyroiditis and sensorineural hearing loss.
- Treatment: preventive – immunization; analgesia and oral hygiene. Settles spontaneously.

Bacterial parotitis

- *Staphylococcus aureus* and *Streptococcus viridans* infection of the parotid gland; results in an inflamed tender unilateral or bilateral parotid swelling.
- Associated: dehydration and poor oral hygiene.
- Affects: postoperative or terminally ill patients.
- Treatment: intravenous fluids, oral hygiene, flucloxacillin 500 mg qds and benzylpenicillin 1.2 g tds i.v., later changing to oral equivalents.

Pleomorphic adenoma (mixed salivary tumour)

Definitions

- Benign encapsulated salivary tumour of mixed epithelial and mesodermal origin.
- Commonest salivary tumour – occurs most often in the parotid gland.
- Affects mainly women >40 years of age.

Clinical features

- Smooth lobulated fixed swelling of one parotid gland.
- Slowly enlarges over years.
- Oral examination may show the tonsil to be displaced inwards.

Investigation

➤ CT/MRI demonstrates extent of the tumour – deep lobe involvement.
➤ Avoid biopsy – can lead to recurrence from needle track seeding.

Treatment

➤ Observation of small non-progressive tumours.
➤ Conservative superficial parotidectomy or excision with a surrounding cuff of normal tissue. Recurrence may occur if excision is incomplete, but very extensive resection may lead to facial nerve palsy.
➤ Conservative total parotidectomy with preservation of facial nerve branches when deep part of the gland is involved.
➤ Radiotherapy is sometimes used to treat recurrence.

Complications

Complications of parotidectomy

- Frey's syndrome: sweating of the skin of the parotid region during eating results from parasympathetic secretomotor fibres severed during surgery growing into the skin. This may resolve over 6 months, otherwise division of the parasympathetic pathway by tympanic neurectomy is necessary.
- Facial nerve injury: particularly weakness of the ipsilateral edge of the mouth from the mandibular branch – avoided by careful preservation at surgery and superficial parotidectomy – but resection of the nerve is necessary for treatment of malignant disease.
- Salivary fistula: uncommon – usually resolves spontaneously.

Warthin's tumour

Definitions

- Benign tumour of parotid lymphoid tissue in lymph nodes of the parotid sheath.
- Occurs exclusively in the parotid.
- Affects: mainly men >50 years of age.

Clinical features

- Small, soft, mobile superficial tumour at the angle of the mandible.
- May occur bilaterally.

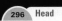

Investigation
➤ CT/MRI demonstrates extent of the tumour.
➤ Histology of excised tumour.

Treatment
➤ May be excised by limited parotidectomy – recurrence may occur.

Adenocystic carcinoma

Definitions
● Malignant tumour occurring in minor salivary glands, and submandibular and sublingual glands.
● Affects: 30–70 years age range; slightly commoner in women.

Clinical features
● Slowly enlarging, hard, fixed swelling of affected gland.
● Facial or trigeminal nerve palsy (page 210) indicates skull base invasion.
● Distant metastases.

Investigation
➤ CT/MRI demonstrates extent of the tumour.

Treatment
➤ Extensive surgical resection without preservation of adjacent nerves.
➤ Prognosis: one-third of patients die within 1 year.

Mucoepidermoid carcinoma

Definitions
● Malignant salivary tumour of mucin-secreting and epidermoid cells.
● Commonest malignant tumour of the parotid gland; also occurs in submandibular and minor glands.

Clinical features

- Hard, fixed swelling of affected gland.
- Facial palsy (page 212) from local invasion in parotid tumours.
- Cervical node metastases.
- Distant metastases.

Investigation

➤ CT/MRI demonstrates extent of the tumour.

Treatment

➤ Extensive surgical resection without preservation of adjacent nerves with neck dissection for involved nodes; sometimes with adjunctive radiotherapy.
➤ Prognosis: up to 70% of cases have 5-year survival; but depends on grade and extent.

Sialolithiasis

Definitions

- Salivary calculi typically occur in the submandibular (Wharton's) duct.
- Affects: mainly middle-aged patients.

Clinical features

- Aching and swelling of the submandibular gland – worse on eating.
- Stone may be palpable, or visible at the duct orifice.
- Stimulation with lemon juice shows no secretion on the affected side.

Investigation

➤ Plain X-rays may show the calculus.
➤ Sialography confirms diagnosis.

Treatment

➤ Surgical removal of stones by marsupializing the duct.

NECK

Sternomastoid tumour of infancy

Definitions

- Organizing haematoma and subsequent fibrosis of sternomastoid muscle.
- Aetiology: birth trauma – association with breech presentation.

Clinical features

- Sternomastoid tumour at birth.
- Torticollis: the head is held to one side because of contraction or contracture of one sternomastoid muscle – which becomes more prominent on attempting to straighten the head.

Investigation

➤ Clinical diagnosis.

Treatment

➤ Heat.
➤ Physiotherapy.
➤ Surgical lengthening – rarely required.

Rhabdomyosarcoma of sternomastoid

Definitions

- Rare malignant tumour of sternomastoid muscle.

Clinical features

- Sternomastoid tumour in adult.

Investigation

➤ Surgical biopsy – histology.

Treatment
➤ Local resection – frozen section to demonstrate clear margins.
➤ Radiotherapy with chemotherapy.
➤ Prognosis: 70% 5-year survival.

Laryngocoele (page 291)

Pharyngocoele (page 288)

Goitre (page 307)

Carotid and subclavian aneurysm
(page 551)

Superior vena cava syndrome

Definitions
● Obstruction of the superior vena cava by:
  – Mediastinal mass
  – Fibrosis
  – Thrombosis
  – Tumour invading the vein.

Clinical features
● Distended veins over the head and neck.
● Collateral veins across the chest.
● Swelling of face, neck and arms.
● Peri-orbital oedema.
● Chemosis.

Investigation
➤ Chest X-ray – mediastinal widening.
➤ CT/MRI – delineates mass.
➤ Venography – identifies level of obstruction.

Treatment
➤ Heparin 5000 units i.v. bolus, then infusion of 2000 units/hour adjusted according to daily activated partial thromboplastin time – continue until oral

➔

anticoagulation is stabilized; warfarin 10 mg daily orally for first 2 days, then maintenance dose to keep international normalized ratio at 2.5.
➤ Radiologically placed stents.
➤ Treat underlying mediastinal tumour – radiotherapy or surgery.

Cystic hygroma

- A congenital cystic lymphatic malformation in the root of the neck.
- Large cystic hygromas may obstruct delivery, or cause swallowing or respiratory difficulty, although smaller cases may not become apparent until adolescence.
- Investigation: CT or MRI.
- Treatment: aspiration and injection of sclerosant (or hot water) for smaller cases, otherwise surgical excision.

Cervical lymphadenopathy

Acute inflammatory lymphadenopathy

Definitions

- Commonest cause of cervical lymphadenopathy.
- Aetiology:
  - Tonsillitis, pharyngitis, laryngitis, parotitis, dental abscess
  - Furuncle or abscess, infected wounds, infected skin malignancy
  - Infectious mononucleosis – glandular fever
  - Toxoplasmosis
  - Cytomegalovirus
  - Actinomycosis
  - Lyme disease
  - Bubonic plague
  - Rickettsial infections.

Clinical features

- Firm, tender nodes.

- Tonsillitis particularly affects the tonsillar node at the angle of the mandible.
- Features of the underlying condition.

Investigation

According to clinical picture:

➤ Throat swab – group A streptococcus most likely cause of tonsillitis (in <5 years age group, viral aetiology)
➤ Monospot test – detects 85% of cases of infectious mononucleosis
➤ Enzyme-linked immunosorbent assay tests – specific immunological tests for infectious mononucleosis, cytomegalovirus, toxoplasmosis
➤ Cytomegalovirus isolation from saliva
➤ Histology of lymph node – identifies toxoplasma
➤ Fine-needle aspiration (FNA) – filamentous branched Gram-positive bacteria in actinomycosis.

Treatment
➤ Treatment of underlying infection.

Tuberculous lymphadenitis

Definitions

- Secondary to tonsillar infection.
- Aetiology:*Mycobacterium bovis* from unpasteurized milk, rarely pulmonary tuberculosis.
- Affects mainly immigrants from area of high prevalence.

Clinical features

- Progressive stages:
  - Solid node
  - Fluctuant mass
  - Collar-stud abscess
  - Discharging sinus.

Investigation

➤ Lymph node biopsy:
  – Histology – granulomas with caseous necrosis, organisms rarely identified
  – Microbiology – tuberculosis culture positive in 70%.
➤ Chest X-ray – rarely paratracheal lymphadenopathy or primary focus.
➤ Mantoux/Heaf test:
  – Negative – excludes tuberculosis
  – Positive – not diagnostic, may simply indicate immunity.
➤ Trial of treatment – if clinical suspicion is strong in spite of negative investigations.

Treatment

➤ Isoniazid 300 mg and rifampicin 450–600 mg daily orally for 6 months; pyrazinamide 1.5–2.0 g and ethambutol 15 mg/kg daily orally for the first 2 months.
➤ Surgical drainage/excision – often necessary for diagnosis but may cause chronic sinus.

Rare causes of chronic cervical lymphadenitis

● Sarcoidosis, histiocytosis X and cat-scratch disease.

Lymphomas

Definitions

● Lymphomas are divided into Hodgkin's and non-Hodgkin's disease.
● A malignant proliferation of lymphocytes in the reticuloendothelial system.

Hodgkin's disease

● Affects young adults; twice as common in men.
● Has a bimodal age presentation: early peak at 20–30 years and a later peak over the age of 50 years.
● Associated: chromosomal abnormalities and Epstein–Barr virus infection.

Clinical features

- Large, painless, rubbery cervical or axillary nodes.
- Constitutional symptoms: malaise, weight loss and pyrexia – night sweats.
- Superior vena cava syndrome – may result from mediastinal node involvement.
- Ann Arbor classification:

    I   Single node region or extralymphatic site

    II Two or more node regions on one side of the diaphragm; or single node region and one extralymphatic site on one side of the diaphragm

    III Node regions on both sides of the diaphragm

    IV Diffuse involvement of one or more extralymphatic sites.

    Each stage is divided into:

    – a = no systemic symptoms

    – b = systemic symptoms.

Investigation

➤ Lymph node biopsy and histology – abnormal mononuclear cells, Reed–Sternberg binucleate cells.

Histological variety	Survival at 5 years (%)
Lymphocyte predominant	80–85
Nodular sclerosing	70–80
Mixed cellularity	50–60
Lymphocyte depleted	40–50

➤ Bone marrow aspirate and trephine – usually normal, infiltrated in stage IVb.

➤ Chest X-ray/CT chest – staging.

Treatment

➤ Ia/IIa – radiotherapy.

➤ Ib/IIb – chemotherapy.

➤ IIIa – radiotherapy or chemotherapy.

➤ IIIb, IVa, IVb – chemotherapy.

➤ Chemotherapy is given as a combination of agents in monthly cycles on 6–8 occasions.

➤ Prognosis:

    – Low grade disease 80–90% 5-year survival

    – High grade disease 40–50% 5-year survival.

Non-Hodgkin's disease

Definitions

- Is a malignant proliferation of lymphocytes in the reticuloendothelial system: clinical and histological features distinguish a group of conditions termed non-Hodgkin's lymphomas.
- Mostly affect 60–80 years age group.

Clinical features

- Lymphadenopathy with no clear anatomical pattern.
- Marrow infiltration – anaemia, pancytopenia.
- Splenomegaly.
- Symptoms from involvement of extranodal sites:
  - Facial swelling – Burkitt's lymphoma (page 132)
  - Dyspeptic symptoms – gastric lymphoma
  - Intestinal obstruction – small bowel lymphoma.

Investigation

- ➤ Lymph node or extranodal site biopsy and histology – lymphocyte infiltration without characteristic changes of Hodgkin's; histological types range from low grade/centrocytic – lymphocytes are arranged in follicles – to high grade/lymphoblastic – diffuse lymphocyte infiltration.
- ➤ Bone marrow aspirate and trephine (multiple sites) – may be infiltrated.
- ➤ Full blood count – anaemia if extensive marrow involvement.
- ➤ Chest X-ray/CT chest – staging.

Treatment

Low grade:

- ➤ No treatment – if asymptomatic
- ➤ Combination chemotherapy – for symptom control
- ➤ Radiotherapy – localized types.

High grade:

- ➤ Combination chemotherapy.

➔

Prognosis depends on grade and stage, with variable survival:

➤ Low grade lymphomas – less aggressive, but less responsive to treatment
➤ High grade lymphomas – more aggressive, but more responsive to treatment.

Myeloma (page 642)

Secondary carcinoma

Definitions

- Pathology:
  - Squamous carcinoma of the upper aerodigestive tract – most common.
  - Skin tumours of head and neck – less common.
  - Medullary thyroid carcinoma – rare.
- Affects mainly males >50 years of age.
- Aetiology: heavy smoking, alcohol intake, chewing of tobacco and betel nut.

Clinical features

- Small, hard node.
- Examination of the oral cavity and salivary system.
- Indirect laryngoscopy and flexible nasopharyngeal endoscopy.

Investigation

➤ FNA – identifies squamous carcinoma, melanoma and thyroid carcinoma.
➤ Biopsy tongue base and piriform sinus – if no primary site identified.
➤ Chest X-ray – bronchogenic primary.

Treatment

➤ Radiotherapy.
➤ Block dissection of neck and radiotherapy.
➤ Resection of primary tumour.

Branchial cyst

- A branchial arch remnant forming a congenital cyst; usually first noticed in young adults as a fluctuant swelling between the carotid sheath and sternomastoid muscle. It does not usually transilluminate – contains cholesterol crystals.
- Infected cysts – tender, hard, inflammation of skin.
- Surgical excision of the cysts and any associated track – multiple step incisions may be needed.

Branchial fistulae

- A branchial arch remnant noticed at or soon after birth as a discharging orifice at the anterior border of the lower part of the sternomastoid muscle – the associated tract opens into the tonsillar fossa.
- Intermittent infection causes discharge.
- Treatment: surgical excision of the whole track – multiple step incisions may be needed.

Branchial sinus

- A branchial arch remnant with only an external opening – may be present at birth, or follow drainage of an infected cyst.
- Treatment: surgical excision of the whole track – multiple step incisions may be needed.

Thyroglossal cyst, sinus and fistula
(page 317)

Sublingual dermoid

- Congenital cystic inclusions of ectoderm.
- Opaque white swelling the floor of the mouth, or beneath the chin.
- Treatment is by enucleation, via either the mouth or through an incision beneath the chin.

Plunging ranula

- Retention cyst of a sublingual salivary gland.

- Presents as a swelling in the floor of the mouth, or the digastric triangle of the neck.
- A transilluminable blue-tinged swelling is visible to one side of the frenulum linguae.
- Treatment is by marsupialization under lingual nerve block: the roof of the cyst is excised, and the cavity packed with gauze soaked in Whitehead's varnish.

Carotid body tumour (page 550)

THYROID

Euthyroid goitre

Definitions

- Swelling of the thyroid gland without disturbance of thyroid function.
- Aetiology:
  - Smooth goitre:
    - Iodine deficiency – in 'soft' water areas, e.g. Derbyshire, UK (endemic goitre)
    - Congenital defects of thyroxine synthesis
    - Goitrogens
    - Physiological demand (e.g. puberty, pregnancy).
  - Multinodular goitre:
    - Disordered metabolism.
  - Other types:
    - Malignancy
    - Hashimoto's thyroiditis
    - Riedel's thyroiditis
    - De Quervain's thyroiditis
    - Thyroid amyloidosis.

Clinical features

- Swelling in lower anterior neck.
- Moves upwards on swallowing.
- Smooth or nodular.

Investigation

➤ Serum thyroid-stimulating hormone (TSH)/
  tri-iodothyronine (T_3)/thyroxine (T_4):
  – Normal TSH – euthyroid
  – Low TSH/raised T_3 – hyperthyroidism
  – Raised TSH/low T_4 – hypothyroidism.
➤ Ultrasound – differentiates cysts/nodules/possible
  adenomas or carcinomas.
➤ Chest X-ray/thoracic outlet X-ray – retrosternal
  extension.
➤ FNA – malignancy.
➤ Thyroid antibodies – thyroiditis.

Treatment

Diffuse goitre:

➤ Iodized table salt – prevents endemic cases
➤ Eliminate goitrogens
➤ Thyroxine 100 µg daily orally – suppresses TSH,
  causing regression in 70%.

Multinodular:

➤ Subtotal thyroidectomy.

Thyrotoxicosis

Definitions

● Condition resulting from the effects of excessive
  circulating thyroxine.
● Aetiology:
  – Autoimmune (Graves' disease)
  – Toxic adenoma (Plummer's disease)
  – Excessive thyroxine replacement.
● Less commonly:
  – Thyroiditis (page 314)
  – Metastatic thyroid carcinoma (page 313)
  – Struma ovarii
  – TSH-secreting pituitary tumour
  – Choriocarcinoma
  – Hydatidiform mole
  – Neonatal thyrotoxicosis.

Clinical features

Symptoms:

- Weight loss
- Diarrhoea
- Irregular menstruation
- Heat intolerance
- Sweating
- Weakness
- Palpitations.

Signs:

- Tremor
- Myopathy
- Tachycardia
- Atrial fibrillation
- Lid-lag and proptosis
- Exophthalmic ophthalmoplegia in rare severe cases – limitation of eye movement at extremes of gaze
- Corneal and optic nerve damage in rare severe cases – sight loss
- Goitre with a bruit over the superior thyroid artery.

Investigation

➤ Serum $TSH/T_3/T_4$:
  - Low TSH/raised T_3 – overactivity of the thyroid gland or excessive thyroxine replacement therapy
  - Raised TSH and T_3 – TSH-secreting pituitary tumour.
➤ Isotope scanning – identifies toxic adenoma, or site of overactivity in a nodular goitre.
➤ Electrocardiograph – tachycardia/atrial fibrillation.
➤ Chest X-ray/thoracic outlet X-ray – retrosternal extension.
➤ FNA – malignancy.
➤ Thyroid antibodies – thyroiditis.

Treatment

Graves' disease:

➤ Children:
  - Carbimazole 250 μg/kg tds orally for up 2 years.

➔

➤ <40 years of age:
  – Carbimazole 15–40 mg daily orally until euthyroid, then 5–15 mg daily orally for 6 months
  – Propranolol 40 mg daily orally – added in severe cases
  – Bilateral subtotal thyroidectomy – for relapse 65%.
➤ >40 years of age:
  – ^{131}I 200–600 MBq once orally; stop antithyroid drugs 4 days beforehand, and re-start 7 days afterwards; later (usually a few months) – when activity of the gland ceases – stop antithyroid drugs and commence thyroxine replacement.

Preparation for thyroid surgery:

➤ Carbimazole 30–40 mg daily orally, reducing to 5 mg after 12 weeks; and propranolol 40 mg daily orally
➤ Plan surgery only when euthyroid
➤ Lugol's iodine 30 minims (drops) tds orally, or potassium iodide 60 mg tds orally for 2 weeks prior to surgery – to reduce the vascularity of the gland.

Exophthalmos:

➤ Sleep in upright position
➤ Methylcellulose eyedrops
➤ Lateral tarsorrhaphy – severe cases
➤ Prednisolone and orbital decompression – severe cases where sight is threatened.

Toxic nodular goitre:

➤ Antithyroid drugs (see above)
➤ Subtotal thyroidectomy.

Toxic adenoma:

➤ Antithyroid drugs (see above)
➤ Unilateral thyroid lobectomy or ^{131}I.

Thyrotoxicosis in pregnancy:

➤ Propylthiouracil – crosses placenta less than carbimazole
➤ Subtotal thyroidectomy – safe in the second trimester
➤ Radioactive iodine is contraindicated – crosses the placenta and damages fetal thyroid.

Neonatal hyperthyroidism:

➤ Antithyroid drugs (see above)
➤ Resolves within 1–2 months.

Complications

- Acute upper airway obstruction from haematoma – requires intubation and evacuation of haematoma.
- Recurrent laryngeal nerve injury – transient 2–4% of cases, permanent 1%.
- Hypocalcaemia:
  - Measure corrected serum calcium in the first few days after surgery, and again at 6 weeks
  - Transient – 10 mL of 10% calcium gluconate i.v.
  - Permanent – vitamin D (1α-hydroxycalciferol) 1–2 µg/day.
- Hypothyroidism:
  - Measure T_4/TSH at 6 weeks after surgery, and then at 6-month intervals for at least 2 years
  - Eventually affects 50% of patients.
- Recurrent hyperthyroidism 4% – antithyroid drugs in patients <40 years, ^{131}I in patients >40 years of age.
- Thyroid crisis.

Thyroid crisis

Definitions

- Life-threatening exacerbation of hyperthyroidism.
- Aetiology: release of thyroxine during surgery in inadequately prepared patient.

Clinical features

- Distress.
- Dyspnoea.
- Tachycardia.
- Hyperpyrexia.
- Restlessness.
- Confusion.
- Delirium.
- Vomiting and diarrhoea.

Investigation

➤ Clinical diagnosis.

Treatment

- ➤ Intravenous fluids.
- ➤ Ice packs.
- ➤ Oxygen.
- ➤ Digoxin up to 1 mg i.v. over 2 hours.
- ➤ Diazepam 5 mg tds orally or rectally for sedation.
- ➤ Hydrocortisone 500 mg i.v.
- ➤ Carbimazole 15–20 mg qds orally.
- ➤ Lugol's iodine 0.3 mL tds orally.
- ➤ Propranolol 1–2 mg i.v. – half-hourly until symptoms controlled.
- ➤ Plasmapheresis – severe unresponsive cases.

Malignant goitre

Types:

- Papillary carcinoma
- Follicular carcinoma
- Anaplastic carcinoma
- Malignant lymphoma
- Medullary carcinoma.

Associations:

- Lymphomas – long-standing Hashimoto's thyroiditis
- Medullary carcinoma – multiple endocrine neoplasia (MEN) IIa and IIb.

Clinical features

- Goitre with pain or discomfort.
- Hoarseness – recurrent laryngeal nerve involvement.
- Horner's syndrome – invasion of the cervical sympathetic chain.
- Cervical lymphadenopathy.

Investigation

- ➤ Isotope scan of thyroid – a solitary 'cold' nodule is suggestive.
- ➤ Bone scan – screening for metastases.
- ➤ Chest X-ray – screening for metastases.
- ➤ FNA – cannot distinguish follicular adenoma from carcinoma.

Treatment

Papillary carcinoma:

➤ Total thyroid lobectomy with clearance of pretracheal and paratracheal nodes
➤ Subsequent total thyroidectomy – if histology demonstrates extracapsular disease
➤ Subsequent excision of node metastases that develop later
➤ Thyroxine 100–200 μg daily orally.

Follicular carcinoma:

➤ Total thyroid lobectomy
➤ Subsequent total thyroidectomy – if histology demonstrates invasive carcinoma.

Metastases of papillary or follicular carcinoma:

➤ ^{131}I therapy:
  – Thyroxine is stopped 2 weeks beforehand
  – ^{131}I 2–5 mCi (555 MBq = 15 mCi) is administered and uptake assessed at 24 hours – >1% indicates metastatic disease
  – ^{131}I 150–200 mCi – if metastatic disease was demonstrated
  – Repeat assessment and treatment at 6 months.

Anaplastic (poorly differentiated) carcinoma:

➤ Radiotherapy and chemotherapy (doxorubicin)
➤ Prognosis: death within 6 months.

Medullary carcinoma:

➤ Total thyroidectomy with clearance of paratracheal and upper mediastinal nodes and sampling of carotid sheath nodes
➤ Subsequent radical neck dissection – if nodes are involved on sampling.

Rare goitres and thyroiditis

Definitions

Hashimoto's thyroiditis:

• Autoimmune.

Riedel's thyroiditis:

- Fibrous replacement of the gland
- Associated with retroperitoneal fibrosis.

De Quervain's thyroiditis:

- Postviral.

Clinical features

Hashimoto's thyroiditis:

- Firm goitre
- Postmenopausal females.

Riedel's thyroiditis:

- Firm 'woody' goitre.

De Quervain's thyroiditis:

- 'Flu-like' illness with a tender goitre.

Investigation

➤ Serum TSH/T_3/T_4:
  - Hashimoto's thyroiditis – late hypothyroidism
  - De Quervain's thyroiditis – early hypothyroidism.
➤ Ultrasound – may exclude common nodular goitre.
➤ FNA:
  - Assists differentiation from malignancy
  - Riedel's thyroiditis usually gives acellular specimen.
➤ Thyroid antibodies – antithyroglobulin and antimicrosomal autoantibodies in Hashimoto's thyroiditis.

Treatment

Hashimoto's thyroiditis:

➤ Thyroxine and prednisolone may produce remission
➤ Thyroidectomy – suspicion of malignancy.

De Quervain's thyroiditis:

➤ Three-quarters of cases recover spontaneously.
➤ Thyroxine – if persists.

➤

Riedel's thyroiditis:

➤ Thyroidectomy – suspicion of malignancy and relief of
   tracheal compression.

Solitary thyroid nodule

Definitions

- Pathology:
  - Part of multinodular goitre 50%
  - Adenoma
  - Carcinoma.
- Associated: thyrotoxicosis – 'toxic adenoma'.

Clinical features

- Palpable nodule in the thyroid – moves upwards on
  swallowing.

Investigation

➤ Ultrasound:
  - Solitary nodule vs multinodular goitre
  - Solid vs cyst.
➤ FNA:
  - Resolves vs residual
  - Benign vs malignant.
➤ Serum TSH – euthyroid vs hyperthyroid.
➤ Isotope scanning:
  - 'Hot' nodules – toxic adenoma
  - 'Cold' nodules – carcinoma.
➤ Intra-operative frozen section – determines extent of
  surgery.

Treatment

➤ Observe – benign euthyroid nodule.
➤ Antithyroid drugs – benign toxic nodule.
➤ Thyroid lobectomy – suspicious, residual on aspiration
  and unresponsive toxic nodule.
➤ Radical thyroidectomy – malignant.

Hypothyroidism

Definitions

- Condition resulting from the effects of a lack of circulating thyroxine
- Aetiology:
  - Adult hypothyroidism (myxoedema):
    - Thyroidectomy or radioiodine treatment
    - Hashimoto's thyroiditis
    - Antithyroid drugs.
  - Neonatal cases (cretinism):
    - Agenesis of the thyroid.

Clinical features

Adult hypothyroidism (myxoedema).

- Symptoms:
  - Cold intolerance
  - Lethargy
  - Weight gain
  - Constipation.
- Signs:
  - Obesity
  - Puffiness of the face/eyelids
  - Dry hair and skin
  - Pretibial oedema
  - Alopecia (characteristically lateral one-third of eyebrows)
  - 'Croaky' voice
  - Bradycardia
  - Anaemia
  - Carpal tunnel syndrome
  - Polyneuritis
  - Cerebellar syndrome
  - Myopathy
  - Delayed ankle-jerks
  - Psychiatric disturbances.

Neonatal cases (cretinism):
  - Retardation of physical and mental development
  - Large tongue
  - Distended abdomen
  - Umbilical hernia

- Dry hair and skin
- Delayed growth and bone maturation.

Investigation
➤ Serum TSH – raised.
➤ Serum T_3/T_4 – low.

Treament
➤ Thyroxine 100–150 µg daily orally (elderly commence with one-fifth dose, building up over 2 months to avoid cardiac complications).

THYROGLOSSAL TRACT

Thyroglossal sinus and cyst, and ectopic thyroid

Definitions
Abnormalities of the thyroglossal tract:

- Ectopic thyroid tissue
- Thyroglossal cyst or sinus.

Clinical features
- Swelling or sinus.
- Midline of the neck.
- Moves upwards on protrusion of the tongue.

Investigation
➤ Clinical diagnosis.
➤ Ultrasound, CT or MRI may assist delineation.
➤ Radioisotope scan – ensures that ectopic thyroid is not the only functioning thyroid tissue.

Treatment
➤ Surgical excision of the whole thyroglossal tract, from the base of the tongue to the hyoid bone – the body of which is resected.

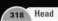

PARATHYROIDS

Hyperparathyroidism

Definitions

Primary hyperparathyroidism:

- Increased parathyroid hormone (PTH) secretion
- Aetiology:
  - Parathyroid adenoma
  - Parathyroid hyperplasia in MEN IIa.

Secondary hyperparathyroidism:

- Compensatory parathyroid hyperplasia in chronic renal failure.

Tertiary hyperparathyroidism:

- Excessive PTH secretion in chronic renal failure after renal transplantation.

Clinical features

Primary hyperparathyroidism:

- Incidental hypercalcaemia
- Renal calculi
- Peptic ulceration (from increased gastrin secretion)
- Pancreatitis
- Radiological bone changes
- Corneal keratopathy
- Psychiatric symptoms – behavioural change, dementia or psychosis.

Secondary hyperparathyroidism:

- Features of chronic renal failure.

Tertiary hyperparathyroidism:

- As primary.

Investigation

➤ Calcium (corrected serum level) – repeated measurements:
  - Primary and tertiary hyperparathyroidism – hypercalcaemia
  - Secondary hyperparathyroidism – hypocalcaemia.

➜

➤ Serum PTH level – three measurements:
  – Primary or tertiary hyperparathyroidism – raised PTH with hypercalcaemia
  – Secondary hyperparathyroidism – raised PTH with reduced serum calcium suggests.
➤ Serum Cl/PO_4 – chloride levels are raised and phosphate levels are reduced in primary hyperparathyroidism.
➤ Urinary Ca – 24-hour urinary calcium excretion is raised in primary hyperparathyroidism.
– Serum alkaline phosphatase (skeletal) – raised in primary hyperparathyroidism.
➤ Urinary adrenaline metabolites – to screen for phaeochromocytoma (MEN IIb).

Treatment

Primary hyperparathyroidism:

➤ Surgical exploration of the neck and frozen section
➤ Adenoma – excision
➤ Hyperplasia all four glands – remove three and a half glands
➤ No cause identified – selective venous catheterization with PTH assay.

Secondary hyperparathyroidism:

➤ Management of chronic renal failure (page 496)
➤ Calcium up to 1.5 g daily orally
➤ Cholecalciferol (1-α-hydroxyvitamin D_3) 50 000 units daily orally.

Tertiary hyperparathyroidism:

➤ Total parathyroidectomy with autotransplantation into an arm muscle – accessible if problems persist.

After surgery:

➤ Calcium up to 1.5 g daily orally
➤ Cholecalciferol (1-α-hydroxyvitamin D_3) 50 000 units daily orally.

Hypoparathyroidism

Definitions

- Complicates 1% of thyroid surgery.
- Aetiology: excision, trauma or ischaemia of the parathyroids.

Clinical features

- Paraesthesiae of the face, fingers or toes.
- Abdominal cramps.
- Chvostek's sign – facial twitching elicited by tapping over the facial nerve.
- Trousseau's sign – carpal spasm on arterial occlusion of the forearm by a sphygmomanometer cuff inflated at 200 mmHg for 5 minutes.

Investigation

➤ Serum Ca and PTH – both serum calcium and PTH levels are low.
➤ Electrocardiograph – prolonged Q-T interval.

Treatment

Acute:

➤ 20 mL of 10% calcium gluconate i.v. 4-hourly until calcium levels rise.

Maintenance:

➤ Calcium up to 1.5 g daily orally.
➤ Calciferol (vitamin D_2) up to 100 000 units daily orally.

BREAST DISEASES

BENIGN CONDITIONS

Developmental anomalies

Definitions

- Non-development of the breast following puberty.

- Breast hypoplasia (Poland's syndrome when associated with malformation of the pectoral muscle).
- Supernumerary breasts and/or nipples.

Clinical features

- Supernumerary nipples and breasts occur along the nipple line, which extends from the axilla to the pubis.
- Become active during lactation.

Treatment

➤ Accessory breasts may be removed.
➤ Non-development or hypoplasia requires reconstruction with prosthetic implants and/or myocutaneous flaps.

Breast hypertrophy

Definitions

- Benign condition of uncertain causation.
- Unilateral or bilateral, affecting the young woman or the adolescent (virginal hypertrophy).

Clinical features

Breasts are large and pendulous, with dragging discomfort/pain and difficulty with breast support.

Treatment

➤ Reduction mammoplasty.

Gynaecomastia

Definitions

- Enlargement of the breast disc in the male.
- Found in adolescence, when it is usually idiopathic and transient.
- In chronic liver disease.
- Associated with:
  - Oestrogenic activity
  - Drug-induced (H_2 receptor antagonists, digoxin, spironolactone, antipsychotic drugs)
  - Testicular tumours.

Clinical features

- Breast pain.
- Enlargement of the breast disc.
- Psychosocial affectation with body image.

Investigation

- Ultrasound scan.
- Fine-needle cytology.
- Endocrine testing is rarely needed.

Treatment

➤ Resolves following pubertal development or on resolution of liver disease.
➤ Subcutaneous mastectomy, where the condition persists, is cosmetically unacceptable or painful.

Benign breast change

(Fibroadenosis; fibrocystic change, aberrations of normal development and involution.)

Definitions

- Affects 1 in 3 women.
- Associated with abnormal sensitivity to oestrogen and progesterone.
- Characterized by adenosis, fibrosis and/or cyst formation.
- Confined to one or more segments of one or both breasts.
- May be associated with epithelial hyperplasia.

Clinical features

- Non-cyclical breast discomfort/pain with/without swelling or nodularity.
- Nodularity/cysts may be palpable and tender.

Investigation

➤ Ultrasound scan for a palpable lesion in patients <35 years of age.
➤ Mammography in patients >40 years of age.

➔

> Pneumocystogram of recurring cysts post aspiration.
> Core needle or excision biopsy of residual palpable lesion post aspiration.

Treatment

> Reassurance and symptomatic measures.
> Stop hormonal contraception or replacement therapy.
> Evening primrose oil caps 40–160 mg twice or thrice daily for 3 months.
> Starflower oil or danazol capsules 100–300 mg daily for 3–6 months for severe symptoms.
> Aspirate cysts that are >2 cm in size or if symptomatic.

Breast involution

Definitions

Changes are caused by:

- Menopause
- Lobular involution (apocrine change, adenosis, fibrosis and microcyst formation)
- Ductal involution (periductal round cell infiltration leading to periductal mastitis and epithelial hyperplasia).

Clinical features

- Breast nodularity.

Investigation

> Significant imaging abnormalities are rare.
> Image-guided core needle or excision biopsy may be required for histological reassurance.

Treatment

> Reassurance.

Fibroadenoma

Definitions

- A focal area of lobular stromal hyperplasia with epithelial proliferation.

- Associated with abnormal oestrogen/progesterone levels.
- May be multiple or become large (giant fibroadenoma).

Clinical features

- Discrete, firm, mobile lump ('breast mouse').

Investigation
➤ Ultrasound scan.
➤ Fine-needle cytology/core needle biopsy.

Treatment
➤ <35 years of age: reassurance; stop hormonal contraception; usually resolve.
➤ >35 years of age: excision biopsy.

Phillodes tumour

- Histologically more cellular than fibroadenoma, with nuclear pleomorphism and mitoses.
- Tends to recur following excision.
- Slight potential for malignant change (sarcoma).

Treatment
➤ Wide local excision.

Mondor's disease (superficial thrombophlebitis)

- May occur spontaneously or following surgery.
- The thrombosed vein is usually visible and felt as a cord-like thickening beneath the skin.
- Self-resolving.

Duct papilloma

Definitions

- Arise as epithelial-covered fibrovascular cores in lactiferous ducts.

Clinical features

- Bloody nipple discharge from a single duct.
- Palpable lump beneath the areola.

Investigation

➤ Ultrasound scan may identify a small intra-duct lesion.

Treatment

➤ Microdochectomy or major (total) duct excision.

Periductal mastitis (duct ectasia)

Definitions

- Dilated ducts containing inspissated secretions.
- Found in older women.
- Associated with cigarette smoking.

Clinical features

- Nipple discharge associated with underlying palpable nodularity.

Treatment

➤ Total duct excision.

Granulomatous lobular mastitis

- Presents as a tender lump as a result of a chronic inflammatory reaction.
- Needle biopsy is diagnostic.
- Difficult to treat as it is associated with poor healing following excision, with a tendency to recur.

Eczematous conditions

Definitions

- May be associated with a generalized rash.
- Involves the areola and the surrounding skin (rarely the nipple).

Clinical features

- An itchy, red rash, which may be scaly with no skin erosion.

Treatment

➤ 1% hydrocortisone topical cream for 4 weeks.
➤ Poor response suggests Paget's disease requiring biopsy.

Fat necrosis

Definitions

- Usually results from blunt trauma.
- Leads to an organizing haematoma or fat necrosis.

Clinical features

- May present as a firm mass.

Investigation

➤ Clinical examination, breast imaging and fine-needle cytology (triple assessment) and core-needle biopsy if indicated.

Treatment

➤ Reassurance.

Acute/chronic inflammation

Abscess formation

Definitions

- Associated with cracked nipple during lactation (infection from oral pathogens from infant, *Staphylococcus aureus*).
- Non-lactational breast abscesses found in smokers (associated with periductal mastitis) and tend to recur.
- In postmenopausal women, inflammatory carcinoma must be excluded.

Clinical features

- Pain, peri-areolar redness, warmth and swelling.
- May be fluctuant.
- Axillary adenitis.

Investigation

➤ Ultrasound scan or mammography (in chronic abscess).
➤ Fine-needle/core-needle biopsy (when in doubt as to causation).

Treatment

➤ Early inflammatory stage resolves on broad-spectrum antibiotic therapy.
➤ Aspirate pus with wide-bore needle under broad-spectrum antibiotic cover.
➤ Repeated aspirations may be required for resolution.
➤ Incisional drainage is reserved for recurrent or complicated abscesses.
➤ Spontaneous discharge of pus if untreated, resulting in a mammary fistula.

Sclerosing adenosis

- Proliferative lesion of the breast lobule.
- Architectural distortion on mammography.
- Benign on image-guided core-needle biopsy.

Radial scars (complex sclerosing lesions)

- Secretory ductules radiating from an area of collagenous (hyalinized) fibrous tissue.
- Architectural distortion on mammography.
- Benign; may require image-guided core-needle biopsy confirmation.

Mammary fistula

Definitions

- An abnormal communication between lactiferous ducts and the exterior.

- An infrequent complication of acute periductal mastitis and abscess drainage.

Clinical features

- Found usually at the areolar margin or at the lateral edge of a drainage scar.

Investigation

➤ Fistulogram defines the tract and the site of communication with the breast duct(s).

Treatment

➤ Fistulectomy with major duct excision (as surrounding ducts are usually affected by periductal mastitis).

Tuberculosis

Definitions

- From haematogenous spread or extension from an infective focus in the pleural cavity.

Clinical features

- Presents as a cold abscess, sinus, ulcer or a contracted breast.

Investigation

➤ Mammography shows extensive inflammatory reaction of the breast.

Treatment

➤ Surgical exploration of the sinus and abscess drainage.
➤ Systemic antituberculous therapy.
➤ Mastectomy for extensive breast involvement.

Breast screening and assessment

Definitions

- Mammographic screening of the female population aged 51–70 years performed at 3-yearly intervals.

- Women with screen-detected abnormalities are recalled for further assessment.
- Abnormal results are discussed at the MDT meeting to establish diagnosis and advice on management.

BREAST CANCER

In-situ carcinoma

Definitions

- Malignant proliferation of cells confined to within the basement membrane, as in the duct lumen in ductal carcinoma in situ (DCIS) or lobular units in lobular carcinoma in situ (LCIS).

Clinical features

- Usually asymptomatic.

Investigation
➤ Detected on mammography.
➤ Stereotactic core-needle biopsy.

Treatment
➤ DCIS is premalignant, requiring wide local excision and tamoxifen therapy.
➤ LCIS is regarded as a risk factor rather than a premalignant condition for lobular carcinoma, requiring surveillance.

Primary breast carcinoma

Definitions

- A systemic disease that originates in the breast.
- Divided into cancers of no special type (>80% of cancers) and others.
- 'No special type' tumours are invasive ductal and lobular carcinoma.

- Paget's disease of the nipple is a subepidermoid carcinoma arising in the nipple areolar complex that invades the breast.

Clinical features

- 80% of symptomatic lesions present as a palpable lump, with nipple retraction or bloodstained discharge.
- An axillary mass or Paget's disease are less common presentations.

Investigation

➤ Diagnosed at first clinic visit by triple assessment (palpation, breast imaging and fine-needle cytology).
➤ Core-needle biopsy (image-guided) is required in equivocal findings.
➤ Non-palpable and asymptomatic lesions are detected during population screening.

Clinical staging [tumour (size), (lymph) node (involvement), metastasis (TNM classification)]

Clinical stage	T	Tumour size (cm)	N	Axillary nodes	M	Distant spread
1 Early disease: confined to breast	T_1	<2	N_0	Non-palpable	M_0	No metastases
2 Early disease: with axillary nodal spread	T_2	2–5	N_1	Mobile nodes	M_0	
3a Locally advanced disease	T_3	>5	N_2	Fixed nodes	M_0	
3b Chest wall and other nodal spread	T_4	Skin/chest wall involvement	N_3	Ipsilateral internal mammary nodes	M_0/M_1	
4 Advanced disease: extension beyond breast/chest wall					M_0/M_1	

Treatment

Surgery is aimed at local control when removal of the tumour would effect a cure or improve prognosis:

➤ Wide (complete) local excision removes small (<5 cm) tumours followed by radiotherapy to the conserved breast

➤ Simple mastectomy is for large (>5 cm) tumours, or those involving the chest wall or with skin involvement exceeding the size of the tumour

➤ Axillary surgery, in the form of a node sampling (four or more nodes required to stage the disease) or a clearance (removing all nodes from behind the pectoralis minor muscle and below the level of the axillary vein), is performed to remove metastatic axillary disease.

Surgery for breast malignancy

Operation	Indications	Advantages	Disadvantages
Wire-guided excision biopsy	Screen-detected lesions	Complete excision of small cancers through a small incision	Dislodgement of the wire may render biopsy difficult
Wide local excision	Tumours <5 cm, away from NAC DCIS	Breast conserved; Good cosmesis when <11% of tissue removed	Postoperative breast radiotherapy is usually indicated Poor cosmesis unless the defect is filled by tissue transposition
Simple mastectomy	Tumours >5 cm, tumours involving the NAC, the chest wall or skin involvement exceeding the size of the tumour	Local recurrence unusual	External prosthesis or breast reconstruction required
Subcutaneous or skin-sparing mastectomy	Premalignant conditions, widespread DCIS, LCIS and small central tumours	Cosmetically pleasing reconstruction	Requires close surveillance

(Continued)

(Continued)

Operation	Indications	Advantages	Disadvantages
Sentinel node biopsy	For nodal status	Minimal surgery with reduced morbidity; detailed histology	Errors in nodal localization
Axillary node sampling	All infiltrating tumours; High-grade DCIS	Four node sampling correlates well with clearance in disease staging	Requires axillary radiotherapy or surgical clearance if nodes are involved
Axillary clearance performed during primary surgery or as a delayed procedure	Early infiltrating tumours of any histological type Not for in-situ disease	Avoids axillary radiotherapy; Controls axillary disease	Upper limb swelling, paraesthesiae, reduced shoulder movement and strength; predisposes to limb sepsis

Complications

Wound	Nerve injuries	Shoulder and arm
Bruising	Intercostobrachial nerve	Stiffness
Haematoma	Long thoracic nerve of Bell	Weakness
Infection		Swelling
Dehiscence	Nerve to lattissimus dorsi	Paraesthesiae

Prognosis of breast cancer following primary surgical treatment is dependent on tumour size, type and grade, the extent of axillary disease, evidence of vascular invasion, hormonal (oestrogen and progesterone) receptor status and the presence of oncogene *Her-2*.

The Nottingham Prognostic Index (NPI), based on the first three criteria, is expressed as:

$$NPI = 0.2 \times (\text{tumour size (cm)}) + \text{grade } (1–3)^\star + \text{nodal score } (1–3)^\#:$$

Good <3.4	>85%	10-year survival
Moderate = 3.41–5.40	50–70%	10-year survival
Poor >5.4	20%	10-year survival

*Tumour grades are: 1, low; 2, intermediate; and 3, high.
#Nodal scores are: 1, none; 2, one to three; 3, more than three nodes with tumour.

Adjuvant treatment

Reserved for advanced disease: tumour >2 cm; grade II or III; lymphovascular invasion, lymph nodal involvement; NPI >3.4.

Neo-adjuvant chemo-endocrine or radiotherapy is used to downstage locally advanced disease prior to surgery.

Radiotherapy

Indications

- To conserved breast – reduces incidence of local recurrence.
- To chest wall – palliates chest wall/internal mammary nodal involvement.
- To axilla – eradicates/palliates nodal disease (alternative to surgery).
- To supraclavicular fossa – palliates nodal disease.

Side-effects

- Skin reaction; tiredness; lethargy.
- Axillary irradiation: lymphoedema of arm and shoulder weakness.
- Cardiac and lung damage.

Endocrine therapy

- More effective in oestrogen- and/or progesterone-sensitive tumours.
- Consists of anti-hormone therapy or gonadal ablation.
- Usually given in combination with other treatment modalities.
- Prevents/delays distant metastases.
- Prolongs survival.
- Drugs used: tamoxifen 20 mg, anastrozole 1 mg or letrozole 2.5 mg daily.

Side-effects

- Hot flushes.
- Gastrointestinal symptoms.

- Vaginal dryness.
- (Tamoxifen: visual changes, uterine tumours).

Chemotherapy

Objectives:

- Extend disease-free interval
- Prolong survival
- Protect contralateral breast
- Neo-adjuvant therapy to downstage locally advanced tumours
- Prophylaxis in premenopausal women with good prognosis tumours.

Cytotoxic agents are used in the following combinations:

- Cyclophosphamide, methotrexate, 5-fluorouracil 4 to 5 5-weekly cycles
- Epirubicin, cyclophosphamide, 5-fluorouracil 5 to 6 5-weekly cycles
- Docetaxel either alone or in combination with an anthracycline (doxo-rubicin/epirubicin).

Side-effects:

- Hair loss
- Gastrointestinal symptoms (nausea, vomiting, diarrhoea)
- Malaise
- Blood dyscrasias (agranulocytosis, aplastic anaemia)
- Susceptibility to infections.

Surveillance (following treatment)

Follow-up is influenced by clinical need; for example, following treatment of a 2 cm lesion, visits are:

year 1	3 monthly
year 2	6 monthly
years 3–5	9–12 monthly with chest X-ray, full blood count, serum Ca^{2+} and liver function tests (LFTs)

Surveillance mammography is undertaken:

- Annually of the conserved breast
- Biennially of the contralateral breast after mastectomy.

Surveillance may cease after 5 years in the absence of recurrence or adverse features. Patients may then enrol in or return to breast screening.

Recurrence

Tumour recurrence requires re-staging of the disease with:

- Chest X-ray
- Liver ultrasound scan
- Radioisotope bone scan
- Liver function tests.

Local recurrence is effectively treated by local measures:

- Surgery
- Radiotherapy.

Systemic recurrence is incurable but may be effectively palliated:

- Change endocrine therapy
- Revise chemotherapy to include an anthracycline and a taxane (docetaxel/pacetaxel)
- Gene-specific targeted therapy: HER2 (neu or c-erb B2) positive tumours respond to trastuzumab (herceptin).

Advanced carcinoma

Definitions

- Stage III (locally advanced).
- Stage IV (metastatic disease).

Clinical features

Usually symptomatic and may present with:

- Skin nodules
- Skin oedema (peau d'orange)
- Skin ulceration
- Large (>4 cm) primary
- Distant metastases.

Treatment

Aims are palliative, to control disease symptoms, improve the quality of and to prolong life:

➤ Limited surgery, radiotherapy, chemotherapy or gene-targeted therapy may be used.

Adjuvant therapy for site-specific complications:

➤ Chest wall/skin involvement: radiotherapy ± surgical excision ± reconstruction
➤ Liver/bone involvement: anthracycline therapy with doxetaxol or trastuzumab
➤ Bone pain: radiotherapy with oral sodium clodronate 1.6–3.2 g daily
➤ Brain metastases: surgery if localized.

Endocrine agents, anastrozole or letrozole may be included for hormone-sensitive tumours.

AXILLA

Axillary abscess

Definitions

● Infection of hair follicles or sweat glands caused by shaving and possibly poor hygiene.

Clinical features

● Painful, tender axillary swelling with minimal constitutional symptoms.
● Swelling may be fluctuant or indurated.

Treatment

➤ Wide-bore needle aspiration under broad-spectrum antibiotic cover (repeated aspirations may be required).
➤ Incision and drainage is traditional and effective.
➤ Excision of the abscess under antibiotic cover is reserved for recurrent or complicated abscesses.

THORAX

PULMONARY DISEASE AND THORACIC TRAUMA

Pulmonary infection

Lung abscess

Definitions

- Localized area of suppuration and cavitation in the lung.
- Most commonly resulting from aspiration – dysphagia, impaired consciousness (alcohol, fits, stroke, head injury).
- Poor oral hygiene.
- Infectious material gravitates to dependent segments of lung.
- Other causes include pulmonary infarction, trauma, bronchial obstruction, necrotizing pneumonia.
- Opportunistic infection in immunocompromised patients associated with *Staphylococcus aureus*, *Pseudomonas* spp., *Proteus* spp., *Escherichia coli* and *Klebsiella* spp.

Clinical features

- Periodic symptoms reflect intermittent discharge of abscess by erosion into an adjacent bronchiole.
- Typical history of upper respiratory tract infection with fever, tachycardia, chest pain.
- Followed by haemoptysis and purulent sputum when bronchocavitary fistula is formed.
- If abscess contents are completely evacuated, the lung can expand and the cavity is obliterated.
- Failure of the cavity to discharge completely results in chronic abscess.

Investigation

➤ Chest X-ray:
  – early abscess appears as area of consolidation

➡

– cavitation with air–fluid level appears 10–14 days after onset of cough, fever and chest pain.
➤ Computerized tomography (CT) scan.
➤ Bronchoscopy – obtain material for culture, exclude foreign body or neoplasm, identify involved bronchial segment.

Treatment
➤ Identify infectious organism.
➤ Prolonged antibiotics (6–8 weeks).
➤ Physiotherapy and postural drainage.
➤ Bronchoscopy (suction drainage).
➤ Percutaneous drainage reserved for extremely ill patients who cannot withstand any other procedure.
➤ Surgical treatment: definitive resection of involved lung parenchyma by lobectomy or segmentectomy. Indicated for:
  – Unsuccessful medical therapy
  – Suspicion of carcinoma
  – Significant haemoptysis
  – Empyema
  – Bronchopleural fistula.

Complications
● Majority of patients respond to medical treatment; 10–15% require surgery.
● Before antibiotics, mortality 30%.
● Currently mortality 5%; higher in patients with opportunistic infection.
● Operative mortality up to 10%.

Bronchiectasis

Definitions
● Suppurative disease of lung characterized by dilatation of the bronchi.
● Congenital factors (uncommon):
  – Congenital cystic bronchiectasis
  – Immunoglobulin A deficiency
  – Hypogammaglobulinaemia

- – Alpha-1 antitrypsin deficiency
  - – Cystic fibrosis
  - – Kartagener's syndrome.
- Acquired factors (more common):
  - – Infection (most common cause)
  - – Bronchial obstruction – tumour, foreign body, mucous plug, extrinsic compression by enlarged lymph node
  - – Middle-lobe syndrome (secondary bronchial obstruction as a result of fibrosis following infection with histioplasmosis)
  - – Tuberculosis (TB)
  - – Acquired hypogammaglobulinaemia.
- Pathology – three types:
  - – Cylindrical: dilated bronchi of regular outline
  - – Varicose: greater dilatation and irregularity
  - – Saccular or cystic: dilatation increases towards the periphery.
- Typically affects distal bronchi which have less cartilage.
- Most commonly within basal segments of lower lobe.
- Bilateral in 30%.

Clinical features

- Recurrent chest infection with copious foul-smelling sputum.
- Haemoptysis is common in adults.
- Signs include dullness to percussion over the affected segment and coarse crackles.

Investigation

➤ Chest X-ray non-specific.
➤ CT scan (high-resolution) diagnostic – features include lack of bronchial tapering, bronchial dilatation and wall thickening, bronchi visualized in lung periphery.
➤ Bronchoscopy – identify affected segments, foreign bodies, neoplasm, obtain material for culture.

Treatment

➤ Prevent and control infection.
➤ Coughing, chest physiotherapy and postural drainage.

➜

➤ Bronchoscopy to clear secretions.
➤ Surgery indicated if failed medical therapy with localized disease: resection of affected lung parenchyma by lobectomy or segmentectomy.

Complications

● Surgical mortality <1%.

Carcinoma of the bronchus

Definitions

● Commonest malignancy in UK.
● Incidence 40 000 new cases per year in UK; 30 000 deaths per year; <10% suitable for curative surgery.
● Commoner in men but incidence falling in men and increasing in women, reflecting changes in smoking habits.
● Aetiology:
   – Primary risk factor is smoking (85–90% of lung cancers are smoking related)
   – Occupational risk with asbestos exposure (5%).
● Cell types:
   – Non-small-cell lung cancer (NSCLC) – commonest (75–80%); see below
   – Small-cell lung cancer (SCLC) – (up to 25%)
   – Carcinoid – uncommon (2–5%), low-grade tumours.
● **NSCLC:**
   – **Adenocarcinoma** – incidence increasing, more common in women, usually peripheral and metastasize early, associated with skip metastasis to mediastinal lymph nodes; subtype is **bronchoalveolar carcinoma**, which is often multicentric
   – **Squamous cell carcinoma** – incidence falling, more often arise centrally, and spread within thorax
   – **Large-cell carcinoma** – histological diagnosis of exclusion.
● **SCLC:**
   – Rapid growth
   – Majority have metastases at time of diagnosis

- Greater responsiveness to chemotherapy and radiotherapy.

- **Staging:**
  - International Tumour, Nodes, Metastases (TNM) Staging System, 1997 (see table)
  - Tumour (T) staging reflects tumour size, airway location and local invasion
  - Node (N) staging describes intrathoracic and supraclavicular lymph node spread
  - Metastasis (M) staging reflects presence or absence of distant spread
  - Stage I and II disease is resectable; stage IIIA disease may be resectable; stages IIIB and IV disease are not resectable.

International TNM Staging System for Lung Cancer (1997)

Stage	TNM classification
IA	**T1 N0 M0**
	(T1 = tumour ≤3 cm size, peripheral, no local invasion)
IB	**T2 N0 M0**
	(T2 = tumour ≥3 cm size, ≥2 cm from carina or invading visceral pleura)
IIA	**T1 N1 M0**
	(N1 = metastasis to ipsilateral intrapulmonary, peribronchial or hilar nodes)
IIB	**T2 N1 M0 or T3 N0 M0**
	(T3 = tumour of any size in main bronchus ≤2 cm from carina or invading chest wall, diaphragm, mediastinal pleura or parietal pericardium)
IIIA	**T3 N1 M0 or T1–3 N2 M0**
	(N2 = metastasis to ipsilateral mediastinal or subcarinal nodes)
IIIB	**T4 N0–2 M0 or T1–4 N3 M0**
	(T4 = satellite nodules within same lobe of lung as primary; invasion of trachea, carina, mediastinum, vertebrae; malignant pleural or pericardial effusion) (N3 = metastasis to contralateral mediastinal or hilar nodes or to supraclavicular or scalene nodes)
IV	**T1–4 N0–2 M1**
	(M1 = distant metastasis; tumour nodules in non-primary lobes of lung)

Clinical features

- Cough most common symptom ± haemoptysis, breathlessness.

- May present as slowly resolving chest infection or as asymptomatic finding on chest X-ray.
- Poor prognostic symptoms include pain, hoarse voice, anorexia and weight loss; these imply advanced disease.
- Pleural effusion may be the result of malignant pleural involvement.
- Paraneoplastic syndromes: Cushing's, syndrome of inappropriate ADH secretion, parathyroid-like hormone secretion, hypertrophic pulmonary osteoarthropathy.

Investigation

➤ Objectives of investigations: diagnosis, staging, assessment of suitability of tumour for resection and of fitness for surgery.
➤ Chest X-ray.
➤ Diagnostic investigations:
  – Tissue diagnosis required to plan treatment
  – Sputum cytology may be helpful but is not diagnostic
  – Bronchoscopy – establish diagnosis and assess suitability for resection
  – CT-guided fine-needle aspiration and biopsy
  – Surgical biopsy.
➤ Staging investigations:
  – CT scan: chest (lung and mediastinal windows) and abdomen (including liver and adrenal glands)
  – Positron emission tomography (PET) scan based on increased glucose uptake in tumour cells; useful to distinguish benign from malignant lung nodules and to demonstrate tumour spread
  – Surgical staging: mediastinoscopy, anterior mediastinotomy, thoracoscopy (for biopsy of mediastinal lymph nodes, also assessment of pleural disease with thoracoscopy)
  – Assessment of distant spread: bone scan, CT brain (not routinely performed).
➤ Respiratory function tests assess fitness for surgery:
  – **Spirometry** is most important and easily performed: forced expiratory volume in 1 second (FEV_1) >1.5 L is adequate for lobectomy; FEV_1 >2 L is adequate for pneumonectomy

→

- **Gas transfer factor** readily available but more time-consuming to test than spirometry alone; important in patients where spirometry is inadequate, breathlessness greater than expected from spirometry, or in those with interstitial lung disease
- **Oxygen saturations:** $SpO_2 > 90\%$ at rest, on room air is sufficient
- **Exercise testing** is indicated with borderline respiratory function (shuttle walk test consisting of 25 shuttles of 10 m each is most reproducible)
- **Quantitative isotope perfusion scan** may be useful in assessing suitability for pneumonectomy with borderline respiratory function.
➤ Assessment of cardiovascular fitness:
- 12-lead electrocardiograph (ECG) mandatory
- Echocardiogram if any cardiac murmur audible
- Previous myocardial infarction (within 6 months) or uncontrolled heart failure or arrhythmia require formal cardiology assessment if surgery is planned
- Surgery should not be performed within 6 weeks of a myocardial infarct.

Treatment

➤ **Surgery** with curative intent:
- **Anatomical** resection (lobectomy, bilobectomy or pneumonectomy) preferred
- **Sublobar** resection (wedge or bronchopulmonary segment) suitable for peripheral lesions, reserved for elderly patients or those with borderline lung function
- **Bronchoplastic** resection ('sleeve resection') for selected cases where endobronchial tumour or upper lobe tumour can be resected with preservation of uninvolved lung by reconstruction of the bronchus.
➤ **Radiotherapy:**
- Radical or palliative
- For patients unfit for surgery or with stage III disease

➜

- – Treatment may be limited by poor respiratory reserve, therefore dose and toxicity must be considered when planning treatment
- – Contraindications to radical radiotherapy: poor cardiopulmonary reserve, malignant effusion, active chest infection, stage IV disease.

➤ **Chemotherapy:**
  - – Multidrug regimens used, usually cisplatin based
  - – May be neoadjuvant (administered before surgical resection), adjuvant (administered after surgical resection) or palliative
  - – Neoadjuvant chemotherapy confined to clinical trials at present
  - – Adjuvant chemotherapy limited by poor patient tolerance following thoracotomy; no clear proven benefit as yet.

➤ **Palliative care:**
  - – Treat symptoms
  - – Radiotherapy good for symptomatic relief of cough, chest pain, breathlessness, superior vena caval obstruction
  - – Palliative chemotherapy of most benefit when good performance status, minimal weight loss, low tumour bulk.

Complications

- Mean survival of untreated lung cancer is 6 months.
- Operative mortality: lobectomy up to 4%; pneumonectomy up to 8%.
- Complications of thoracotomy and lung resection include: atelectasis, sputum retention and lobar collapse, air leak, bronchopleural fistula, pneumonia, empyema, myocardial infarction, atrial fibrillation, pulmonary embolism (PE), chronic post-thoracotomy pain, prolonged respiratory insufficiency.
- 5-year survival after lung resection reflects stage of disease: stage I 70%, stage II 50%, stage IIIA 30%.
- Failure after surgical resection is caused by local recurrence in 20%, distant metastasis in 80%.

- Sublobar resection (wedge resection or segmentectomy) is associated with higher local recurrence rate and shorter long-term survival than lobectomy.
- Radical radiotherapy achieves up to 15–20% 5-year survival in stage I–II disease, and 3–10% 5-year survival in stage III disease.

Pulmonary embolism (page 76)

Definitions

- Emboli usually arise from thrombosis in large systemic veins (iliac and femoral).
- Virchow's triad for pathogenesis of venous thrombi:
  - Stasis of blood
  - Injury to vessel intima
  - Hypercoagulability.
- Risk factors: surgery, trauma, heart failure, stroke, systemic infection, carcinomatosis, pregnancy, clotting disorder (thrombophilia).
- Effects result from mechanical occlusion, therefore symptoms and signs reflect size of embolus.
- Obstruction of a large pulmonary artery raises pulmonary artery pressure, resulting in acute right heart pressure loading and reduced left heart filling. As right ventricle fails and dilates, the interventricular septum is displaced, thus further impairing left heart filling.
- Reflex responses include bronchoconstriction and pulmonary vasoconstriction.

Clinical features

- Symptoms are not specific to PE: breathlessness, pleuritic chest pain, haemoptysis.
- Classic signs are uncommon: cyanosis, tachypnoea, tachycardia, loud second heart sound, gallop rhythm, pleural rub.
- Often tachycardia is the only obvious clinical sign.
- Massive PE presents with shock/pulseless electrical activity.
- Total obstruction of main pulmonary artery causes sudden death.
- There may be evidence of venous thrombosis (page 583).

Investigation

➤ **Chest X-ray** is often normal in early stage; some days later may reveal linear atelectasis, raised hemidiaphragm, prominent pulmonary artery, pleural effusion.
➤ **ECG** is often non-specific. Characteristic changes are: sinus tachycardia, right axis deviation (dominant S-wave in lead V_1) with a Q-wave and inverted T-wave in V_3 (the $S_1Q_3T_3$ pattern), right ventricular strain (inverted T-waves in leads V_{1-4}), right bundle branch block. It may also reveal supraventricular arrhythmia.
➤ **Pulse oximeter** may show oxygen desaturation.
➤ **Arterial blood gas** may reveal hypoxaemia and hypocarbia (with large PE).
➤ **Ventilation–perfusion scan** is a useful non-invasive test to demonstrate mismatch of ventilation and perfusion.
➤ **Spiral CT pulmonary angiogram** is definitive for diagnosis.

Treatment

➤ **Prophylaxis**, e.g. low-molecular weight heparin and compression stockings for hospital in-patients.
➤ **Resuscitation**, including volume replacement to increase venous return.
➤ **Anticoagulation** with heparin and warfarin. Duration of long-term anticoagulation is controversial; guidelines suggest 3 months for first episode of thromboembolism, 1 year for recurrence, indefinite if history of three or more events, or of proven thrombophilia.
➤ **Thrombolysis** accelerates resolution of haemodynamic disturbance; reserved for critically ill patients.
➤ **Pulmonary embolectomy** is reserved for selected patients where significant haemodynamic compromise precludes delay for thrombolysis, or where thrombolysis is ineffective or contraindicated. High-risk procedure but may be life-saving.
➤ **Caval filter** is indicated for patients with recurrent PE despite anticoagulation.

Complications

- 10% of PE fatal in first hour.
- Mortality for treated PE is 8%.
- Operative mortality for pulmonary embolectomy is 50%.

Pleural disease

Pneumothorax

Definitions

- Air within pleural space, between visceral and parietal pleura.
- **Primary spontaneous:** associated with young adults of aesthenic build, unknown aetiology, no underlying lung disease, histology reveals subpleural bullae in upper lobes.
- **Secondary spontaneous:** tends to occur in older patients; associated with underlying disease, e.g. chronic obstructive pulmonary disease, interstitial lung disease, infection, neoplasm, Marfan's.
- **Secondary** pneumothorax: traumatic, iatrogenic.
- Pressure gradient between intrabronchial pressure (-1 to -3 mmHg in inspiration, $+1$ to $+5$ mmHg in expiration) and intrapleural pressure (-8 to -9 mmHg in inspiration, -3 to -6 mmHg in expiration) holds visceral pleura against parietal pleura.
- Pneumothorax occurs as a result of disruption of either pleural surface, resulting in loss of negative intrapleural pressure and collapse of the lung.
- If pleural disruption seals **(closed pneumothorax)**, pneumothorax is stable.
- If pleural disruption remains open **(open pneumothorax)**, pressures equalize between communicating spaces, resulting in loss of intrathoracic pressure and ineffective respiratory effort.
- **Tension pneumothorax** occurs when pleural disruption opens in inspiration but not in expiration (valve effect); increasing positive intrapleural pressure results in mediastinal shift, thus interfering

with venous return to the heart and decreasing cardiac output.
- Recurrent spontaneous pneumothorax associated with smoking (in patients who have not had treatment to prevent recurrence – see below).

Clinical features

- Consequences depend on the size of pneumothorax, presence of tension and condition of the underlying lung.
- May be asymptomatic; pain is the most frequent complaint; breathlessness.
- Small pneumothorax may not show any abnormal signs.
- Classic signs are reduced chest wall excursion on affected side, hyperresonance to percussion, reduced/absent tactile vocal fremitus, reduced/absent breath sounds.
- **Tension pneumothorax:** severe breathlessness and cardiovascular collapse/pulseless electrical activity; pallor/cyanosis, distended neck veins/raised jugular venous pressure (JVP), mediastinal deviation away from affected side (trachea and apex beat deviated), weak pulse, tachycardia, hypotension, hyperresonance, absent breath sounds unilaterally.

Investigation

➤ Chest X-ray demonstrates air in pleural space; should never be performed before treatment of suspected tension pneumothorax.
➤ 'Small' = visible rim <2 cm between lung margin and chest wall.
➤ 'Large' = visible rim >2 cm between lung margin and chest wall.
➤ CT scan if:
  – Secondary spontaneous pneumothorax (to define cause and assess state of other lung)
  – Pneumothorax obscured by surgical emphysema
  – Suspicion of aberrant chest tube position
  – To differentiate from complex bullous lung disease.

Treatment

➤ Tension pneumothorax requires immediate decompression with large-bore cannula of adequate length inserted into the second intercostal space in midclavicular line; followed by definitive intercostal tube drainage.

➤ Observation only: small closed primary pneumothorax, if not breathless.

➤ Aspiration: small closed primary pneumothorax if breathless, large closed primary pneumothorax, small closed secondary pneumothorax if not breathless.

➤ Aspiration can be repeated once in primary pneumothorax if patient still symptomatic.

➤ Intercostal tube drainage: failed aspiration, secondary pneumothorax, open pneumothorax, tension pneumothorax.

➤ Persistent air leak or failure of the lung to re-expand should be referred for specialist opinion (respiratory physician/thoracic surgeon).

➤ Indications for pleurodesis:
  – Persistent air leak (>5 days)
  – Persistent pneumothorax despite chest drain
  – Recurrent spontaneous pneumothorax (second episode)
  – Previous contralateral pneumothorax
  – Bilateral spontaneous pneumothorax.

➤ Chemical pleurodesis: reserved for patients unwilling or unfit for surgery, usually elderly patients with secondary spontaneous pneumothorax; talc most effective; alternatives are tetracycline and bleomycin.

➤ Surgical pleurodesis: open thoracotomy and pleurectomy has lowest recurrence rate; thoracoscopy [video-assisted thoracoscopic surgery (VATS)] with pleural abrasion or with talc pleurodesis also effective.

➤ Talc pleurodesis is to be avoided in young patients as it makes thoracotomy in later life very problematic.

➤ With surgery, resection of macroscopic bleb or apex of upper lobe is associated with lower recurrence rate in primary spontaneous pneumothorax (because of underlying subpleural bullous disease).

Complications

- First-time primary spontaneous pneumothorax is associated with 10% recurrence rate; after one recurrence, 50% recur again.
- Thoracoscopy is safe, low-risk surgery, and preferable to thoracotomy as first-line surgery for pneumothorax. Advantages include less postoperative pain and more rapid recovery and rehabilitation.
- Recurrence rates after surgery: open pleurectomy <1%, VATS pleural abrasion 2%, VATS talc pleurodesis 5%.

Pleural effusion

Definitions

- Accumulation of fluid in the pleural space.
- Pleural physiology:
  - Pleural space contains 2–3 mL of fluid with protein content of 1.5 g/100 mL
  - Hydrostatic pressure in parietal pleura = systemic capillary pressure (30 cmH$_2$O) + negative pleural pressure (5 cmH$_2$O); opposing pressure = colloid osmotic pressure of blood (34 cmH$_2$O) – colloid osmotic pressure of pleural fluid (8 cmH$_2$O); therefore net pressure gradient of 9 cmH$_2$O across parietal pleura moves fluid from parietal pleura into pleural space.
- Pleural fluid accumulates when:
  - Hydrostatic pressure rises, e.g. congestive heart failure
  - Capillary permeability increases, e.g. pleuritis, pneumonia
  - Colloid osmotic pressure falls, e.g. hypoalbuminaemia
  - Intrapleural pressure falls (becomes more negative), e.g. lobar collapse, atelectasis
  - Lymphatic drainage impaired, e.g. malignancy, irradiation.
- Classified as transudate (accumulation as a result of changes in hydrostatic and osmotic pressures) or exudate (accumulation as a result of changes in capillary permeability or lymphatic drainage).

Clinical features

- Chest pain:
  - Pleuritic pain – sharp, stabbing, eased with quiet inspiration, intensified by deep inspiration; fades as effusion enlarges
  - Constant dull ache – usually associated with tumour.
- Breathlessness.
- Signs: reduced chest expansion on affected side, dullness to percussion, reduced tactile vocal fremitus, diminished breath sounds. May be signs of underlying disease (e.g. heart failure, infection, malignancy).

Investigation

➤ Pleural aspiration – fluid sent for biochemical analysis, cytology, microbiology analysis (Gram stain, Ziehl–Neelsen stain, culture).
  - Protein and lactate dehydrogenase (LDH) determination – to distinguish transudate from exudate.
  - Light's criteria (1972) – pleural effusion is an exudate in one or more of the following:
    - Pleural fluid protein/serum protein ratio >0.5
    - Pleural fluid LDH/serum LDH ratio >0.6
    - Pleural fluid LDH $>$ two-thirds of upper limit of normal for serum LDH.
  - pH <7.2 implies bacterial contamination (pH of pleural fluid normally parallels pH of arterial blood).
  - Amylase raised in oesophageal rupture, acute pancreatitis, ruptured pancreatic pseudocyst.
  - Raised haematocrit suggests trauma, lung infarct or malignancy.
  - Lymphocytosis is common in malignancy and in TB.
  - Cytology positive for malignant effusions in 60% – with negative cytology, aspiration should be repeated if malignancy suspected (positive in 90% after three sequential aspirates).
➤ Diagnostic imaging:
  - Chest X-ray – posteroanterior and lateral
  - Ultrasound scan – visualise septae within effusion; guide to drainage
  - CT scan – should be performed in all undiagnosed pleural exudates; demonstrates size and position of a loculated effusion, pleural thickening, malignancy, state of other lung.

➔

➤ Pleural biopsy – needle biopsy useful in diagnosis of TB and malignancy (diagnostic yield better with CT guidance in malignancy as often localized pleural disease, whereas TB is generalized).

➤ Thoracoscopy when diagnosis still unclear (90% diagnostic).

Treatment

➤ No intervention if small or asymptomatic.

➤ Large effusions should be drained for symptomatic relief.

➤ Transudate – treat underlying cause.

➤ Infected effusion (page 353 Empyema).

➤ Malignant effusion:
  – Thoracocentesis: first-line treatment for symptomatic patient; recommended not to aspirate >1.5 L on a single occasion (theoretical risk of re-expansion pulmonary oedema in spontaneously breathing patient); 100% of malignant effusions recur within 1 month of aspiration
  – Radiotherapy and chemotherapy may control effusion if tumour responds to treatment
  – Intercostal chest drain with chemical pleurodesis to obliterate pleural space
  – Surgery: thoracoscopic talc pleurodesis is superior to chemical pleurodesis and preferable if the patient is willing and able to undergo surgery
  – Pleuroperitoneal shunt if pleurodesis fails or there is a trapped lung (decortication may help in some instances).

Complications

● Prognosis reflects underlying cause of effusion.

● Thoracocentesis should not be repeated because of risks of hypoproteinaemia, empyema, pneumothorax, bronchopleural fistula, fluid loculation.

● With recurrent effusion, consider thoracoscopic drainage and pleurodesis.

● Low complication rates with thoracoscopy.

● Risk of malignant seeding at skin sites of aspiration, chest drain insertion or surgical wounds with mesothelioma – managed by prophylactic irradiation.

Empyema

Definitions

- Pus in the pleural space.
- Most commonly postpneumonic; postoperative empyema is uncommon with antibiotic prophylaxis (e.g. postpneumonectomy with bronchopleural fistula).
- Three phases:
  - **Exudative/acute** (0–2 weeks) – pleural fluid has low viscosity, low cellular content, low white blood cell count and LDH, normal glucose and pH; lung expandable
  - **Fibrinopurulent/transitional** (2–6 weeks) – more turbid fluid, increased white blood cell count, LDH rises, pH <7.2, fibrin deposition limits extension of effusion and begins to trap lung
  - **Organizing/chronic** (>6 weeks) – organized fibrous pleural peel; frankly purulent fluid in pleural cavity.

Clinical features

- Symptoms similar to those of underlying infection – unwell, malaise, fever, productive cough, pleuritic chest pain.
- Signs of pleural effusion (page 351).

Investigation

➤ Pleural aspiration.
➤ Chest X-ray.
➤ Ultrasound scan can distinguish fluid from consolidation.
➤ CT scan essential to identify complex, multiloculated empyema for surgical intervention.

Treatment

➤ Objectives of treatment: treat infection, evacuate fluid, re-expand lung and obliterate pleural dead space.
➤ Antibiotics only if small parapneumonic effusion and no evidence of empyema.

➜

> ➤ Intercostal chest drain – effective in acute phase, indicated when empyema is confirmed by any of these:
>   – Frankly purulent or turbid pleural fluid
>   – pH <7.2
>   – Positive Gram stain or culture
>   – Large effusion
>   – Poor clinical progress despite antibiotics.
> ➤ Percutaneous intrapleural fibrinolysis may improve drainage of fibrinopurulent empyema.
> ➤ Thoracoscopy is more effective than fibrinolysis in treatment of fibrinopurulent empyema with regard to debriding pleural space and achieving effective drainage.
> ➤ Thoracotomy and decortication indicated for chronic empyema with trapped lung, to remove thickened visceral pleural cortex and re-expand underlying lung.

Complications

- Faster postoperative recovery with thoracoscopy.
- 30% conversion rate from thoracoscopy to thoracotomy and decortication.
- Decortication associated with significant morbidity from bleeding and postoperative air leak and mortality risk up to 10%.

Mesothelioma

Definitions

- Primary tumour of pleura.
- Uncommon (1300 per year) but incidence increasing.
- Associated with long-term asbestos exposure; long latent period.
- 20% sarcomatous; 50% epithelioid; 30% mixed epithelioid and sarcomatous.
- No clear consensus on best approach to staging; simplest is Butchart Staging System; more detailed staging system is the International Mesothelioma Interest Group TNM Staging System.

The Butchart Staging System for Malignant Mesothelioma (1976)

Stage	Description
I	Tumour confined within capsule of ipsilateral pleura, lung, pericardium and diaphragm
II	Tumour invades chest wall or mediastinum: oesophagus, heart, opposite pleura. Positive intrathoracic lymph nodes
III	Tumour invades through diaphragm to peritoneum. Positive lymph nodes outside the chest
IV	Distant blood-borne metastases

Clinical features

- Chest pain.
- Breathlessness.
- Pleural effusion (page 350).

Investigation

➤ Chest X-ray.
➤ CT scan.
➤ Magnetic resonance imaging (MRI) may provide more detail about chest wall invasion.
➤ Pleural fluid for cytology (30% diagnostic).
➤ Pleural biopsy (CT-guided needle biopsy or thoracoscopic).
➤ Immunohistochemistry may be required to distinguish mesothelioma from metastatic adenocarcinoma.

Treatment

➤ Key management issues:
  - Management of pleural effusion
  - Radiotherapy
  - Chemotherapy
  - Surgery for resectable disease
  - Palliative care
  - Compensation.
➤ Staging essential for:
  - Selection of patients for surgery
  - Prognosis
  - Clinical trials.

➔

- Surgery:
  - Thoracoscopic talc pleurodesis is currently the operation of choice for management of pleural effusion
  - Thoracoscopic pleurectomy can achieve reduction in tumour bulk and effective prevention of recurrent effusion, but the benefit over pleurodesis is not established at present
  - Radical surgery (extrapleural pneumonectomy) is reserved for patients with low-volume stage I disease and epithelioid tumour who are able to tolerate major surgery
  - Role of radical surgery unproven at present.
- Radiotherapy:
  - Recommended for patients with pain or chest wall mass
  - Pain relief in 50%
  - Reduction in size of palpable masses in 50%
  - Prophylaxis against chest wall implantation following invasive procedures (untreated risk 10%; risk after radiotherapy 0%)
  - Breathlessness not relieved.
- Chemotherapy:
  - Many agents tried, with 10–20% response rate
  - No published trials to demonstrate effect on symptoms or survival
  - Should be offered in the context of a clinical trial.
- Palliative care for relief of pain, breathlessness, cough, anorexia, weight loss, fatigue, sweating.
- Compensation:
  - Diagnosis and causation must be established
  - Industrial Injuries Disablement Benefit from Department of Social Security
  - Common law claim for damages from firm(s) where exposure occurred.

Complications

- Epithelioid tumours associated with better prognosis.
- Mean survival 8–14 months.
- Prognosis worse with peritoneal involvement; mean survival 7 months in this group.

- Operative mortality of pleuropneumonectomy is high: where few cases are performed, operative mortality may be as high as 30%; experienced centres (USA) report operative mortality of up to 10%.
- 5-year survival after extrapleural pneumonectomy is 15%.
- Mortality and morbidity with thoracoscopic surgery in mesothelioma is 1.5%.

Mediastinal masses

Definitions

- Mediastinum is defined by the thoracic inlet superiorly, diaphragm inferiorly, sternum anteriorly, vertebral column posteriorly and parietal pleura laterally.
- Subdivided into superior (above the sternal angle of Louis and the lower border of T4 vertebra), anterior (anterior to pericardium), middle (defined by the anterior and posterior pericardial reflections) and posterior compartments.
- Mediastinal masses may occur as a result of local or systemic disease.
- Localized conditions include infection, haemorrhage, aneurysms, primary tumours and congenital cysts.
- Systemic disease includes disseminated malignancy, granulomas, systemic inflammatory conditions.
- Up to 40% of mediastinal masses in adults are caused by malignant tumour; in children, up to 75% are benign.
- 50% of mediastinal tumours are located in the anterior mediastinum.
- The following may present as an anterior mediastinal mass:
  - Thymoma (most common anterior mediastinal tumour; second to neurogenic for whole mediastinum)
  - Lymphoma
  - Germ cell tumour (e.g. teratoma, seminoma)
  - Intrathoracic thyroid gland

- Ascending aortic aneurysm
- Post-stenotic dilatation of ascending aorta (in aortic stenosis).
- Middle mediastinal masses include:
  - Pericardial cyst
  - Bronchogenic cyst
  - Lymphoma.
- Posterior mediastinal masses may be:
  - Neurogenic tumour (commonest mediastinal tumours, arising from sympathetic ganglia or intercostal nerves, e.g. neuroblastoma, neurilemmoma, neurofibroma)
  - Bronchogenic cyst
  - Enteric cyst
  - Descending aortic aneurysm
  - Coarctation of the aorta
  - Oesophageal lesions (e.g. diverticula, tumour, hiatus hernia).

Clinical features

- Diverse clinical presentations, reflecting multiplicity of conditions.
- Up to one-third of patients are asymptomatic, with mass detected on routine chest X-ray; more commonly with benign mass.
- Symptoms may be the result of local mechanical effects (more common with malignant tumours), or systemic (reflecting underlying disease).
- Common complaints are of chest pain, cough and fever.
- Paraneoplastic syndromes are not uncommon.
- Superior vena cava (SVC) syndrome:
  - SVC obstruction caused by compression, invasion or thrombosis
  - Most commonly caused by malignant neoplasm involving superior mediastinum
  - Increased venous pressure results in oedema of head, neck and upper extremities; distended neck veins, dilated collateral veins over upper body; cyanosis, headache, confusion
  - Signs may develop slowly or present strikingly with sudden occlusion.

Investigation

➤ Chest X-ray (postero-anterior and lateral) defines location, size, density and calcification.
➤ CT scan (contrast-enhanced) or MRI provide detailed information on relation of mass to surrounding structures; good guide to resectability.
➤ Echocardiography may be useful with middle mediastinal masses.
➤ Serology in adult males with anterior mediastinal mass: alpha-fetoprotein and beta-human chorionic gonadotrophin.
➤ Biopsy:
  – Fine-needle biopsy diagnostic in up to 90% of cases
  – Mediastinoscopy (for lesions of the middle mediastinum around the lower trachea and carina)
  – Mediastinotomy (for lesions of the anterior mediastinum)
  – Thoracoscopy or thoracotomy (for lesions of the posterior mediastinum).

Treatment

➤ Precise histological diagnosis is essential to determine optimal treatment.
➤ Not all mediastinal masses are treated by surgery; however, resectable lesions should be excised.
➤ Anterior mediastinal masses are approached by median sternotomy.
➤ Middle and posterior mediastinal masses are approached by posterolateral thoracotomy.
➤ In selected patients, resection may be possible by thoracoscopic surgery.

Complications

● Prognosis and surgical complications reflect underlying disease.
● Care must be taken to identify systemic syndromes (e.g. myasthenia gravis, malignant hypertension, hypercalcaemia, thyrotoxicosis), in order to avoid potentially serious postoperative complications.

Thoracic injuries

- Blunt or penetrating.
- Common cause of trauma deaths (25%).
- Blunt chest injury occurs in 25% of road traffic accidents.
- Pathophysiology: **impaired ventilation** and **lung injury** result in hypoxaemia and hypercarbia (respiratory acidosis); **hypovolaemia** results in hypotension and tissue hypoperfusion, leading to tissue hypoxia and metabolic acidosis.
- Life-threatening injuries include:
  - Airway obstruction/large airway injury
  - Tension pneumothorax
  - Large haemothorax
  - Sucking chest wound
  - Flail chest
  - Cardiac tamponade
  - Lung contusion
  - Myocardial contusion
  - Aortic transection.
- Common injuries include rib and sternal fracture.
- Injury to major airways is rare.
- Immediate management involves resuscitation (Airway–Breathing–Circulation), oxygen and identification and treatment of immediately life-threatening injuries.
- Many conditions are manageable with chest drainage and do not require thoracotomy.
- Indications for emergency thoracotomy:
  - Penetrating chest injury with haemodynamic instability
  - Pulseless electrical activity: a state where there is ECG evidence of electrical activity in the heart, yet no cardiac output.
- Contraindications for emergency thoracotomy:
  - Blunt trauma
  - Pulseless with no electrical activity.
- Complications of chest trauma include acute respiratory distress syndrome (ARDS), infection and thromboembolism.

Airway obstruction or injury

- Obstruction of or injury to larynx, trachea or major bronchus.
- Airway obstruction associated with fractures of mid-face and mandible or neck injury.
- Larynx or trachea may be injured with cervical trauma.
- Signs include hoarseness, stridor, surgical emphysema.
- Tracheal or bronchial injury may be associated with pneumothorax or pneumomediastinum.
- First priority of management is to secure and maintain airway.
- Operative repair indicated.

Tension pneumothorax

- A clinical diagnosis.
- Continued massive air leak after drainage of a tension pneumothorax suggests major bronchial tear; urgent thoracotomy indicated.

Large haemothorax

- 1500 mL of blood in chest cavity.
- Occurs with blunt or penetrating trauma.
- Results in hypovolaemia and hypoxia.
- Signs of shock with pleural effusion.
- May cause tension haemothorax – neck veins may be empty or distended.
- Resuscitate by replacing blood volume and decompressing chest cavity using large-bore intercostal chest drain.
- Continued blood loss after initial drainage (>100 mL/hour for 4 hours) requires urgent thoracotomy.
- Residual haemothorax that fails to drain requires surgical evacuation.

Sucking chest wound

- Large, open defect of the chest wall.
- Results in open pneumothorax.
- Impairs ventilation, leading to hypoxia.
- Initial management: occlusive dressing and intercostal chest drain insertion.
- Definitive treatment: surgical closure of defect.

Flail chest

- Crushing injury.
- Loss of bony continuity of the thoracic cage: fractures of two or more ribs twice each create a free-floating (flail) segment of chest wall.
- More serious variant is when ribs or costal cartilages are fractured on either side near the sternum, rendering the sternum flail.
- Free-floating flail segment disrupts normal chest wall movement: sucked in during inspiration and driven out during expiration; breathing is therefore paradoxical. Air is shunted from the injured to the uninjured side and back again, rather than being exhaled, leading to progressive accumulation of carbon dioxide.
- Pain further impairs chest wall movement.
- Loss of effective cough results in accumulation of tracheobronchial secretions.
- Flail segment may be associated with significant underlying lung injury.
- Respiratory embarrassment occurs as a result of a combination of pain, paradoxical chest wall motion and underlying lung contusion. Increasing hypoxia and carbon dioxide retention result in increased dyspnoea and more pronounced paradoxical movement, with worsening respiratory failure.
- Chest X-ray may reveal multiple rib fracture.
- Therapy includes administration of oxygen, adequate ventilation, careful fluid resuscitation, analgesia (best with thoracic epidural).
- Mechanical ventilation may be required.

Cardiac tamponade

- Most commonly results from a penetrating injury.
- Consider cardiac injury with penetrating chest injury medial to nipple/scapula or subxiphoid.
- Consider tamponade when faced with pulseless electrical activity in the absence of hypovolaemia or tension pneumothorax.

Lung contusion

- Trauma leading to haemorrhage into lung parenchyma or microvascular injury.
- May occur to varying degree with any chest trauma.
- Results in impaired oxygenation, leading to hypoxaemia and shunting.
- Insidious onset; diagnosis difficult.
- Chest X-ray may reveal patchy pulmonary infiltrates.
- Low threshold for mechanical ventilation.

Myocardial contusion

- Diagnosis difficult; key is history of mechanism of injury.
- ECG may mimic myocardial infarction, with elevation of cardiac enzymes.
- Coronary artery injury may result in myocardial infarction.
- Risk of sudden arrhythmia resulting in pump failure.
- Patients with evidence of myocardial contusion should be monitored for at least 48 hours.
- Echocardiography is indicated for suspected tamponade or if there is an audible murmur.

Aortic transection

- Transection usually occurs at the junction between the mobile aortic arch and the fixed descending aorta (just distal to the left subclavian artery and ligamentum arteriosum) as a result of shear forces from a sudden deceleration injury.
- Often fatal at scene.
- Survivors usually have aortic laceration with intact adventitia.
- Symptoms and signs not specific.
- Diagnosis from history and investigations.
- Suspicious chest X-ray is indication for further investigation (CT scan or aortogram).
- Chest X-ray findings in aortic transection:
  - Wide mediastinum
  - Fractured first and/or second rib
  - Loss of aortic knuckle

- Loss of space between aortic knuckle and pulmonary artery
- Pleural cap
- Tracheal deviation to right
- Left main bronchus depressed
- Right main bronchus elevated and shifted to right
- Oesophageal deviation.
- Initial management: resuscitation and careful blood pressure control.
- Definitive treatment: prompt surgical repair of thoracic aorta with interposition graft.

Rib fractures

- Most common form of chest injury.
- Clinical rather than radiographic diagnosis.
- Pain with respiration.
- Localized tenderness to palpation.
- Managed with analgesia.

Sternal fractures

- Classically steering wheel or seat belt injury.
- Degree of injury ranges from anterior table fracture to severely displaced fracture.
- Managed primarily with analgesia.
- Monitor patients with suspected myocardial contusion.

CARDIAC CONDITIONS

Ischaemic heart disease

Definitions

- The most important cause of death in the developed world.
- Men more often affected; women equally affected after menopause.
- Pathology: coronary artery stenosis – atheromatous plaque causes narrowing or obliteration of vessel lumen; sudden and complete obstruction occurs as a result of acute thrombosis.

- Aetiology – risk factors include:
  - Family history of coronary artery disease
  - Diabetes mellitus (type 1 or type 2)
  - Hypercholesterolaemia (>6.5 mmol/L or treated)
  - Hypertension (>140/90 mmHg or treated)
  - Hypothyroidism
  - Smoking
  - Obesity
  - Advancing age.
- Ischaemia of myocardium may occur in the absence of coronary artery stenosis secondary to:
  - Left ventricular hypertrophy, e.g. hypertension, hypertrophic cardiomyopathy
  - Aortic stenosis
  - Low cardiac output
  - Anaemia.

Clinical features

- **Angina pectoris:** pain derived from the heart itself when the oxygen demand of the myocardium exceeds supply:
  - Strangulating pain felt retrosternally (contrasting with the crushing pain of infarction): it may radiate to the arm, jaw, or neck
  - Commonly exacerbated by exercise and cold weather; relieved by rest and by sublingual nitrates
  - May occur after eating
  - May occur at night and wake the patient from sleep (nocturnal angina)
  - May be atypical, e.g. presenting as epigastric pain.
- **Angina status** defined by the Canadian Cardiovascular Society (CCS):
  - CCS0: no angina
  - CCS1: angina only with strenuous, rapid or prolonged exertion
  - CCS2: slight limitation of ordinary activity
  - CCS3: marked limitation of ordinary physical activity
  - CCS4: unable to perform any physical activity without pain; rest pain.
- Can present as **breathlessness (dyspnoea)**, **congestive heart failure** without angina, **arrhythmia**, **asymptomatic** abnormal ECG, **sudden death**.

- Dyspnoea status defined by the New York Heart Association (NYHA):
  - NYHA I not limited by cardiac disease; asymptomatic
  - NYHA II: slight limitation of ordinary physical activity; comfortable at rest
  - NYHA III: marked limitation of physical activity; symptoms with less than ordinary activity; comfortable at rest
  - NYHA IV: unable to perform any physical activity without discomfort; symptoms at rest.
- Pain at rest lasting longer than a few minutes and associated with nausea or vomiting may signify an acute coronary syndrome [**unstable angina** or **myocardial infarction** (MI)].
- Clinical examination usually unremarkable. May be evidence of anaemia, high cholesterol, high blood pressure, or signs of aortic stenosis (page 369).

Investigation

➤ **Chest X-ray:**
  - May reveal cardiomegaly
  - Detects incidental pathology.
➤ **12-lead ECG:**
  - Establish rhythm
  - ST-segment changes are important in acute ischaemia (ST-segment depression) or infarction (classically ST-segment elevation may not always be apparent, as in non-ST-elevation MI – 'NSTEMI')
  - Evidence of previous MI (Q-waves in infarct territory, or inverted T-waves in 'subendocardial' or 'non-Q' MI)
  - Signs of recent severe ischaemia
  - Features of left ventricular hypertrophy – left axis deviation, voltage changes of deep S-wave in V_{1-2} and tall R-wave in V_{5-6}, inverted T-waves V_{5-6}.
➤ **Stress ECG/exercise test:**
  - Most commonly treadmill stress test with standard protocol (Bruce)
  - Detects ST-segment changes during exercise

➤

- Not good for screening or diagnosis – high incidence of non-specific changes result in false positive, particularly in women
- Important in risk stratification of patients in whom diagnosis established
- Contraindicated in unstable angina and for patients with poor cardiac reserve.

➤ **Echocardiography:**
  - Assess resting left ventricular function
  - Detect concomitant valve disease.

➤ **Nuclear imaging:**
  - Ventriculography [multigated acquisition scanning (MUGA scan)] or myocardial perfusion scintigraphy (thallium scan)
  - **Ventriculography** performed using technetium-99m ($^{99}Tc^m$)-labelled blood, demonstrates left ventricular ejection fraction and wall motion abnormalities
  - **Myocardial perfusion scan** performed using thallium-201 (^{201}Tl): administered at peak effort during stress testing and taken up by non-ischaemic myocardium, then redistributes to all viable myocardium after 4 hours at rest, thus demonstrating areas of reversible ischaemia.

➤ **Coronary angiography:**
  - Provides detailed anatomy of the coronary arteries
  - Extent and distribution of disease predicts outcome
  - Important for risk stratification and essential for planning interventional treatment.

Treatment

➤ Objectives are to improve patient survival and enhance quality of life.
➤ **Medical therapy:**
  - For mild to moderate symptoms and low-risk disease
  - Improves exercise tolerance and quality of life
  - Low-dose aspirin and combination therapy with two anti-anginals (beta blockers, calcium antagonist, long-acting nitrate or potassium-channel opener) is most effective.

➔

- Refer for further assessment when symptoms are severe, unstable or rapidly progressive.
- **Percutaneous intervention (PCI):**
  - Coronary angioplasty ± stenting
  - Effective symptomatic relief
  - 25% develop restenosis within 6 months
  - 1 in 6 requires further PCI or coronary artery bypass graft surgery (CABG).
- **CABG:**
  - Improves both survival and quality of life in selected patients (moderate to high risk with medical therapy)
  - Indicated also for prognostic (survival) benefit in selected asymptomatic patients
  - Significant survival benefit (compared with medical therapy) seen with left main stem disease (stenosis >50%), left main stem equivalent (≥70% stenoses of proximal left anterior descending artery and proximal circumflex artery), proximal three-vessel disease (stenoses >50%) and proximal one-vessel or two-vessel disease, including disease of the left anterior descending artery (stenoses >50%)
  - With proximal two-vessel or three-vessel disease, survival benefit is greater in patients with impaired left ventricular (LV) function (LV ejection fraction <50%).
- **Risk factor management.**

Complications

- Mortality 20% at 5 years with medical therapy for high risk coronary artery disease.
- Procedure-related mortality for PCI <1%, for CABG 2–4% overall (modified by risk stratification, e.g. Parsonnet, Euroscore).
- Other major complications of surgical revascularization: cerebral – stroke 2%, reversible neuro-psychological deficit; systemic inflammatory response; perioperative infection – mediastinitis (<1%); arrhythmia [atrial fibrillation (AF) 30%]; reversible renal dysfunction.

Valve disease

Aortic stenosis

Definitions

- Obstruction of left ventricular outflow:
  - Valve stenosis – congenital: bicuspid valve, other malformation; acquired: degenerative calcification, rheumatic heart disease
  - Subvalvular stenosis – congenital, hypertrophic obstructive cardiomyopathy
  - Supravalvular stenosis – congenital (rare).
- Normal adult valve area 3–4 cm^2; significant change in circulation occurs only when valve area reduced to 25% of normal size.
- Outflow obstruction results in systolic **pressure overload** and concentric **left ventricular hypertrophy**. LV compensation generates transvalvular pressure gradient.
- As compensatory mechanisms fail, wall stress (afterload) increases, LV ejection fraction decreases and ventricle dilates.

Clinical features

- Initially asymptomatic; long latent period.
- Symptoms: angina (page 365), syncope (more sinister), heart failure (breathlessness, fatigue).
- Signs: slow-rising, small volume pulse; left ventricular heave; systolic thrill over aortic area (second intercostal space to R of sternum); harsh ejection systolic murmur radiating to neck (loudest in expiration); paradoxical split second heart sound.

Investigation

- ➤ **12-lead ECG and chest X-ray**.
- ➤ **Echocardiography:**
  - Diagnosis
  - Assessment of severity by valve area (mild >1.5 cm^2, moderate >1.0–1.5 cm^2, severe ⩽1.0 cm^2), transvalvular flow and pressure gradient (severe >50 mmHg)

➜

- Evaluate LV function and dimensions
- Follow-up of asymptomatic patients
- Stress echocardiography may be useful in symptomatic patients with impaired LV function and mild–moderate gradient, to assess ventricular response to dobutamine stress and thus potential for recovery of LV function in patients being considered for surgery.

➤ **Cardiac catheterization:**
- Coronary angiography in symptomatic patients over 40 years old.

➤ **Exercise testing:**
- Asymptomatic severe aortic stenosis: exercise testing for objective evidence of whether or not symptoms occur, to determine whether surgery is indicated.

Treatment

➤ No specific medical therapy available.
➤ Restrict physical activity according to severity of stenosis.
➤ Antibiotic prophylaxis to prevent infective endocarditis, e.g. to cover dental treatment.
➤ Asymptomatic patients: serial echocardiography to monitor progression of stenosis.
➤ Symptomatic patients: aortic valve replacement (AVR) (balloon valvotomy in selected patients).
➤ AVR also indicated if undergoing CABG or other heart valve surgery.
➤ Inoperable patients managed symptomatically (anti-anginals, anti-arrhythmics, diuretics, angiotensin-converting enzyme inhibitors).

Complications

- Average survival after symptoms develop is 2–3 years.
- Surgical mortality 2% (other risks see complications of CABG, page 368).
- Long-term morbidity and mortality after AVR 2% per year.

Aortic regurgitation

Definitions

- Failure of coaptation of valve cusps as a result of aortic root dilatation or aortic valve cusp abnormality.
- Root dilatation:
  - Idiopathic
  - Myxomatous
  - Marfan's syndrome
  - Ascending aortic dissection.
- Valve cusp abnormality:
  - Congenital (bicuspid)
  - Calcific degeneration
  - Rheumatic heart disease
  - Infective endocarditis.
- Pathophysiology differs between sudden, acute aortic regurgitation (AR) and chronic AR.
- **Acute severe AR:** sudden increase in end-diastolic volume results in dramatic increase in LV end-diastolic pressure. LV unable to compensate acutely, so stroke volume falls, heart rate rises to compensate.
- **Chronic AR:** increase in end-diastolic volume results in increased chamber compliance, allowing increase in volume without increase in pressure. Volume loading results in LV dilatation and increased stroke volume. Symptoms develop when compensatory mechanisms fail and ejection fraction falls below normal.

Clinical features

- **Acute severe AR:** pulmonary oedema and/or cardiogenic shock, ventricular arrhythmia.
- **Chronic AR:** asymptomatic during compensatory phase; symptoms include breathlessness, angina, heart failure.
- Signs: collapsing 'water hammer' pulse, Corrigan's sign (when the large volume carotid pulse is visible in the neck), LV heave, early diastolic murmur, Austin–Flint murmur (mid-diastolic murmur produced when the flow of blood back into the LV partially closes and obstructs the mitral valve), ejection systolic murmur.

Investigation

➤ **12-lead ECG and chest X-ray**.
➤ **Echocardiography:**
  – Diagnosis
  – Valve morphology
  – Aortic root size and morphology
  – Evaluate LV function and dimensions
  – Assess severity of AR
  – Follow-up of asymptomatic patients.
➤ **Cardiac catheterization:**
  – Aortogram: anatomy of aortic root, severity of AR
  – Ventriculogram: LV dilatation and function
  – Coronary angiography for surgical candidates.
➤ Exercise testing to assess patients with equivocal symptoms.

Treatment

➤ **No treatment:** mild to moderate AR, normal LV function, normotensive.
➤ **Serial testing** clinical assessment and echocardiography.
➤ **Antibiotic prophylaxis** to prevent infective endocarditis.
➤ **Medical therapy:** vasodilator therapy to reduce systolic blood pressure, improve forward stroke volume and reduce regurgitant volume:
  – Asymptomatic patients with severe AR, LV dilatation and normal systolic function
  – Asymptomatic patients with systemic hypertension
  – Short-term therapy for patients awaiting AVR
  – Symptomatic AR and/or LV dysfunction when surgery is contraindicated for other reasons.
➤ **Surgery: aortic valve replacement/aortic root replacement:**
  – Acute severe AR
  – Symptomatic chronic AR: breathlessness NYHA class III or IV; angina CCS2 or greater
  – Chronic AR where exercise testing provokes symptoms or abnormal LV response

➜

- Asymptomatic chronic AR with subnormal LV ejection fraction at rest
- Asymptomatic chronic AR with LV end-systolic diameter >55 mm (normal range 25–41 mm) or LV end-diastolic diameter >75 mm (normal range 35–55 mm)
- If undergoing CABG or other heart valve surgery
- Root replacement if aortic root >50 mm on ECG.

Complications

- 1 in 4 asymptomatic patients with LV systolic dysfunction develop symptoms within 1 year.
- Mortality rate in symptomatic patients >10% per year.

Mitral stenosis

Definitions

- Obstruction to LV inflow.
- Congenital (rare)/acquired (rheumatic heart disease).
- Rheumatic heart disease causes mitral valve leaflet thickening and calcification, commissural fusion, chordal fusion resulting in reduced mitral valve orifice.
- Female:male = 2:1.
- Normal mitral valve area 4–5 cm^2.
- Symptoms develop when valve area <2.5 cm^2.
- Reduction in mitral valve area generates diastolic transmitral gradient, resulting in pressure-loading of left atrium; leads to increased pulmonary venous pressure, pulmonary oedema, pulmonary arterial hypertension, increased load on right ventricle.
- As stenosis progresses, cardiac output falls.

Clinical features

- Initially asymptomatic. Long latent period of 20–40 years from onset of rheumatic fever; mean age of patient at presentation 40–60 years.

- Symptoms:
  - Breathlessness progresses with increasing left atrial (LA) pressure: initially on exertion when valve area 1.5–2.5 cm^2, progressing to orthopnoea, paroxysmal nocturnal dyspnoea, pulmonary oedema. Becomes less prominent with development of pulmonary hypertension
  - Pulmonary hypertension and low cardiac output cause fatigue
  - AF
  - Systemic embolus.
- Signs:
  - Cardiovascular – AF, small pulse, jugular venous pressure (JVP) may be raised, 'tapping' apex beat (palpable first, mitral, heart sound), right ventricular (RV) heave with pulmonary hypertension, loud first heart sound, opening snap, low-pitched rumbling mid-diastolic murmur (sometimes with presystolic accentuation) at the apex
  - Chest – inspiratory crackles
  - Abdomen – hepatomegaly, ascites; peripheral oedema.

Investigation

➤ **ECG:** heart rate, rhythm, P-mitrale, RV hypertrophy.
➤ **Chest X-ray:** cardiothoracic ratio, LA dilatation, pulmonary oedema.
➤ **Echocardiography:**
  - Diagnosis
  - Assess mitral valve morphology
  - Assess haemodynamic severity: mitral valve area, gradient, pulmonary artery pressure
  - Assess RV size and function
  - Examine other heart valves
  - Follow-up.
➤ **Cardiac catheterization:**
  - Assess severity of mitral stenosis (MS)
  - Measure LV, LA and pulmonary artery (PA) pressures
  - Coronary angiography.

Treatment

➤ **Non-invasive:**
  - Asymptomatic patient in sinus rhythm: no treatment
  - Reduce physical activity if greater than mild MS
  - Antibiotic prophylaxis to prevent infective endocarditis
  - Salt restriction and diuretic for pulmonary oedema
  - Anti-arrhythmic drugs, cardioversion and anticoagulation for AF
  - Serial testing by clinical assessment and echocardiography.

➤ **Valvotomy:**
  - Surgical or percutaneous
  - NYHA II–IV with moderate to severe stenosis (mitral valve (MV) area $\leqslant 1.5$ cm^2)
  - Asymptomatic patients with pulmonary hypertension (PA systolic pressure >50 mmHg at rest)
  - Successful outcome requires favourable valve morphology: pliable and non-calcific valves with minimal fusion of subvalvular apparatus
  - Contraindicated in presence of mitral regurgitation (MR)
  - Percutaneous valvotomy results in doubling of valve orifice and 50% reduction in transmitral gradient; contraindicated in presence of LA thrombus.

➤ **Mitral valve replacement (MVR):**
  - Moderate to severe MS (MV area $\leqslant 1.5$ cm^2) and NYHA III–IV with unfavourable valve morphology for valvotomy
  - Severe MS (MV area $\leqslant 1.0$ cm^2) with pulmonary hypertension, not suitable for valvotomy.

Complications

● 10-year survival of untreated MS:
  - NYHA I–II   >80%
  - NYHA III   50–60%
  - NYHA IV   0–15%.

- – Valvotomy:
  - – Procedural mortality 1–2%
  - – MR in up to 10%; other risks – and of percutaneous balloon valvotomy – cardiac tamponade, thromboembolism
  - – Event-free survival 60% in patients with favourable morphology
  - – Other operative complications as for CABG – see page 368.
- MVR:
  - – Procedural mortality 5% (may be higher, up to 20% – multifactorial)
  - – Other complications: valve thrombosis, valve dehiscence, valve infection, valve malfunction, embolic events
  - – Risk of long-term anticoagulation with mechanical valve.

Mitral regurgitation

Definitions

- Major structural components of the mitral valve are: mitral annulus, valve leaflets (anterior and posterior), chordae tendinae and papillary muscles, and LV.
- Loss of functional integrity of any one or all of these components may result in valve incompetence.
- Causes: degenerative [mitral valve prolapse (2–6% of population), chordal rupture], rheumatic heart disease, ischaemic heart disease, infective endocarditis, collagen vascular diseases, LV dilatation (resulting from ischaemia, cardiomyopathy, myocarditis).
- Regurgitation of stroke volume of LV into LA results in:
  - – Reduced systemic (forward) blood flow
  - – Pressure and volume loading of LA
  - – Volume loading of LV.
- Subsequent effects depend on whether valve insufficiency is acute or chronic.
- When regurgitation is acute (as a result of rupture of a papillary muscle or chorda, or infective endocarditis):
  - – LA volume is small, so pulmonary vascular pressure rises abruptly and pulmonary congestion ensues, with severe hypoxia

- Sudden LV volume overload occurs with reduced stroke volume and cardiac output.
- In chronic insufficiency:
  - LA dilates and accommodates regurgitant volume with low filling pressure
  - LV compensates for volume overload by dilatation and eccentric hypertrophy; total stroke volume is increased by augmented preload and reduced afterload, and normal forward stroke volume is maintained
  - Pulmonary congestion occurs late and reflects loss of LV compensation; LV dysfunction results in further dilatation, increased filling pressure and reduced forward output.

Clinical features

- **Mild insufficiency** usually asymptomatic. Apical systolic murmur is the only physical finding. Mid-systolic click may be audible with prolapsing valve leaflet.
- **Acute severe MR:**
  - History of MI or infective endocarditis
  - Signs of low cardiac output (shock) and pulmonary oedema
  - Third and fourth heart sounds are caused by rapid LV filling.
- **Chronic severe MR:**
  - Initially asymptomatic; onset of symptoms after many years
  - As insufficiency progresses: symptoms of weakness, fatigue, palpitations, breathlessness on exertion
  - With LV failure, symptoms of pulmonary oedema more prominent
  - Prominent apex beat reflects LV enlargement
  - Characteristic murmur is harsh, blowing, apical systolic murmur
  - Severity of insufficiency correlates with pansystolic characteristic of murmur: murmur of mild insufficiency does not extend throughout systole, whereas murmur of severe insufficiency is truly pansystolic
  - Right-sided heart failure with hepatic enlargement and peripheral oedema are late signs and indicate irreversible ventricular dysfunction.

Investigation

➤ **ECG** to establish cardiac rhythm.
➤ **Chest X-ray** demonstrates enlargement of LA and LV.
➤ **Echocardiography:**
  - Assess LA and LV volume
  - Estimate LV ejection fraction
  - Determine severity of regurgitation
  - Establish anatomical basis and mechanism of MR
  - Estimate PA pressure.
➤ **Cardiac catheterization:**
  - Indications: when there is discrepancy between clinical and non-invasive findings regarding severity of MR, or when non-invasive tests are inconclusive regarding severity of MR, LV function or need for surgery
  - Left ventriculography demonstrates regurgitation and LV function
  - Right heart catheterization provides direct measurement of PA pressure and indirect measurement of LA pressure (pulmonary artery wedge pressure) to assess severity of MR
  - Coronary angiography when surgery is indicated: patients over 40 years old, history of angina or MI, risk factors for coronary artery disease, or when ischaemia is thought to be cause of MR.

Treatment

➤ **Acute severe MR:**
  - Non-surgical therapy aims to reduce MR by reducing systemic vascular resistance and LV size, resulting in increased forward flow and reduced pulmonary congestion. Strategies include vasodilators (glyceryl trinitrate or nitroprusside), inotropes (dobutamine) and intra-aortic balloon counterpulsation
  - If infective endocarditis is the cause, identification and treatment of causative organism are essential
  - Surgery (valve repair or replacement) is definitive treatment and may be life-saving.

➔

> **Chronic severe MR:**
  * **Medical therapy:**
    - No treatment for asymptomatic patients
    - Follow-up by clinical evaluation (6-monthly) and echocardiography (annual)
    - Modify physical activity with mildly symptomatic patients or those with LV dilatation or AF
    - Antibiotic prophylaxis to prevent infective endocarditis
    - Salt restriction and diuretic for pulmonary oedema
    - Anti-arrhythmic drugs, cardioversion and anticoagulation for AF.
  * **Mitral valve repair or replacement:**
    - Symptomatic (NYHA II–IV) patients with normal LV function [ejection fraction (EF) >60%, left ventricular end systolic dimension (LVESD) <45 mm]: relieve symptoms and maintain LV function
    - Symptomatic or asymptomatic patients with mild to moderate LV dysfunction (EF 30–60%, LVESD 45–55 mm): improve symptoms and prevent further deterioration of LV function
    - Asymptomatic patients with normal LV function and AF or pulmonary hypertension: preserve LV size and function, prevent further sequelae of chronic MR.
> Inoperable patients managed symptomatically (anti-arrhythmics, diuretics, angiotensin-converting enzyme inhibitors).

Complications

* Mitral valve repair: 2% procedure-related mortality; late cardiac death in <20% at 10 years; re-operation in 10–15% at 10 years.
* Increased risk of surgical mortality associated with:
  - Increasing age and NYHA classification
  - Associated coronary disease
  - Concomitant procedure
  - Raised PA pressure.

Tricuspid valve disease

- Majority of cases are secondary tricuspid regurgitation resulting from RV failure with long-term dilatation of the tricuspid valve annulus.
- Rheumatic tricuspid valve disease is uncommon.
- Tricuspid valve endocarditis is associated with intravenous drug abusers.
- Signs are those of congestive cardiac failure: prominent jugular venous pulsation, liver congestion, ascites and peripheral oedema.
- Surgery for tricuspid valve disease is uncommon in the UK, frequently performed in association with other valve replacements.

Pulmonary stenosis

- Congenital, usually asymptomatic.
- Often present with pulmonary ejection systolic murmur.
- Severe obstruction can cause syncope on exertion.
- Results in RV hypertrophy; failure if long-standing obstruction.
- Treated by balloon dilatation or surgery.

Endocarditis

- Bacterial infection of the endocardium.
- Infective vegetation: endothelial damage results in platelet and fibrin deposition with bacterial multiplication within the platelet–fibrin complex.
- Risk factors: conditions resulting in abnormal flow of blood predisposing to endothelial injury (hence need for antibiotic prophylaxis with dental and/or surgical procedures in such patients):
  – Valvular heart disease
  – Congenital heart disease
  – Prosthetic heart valves
  – Intravenous drug abusers (tricuspid valve endocarditis).
- Clinical features:
  – May be insidious onset – persistent 'flu-like' illness, fever, malaise
  – Followed by progressive congestive heart failure with a murmur

- *Staphylococcus* endocarditis often associated with dramatic and rapid deterioration
- Embolic phenomena – transient ischaemic attack (TIA)/stroke, chest pain, haemoptysis, abdominal pain, splinter haemorrhages, Osler's nodes (cutaneous emboli), haematuria
- Blood tests reveal raised white blood cell count, erythrocyte sedimentation rate and CRP with progressive anaemia.

- Management:
  - Identify causative organism (usually *Streptococcus* spp, *Staphylococcus* spp or Gram-negative organism)
  - Treat with appropriate antibiotics for 6 weeks
  - Serial echocardiography to assess LV function and affected valve(s), and to monitor progress with antibiotic treatment
  - Indications for surgery: persistent sepsis, heart failure, new conduction defect (with aortic root abscess), systemic embolization
  - Surgical mortality in acute endocarditis is as high as 50%.

Rheumatic fever

- 'Allergic' response to infection with Group A haemolytic *Streptococcus* – classically occurs 2–3 weeks after streptococcal throat infection or scarlet fever.
- Protein within bacterial wall triggers excessive immune response, resulting in endothelial injury.
- Important cause of valvular heart disease, affecting mitral valve most commonly.
- Uncommon after 1970 but incidence increasing since late 1980s.
- Clinical features: fever, flitting large joint arthropathy, sinus tachycardia, murmur (usually of MS or AR).
- Echocardiography may reveal non-infective vegetations; in severe rheumatic fever, assess pericardial effusion (with pericarditis), LV size and function (with myocarditis).
- Joints (arthropathy) always return to normal; MS develops over following years.
- Treat with penicillin or erythromycin to eradicate streptococcal infection.

● Patients who have experienced one episode of rheumatic fever are at high risk of recurrence, particularly those with cardiac involvement. Secondary prevention of rheumatic fever with long-term antibiotics is recommended.

Pericardium

Jugular venous pulse

● A measure of right atrial pressure.
● Indicates level of 'filling' of the cardiovascular system.
● Reflects competence of the right heart to accept and deliver blood.
● Defined by three waves (a, c, v) and two negative descents, x and y:
  – **a wave:** produced by atrial systole
  – **x-descent:** occurs when atrial contraction finishes
  – **c wave:** interrupts the x-descent. Small positive deflection caused by displacement of the tricuspid annulus into the right atrium as the RV pressure rises. Synchronous with ventricular systole
  – **v wave:** results from the passive rise in pressure that occurs as venous return continues to the right atrium during ventricular systole
  – **y-descent:** represents the fall in right atrial pressure when the tricuspid valve opens and blood enters the right ventricle.
● The **a wave** is distinguished from the **v wave** by palpation of the carotid artery: the a wave occurs immediately before the carotid pulsation.
● Changes in pressure waves reflect pericardial disease.

Cardiac tamponade

Definitions

● Normally 15–50 mL serous pericardial fluid; intrapericardial pressure 2 mmHg at rest.
● Accumulation of pericardial fluid initially has no haemodynamic effect.

- Haemodynamic compromise depends on volume of pericardial contents and rate at which contents accumulate.
- Pathophysiology reflects impairment of diastolic filling of the heart as a result of pressure exerted by accumulating fluid in the pericardium.
- Right side affected earlier than left; y-descent of JVP is amputated.
- Tamponade may be acute or chronic.
- Acute tamponade resulting from haemopericardium – secondary to trauma or iatrogenic.
- Chronic tamponade caused by accumulation of pericardial effusion secondary to pericarditis (see below), malignancy, connective tissue disorder.

Clinical features

- **Beck's triad:**
  - Raised JVP
  - Low systemic blood pressure
  - Muffled heart sounds.
- **Pulsus paradoxus:**
  - Exaggeration of the normal physiological response during respiration. Deep inspiration causes a reduction in intrathoracic pressure with twofold effect: RV volume increases and blood pools within pulmonary circulation. Overall result is that with inspiration LV diastolic filling falls, resulting in a lower stroke volume. This results in a fall in systolic blood pressure and pulse pressure, normally by less than 10 mmHg
  - In cardiac tamponade fluid within the pericardium exerts its own pressure: the normal physiological response is exaggerated by further compromise of LV filling
  - 'Paradox' is that the heart may still be auscultated, although no pulse is palpable.
- **Acute:** dramatic cardiovascular collapse/shock/pulseless electrical activity; high JVP with pulsus paradoxus.
- **Chronic:** insidious onset of symptoms (malaise) and signs (pallor, sweating, cyanosis, cool peripheries, tachypnoea, tachycardia, high JVP, pulsus paradoxus; cerebral and renal impairment).

Investigation
- ➤ **ECG:** low QRS voltage with large effusion.
- ➤ **Chest X-ray:** enlarged cardiac silhouette with sharply defined left heart border.
- ➤ **Echocardiography:** diagnostic.

Treatment
- ➤ Pericardiocentesis: percutaneous pericardial aspiration, ideally under echocardiographic guidance.
- ➤ Evacuation of as little as 50 mL can result in marked improvement in acute tamponade.
- ➤ Evacuation of haemopericardium/surgical repair.
- ➤ Pericardial window for chronic tamponade.

Pericarditis
- Acute/chronic.
- Inflammatory/infective.
- Causes: idiopathic, viral, pyogenic, tuberculosis, post-MI (Dressler's syndrome), systemic (connective tissue diseases), metabolic (uraemia), neoplastic, postoperative (postpericardiotomy syndrome).
- Symptoms and signs: fever, malaise, pericardial pain (sharp, pleuritic, relieved by sitting forward). Pericardial rub may be audible. With constrictive pericarditis, high JVP – Kussmaul's sign (JVP rises on inspiration) and Friedreich's sign (deep and rapid y-descent reflects abrupt limitation of RV filling).
- Management: non-steroidal anti-inflammatory drugs, treat underlying cause, pericardiocentesis or pericardial window may be required, pericardiectomy for constrictive pericarditis.

Congenital defects of the pericardium
- Pericardial cysts – asymptomatic mass seen on chest X-ray, typically located in costophrenic angle.
- Pericardial diverticula communicate with pericardial sac.

Congenital heart disease

Atrial septal defect

Definitions

- Defect of the interatrial septum; may be simple or complex.
- Male:female = 1:2.
- Aetiology unknown.
- Types of atrial septal defect (ASD):
  - Patent foramen ovale (PFO) (occurs in 10–20% of adults)
  - Secundum ASD (commonest cardiac malformation)
  - Sinus venosus defect
  - Partial anomalous pulmonary venous drainage
  - Primum ASD.
- Communication between left atrium (LA) and right atrium (RA) results in left-to-right shunt as a result of greater compliance of RV. Degree of shunt depends on: size of defect, compliance of RV and LV, relative vascular resistances. Left-to-right shunt results in right heart volume overload. Increase in pulmonary vascular resistance is uncommon and unpredictable, but inevitably lethal.
- In infancy and early childhood defect may close spontaneously; unlikely after the age of 2 years, uncommon after 4 years.

Clinical features

- Usually asymptomatic; children may suffer recurrent chest infections, breathlessness on extreme exertion; in adults, breathlessness on exertion, palpitations, paradoxical emboli, stroke, congestive heart failure.
- Signs: cyanosis (late, as a result of pulmonary hypertension and shunt reversal – Eisenmenger syndrome), AF (adults), RV (parasternal) heave, widely split second heart sound, flow murmurs in tricuspid area (fourth intercostal space, left sternal edge) and in pulmonary area (second intercostal space, left sternal edge); murmurs louder in inspiration because of increased venous return.

Investigation

➤ **ECG:** evidence of RV hypertrophy: right axis deviation, partial right bundle branch block.
➤ **Chest X-ray:** enlarged right heart, prominent pulmonary arteries, pulmonary plethora.
➤ **Echocardiography:**
  - Confirm diagnosis
  - Differentiate type of ASD
  - Characterize for closure (percutaneous/surgical).
➤ **Cardiac catheterization:**
  - Performed in older population to assess pulmonary vascular resistance and to evaluate associated cardiac defects.

Treatment

➤ **ASD closure:** ideally performed at age 2–5 years.
➤ **Indications:**
  - Large left-to-right shunt (defect ≥1 cm diameter, ratio of pulmonary:systemic blood flow ≥1.5:1.0).
  - Small shunt but symptoms secondary to ASD.
➤ Small, asymptomatic shunts require continued follow-up and evaluation every 5 years.
➤ **Contraindications:**
  - Irreversible pulmonary hypertension
  - Congestive heart failure
  - Severe MR.
➤ **Percutaneous ASD closure:**
  - Cardiac catheterization and engagement of specific closure device
  - Suitable for secundum ASD and PFO.
➤ **Surgical closure:**
  - Direct suture or patch repair.

Complications

● Premature death with untreated ASD:
  - Average life expectancy 40 years; 90% mortality by age 60 years.

- Death as a result of heart failure (80–85%) or pulmonary hypertension (15–20%).
- Operative mortality <1%.

Ventricular septal defect

- Hole in interventricular septum; may be primary anomaly or one component within a variety of cardiac anolamies, e.g. tetralogy of Fallot, transposition of the great arteries.
- Results in blood flow from LV to RV; magnitude of left-to-right shunt is key to clinical picture and management.
- Small shunt may be asymptomatic; large shunt results in right and left heart volume overload, presenting as breathlessness, recurrent chest infections, failure to thrive.
- Signs: pink (cyanosis late, in Eisenmenger syndrome – sign of shunt reversal), parasternal heave, loud second heart sound, pansystolic murmur and mid-diastolic flow murmur with moderate to large shunt, signs of heart failure/shock with large ventricular septal defect (VSD).
- Diagnosis confirmed by echocardiography and cardiac catheterization.
- Small VSD may close spontaneously.
- Surgical closure indicated with large VSD, severe symptoms, moderate VSD (causing ≤3:1 shunt) that does not reduce in size over first 5 years of life.
- Contraindications to surgery: small VSD, pulmonary hypertension, Eisenmenger syndrome.
- Complications: infective endocarditis; with moderate to large shunts – pulmonary hypertension, premature death (resulting from heart failure, chest infection).

Patent ductus arteriosus

- Persistence of connection between systemic (distal aortic arch) and pulmonary (left pulmonary artery) circulations following birth, causing left heart volume overload.

- May be asymptomatic or present with failure to thrive, heart failure.
- Signs include continuous murmur (loudest under left clavicle), mitral flow murmur.
- Diagnosis confirmed by echocardiography.
- Presence of clinically detectable patent ductus arteriosus (PDA) is indication for closure.
- Complications of PDA: infective arteritis, aneurysm of ductus, congestive heart failure, progressive pulmonary vascular disease leading to pulmonary hypertension.
- Complications of PDA repair: recurrent laryngeal nerve injury, incomplete closure, recanalization, early complications of thoracotomy.

Tetralogy of Fallot

Definitions

- Tetralogy consists of:
  - RV outflow tract obstruction (pulmonary infundibular stenosis)
  - VSD
  - Right-deviated aorta, overriding the VSD
  - RV hypertrophy.
- Common congenital heart condition, affecting up to 6 in 10 000 births.
- Occurs as a result of unequal division of the conus and truncus arteriosus.
- Key features of pathophysiology are RV outflow tract obstruction and VSD:
  - VSD is usually large
  - Differences in systemic vascular resistance and RV outflow tract obstruction determine size and direction of shunt (right-to-left with severe pulmonary stenosis, left-to-right with minimal stenosis – 'pink tetralogy').

Clinical features

- Cyanosis (blue baby).
- Ejection systolic murmur.

- Continuous murmur in patients with aortopulmonary collaterals.
- Polycythaemia.
- Clubbing.

Investigation

> **Chest X-ray:** 'boot-shaped heart'
> **ECG:** right axis deviation, RV hypertrophy
> **Echocardiography:** to define anatomy
> **Cardiac catheterization:** to assess pulmonary circulation, pressures and resistance, collaterals.

Treatment

> Prostaglandins maintain ductus arteriosus patent, thus maintaining pulmonary blood flow in acutely ill neonate.
> Most patients require surgical intervention; 25% of untreated infants die in first year of life.
> Surgery can achieve either palliation (by systemic to pulmonary shunt or relief of RV outflow tract obstruction) or correction.
> Surgical mortality up to 5%.
> Long-term result of surgery is 90% 5-year survival.

Transposition of the great arteries

- Great vessels reversed: aorta arises from RV, pulmonary artery arises from LV.
- Commonest cyanotic congenital heart defect.
- Occurs as a result of abnormal division of the conus and truncus arteriosus.
- May be coexistent PFO, VSD or PDA.
- Pathophysiology: separate parallel circulations; survival depends on mixing of blood between right and left heart, and cyanosis depends on degree of mixing.
- Signs: cyanosis, congestive heart failure, prominent RV heave, loud heart sounds with single second sound.

Investigation

➤ Chest X-ray: often normal at birth; later egg-shaped heart, narrow cardiac pedicle (aorta and PA), pulmonary plethora.
➤ Echocardiography defines anatomy.
➤ Cardiac catheterization demonstrates atrioventricular connections and coronary anatomy (important consideration for surgical intervention), allows balloon atrial septostomy.

Treatment

➤ If untreated, mortality is 90% within first year.
➤ Short-term measure: balloon atrial septostomy – improve mixing between pulmonary and systemic circulations.
➤ Surgical repair – arterial switch, Rastelli operation or atrial switch (Mustard or Senning operations) – operative mortality 10%.
➤ Long-term outcome after surgery is 90% 5-year survival.

ABDOMEN

ABDOMINAL WALL

Developmental anomalies

Gastroschisis

Definitions

- Absence of the abdominal wall adjacent to the umbilicus with the umbilical cord arising from the edge of the defect.
- Associated with infants of very young mothers.

Clinical features

- Herniation of small and large bowel, stomach and gonads not enclosed in a sac.
- Associated with malrotation and bowel atresias.

Treatment

➤ Protect gut in warm sterile bag; maintain fluid and electrolyte balance.
➤ Gradual reduction of herniated viscera by enclosing in a silastic bag sutured to the margins of the defect followed by repair of the abdominal wall either primarily or with a polypropylene mesh.
➤ Definitive closure once sufficient abdominal wall development.

Exomphalos (omphalocoele)

Definitions

● Caused by failure of the midgut to return to the abdomen during fetal development.
● Incidence: 1:6000 live births.
● It is a midline translucent sac containing any or all abdominal viscera, including the liver with the umbilical cord attached to it.
● Associated with cretinism (congenital hypothyroidism), trisomy 13 chromosomal defect and the Beckwith–Wiedemann syndrome.
● Associated with older mothers.

Clinical features

● A variable-sized thin-walled hernia arising from the centre of the abdomen with the umbilical cord attached close to the apex.
● Sac may rupture during birth.

Treatment

➤ Small sacs are reduced by twisting the cord with firm strapping to hold it in.
➤ Larger sacs may be enclosed in a silastic bag sutured to the edge of the abdominal defect to prevent their rupture, contents being slowly reduced over a period of days or weeks and the defect repaired. Alternately the contents may be enclosed in abdominal skin flaps until the abdomen is sufficiently developed to receive the contents.

ABDOMINAL HERNIAS

Definitions

- Hernias are protrusions of viscera through fascial defects.
- Inguinal hernias are protrusions of abdominal viscera through the inguinal canal. They may be indirect, passing via the deep ring, along the spermatic cord, or direct, emerging through a weakness of the posterior wall of the canal. Both types emerge via the superficial ring, so clinically appear as swellings above and medial to the pubic tubercle. The narrow opening through the abdominal wall is referred to as the neck of the hernial sac. They may extend down to the scrotum – inguinoscrotal hernias. They are much commoner in men than in women (25:1).
- Femoral hernias are protrusions of abdominal viscera through the cribriform fascia covering the saphenous opening in the femoral triangle. They present as a swelling below and lateral to the pubic tubercle. They are small and are at an increased risk of strangulation; they are commoner in women than in men (2.5:1.0).
- Obturator hernias are rare and emerge through the obturator foramen on to the medial aspect of the groin; they are small and susceptible to strangulation.
- Internal hernias occur when a loop of small bowel herniates through a defect in the mesentery, the diaphragm or the pelvic floor.

Clinical features

- External hernia presents as a reducible swelling in the abdominal wall associated with some local discomfort; bowel sounds may be heard and a cough impulse elicited over it.
- Irreducible hernia is painful, and cough impulse and bowel sounds are usually absent over it.
- Strangulation produces severe pain and tenderness with inflammation and oedema of the covering skin.
- In a Richter's hernia a side portion of the bowel wall enters the hernial sac and becomes strangulated (found in femoral and obturator hernias) without signs of bowel obstruction.

Treatment

Inguinal hernias:

➤ Repair (herniorrhaphy) by a variety of methods: mesh repair of the posterior wall of the inguinal canal (Lichtenstein), anatomical approximation of the conjoined tendon to the inguinal ligament (Bassini), or the medial aspect of the conjoined tendon to Cooper's ligament (McVey, suitable for femoral hernias) or a multilayer suture repair (Shouldice).

➤ During operation, the contents of the sac are examined, viable contents reduced and sac excised (herniotomy). Ischaemic bowel is examined after release of the constricting neck of the sac and infarcted (dead) bowel is excised.

➤ Irreducible hernias are operated upon urgently to forestall ischaemic injury, with bowel decompression by nasogastric aspiration and intravenous replacement of fluid and electrolyte loss.

➤ Orchidectomy at the time of repair may be advised in the elderly if the defect is large and the integrity of the posterior wall poor.

➤ In infants and children only herniotomy is performed at the external ring; episodes of incarceration (irreducible without strangulation) are treated by sedation and manual reduction prior to surgery.

Other hernias

● Umbilical hernia in infants and children is herniation through a weak umbilical scar and most regress and disappear by puberty; obstruction or strangulation is rare.

● Incisional hernia is the result of a weakness in the scar of abdominal surgery; contributing factors are wound infection, malnutrition, obesity, postoperative chest infection and abdominal distension; repair is by fascial approximation (keel repair) or by using a polypropylene mesh.

● A Spigelian hernia protrudes between the semilunar line and the lateral rectus border.

- A lumbar hernia is found in the triangle of Petit (between the iliac crest, posterior edge of the external oblique and the anterior edge of the lattisimus dorsi) or through the space bounded by the twelfth rib, serratus posterior inferior and the lateral edge of erector spinae.
- Repair for both is by suture approximation of the bordering fascia or by a mesh overlay.

DIAPHRAGM

Diaphragmatic hernia

Definitions

- The diaphragm is a fibromuscular dome-shaped structure separating the thorax from the abdomen.
- Herniation of abdominal contents into the thorax occurs in congenital defects at the foramen of Morgagni (anterior), the oesophageal hiatus and the foramen of Bochdalek (posterolateral).

Clinical features

- Present soon after birth with respiratory distress.
- Scaphoid abdomen and apparent dextrocardia.

Investigation

➤ Imaging evidence of stomach or bowel in the hemithorax.

Treatment

➤ Urgent nasogastric suction to relieve compression on the thoracic viscera.
➤ Resuscitation followed by surgical repair of the defect.

Traumatic rupture of the diaphragm

Definitions

Small perforations:

- Associated injuries are more significant
- Aetiology: penetrating trauma.

Large radial tear:

- Typically of left hemidiaphragm
- Aetiology: severe blunt abdominal or thoracic trauma.

Clinical features

- Incidental finding on imaging, laparotomy or thoracotomy for associated injuries.
- Bowel sounds in chest.

Investigation

➤ Chest X-ray:
  - Apparently raised hemidiaphragm
  - Apparent gastric dilatation
  - Apparent effusion/collection in lower chest.
➤ Contrast X-rays/chest CT: confirm diagnosis.

Treatment

➤ Surgical repair at laparotomy or thoracotomy.

Eventration of the diaphragm

- A rare condition found in adults and mistaken for an old diaphragmatic rupture or a congenital diaphragmatic hernia.
- Abnormally elevated left hemidiaphragm caused by muscle atrophy or paralysis.
- Minimally symptomatic.
- In the presence of paradoxical breathing, surgical plication of the redundant diaphragm may be indicated.

ACUTE ABDOMEN

Acute intestinal obstruction in the newborn

Congenital atresias

Definitions

- Maldevelopment of segment(s) of bowel resulting in the absence or narrowing of the lumen.

- Causes neonatal bowel obstruction in 1:2000 births.
- Results from antenatal vascular or mechanical events that compromise local blood supply and arrest development.
- Associated with mesenteric abnormality and malrotation causing volvulus.

Clinical features

Small bowel atresia/stenosis:

- Vomiting in the neonate; contains bile if the obstructing septum lies below the duodenal papilla.
- Central abdominal distension in jejunal or ileal obstruction.
- Peritonism suggests vascular compromise.

Investigation

➤ Plain abdominal X-ray: in duodenal obstruction, stomach and proximal duodenum are distended – 'double bubble'; in jejunal and ileal obstruction air–fluid levels may be present.

Treatment

➤ Correct fluid and electrolyte deficits.
➤ Duodenal atresia requires duodenojejunostomy and splinting of the anastomosis with a feeding tube.
➤ Atretic segments in the jejunum or ileum may produce dilated proximal loops that require tapering prior to anastomosis.

Malrotation and neonatal volvulus

Definitions

- Small bowel mesentery is normally fixed at two points: at the duodenojejunal flexure and at the ileocaecal region.
- Arrest of normal rotation leaves the caecum in the left hypochondrium with a band running across and compressing the second part of the duodenum.

- Arrested rotation predisposes to midgut volvulus with the whole small bowel twisting on a narrow mesentery.

Clinical features

- Vomiting with central abdominal distension and dehydration.

Investigation

➤ Plain X-ray of the small bowel gas shows malrotation and level of obstruction.

Treatment

➤ The volvulus is reduced, the transduodenal band (Ladd's band) divided, the duodenum mobilized and the mesentery freed.
➤ Appendicectomy is routinely performed to avoid diagnostic difficulty with appendicitis in the future.
➤ Infarcted bowel necessitates resection.

Meckel's diverticulum

Definitions

- A remnant of the vitello-intestinal tract found on the anti-mesenteric border of the terminal ileum and may extend to the umbilicus as a fistula.
- Rarely it contains ectopic gastric mucosa or a carcinoid tumour.

Clinical features

- Usually an incidental finding at surgery.
- When inflamed, the clinical presentation is similar to that of acute appendicitis.

Investigation

➤ Differential white cell count is raised.
➤ A Meckel's radioisotope scan may reveal acid-producing gastric mucosa.

Treatment

➤ Excision of the inflamed diverticulum.
➤ Presence of gastric mucosa requires the resection of the ileal loop containing the diverticulum to ensure complete excision of all acid-producing mucosa.

Meconium ileus

Definitions

● Associated with cystic fibrosis, with sticky meconium impacting in the terminal ileum.
● Also associated with atresia, volvulus and meconium peritonitis.

Clinical features

● Infant is born with small bowel obstruction, presenting with progressive abdominal distension and bile-stained vomiting.
● A rubbery mass of inspissated meconium may be palpable.

Investigation

➤ Plain X-ray: shows dilated small bowel loops.
➤ Gastrografin enema (in the absence of acute obstruction) shows up the meconium and excludes Hirschsprung's disease.

Treatment

➤ Colonic washouts may restore patency.
➤ Proximal ileum is anastomosed end-to-side to the colon with a distal ileostomy to clear the obstruction.

Bowel obstruction

Definitions

● Dynamic: presents as an emergency and the obstruction may be in the lumen (food bolus, gallstone), the bowel wall (inflammatory stricture, intussusception or tumour) or outside the bowel (adhesions, hernia, volvulus or mesenteric vascular occlusion).

● Adynamic: occurs after abdominal surgery or is secondary to electrolyte imbalance, sepsis, chronic renal failure or retroperitoneal haematoma.

Clinical features

● Acute small bowel obstruction: severe, central colicky abdominal pain with vomiting leading to distension and rapid fluid and electrolyte loss.
● Chronic obstruction usually involves the large bowel with gradual onset of colic in the flanks or the lower abdomen with progressive distension and constipation.
● Subacute obstruction is when there is a partial obstruction with intermittent obstructive signs.
● Strangulation obstruction presents as a severe, persisting pain superimposed on colicky pain of obstruction with signs of peritoneal irritation.
● A competent ileocaecal valve in colonic obstruction may result in a closed loop obstruction with a distended caecum.

Investigation

➤ Plain abdominal X-ray reveals characteristics of the distended bowel from which the level of obstruction is identified.
➤ Contrast-enhanced computerized tomography (CT) scan delineates the type and level of obstruction.

Treatment

➤ Nasogastric decompression of stomach and bowel proximal to the obstruction.
➤ Intravenous fluid and electrolyte therapy and adequate analgesia (inflammatory or infective causes require antibiotics).

➔

> ➤ Emergency surgery is required to relieve the
> obstruction and may involve resection of the affected
> loop of bowel; dilated proximal bowel may require
> surgical decompression before bowel continuity is
> safely re-established (usually by means of a temporary
> stoma covering the anastomosis); in the presence of
> sepsis or poor viability, the proximal and distal bowel
> loops are exteriorized until viability is restored.
> ➤ Postoperative adhesion obstruction usually resolves on
> conservative measures.

Pseudo-obstruction

- Found in chronically ill or bed-ridden patients or
  following fracture of the femoral neck; presents with
  constipation and gradual abdominal distension.
- Autonomic dysfunction inhibits bowel motility
  and is associated with electrolyte or metabolic
  abnormality.
- Gastrografin enema demonstrates unhindered flow
  of contrast up to the caecum and beyond.
- Relief of constipation requires bowel washouts or
  manual evacuation.

Intussusception

Definitions

- Telescoping of a bowel loop into adjoining distal loop,
  typically the terminal ileum into the caecum and colon,
  as a result of increased peristaltic activity.
- An intraluminal lesion (hyperplastic submucosal
  lymphoid tissue or polyp) forms the nidus for the
  intussusception.
- Occurs during weaning in the very young (changes in
  the bowel flora producing lymphoid hyperplasia)
  and as a complication of acquired immunodeficiency
  syndrome-related gastroenteritis or polyps (polyposis
  coli or Peutz–Jeghers syndrome) in adults.
- 80% of incidences occur in patients under 2 years
  of age.

Clinical features

- Sudden onset of colicky abdominal pain with drawing up of legs and vomiting, with hyperactive bowel sounds (in the child).
- Passage of blood-stained mucoid motions ('redcurrant jelly' stools).
- Palpable, mobile abdominal mass that may be also felt rectally.
- Abdominal distension and peritonism are late features.

Investigation

➤ Double-contrast Gastrografin enema ('claw sign' of ileocolic intussusception).
➤ In adults, a contrast-enhanced CT scan of the abdomen or barium enema is confirmatory.

Treatment

➤ The diagnostic enema may be used to reduce the intussusception by hydrostatic pressure (in the child).
➤ Surgical reduction by taxis; bowel resection (right hemicolectomy) if there is gross oedema preventing reduction or vascular compromise.

Volvulus of the bowel

Definitions

- Caused by axial rotation of a loop of bowel, typically the sigmoid colon, but sometimes the caecum if abnormal development results in a large mesentery.
- An unusually large meal and redundant mesentery predispose to volvulus.
- Sigmoid volvulus – typically affects elderly, chronically debilitated patients.

Clinical features

- Colicky abdominal pain with retching or hiccups followed by distension.
- May be intermittently relieved, with sudden passage of flatus and liquid stool.

Investigation

➤ Plain abdominal X-ray may be diagnostic:
  – Large, gas-filled, 'kidney bean-shaped' swelling in the right upper zone: sigmoid volvulus.
  – Large, gas-filled, 'kidney bean-shaped' swelling in the left lower zone: caecal volvulus.

Treatment

➤ Sigmoid volvulus may be relieved at rigid sigmoidoscopy.
➤ Emergency laparotomy and resection of the volvulus for strangulated or recurrent cases.
➤ Gangrenous bowel is exteriorized and resected, with the formation of a 'double-barrel' colostomy (Paul–Mikulicz procedure).

Appendicitis

Definitions

● Appendicitis is the commonest cause of an acute abdomen and is caused by luminal obstruction leading to inflammation and gangrene.
● Associated factors are diets low in residue and high in animal fats, and purgative abuse.
● Complications: an inflammatory mass, abscess or perforation.

Clinical features

● Central abdominal pain that shifts to the right iliac fossa.
● Nausea, anorexia with occasional vomiting and furring of the tongue/fetor oris.
● Low-grade pyrexia 37–38°C.
● Localized tenderness, rebound tenderness and guarding at McBurney's point.
● Compression of left iliac fossa may cause right iliac fossa pain (Rosvig's sign).
● Retrocaecal appendicitis may produce psoas spasm elicited by passive hyperextension of the hip (psoas sign).
● Para-ileal or a pelvic appendicitis may produce diarrhoea and is tender on rectal examination.

- A swinging pyrexia and a palpable, tender swelling suggest an inflammatory mass (phlegmon) or abscess.
- Generalized peritonitis if perforation occurs.

Investigation
➤ Leukocytosis and raised CRP titre.
➤ Urinalysis to eliminate a urinary infection.
➤ Pregnancy test to exclude early pregnancy.

Treatment
➤ Urgent appendicectomy; peritoneal toilet if there is contamination, with parenteral antibiotic therapy (cefuroxime 750 mg 8-hourly or cefoxitin 1–2 g 8-hourly for 5–7 days).
➤ Appendix mass is treated with intravenous fluids, antibiotics and analgesia with 4-hourly observations of vital signs; resolution is usually complete and interval appendicectomy may not be indicated.
➤ Appendix abscess is drained extraperitoneally and may require interval appendicectomy.

Acute mesenteric adenitis
- Inflammation of the mesenteric nodes in infants and children with similar clinical features to acute appendicitis, but is self-limiting.

Intestinal ischaemia (see page 568)

Peritonitis

Definitions
- Inflammation of the peritoneal cavity, which may be localized or generalized and invariably caused by bacterial invasion.
- Infection may be from the bowel (*Escherichia coli*, aerobic/anaerobic *Streptococcus* spp, *Bacteroides* spp, *Clostridium welchii* or *C. perfringens*), from the female genital tract (*Pneumococcus* spp, *Gonococcus* spp), blood-borne (beta-haemolytic *Streptococcus* spp, *Mycobacterium tuberculosis*) or iatrogenic, following surgery or peritoneal dialysis.

- Primary peritonitis is rare and is of uncertain causation (pneumococcal peritonitis).
- Perforated peptic ulcer, perforated diverticular disease, perforated appendicitis, perforated gallbladder; rupture of the bladder or ectopic pregnancy and pancreatitis – these fluids may initially be sterile but quickly become secondarily infected.
- Anastomotic leak.

Clinical features

- Local or general abdominal tenderness with guarding or rigidity, percussion rebound and reduced or absent bowel sounds.
- Localized peritonitis:
  - Malaise, fever, severe constant abdominal pain, worse on movement nausea/vomiting
  - Signs specific to visceral inflammation (e.g. cholecystitis, appendicitis, diverticulitis)
- Generalized peritonitis:
  - Patient is anxious and lies still with severe generalized abdominal pain and nausea or thirst
  - Silent abdomen with generalized tenderness and rigidity
  - Dehydration, confusion, peripheral vascular shutdown, leading to toxaemia and coma.

Investigation

- Raised white blood cell count and CRP titre and fluid and electrolyte derangement.
- Plain X-ray reveals gas or fluid collection outside the viscera and dilated loops of bowel.
- Abdominal ultrasound or CT scan may identify fluid collections and cause of sepsis.

Treatment

- Correct fluid and electrolyte imbalance: monitor fluid replacement with central venous pressure readings and urinary output.
- Adequate parenteral analgesia and broad-spectrum antibiotic therapy.

→

> ➤ Supplemental oxygen therapy with monitoring of arterial blood gases and pH.
> ➤ Surgical control of sepsis (removal of perforated appendix, inflamed or necrotic bowel, closure of a perforation or an anastomotic leak) with peritoneal lavage.
> ➤ Complications: bacterial toxaemia resulting in renal or respiratory failure, residual sepsis, adhesive bowel obstruction and incisional hernia.

Intra-abdominal abscess

- Caused by loculation of infected fluid in a peritoneal recess following surgery (anastomotic leak) or as a result of visceral perforation with localized sepsis, and some tropical infections (page 134).
- May present with minimal constitutional symptoms.
- Often identified on CT in critically ill patients with unexplained fever, sepsis or acidosis.
- May point to the abdominal wall with inflammatory induration of the overlying skin, at a recent surgical wound or drain site, at the diaphragm (subphrenic abscess), vaginal fornix or rectum (pelvic abscess).
- Contrast-enhanced CT scan or a gallium scan of the abdomen defines the site.
- Drainage of the abscess (or collection) by image-guided aspiration per abdomen, per rectum or per vaginam; open surgical drainage may be performed retro-peritoneally when the abscess is adherent to the parietal peritoneum or by entering the peritoneal cavity.

ABDOMINAL TRAUMA

General principles

Definitions

- Aetiology:
  - Blunt trauma: motor vehicle accidents, assaults with blunt weapons
  - Penetrating trauma: knife wound, ballistic injury (page 605).

Clinical features

- Bruising, abrasion, penetrating wounds over the abdomen or lower chest.
- Concealed haemorrhage: splenic, liver and vascular injury:
  - Haemodynamic changes or shock immediately
  - Abdominal distension: dull to percussion
  - Peritonism
  - Generalized or localized tenderness and guarding
  - Bowel sounds absent.
- Peritonitis: gastrointestinal injury:
  - Haemodynamic changes or shock hours afterwards
  - Generalized tenderness and guarding
  - Bowel sounds absent.

Investigation

➤ Intervention without investigation: shock, peritonitis.
➤ Chest X-ray: free gas indicates gastrointestinal injury.
➤ Diagnostic peritoneal lavage.
  - Indications:
    - Uncertain findings
    - Unreliable findings: head injury, alcohol
    - Suspected concealed haemorrhage without abdominal signs
    - Knife wounds where the peritoneum is breached, but without abdominal signs or haemodynamic instability
    - Abdominal CT.
  - Procedure – diagnostic peritoneal lavage:
    - Bladder is emptied with a catheter
    - Lignocaine 1% is infiltrated
    - Vertical midline incision one-third of the way down from the umbilicus two-thirds of the way above the symphysis pubis
    - Dissect down to and open the peritoneum
    - Pass a peritoneal dialysis catheter into the peritoneal cavity
    - Aspirate
    - Run in 1 L of warm saline and leave for 3 minutes
    - Place the bag on the floor and allow the fluid to run out

➜

– 20 mL of the fluid is sent for laboratory analysis.
- Positive result:
  – Visible blood on aspiration
  – Red blood cells $>10^9$/L
  – Bile, bacteria or faecal material.
➤ Abdominal CT.
➤ Explore knife wounds under local anaesthesia or instil water-soluble contrast medium into wound to assess whether peritoneum is breached.

Treatment

➤ Laparotomy.
- Indications in abdominal trauma:
  – Shock
  – Peritonitis
  – Evisceration
  – Ballistic penetrating trauma
  – Free gas on chest X-ray
  – Ruptured diaphragm on chest X-ray or CT
  – Positive peritoneal lavage.
- Action:
  – Pack sites of haemorrhage to allow resuscitation
  – Deal with source of haemorrhage: splenectomy, tie off/suture bleeding vessels
  – Close gastrointestinal lacerations: exteriorize if further breakdown is likely
  – Remove grossly disrupted and non-viable viscera.
- Excessive transfusion need and continued instability:
  – Limit duration of surgery to 1 hour
  – Pack abdomen and cover wound: closure may result in abdominal compartment syndrome
  – Transfer to intensive care for support
  – Second-look laparotomy when stabilized.

Stomach

- Usually injured in penetrating trauma, but, rarely, may rupture in blunt trauma.
- A tear into the lesser sac may be missed.
- Treatment: suture repair at laparotomy.

Duodenum

Definitions

- Rupture of the second part of the duodenum.
- Aetiology: compression by a lap seat-belt during deceleration in a motor vehicle accident.

Clinical features

- Blood in nasogastric tube.
- Peritonitis: may not develop in retroperitoneal injury.
- Unexplained sepsis and ileus.

Investigation

➤ Abdominal X-ray: loss of psoas shadow, retroperitoneal gas.
➤ X-ray/CT with nasogastric tube contrast: may demonstrate a leak.
➤ Abdominal CT: periduodenal haematoma.

Treatment
➤ Surgical repair at laparotomy.

Small bowel

- Usually injured in penetrating trauma, but may also be lacerated in blunt trauma.
- Treatment: suture repair at laparotomy; non-viable areas are resected.

Colon

- Usually injured in penetrating trauma, but may also be lacerated in blunt trauma.
- Treatment:
  - Penetrating wounds may be sutured at laparotomy, often with a proximal defunctioning stoma
  - Non-viable areas are resected and the ends brought out as a double-barrelled colostomy
  - Stomas are usually closed after 6 weeks.

Rectum

- Usually injured in penetrating trauma or severe pelvic fracture.
- Treatment:
  - Surgery to create an end sigmoid colostomy, lavage the rectum and drain the pelvis.
  - Once healing has occurred, further surgery can be undertaken to repair anal sphincters and reverse the colostomy.

GYNAECOLOGICAL EMERGENCIES

Ectopic pregnancy

Definitions

- Implantation of the fertilized ovum outside the uterus, nearly always in the fallopian tube (intraperitoneal implantation is very rare).
- Incidence 1 for every 300 deliveries.
- Associated factors:
  - Pelvic inflammatory disease
  - Intrauterine devices
  - Migration of the ovum towards the corpus luteum on the opposite side
  - Endocrine abnormalities and treatment of infertility.
- Tubal pregnancy usually ends in rupture of the gestational sac and death of the ovum at 8–12 weeks.
- Rupture into the lumen results in tubal abortion with little bleeding.
- Rupture through the tubal wall into the peritoneal cavity results in significant bleeding.
- Rupture into the broad ligament (rare) results in a broad ligament haematoma.

Clinical features

- Severe lower abdominal pain.
- A missed period.
- Signs and symptoms of early pregnancy are usually present.
- 'Vaginal spotting' may be present (dark brown and scanty).

- Initial presentation may be identical to acute appendicitis when right-sided.
- Signs of intraperitoneal haemorrhage:
  - Faintness or dizziness
  - Rapid low volume pulse
  - Hypotension
  - Referred pain to shoulder tip.
- Abdominal examination: tender in an iliac fossa with muscle guarding and rebound tenderness (peritonism).
- Generalized tenderness suggests haemoperitoneum.
- Pelvic examination: extreme tenderness over the gravid tube, uterus, or in the pouch of Douglas.

Investigation

➤ Beta-human chorionic gonadotrophin (HCG) pregnancy test is positive in early pregnancy.
➤ Abdominal ultrasound scan reveals haemoperitoneum and a gestational sac.
➤ Transvaginal scan defines the ectopic pregnancy.
➤ Laparoscopy provides a definitive diagnosis in doubtful cases.

Treatment

➤ Resuscitate if in haemorrhagic shock, with volume expansion by blood transfusion.
➤ Emergency laparotomy and salpingectomy (or salpingo-oophorectomy) controls bleeding.
➤ Conservation of a minimally damaged tube may be attempted under specific conditions but there is an increased risk of further ectopic pregnancies on that side.
➤ Abortion of a tubal pregnancy prior to rupture may be attempted by laparoscopic instillation of mifepristone and prostaglandins through the fimbriated end.

Complications

- Cervical pregnancy: a rare ectopic site with the risk of severe bleeding requiring hysterectomy.
- Ovarian pregnancy: a rare ectopic site with features similar to a tubal ectopic pregnancy.

Acute pelvic inflammatory disease (page 543)

Septic abortion

Definitions

- This is a uterine infection at any stage of an abortion.
- May present as an acute abdomen or with the patient in septic shock.
- Causes:
  - Delay in evacuating the uterus
  - Trauma to the cervix or uterus during non-therapeutic (illegal) abortion.
- Causative organisms: vaginal or bowel commensals (anaerobic coliforms or streptococci, *Bacteroides fragilis, Clostridium welchii*).

Clinical features

- Elicit history of recent abortion.
- Fever with tachycardia.
- Slight vaginal bleeding.
- Pelvic tenderness.

Investigation

➤ Leukocytosis.
➤ Raised CRP.
➤ Cervical and high vaginal smears for culture and sensitivity.
➤ Aerobic and anaerobic blood cultures.

Treatment

➤ Commence systemic broad-spectrum antibiotics.
➤ Uterine curettage to remove infected retained products of conception.
➤ Uterine perforation with peritonitis may require surgical exploration and hysterectomy.
➤ Monitor and support renal function.

Torsion of ovarian pedicle or cyst

Definitions

- Associated with benign follicular cysts or, rarely, with an ovarian tumour.
- A self-limiting condition.
- May cause intraperitoneal bleeding from venous occlusion.

Clinical features

- Subacute presentation: recurrent lower abdominal pain (caused by twisting and untwisting of pedicle).
- Acute presentation: sudden onset of severe lower abdominal pain, nausea and vomiting.
- Differential diagnosis:
  - Acute appendicitis
  - Acute diverticulitis
  - Ectopic pregnancy
  - Acute pelvic inflammation
  - Rupture of ovarian cyst
  - Torsion of a fibroid
  - Ovulation bleeding
  - Endometriosis.

Investigation

➤ Normal white cell count.
➤ Normal CRP.
➤ Abdominal or transvaginal ultrasound scan.
➤ Laparoscopic examination and ovarian biopsy.

Treatment

➤ Symptomatic measures if the cause is benign and non-recurrent.
➤ Removal of the ovary is advised if associated ovarian pathology is suspected.
➤ Rupture of an ovarian cyst is self-limiting.

OESOPHAGUS

Congenital anomalies

Atresia and stenosis

Definitions

- These are anatomical defects of blind oesophageal pouches with or without tracheal communications.
- Present at birth.
- The commonest anomaly is a dilated upper pouch with the distal oesophagus fistulating into the trachea.

Clinical features

- Spluttering and choking during feeds, with coughing and cyanosis.
- Bronchopneumonia results from repeated aspiration of feeds.

Investigation

In the newborn:

➤ Establish oesophageal patency by passing a nasal catheter (8–10 French) into the stomach and aspirating gastric contents (turns litmus paper pink).

➤ Obstruction to the passage of the catheter at 10 cm suggests atresia and instillation of 1 mL of dionosil with screening delineates the proximal pouch (or tracheal fistulation), while air in the stomach indicates fistulation of the lower oesophagus into the trachea.

Treatment

➤ Extrapleural repair through a right thoracotomy with excision of the atretic segment and the fistula.

Complications

- Bronchopneumonia.
- Anastomotic leak resulting in mediastinitis.

Achalasia of the cardia

Definitions

- A developmental motility disorder with functional narrowing of the lower end of the oesophagus and hypertrophy of the circular muscle fibres.
- Results in intermittent chronic obstruction and stasis, leading to oesophagitis.
- Predisposes to malignancy.

Clinical features

- History of progressive dysphagia to solids.
- Fetid flatulence.
- Retrosternal discomfort.
- Episodes of aspiration pneumonia.

Investigation

➤ Plain radiology: absence of gastric 'air bubble'.
➤ Oesophagoscopy or barium swallow: narrowed segment with gross proximal dilatation and stasis.
➤ Oesophageal manometry: uncoordinated peristalsis and poor sphincter relaxation.

Treatment

➤ Hydrostatic (balloon) dilatation of the stenosed segment and oesophageal sphincter under screening to a diameter of 30–40 mm (50% success rate).
➤ Oesophagocardiomyotomy (Heller's operation) by open surgery or laparoscopically: division of the lower oesophageal sphincter extending to 2–3 cm onto the anterior cardia (90% success rate).
➤ Endoscopic botulinum toxin injection provides irreversible neuromuscular blockade in the lower oesophagus (as effective as balloon dilatation).

Oesophageal perforation

Definitions

- Swallowed foreign bodies or corrosives.
- Penetrating wounds.

- Tear in the lower posterior wall during forceful retching or vomiting (Boerhaave's syndrome).
- Iatrogenic injury during endoscopic dilatation or stenting.

Clinical features

Spontaneous tear of the oesophagus produces:

- Severe retrosternal pain leading to shock with rapid, small volume pulse
- Hypotension, pyrexia and rapid, shallow breathing with reduced air entry
- Surgical emphysema in supraclavicular fossae
- Epigastric tenderness (variable)
- Mediastinitis (late manifestation).

Differential diagnosis:

- Myocardial infarction
- Peptic ulcer perforation
- Dissecting thoracic aneurysm
- Volvulus of the stomach.

Investigation

➤ Plain chest radiology: mediastinal emphysema, hydropneumothorax.
➤ Spiral computerized tomography (CT) scan or flexible oesphagoscopy identifies site of tear.
➤ Gastrografin swallow also identifies site with extravasation of contrast into the posterior mediastinum.

Treatment

➤ Small tears with minimal pleural contamination may be safely treated with nasogastric suction, intravenous fluid and antibiotic therapy, and the injury reassessed endoscopically or with a Gastrografin swallow (over 3–5 days).
➤ Larger tears with respiratory compromise and pleural soilage require immediate thoracotomy with closure of the perforation and chest drainage.
➤ Postoperative ventilatory support, parenteral antibiotic therapy and feeding are required.

Dysphagia

Definitions

- Difficulty in swallowing with sensation of slowing or arrest of food bolus in the oesophagus.

Causes are:

- Benign stricture secondary to gastro-oesophageal reflux
- Corrosive stricture
- Carcinoma, adenoma, leiomyoma
- Chagas' disease
- Pharyngeal webs
- Post-traumatic, post-radiation strictures
- Dismotility: achalasia, oesophageal spasm, bulbar palsy, CVAs
- Globus hystericus
- Schatzki's ring – scleroderma
- Extrinsic causes: goitre, pharyngeal pouch, aortic aneurysm, abnormal vessels, mediastinal tumours, para-oesophageal hiatus hernia.

Clinical features

Pain on swallowing (odynophagia) is found in:

- Reflux oesophagitis
- Peptic ulceration of the lower oesophagus
- Infections: candidiasis and herpes simplex and cytomegalovirus
- Diffuse oesophageal spasm (idiopathic)
- Slowly progressive dysphagia or pain is suggestive of carcinoma.

Investigation

➤ Oesophagogastroscopy.
➤ Barium swallow.
➤ Manometry and pH study.
➤ Spiral CT scan may reveal cause of extrinsic compression (carcinoma of the bronchus, hilar lymphadenopathy, left atrial enlargement).

Treatment

Treat underlying pathology:

➤ Benign strictures respond well to dilatation
➤ Malignant strictures: (page 421 Carcinoma of oesophagus)
➤ Mega-oesophagus in Chagas' disease may respond to nifurtimox or benznidazole used in systemic treatment.

Gastro-oesophageal reflux disease

Definitions

- Most sufferers do not have an obvious cause.
- Hiatus hernia: herniation of the intra-abdominal oesophagus and gastro-oesophageal junction into the chest.
- Scleroderma: replacement of circular muscle of the oesophagus with fibrous tissue.
- Diabetes mellitus: autonomic neuropathy producing gastric stasis.
- Obesity.

Oesophagitis and hiatus hernia

Definitions

- Acute inflammation usually results from corrosive ingestion.
- Chronic inflammation of the lower oesophagus results from acid reflux (gastro-oesophageal reflux disease).

Anti-reflux mechanisms preventing gastric contents from entering the oesophagus are:

- Normal oesophageal clearance
- Normal lower oesophageal sphincter function
- Normal gastric clearance.

Sliding hiatus hernia is caused by:

- Incompetence of the physiological sphincter at the cardia
- Shortening of the oesophagus as a result of chronic inflammation, thereby pulling the cardia into the chest

- Degeneration of the crura as a result of ageing
- Increased intra-abdominal pressure and fatty infiltration of the hiatus are probable causes.

Rolling hiatus hernia is caused by:

- A defect in the dome of the diaphragm into which a portion of the stomach herniates; this may produce an intermittent volvulus of the stomach or, rarely, strangulation.

Clinical features

Sliding hiatus hernia:

- Dyspepsia with epigastric and/or retrosternal pain radiating to the back or neck
- Heartburn, water-brash and dysphagia
- Symptoms are exacerbated when the patient is lying flat.

Rolling hiatus hernia:

- Does not produce reflux oesophagitis, as the competence at the cardia is unimpaired
- Symptoms are from pressure effects on lung or mediastinum
- Volvulus of the herniated part of the stomach may produce epigastric or chest pain radiating to the upper back.

Investigation

➤ Upper gastrointestinal endoscopy: identifies the cause (except in motility disorder) and provides mucosal biopsy.
➤ Barium swallow and meal in the head-down position demonstrates either hernia.
➤ Normochromic, normocytic anaemia may be present.
➤ Faecal occult bloods may be positive.

Treatment

The vast majority of cases respond to non-surgical measures.

➤ Weight reduction.
➤ Small, frequent meals.

→

- ➤ Postural advice.
- ➤ Oral alginates (Gaviscon 1–2 tablets chewed at night) reduces acid reflux for mild symptoms.
- ➤ Long-term H_2 receptor blockade (ranitidine 300 mg at night for 8–12 weeks) or intermittent proton pump inhibition (omeprazole 20 mg daily for 4 weeks) controls symptoms in more severe disease.
- ➤ Correct anaemia.
- ➤ Sliding hernia: anti-reflux surgery is reserved for intractable or progressive disease; it ensures at least 4 cm of terminal oesophagus is prevented from herniating back into the chest, restores the gastro-oesophageal angle and reduces the laxity of the hiatus. The higher intra-abdominal pressure then closes this segment of the oesophagus, thus preventing the reflux of gastric juice. Surgery may be through the chest (Belsey Mark IV operation), through the abdomen or laparoscopically (Nissen fundoplication or the Hill repair).
- ➤ Rolling (para-oesophageal) hernia, even when asymptomatic, must be surgically reduced and the defect in the diaphragm repaired because of the risk of acute dilatation or volvulus and strangulation of the herniated part of the stomach.

Complications

Oesophageal stricture resulting from reflux oesophagitis:

- Most patients are old and frail and carcinoma must be excluded
- These strictures respond well to dilatation
- Anti-reflux surgery following dilatation is rarely required.

Barrett's oesophagus:

- Is the presence of columnar lined epithelium in >3 cm of the distal oesophagus
- May present as a benign stricture or an ulcer
- Is associated with chronic gastro-oesophageal reflux disease
- High grade dysplasia may progress to adenocarcinoma and is an indication for oesophagectomy.

Chronic oesophageal obstruction

Definitions

- Extrinsic causes: para-oesophageal hernia, mediastinal lesions (thymic tumour, thoracic aneurysm, hilar adenopathy, left atrial dilatation).
- Lesions in the wall: scleroderma, aganglionosis, benign and malignant strictures, diverticulae, Chagas' disease.
- Luminal causes: swallowed foreign body, post-cricoid web.

Clinical features

- Dysphagia of varying severity.

Treatment
➤ Treat as per cause.

Oesophageal web (Plummer–Vinson syndrome)

Definitions

- Affects middle-aged women.
- Is a post-cricoid oesophageal mucosal web associated with iron-deficiency anaemia.
- Is premalignant in long-standing disease.

Clinical features

- Progressive difficulty in swallowing.
- Severe retching spells.
- Fear of choking.
- Smooth, pale tongue.
- Angular stomatitis.
- Koilonychia.

Investigation
➤ Hypochromic (iron-deficiency) anaemia precedes symptoms.
➤ Achlorhydria may be present.
➤ Oesophagoscopy or barium swallow identifies the lesion.

Treatment
➤ Dilatation of the web.
➤ Oral iron therapy.
➤ A balanced diet.

Oesophageal ring

Definitions

● Schatzki's ring is an idiopathic fibrous constriction ring at the squamocolumnar junction of the lower oesophagus.

Clinical features

● Dysphagia.

Treatment
➤ Endoscopic dilatation.
➤ Control of reflux with posture and oral alginates.

Carcinoma

Definitions

● Incidence: highest in USA, Middle East, India and parts of China and Russia (6:100 000).
● Squamous carcinoma (95% of all cases occurring in upper and middle oesophagus).
● Adenocarcinoma (mainly lower oesophagus) arising in a Barrett's oesophagus (5% of all cases).
● Manifests as an annular, stenosing, ulcerating or, rarely, a friable fungating lesion.
● Dissemination:
  – Lymphatic (mediastinal and supraclavicular nodes)
  – Blood (liver and bone)
  – Direct extension to neighbouring structures (trachea, bronchus, lung or aorta).
● 70% of patients have extraoesophageal dissemination at diagnosis.

Clinical features

● Retrosternal discomfort.
● Dysphagia progressing from solids to liquids.

- Regurgitation.
- Haematemesis.
- Retrosternal pain is usually a late manifestation.
- Malnutrition and weight loss.

Investigation

➤ Barium swallow.
➤ Oesophagoscopy and biopsy for confirmation.
➤ Endoluminal ultrasonography and liver CT scan for disease staging.
➤ Bronchoscopy to exclude fistulation of middle third growths into the bronchial tree.

Treatment

➤ Oesophageal resection (total or subtotal) with restoration of continuity with gastric, colonic or jejunal interposition, performed through abdominothoracic, three phase (cervical, thoracic, abdominal) or transhiatal (abdominocervical) approaches.
➤ Primary radiotherapy for squamous carcinoma is a non-surgical option in the medically unfit.
➤ Palliation for advanced disease is by oesophageal intubation, endoluminal laser therapy and/or chemoradiotherapy.

Oesophageal varices

Definitions

- Portal hypertension produces varices at the gastro-oesophageal junction and the anorectum where there is communication between portal and systemic circulations.
- Gastro-oesophageal varices are clinically significant as they cause life-threatening haemorrhage.

Clinical features

- Haematemesis and/or melaena.
- Clinical evidence of portal hypertension.
- Stigmata of liver disease.

Investigation

➤ Oesophagoscopy or barium swallow is diagnostic.
➤ Gastroduodenoscopy excludes other causes of upper gastrointestinal haemorrhage.

Treatment

Non-bleeding varices:

➤ Endoscopic sclerotherapy or banding of varices
➤ Long-term lowering of venous pressure with propranolol 40–80 mg once or twice daily.

Acute haemorrhage:

➤ Endoscopic balloon tamponade of bleeding varices
➤ Splanchnic venoconstriction by intravenous infusion of vasopressin (or somatostatin) 20 units over 15 minutes.

Uncontrolled haemorrhage:

➤ Oesophageal transection or devascularization
➤ Portosystemic shunt surgery provides long-term palliation in patients with Child's A and B liver function gradings.

STOMACH AND DUODENUM

Gastric physiology

Definitions

● Vomiting (emesis) is a sequence of events coordinated by the vomiting trigger zone in the medulla: anorexia, nausea, salivation, retching, reverse peristalsis with strong contractions of the diaphragm and abdominal wall, thereby extruding the stomach contents.
● Vagotomy (surgical division of the vagus) reduces acid secretion, gastric emptying, bile and pancreatic secretions and increases faecal fat excretion; may result in the postvagotomy syndrome of dumping and diarrhoea.

Hypertrophic pyloric stenosis

Definitions

- Affects neonates and infants (incidence of 3–4:1000).
- Produces intermittent gastric outlet obstruction as a result of hypertrophy of the circular muscle fibres of the pylorus.

Clinical features

- Visible upper abdominal peristalsis on feeding.
- 'Projectile' vomiting following feeds.
- Vomitus is not bile-stained.
- Palpable abdominal swelling after feeds.
- Dehydration and weight loss are present when diagnosis is delayed.

Investigation

Imaging is unnecessary.

Treatment

Pyloromyotomy (Ramstedt's operation):

➤ Through a small incision in the right upper quadrant, the pylorus is exposed and the hypertrophied circular muscles divided, care being taken not to breach the pyloric mucosa.

Duodenal atresia

Definitions

- Results in stenosis of the duodenum at the point of fusion of the foregut and midgut, close to the ampulla of Vater.

Clinical features

- Bile-stained vomitus from birth.
- Rapid weight loss.

Investigation
➤ 'Double bubble' appearance on plain radiology (contrast imaging is rarely required).

Treatment
➤ Duodenojejunostomy: side-to-side anastomosis of the first part of the duodenum with the proximal jejunum, with temporary stenting with a fine feeding tube to ensure anastomotic patency.

Volvulus of the stomach

Definitions
● Rotation of the stomach occurs around its two fixed points (cardia and pylorus) when associated with eventration of the diaphragm (rotation of the greater curvature with attached transverse colon is upwards into the lax diaphragmatic dome).
● Volvulus may also occur in a rolling hiatus hernia when part of the stomach becomes trapped in the diaphragmatic defect.

Clinical features
● Intermittent upper abdominal discomfort or pain or a feeling of fullness after meals.
● Epigastric pain radiating into the back of the chest accompanied by retching.

Investigation
➤ Barium meal to confirm diagnosis.

Treatment
➤ Should be repaired electively to prevent obstruction and strangulation.
➤ Surgical reduction of volvulus with fixing of the greater curvature to the duodenojejunal flexure; in the case of a hiatal defect, the hernia is reduced and the defect repaired.

Gastric foreign bodies and bezoars

Definitions

- Swallowed foreign bodies are usually household items or toys and may have sharp edges.
- Stomach bezoars are rare and are associated with psychiatric illness; these may be hair balls (trichobezoars), vegetable concretions (phytobezoars) or industrial setting agents and cement (silicobezoars).

Clinical features

- Upper abdominal discomfort or pain with dyspepsia.
- Gastric outlet or small bowel obstruction.

Investigation

➤ Most foreign bodies are radio-opaque and their shape, size and position are visualized on plain radiology.
➤ Organic bezoars are visualized endoscopically.

Treatment

➤ Small foreign bodies or bezoars found in the stomach may be removed endoscopically.
➤ Large objects or those with sharp surfaces require urgent gastrotomy and removal because of the risk of obstruction or perforation.

Gastritis

Definitions

- Acute gastritis: a mild transient mucosal inflammation caused by alcohol or non-steroidal anti-inflammatory agents; erosive gastritis occasionally bleeds.
- Chronic gastritis:
  - Type A: affects the cardia and is mediated by autoantibodies producing atrophic gastritis (associated with pernicious anaemia and gastric cancer)
  - Type B: affects the pylorus and the antrum and is usually the result of *Helicobacter pylori* infection.

Clinical features

- Non-specific dyspepsia, haemorrhage.

Investigation

➤ Upper gastrointestinal endoscopy and mucosal biopsy.

Treatment

➤ Short-term H_2 receptor antagonists or proton pump inhibition following endoscopic diagnosis.
➤ Bleeding from gastric erosions is treated with bed rest, sedation and intravenous omeprazole therapy; cold saline gastric lavage may be tried.
➤ Rarely, subtotal or total gastrectomy is resorted to in catastrophic bleeding from extensive erosive gastritis.

Gastric ulcer

Definitions

- Aetiology: disruption of the gastric mucosal barrier.
- Associated factors: smoking, alcohol consumption, *H. pylori* infection and bile reflux; ingestion of aspirin and non-steroidal anti-inflammatory agents.
- Incidence: male:female ratio of 3:1.
- Acute ulcers usually undergo spontaneous healing but occasionally bleed, perforate or become chronic.
- Stress ulcers: acute gastric erosions, usually in critically ill patients (following major trauma, burns or major surgery).
- Chronic gastric ulcers carry a 5% incidence of malignant change.

Clinical features

- Acute ulcer: bleeding diathesis with haematemesis.
- Chronic ulcer: dyspeptic periodicity with epigastric pain, weight loss and anaemia, vomiting or melaena.

Investigation

➤ Upper gastrointestinal endoscopy with biopsy of ulcer edge for histology and *H. pylori* testing.

Treatment

➤ Medical: triple therapy for *H. pylori* eradication: lansoprazole 30 mg twice daily, clarithromycin 500 mg twice daily, amoxycillin 1 g twice daily (or metronidazole 400 mg twice daily) for 7–14 days. For uncomplicated ulcer: H_2 receptor blockade (cimetidine 400 mg twice daily or ranitidine 150 mg twice daily for 6 weeks) or proton-pump inhibition (omeprazole 20 mg twice daily or lansoprazole 30 mg daily for 6-8 weeks).

➤ Ulcer bleeding may be controlled by cold saline lavage, endoscopic submucosal adrenaline injection, hot probe application or laser photocoagulation.

➤ Surgery is reserved for non-healing or penetrating ulcer, gastric outlet obstruction, hourglass deformity, haemorrhage, perforation or fistulation.

➤ Emergency surgery: a bleeding ulcer is underrun or a perforation oversewn with an omental patch and peritoneal lavage.

➤ Elective surgery: an anti-ulcer procedure consists of vagotomy (truncal or selective) and drainage (pyloroplasty or gastrojejunostomy) or partial gastrectomy.

Chronic duodenal ulcer

Definitions

● Male:female ratio 2–3:1.
● More common than gastric ulcer (four or more times as frequent depending on the community surveyed).
● Situated usually in the first part of the duodenum; anterior ulcers may perforate and posterior ulcers may penetrate into the underlying pancreas or erode into a vessel (branches of the gastroduodenal or pancreatoduodenal arteries).

Causes:

• Gastric acid hypersecretion resulting from vagal stimulation (stress/anxiety states)
• Lifestyle factors: irregular meals, smoking, alcohol consumption

- A larger than normal parietal cell mass, blood group O and *H. pylori* infection
- Endocrine causes: gastrin-secreting pancreatic tumour (Zollinger–Ellison syndrome), multiple adenoma syndrome and hyperparathyroidism.

Clinical features

- Marked dyspeptic periodicity with epigastric pain.
- Normal appetite with no weight loss.
- Melaena and haematemesis.

Complications:

- Haemorrhage
- Perforation
- Gastric outlet obstruction (pyloric stenosis).

Investigation

➤ Upper gastrointestinal endoscopy and mucosal biopsy as indicated.
➤ Barium meal examination.

Treatment

Control of acid secretion:

➤ Virtually all duodenal ulcers heal on H_2 receptor blockade or proton-pump (H^+/K^+ ATPase) inhibition; treatment is continued until endoscopic confirmation of healing (drugs and dosages as for gastric ulcer therapy)
➤ Prolonged or 'interval' therapy with nocturnal dosage to prevent relapse is popular
➤ Triple therapy is indicated in the presence of *H. pylori* infection in duodenal mucosal biopsies
➤ Ulcer haemorrhage is treated by submucosal adrenaline injections, laser photocoagulation or heater probe coagulation.

Surgery:

➤ Anti-ulcer surgery is indicated for failed medical therapy (or inability to tolerate long-term drug therapy) and for complications of bleeding, pyloric stenosis or perforation

➡

> ➤ Operations are truncal vagotomy and drainage procedure (pyloroplasty or gastrojejunostomy), selective vagotomy or antrectomy
> ➤ Perforation requires emergency laparotomy, omental patch, closure of perforation and peritoneal lavage
> ➤ Haemorrhage is controlled by underrunning of the ulcer base; uncontrolled bleeding from a posterior penetrating ulcer may require a partial gastrectomy
> ➤ Ulcer re-bleeding while on medical therapy requires early surgical assessment, as mortality rises when surgery is delayed.

Complications

Complications following surgery for gastric and duodenal ulcers:

* Early: anastomotic haemorrhage, duodenal fistula, stomal obstruction leading to bilious vomiting; paralytic ileus and acute pancreatitis
* Post-gastrectomy (early and late dumping) syndromes consist of abdominal and vasomotor symptoms as a result of rapid gastric emptying and reduced absorption of nutrients. They are associated with abnormal glucose metabolism resulting in an initial transient hyperglycaemia followed by hypoglycaemia lasting up to 4 hours
* Bilious vomiting
* Nutritional syndromes: diarrhoea, malabsorption, steatorrhoea, weight loss, iron-deficiency and megaloblastic anaemias.

Mallory–Weiss syndrome

Definitions

* Linear mucosal tear in the region of the cardia from prolonged retching or vomiting.

Clinical features

* Prolonged vomiting of gastric contents (from alcohol consumption or vertigo) followed by profuse haematemesis.
* Hypovolaemia or hypovolaemic shock.

Investigation

➤ Upper gastrointestinal endoscopy confirms mucosal tear and active bleeding.

Treatment

➤ Resuscitate with rapid replacement of blood loss and sedate with intravenous morphine.
➤ Persisting haemorrhage requires gastrotomy and suture of laceration.

Zollinger–Ellison syndrome (page 484)

Adenocarcinoma of the stomach

Definitions

- Aetiology:
  - Mucosal dysplasia, gastric polyps and adenomas.
  - Dietary carcinogens (nitrosamines), high salt intake.
  - Pernicious anaemia and blood group A.
  - Chronic *H. pylori* infection and type B gastritis.
  - Peptic ulcer surgery is associated with threefold to fourfold increased incidence of gastric cancer.
- Commonest site: prepyloric region.
- Male:female ratio is 3:1 (highest incidence: Japan, China, Chile and Iceland).
- Early cancers (confined to the mucosa and submucosa) are picked up on population screening in communities with a high incidence (Japan).
- Advanced cancers are ulcerating, nodular or infiltrating (linitus plastica) lesions.
- Spread: direct extension to adjacent organs, lymphovascular permeation and transperitoneal seeding.

Clinical features

- Insidious onset with non-specific dyspepsia, general malaise, anorexia and anaemia.
- Advanced cancers (invasion of muscle coat and beyond) present with epigastric mass, pain or symptoms of gastric outlet obstruction.
- Hepatomegaly and ascites are late manifestations.

Investigation

➤ Upper gastrointestinal endoscopy and biopsy to include submucosal tissue (all patients with dyspeptic symptoms must undergo endoscopy prior to treatment).

➤ Barium meal examination defines diffusely infiltrative submucosal lesions (linitus plastica) where there is little mucosal involvement.

➤ Gastric secretory studies reveal associated hypo-chlorhydria or achlorhydria.

➤ CT and endoscopic ultrasound scans stage the disease.

➤ Laparoscopy (and laparoscopic ultrasound scan) also used for disease staging and to assess tumour resectability.

Treatment

Surgery:

➤ Curative resection involves some form of gastrectomy and splenectomy with en bloc removal of perigastric lymph nodes, which provide disease staging (early mucosal lesions have an 80% and advanced lesions a 5–30% 5-year survival).

➤ Local recurrence in the stomach bed following gastrectomy requires further surgery or radiotherapy.

➤ Advanced disease causing obstruction may be palliated with endoluminal stenting, laser or argon beam therapy or surgical by-pass (high gastrojejunostomy).

➤ Chemotherapy is palliative.

Gastric lymphomas

● Usually solitary, seen in the immune-suppressed and AIDS sufferers.

● Extranodal non-Hodgkin's lymphoma [gastric mucosa associated lymphoid tissue (MALT) lymphoma] seen mainly in the elderly.

● Treated by total gastrectomy or chemoradiotherapy (depending on patient fitness).

Gastric carcinoid tumours

- Rare (associated with pernicious anaemia) and have a high potential for invasion and metastasis.
- Gastrectomy is the treatment of choice.

Leiomyosarcoma and neuro-fibrosarcoma of the stomach

- May present with massive haematemesis and/or melaena and barium imaging is diagnostic.
- Partial gastrectomy is the treatment of choice (better prognosis than for carcinoma).

Fibrosarcoma

- Fibrosarcoma arises from the subserosa of the stomach, is the least malignant and usually presents as a palpable mass.

Gastric surgery for morbid obesity

Definitions

- Morbid obesity is defined as body mass index (weight in kg/height in m^2) >45 or 45 kg over the ideal weight for height, age and sex.

Clinical features

- Rotund appearance with cumbersome walk and outward swing of the lower limbs.

Investigation

➤ Investigations to exclude treatable endocrine disorders and obesity-associated diseases.

Treatment

➤ Various non-surgical methods of controlling weight gain (dietary regimens, psychotherapy, wiring of jaws and alternative medicine).
➤ Vertical banded gastropexy (on failure of the above) (mean weight loss is within 30% of the ideal weight).

Gastrinomas (page 484)

BOWEL

Diverticular disease

Definitions

- Diverticula (small out-pouchings of the colonic mucosa through the muscle coat) are present, which become inflamed and produce muscle spasm.
- Occurs throughout the colon but most commonly in the sigmoid colon.
- Common with increasing age in Western communities and is associated with low-residue diet and reduced faecal bulk.

Clinical features

- Low abdominal pain, fever and malaise with abdominal tenderness or palpation of a tender inflammatory mass.
- Localized or generalized peritonitis in an ill patient would suggest perforation or abscess formation.

Investigation

➤ Leukocytosis with a raised CRP titre.
➤ Plain abdominal X-ray is non-specific and may show constipated colonic loops.
➤ Abdominal ultrasound or contrast-enhanced computerized tomography (CT) scan may confirm an inflammatory mass or abscess.

Treatment

➤ Most resolve on fluid and antibiotic therapy (cefuroxime 750 mg and metronidazole 500 mg 8-hourly) with bed rest.
➤ Follow-up colonoscopy or barium enema to confirm diverticular disease and to exclude colonic malignancy.
➤ Peritonitis suggesting perforation necessitates immediate laparotomy and Hartmann's procedure

→

(proximal colostomy and oversewing distal colon at level of pelvic floor) with resection of the affected bowel, peritoneal lavage and drainage.
➤ A pelvic abscess is drained under image-guidance with antibiotic cover.

Congenital megacolon (Hirschsprung's disease)

Definitions

- An aganglionic segment of the colon at or above the peritoneal reflection producing a functional obstruction (absence of ganglion cells in Auerbach's plexus).
- Chronic large bowel obstruction presents in early infancy (those with a very short aganglionic segment may present later in childhood or, rarely, in adulthood).

Clinical features

- Progressive constipation and abdominal distension with failure to thrive.

Investigation

➤ Contrast barium enema reveals a narrowed rectosigmoid colon with distension of the proximal bowel.
➤ Rectal mucosal biopsy is confirmatory.

Treatment

➤ Surgical 'pull-through procedure' with a proximal 'covering' stoma.

Inflammatory bowel disease

Crohn's disease

Definitions

- A chronic, relapsing inflammatory disease of the mucosa and submucosa of the gastrointestinal tract, with a rising incidence (5000 new cases per year in the UK).

- Postulated cause: chronic bowel infection caused by *Mycobacterium avium paratuberculosis* subspecies.
  - Endemic in farm animals; transmitted through milk and faeces (water contamination)
  - Identified in inflamed bowel by DNA extraction and prolonged culture
  - Initiates immune dysfunction and a neuritis (Auerbach's plexus).
- Principally affects the ileum, colon and anal canal, with an unpredictable clinical course and frequent relapses.
- Complications: abscess, fistula and stricture formation.
- Characterized by transmural inflammation, skip lesions, non-caseating granulomas, fissures and fistulae with eventual healing with stricture formation.

Clinical features

- Acute presentation: cramping abdominal pain and distension, diarrhoea with the passage of mucus or blood, low-grade fever, anorexia, fatigue and weight loss.
- Chronic disease: poor appetite, malaise, bowel cramps, anaemia and weight loss.
- Perforation is rare and presents with localized or diffuse peritonitis.
- Disease progression: leads to adhesion obstruction, abscess or fistulae formation.
- Anal disease presents as peri-anal sepsis in the form of anal abscess, anal fissure or fistula in ano.

Investigation

➤ Anaemia, leukocytosis, raised erythrocyte sedimentation rate (ESR) and CRP, electrolyte and liver function derangement.
➤ Procto-sigmoidoscopy and colonoscopy reveal mucosal inflammation, ulceration or skip lesions.
➤ Small bowel enema may show 'cobblestone' or 'pipe stem' features of mucosal oedema or ulceration or segmental narrowing.
➤ Barium enema may show inflammatory changes of the colon with abscess or fistulae formation.
➤ CT scan may show intra-abdominal abscess or fistulation.

Treatment

➤ The acute inflammatory phase requires fluid, electrolyte and antibiotic therapy, with the correction of anaemia and hypoalbuminaemia.
➤ Treated with mesalazine 1200–2400 mg daily in divided doses with/without prednisolone 20–40 mg daily and metronidazole 500–800 mg tds for 5–10 days.
➤ Nutritional support in the form of elemental diet or parenteral feeding.
➤ Azathioprine, cyclosporin and infliximab (a monoclonal antibody inhibiting tumour necrosis factor alpha) for severe refractory disease and for the treatment of fistulae.
➤ Experimental treatment of *Mycobacterium avium paratuberculosis* with clarithromycin and rifabutin over a period of 4–6 months.
➤ Surgery:
  – For disease progression despite medical therapy and requires conservative resection of diseased bowel
  – For complications such as obstruction, stricture, abscess and fistula formation or perforation: toxic dilatation or peri-anal disease; strictureplasty for multiple strictures to conserve bowel length
  – Proctocolectomy with ileostomy for widespread, unremitting colonic disease
  – Drainage for abdominal or peri-anal abscess.

Long-term complications

● Amyloidosis: presents with proteinuria, hepatosplenomegaly.
● Gallstones: as a result of bile salt malabsorption.
● Malignancy: increasing risk after 10 years (as in ulcerative colitis) requires 3-yearly surveillance colonoscopy.

Ulcerative colitis

Definitions

● A chronic non-specific inflammatory disease of the large bowel that usually starts in the rectum and proceeds proximally, involving the mucosa and submucosa with multiple ulcers, pseudopolyps and crypt abscesses.

Clinical features

- Crampy lower abdominal pain.
- Recurrent episodes of mucoid/bloody diarrhoea.
- In fulminant disease: fluid, electrolyte and protein depletion with pyrexia, tachycardia and rapid weight loss.
- Acute toxic dilatation of the colon (toxic megacolon) leads to ischaemia and perforation.

Investigation

➤ Leukocytosis and raised CRP.
➤ Plain abdominal radiology may show a dilated colon.
➤ Colonoscopy reveals the extent and severity of the disease.
➤ Barium enema may show 'cobblestoning' or 'thumb printing' of the colonic mucosa indicating inflammation and ulceration.

Treatment

➤ Fluid and electrolyte replenishment with systemic broad-spectrum antibiotic therapy (cefuroxime 750 mg 8-hourly and metronidazole 500 mg 6-hourly) for infection control.
➤ Mesalazine 1200–2400 mg daily in divided doses and prednisolone 20–40 mg daily orally; mesalazine may be reduced to a maintenance dose and the prednisolone given as a retention enema.
➤ Relapses may require oral azathioprine (2.0–2.5 mg/kg daily), mercaptopurine (1.0–1.5 mg/kg daily) or cyclosporin A.
➤ Surgery is indicated for unremitting or fulminating disease leading to toxic dilatation or haemorrhage and for stricture formation; procedures are: proctocolectomy with ileo-anal pouch or total colectomy with ileorectal anastomosis (requires surveillance of the retained rectum).
➤ Long-standing disease (>10 years) requires 3-yearly colonoscopic or barium enema surveillance because of an increased cancer risk.

Small bowel tumours

Definitions

- Rare tumours: non-Hodgkin's lymphoma (in the elderly), hamartoma and carcinoid, sarcoma (Kaposi's in the HIV patient) and adenocarcinoma (in the immunosuppressed).

Clinical features

- Presents as an acute or subacute small bowel obstruction and the tumour may form the nidus of an ileocolic intussusception.

Investigation

➤ Plain abdominal radiology to confirm bowel obstruction.
➤ Double contrast small bowel enema delineates the lesion.

Treatment

➤ Resection of the loop of bowel containing the lesion with the mesentery.
➤ A right hemicolectomy may be required for an intussusception involving the proximal colon.
➤ Prognosis depends on the type of tumour, extension without the bowel and the presence of nodal or liver metastases.

Carcinoid syndrome

Definitions

- Carcinoid syndrome is associated with carcinoid tumours that are usually found in the midgut and occasionally in the foregut. They are regarded as malignant and survival is related to the extent of liver involvement:
  - Gastric carcinoids are found in the fundus and body of the stomach and present with chronic atrophic

gastritis, achlorhydria and pernicious anaemia, diagnosis is by endoscopy and biopsy
- Midgut carcinoid (argentaffinomas) are found in the appendix in 80% of instances and these are invariably benign; those found in the distal ileum and caecum may produce large amounts of serotonin and predispose to valvular heart disease and heart failure and have a tendency to metastatic spread
- Hindgut carcinoids usually present with colonic obstruction, bleeding or a palpable pelvic mass
- Bronchial carcinoids may produce adrenocorticotropic hormone or growth hormone-releasing hormone and give rise to features of Cushing's syndrome or acromegaly.

Clinical features

- Hot flushes, diarrhoea, bronchial spasm and hypotension.
- Hepatomegaly (in the presence of liver metastases).

Investigation

➤ Elevated urinary levels of the serotonin metabolite 5-hydroxyindole acetic acid.
➤ CT, magnetic resonance imaging and ultrasound scans image the primary lesion and metastatic deposits in the liver or mesentery.
➤ Positron emission tomography has recently been used in tumour localization.

Treatment

➤ Resection of the primary tumour and the regional lymphatics (extended right hemicolectomy for ileal and caecal lesions).
➤ Postoperative adjuvant therapy with somatostatin analogue (octeotride 50–200 µg subcutaneously once, twice or three times daily for 1 week) and alpha-interferon produces good remission in midgut carcinoids.

Colorectal carcinoma

Definitions

- Adenocarcinomas account for 98% of colonic cancers and are staged according to disease extension – Dukes' staging:
  - A: tumour confined to the submucosa (best prognosis)
  - B1: tumour penetrating into but not through the muscle coat
  - B2: tumour penetrating the colonic wall but without nodal metastases
  - C: tumour with mesenteric lymph nodal involvement
  - D: with liver, lung or bone metastases (worst prognosis).
- Sites: rectum 50%, sigmoid colon 25%, caecum and ascending colon 12.5%.
- High incidence in Western communities with a male:female ratio of 2:1, with increasing incidence after the fifth decade of life.
- <5% of cases are hereditary and linked to familial polyposis and non-polyposis syndromes.
- Associated with dietary factors: high intake of animal products and low residue.

Clinical features

- Recent alteration in bowel habit with the passage of blood (melaena) or mucus.
- Fresh rectal bleeding, sense of incomplete emptying and/or tenesmus with spurious diarrhoea are suggestive of rectal cancer.
- Crampy abdominal pain, obstructive symptoms, abdominal mass or ascites are late features signifying advanced colonic tumour.
- Peritonitis or abscess formation as a result of tumour perforation of the bowel wall.

Investigation

➤ Rectal examination and rigid or flexible sigmoidoscopy and mucosal biopsy diagnose cancer of the rectum and sigmoid colon.

➜

➤ Colonoscopy or barium enema visualizes proximal lesions, including the caecum, and must be performed to exclude synchronous cancers when investigating distal lesions.
➤ Endoluminal rectal ultrasound scan assesses local invasion of a rectal tumour.
➤ Liver ultrasound or CT scans for liver metastases.
➤ Carcino-embryonic antigen titres may be raised and act as a useful marker for post-treatment surveillance.

Treatment

➤ Resection of tumour containing loop of colon (right or left hemicolectomy, transverse colectomy or sigmoid colectomy) with the mesocolon.
➤ Rectal carcinoma is treated by anterior restorative resection or by abdominoperineal excision of the rectum with total mesorectal excision (the former is a sphincter-saving procedure).
➤ Neo-adjuvant pelvic radiotherapy may downstage rectal tumours prior to surgery.
➤ Adjuvant chemotherapy: irinotecan and 5-fluorouracil for Dukes' B2, C and D tumours.
➤ Adjuvant radiotherapy is currently being assessed.
➤ Obstructing or perforating tumours of the colon require emergency colonic resection with a covering stoma and are usually advanced (Dukes' C and D).
➤ Endoscopic placement of self-expanding metal stents for obstructive or advanced disease for palliation or prior to surgery is being assessed.
➤ Solitary liver or lung metastases may be resected with a small survival benefit.
➤ Recurrent tumour is detected on surveillance colonoscopy or barium enema and staging investigations are performed before treatment.
➤ Three-yearly colonoscopic or barium enema surveillance is advocated following treatment.

Colorectal cancer syndromes

Diagnosed by careful evaluation of family history.

- Familial adenomatous polyposis:
  - Autosomal dominant with offspring of affected individuals at 50% risk of being gene carriers
  - All gene carriers develop polyps by the age of 40 years
  - Characterized by >100 tubulovillous adenomas in the colon
  - Malignant transformation inevitable if polyps are left untreated.
- Hereditary non-polyposis colon cancer syndromes:
  - Autosomal dominant transmission
  - Associated with extracolonic tumours (Lynch syndrome).
- Colonoscopic screening 3-yearly is recommended.

Colonic polyps

Definitions

- These are pedunculated or sessile and are of three histological types:
  - Tubular: most common with low malignant potential (<5%)
  - Tubulovillous: intermediate potential for malignancy
  - Villous: increased potential for malignant change (40%).

Clinical features

- Alteration in bowel habit and/or rectal bleeding.

Investigation

➤ Colonoscopy or barium enema.

Treatment

➤ Colonoscopic snaring of pedunculated polyps and resection of the bowel containing large sessile polyps.

➜

> ➤ Recurrent villous tumours of the rectum require low anterior resection or laser/argon beam therapy in those unfit for surgery.
> ➤ Surveillance: fewer than three polyps 1 cm or less in size with no villous component require no follow-up; multiple or larger polyps and those with a villous component require 3-yearly and then 5-yearly colonoscopy or barium enema.

Radiation enteritis

Definitions

- Damage to small and/or large bowel from radiotherapy for the treatment of visceral cancer.
- Combination of external beam and intracavitary pelvic irradiation is the most frequent cause.
- Radiation damage is irreversible.

Clinical features

- Mucosal stem cell damage results in transient or persistent diarrhoea and malabsorption.
- Vascular injury leads to bleeding, perforation or fistula.
- Episodes of abdominal pain with signs of obstruction result from fibrosis and stricture formation.
- Diagnosis is usually delayed as symptoms of weight loss, anorexia, abdominal pain or diarrhoea are assumed to be a result of recurrence of the original cancer.

Treatment

> ➤ When mucosal damage is limited, symptoms are controlled by symptomatic measures and nutritional supplementation.
> ➤ Surgical resection of irradiated bowel ensuring healthy anastomosis, otherwise the resected ends must be exteriorized.
> ➤ Fistulae may require excision and interpositioning of viable omentum between epithelial surfaces.

Anal canal

Anorectal malformations

Definitions

- Malformations of the anorectum are the result of defective fusion of the rectum with the anal canal.

Clinical features

Imperforate anus:

- Low anomalies:
  - Epithelial covering or stenosis of the anus or the anal canal; there is usually a tiny opening in the perineum with meconium staining indicating the site of the covered or stenosed anus; occasionally there may be an ectopic anal opening in the perineum or vulva.
- High anomalies:
  - Caused by anorectal atresia; the rectal pouch is situated at or above the pelvic floor with a fistulous communication with the urinary bladder, prostatic or bulbar urethra in boys and with the vestibule or vagina in girls
  - Usually associated with other congenital anomalies.

Introducing a rectal thermometer during the first neonatal examination reveals the anomalies.

Investigation

Assessment of anomaly:

➤ An 'upside-down' plain abdominal radiograph with a radio-opaque marker taped to the anal dimple; the relation of the distal bowel gas to the pelvic floor and marker indicates the extent of the atretic segment.

Treatment

➤ Low anomalies:
  - Covered or ectopic anus requires opening or a cut-back procedure
  - Anal stenosis requires regular dilatation.

➤

> ➤ High anomalies:
> – Early surgery in the form of a 'pull-through' procedure
>   with excision of the fistula and a covering stoma
> – Postoperative anal dilatation and bowel training.

Anal fissure

Definitions

- An unhealed tear in the anal mucosa, caused by trauma
  or ischaemic injury to the lower anal mucosa, usually in
  the posterior midline.
- Associated with chronic constipation, Crohn's and
  sexually transmitted disease.

Clinical features

- There is severe pain on defecation with slight discharge
  or bleeding.
- Examination of the anus requires 5% lignocaine gel
  application; severe discomfort requires examination
  under anaesthesia.
- The fissure is a boat-shaped ulcer with surrounding
  inflammatory induration. The floor is formed by the
  internal anal sphincter and a skin tag (sentinel pile)
  may be present at its base.

Treatment

➤ Acute fissures are treated with bd topical 0.2% glyceryl
  trinitrate (GTN) ointment.
➤ Lateral sphincterotomy to the depth of the fissure
  (partial division of the internal anal sphincter) may be
  required if not healed by GTN after 4 weeks.
➤ Chronic fissures require fissurectomy and
  sphincterotomy, with histology of the excised fissure.
➤ Botulinum toxin A injection may be effective.

Anorectal abscesses

Definitions

- An infection in an anal gland resulting in a crypt
  abscess in the dentate line enlarging to form an anal

abscess, which may extend into the ischiorectal space to form an ischiorectal abscess.

- Infecting organisms are *Escherichia coli* and *Staphylococcus aureus* with occasional *Bacteroides* spp, *Streptococcus* spp and *Proteus* spp.

Clinical features

- Peri-anal abscess (60% incidence) presents at the anal verge as an acutely tender cystic swelling.
- Ischiorectal abscess (30% incidence) is an extension laterally of an intermuscular (intersphincteric) abscess presenting as a tender brawny swelling in the ischiorectal fossa with fever, malaise and pain.

Treatment

➤ Surgical deroofing, drainage and curettage of the abscess cavity under a general anaesthetic and broad-spectrum antibiotic cover (early and adequate surgery may prevent subsequent development of a fistula).

➤ Abscess cavity that fails to heal and continues to discharge should be examined under anaesthesia for a fistulous opening into the anal canal.

Fistula in ano

Definitions

- An inflammatory tract lined by granulation tissue extending from the anorectal mucosa to the peri-anal skin.
- Recurrent infection of the tract produces an intermittent or continuous discharge with associated peri-anal discomfort or pain.
- The internal opening may be above (high fistulae) or below (low fistulae) the anorectal ring (puborectalis muscle).

Clinical features

- Persistent seropurulent discharge causes irritation and inflammation of peri-anal skin.

- Goodsall's rule: anterior fistulae are usually direct and single and open on to the anterior peri-anal skin; posterior fistulae may have multiple external openings with tortuous tracts but have a single internal opening, usually in the posterior midline.
- The internal opening may be palpable or visualized on proctoscopy.
- Granulomatous infections, Crohn's disease or colloid carcinoma of the rectum may present as a fistula; tissue biopsy is necessary to establish the underlying pathology.

Treatment

➤ Low fistulae are laid open using a malleable probe-pointed director and wound edges are trimmed and left to granulate (excised tissue for histology); anal dilatation with dilators prevents stenosis.

➤ Intersphincteric and trans-sphincteric fistulae usually have a low internal opening but the tract may extend above the pelvic diaphragm, with the danger of conversion to a high fistula during probing.

➤ High fistulae: following identification of the internal opening a seton (non-absorbable suture) is tied around the fistula to facilitate drainage and resolution of the surrounding inflammation; a diverting colostomy is performed, followed by excision of the fistula and primary repair of the anorectal ring.

Haemorrhoids

Definitions

- Haemorrhoids are engorgements of venous plexuses within enlarged and prolapsed anal cushions and are located above (internal) or below (external) the dentate line.
- It is a common condition, with hereditary predisposition, and is associated with chronic constipation and purgative use.
- Haemorrhoids are found in three sites (3, 7, and 11 o'clock in the lithotomy position – patient lying on back with legs up).

Clinical features

- Haemorrhoids present with bleeding, mucous discharge or faecal soiling, peri-anal itching and discomfort.
- Internal haemorrhoids are impalpable (unless thrombosed) and are classified as:
  - 1st degree (bleed but do not prolapse)
  - 2nd degree (prolapse on defecation but are self-reducing)
  - 3rd degree (prolapse and require manual reduction).
- Strangulation is caused by obstructed venous return in prolapsed haemorrhoids with swelling and severe pain and may lead to thrombosis and ulceration.

Treatment

- ➤ Topical anaesthetic applications and suppositories with stool softeners provide good symptomatic relief.
- ➤ 1st degree haemorrhoids: sclerotherapy or photocoagulation.
- ➤ 2nd degree haemorrhoids: rubber band ligation or cryosurgery.
- ➤ Associated internal sphincter spasm responds to topical application of nitroglycerine, botulinum toxin injection or anal stretch under general anaesthesia.
- ➤ 3rd degree haemorrhoids: haemorrhoidectomy (Morgan and Milligan), where the pedicle is dissected free of the internal sphincter, transfixed or stapled and excised with preservation of mucocutaneous bridges between pedicles to promote re-epithelialization and prevent anal stenosis.

Pruritus ani

- A persistent itching localized to the anus and the peri-anal skin, and may extend into the introitus in the female.
- It is usually a symptom of an underlying dermatosis, resulting in contact sensitivities to various topical applications; other skin lesions include eczema, allergies and drug reactions, psoriasis, lichen planus, urticaria, miliaria rubra (prickly heat) and dermatitis herpetiformis.

- Rarely, it is related to anorectal pathology, and may occur with piles, fissures, fistulae, warts, Crohn's disease, solitary ulcer, villous adenoma/carcinoma of the rectum and anus, and lesions producing an anal discharge, such as paraffin laxatives, sphincter malfunction and rectal prolapse.
- Infections include sexually transmitted diseases and fungal infections; it is also associated with scabies, fleas, lice and threadworms.
- Additional problems in women include candida infection (thrush), *Trichomonas vaginalis* and urinary leakage from a cystocele or an ectopic ureter.
- Local problems may be accentuated by excessive sweating, poor hygiene and psychological conditions.
- Every baby develops a nappy rash at some point as a result of contact with urine and faeces, but this may also be fungal or a reaction to an emollient.
- Generalized causes of itching that may present as pruritus ani include: obstructive jaundice, diabetes mellitus, hypoparathyroidism and hyperparathyroidism, myeloproliferative disorders, lymphoma, leukaemia and other malignancies, polycythaemia, anaemia and chronic renal failure.

Treatment

➤ Treatment is of the cause, and of secondary bacterial and fungal infection.
➤ Stopping the itch is difficult: regular nail cutting reduces damage; bandaging the hands and restraint at night can help with children.
➤ Cooling helps: calamine lotion is effective in this respect.
➤ Avoid very dry or soggy skin. If sweat or discharge produce the latter effect, regular washing is needed, using soap substitutes or, if soap is used to produce effective cleaning, ensure it is completely washed away.
➤ Adding oil to bath water and emollients after, helps to keep skin supple and avoid drying out.
➤ The side-effects of medication, such as antihistamines, are usually unacceptable; steroids may be needed to reduce inflammatory changes.

Anal warts

Definitions

- Papillomas of the peri-anal skin (anal condylomata) associated with sexually transmitted viral infection (human papilloma virus).
- Rare predisposition to anal cancer.

Clinical features

- Itchy, rubbery, cauliflower-like growths in peri-anal skin.

Treatment

➤ Topical self-treatment with podophyllotoxin (0.5% solution or 0.15% cream) or imiquimod (5% cream); clearance is achieved in 1–6 months.

➤ Ablation with cryosurgery or electrosurgery achieves quick and effective clearance.

➤ Advise use of barrier protection with new sexual contacts.

Anal carcinoma

Definitions

- Tumours arising in the anal canal are adenocarcinomas (70%) and tumours arising in the anal verge are squamous cell carcinomas (30%).
- Predisposing conditions: radiation damage (treatment of pruritus ani), HIV infection, anal warts, peri-anal Crohn's disease and chronic fistulae.

Clinical features

- Usually presents in the sixth and seventh decades of life with rectal bleeding, mucous discharge, tenesmus, the sensation of a lump in the anus or a change in bowel habit.
- Rarely, presents with a groin mass as a result of metastatic nodal spread.
- Rectal examination reveals an ulcerating, polypoid or haemorrhagic lesion in the anal canal or verge.

Investigation
➤ Proctoscopy and biopsy confirms the diagnosis.
➤ Colonoscopy or barium enema is performed to exclude synchronous colonic tumours or polyps.

Treatment
➤ Abdominoperineal mesorectal excision of the anorectum with an end colostomy.
➤ Groin dissection is reserved for clinically involved inguinal nodes.
➤ Radiotherapy and chemoradiation is being assessed as neoadjuvant treatment, with surgery being reserved for residual disease.
➤ Endo-anal excision usually suffices for small squamous tumours of the anal verge in the frail and the elderly.

STOMAS

Definitions
● Feeding stomas are sited in the stomach or proximal jejunum.
  – Feeding gastrostomy: placement of a feeding catheter into the stomach through an abdominal incision (Stamm) or by endoscopic visualization (percutaneous endoscopic gastrostomy)
  – Feeding jejunostomy: a fine balloon catheter or T-tube is secured in the bowel lumen through a midline incision.
● Effluent stomas are in the terminal ileum or colon. Indications:
  – To protect a distal anastomosis
  – To defunction a diseased colon
  – Following bowel resection (in Hartmann's procedure or abdominoperineal resection).
● Temporary stomas are in the form of a loop ileostomy or loop colostomy that is later closed.
● A mucous fistula is when the distal (defunctioned) loop of colon is exteriorized.

- Permanent stomas are an end ileostomy following a panproctocolectomy or an end colostomy following an abdominoperineal resection of the rectum.
- Tube caecostomy is used to irrigate unprepared obstructed bowel during surgery and to protect the anastomosis [a large balloon catheter (26–28 French) is introduced into the caecum and brought out through the abdominal wall].

Stomal siting

- Optimal site must be defined pre-operatively (with the stoma therapist).
- The patient must be able to visualize the site for stoma care.
- It should not be sited too close to the surgical wound (risk of wound contamination), near bony prominences, skin folds, umbilicus or scars (poor bag fitting results in leakage).

Complications

- Metabolic (ileostomy): fluid and electrolyte loss, chronic normochromic, microcytic anaemia, vitamin B_{12} deficiency (megaloblastic anaemia), cholelithiasis (caused by loss of bile salts), urolithiasis (uric acid stones).
- Prolapse, retraction, ischaemia, stenosis, parastomal hernia and skin excoriation (may require surgical revision or stoma resiting).

ABDOMINAL SARCOMAS

Definitions

- Arise from the abdominal wall or from the connective tissue of the gastrointestinal tract or urinary bladder.
- 25% of sarcomas are retroperitoneal.
- Histologically they are low, medium and high grade.
- Slow-growing 'pushing' tumours, highly vascular and non-invasive.
- Usually >7 cm in size on diagnosis.
- Do not usually invade abdominal viscera.

Clinical features

- Minimally symptomatic.
- Occasionally painful abdominal swelling.

Investigation

➤ CT abdominal scan.
➤ Chest radiology (to exclude lung metastases): imaging usually reveals a fatty mass; may be mistaken for an abscess or haematoma.
➤ Image-guided core-needle biopsy provides a definitive pre-operative diagnosis.

Treatment

➤ Surgical excision (radical surgery not indicated as recurrence is inevitable).
➤ Pre-operative radiotherapy or tumour embolization reduces tumour vascularity and may 'downstage' lesion.
➤ Excision of abdominal wall lesions may require myocutaneous flap reconstruction.
➤ Postoperative radiotherapy.
➤ Regional perfusion with tumour necrosis factor or melphalan applicable to limb lesions.

Intra-abdominal desmoid tumours

- Intra-abdominal desmoid tumours are benign and do not require surgery.

LIVER

Definitions

- Liver receives a dual blood supply from the portal vein (70%) and hepatic artery (30%) with a resting blood flow of 1500 mL/min and a normal portal pressure of 8–12 mmHg.
- Blood enters each lobule from the portal triads in the periphery and drains into the central vein.

- The liver is the most important source of metabolic energy (anabolic and catabolic) and of body heat production.
- It carries out immunological, bactericidal and detoxifying functions and stores vitamins B_{12} and A, copper and iron.
- Bile is conjugated in the hepatocytes (contains bile salts, phospholipids, cholesterol and fatty acids) and is secreted into the biliary tree; it emulsifies dietary fat in the jejunum prior to absorption.

Liver failure

Definitions

- Failure of one or more of the above functions caused by disease states producing inflammation, fibrosis, necrosis or infiltration/replacement of normal liver parenchyma.
- It may be acute following:
  - Fulminating infections (hepatitis virus A, B C, D and E, herpes simplex virus or bacterial)
  - Drug reactions or overdose (paracetamol, halothane, antidepressants, non-steroidal anti-inflammatory agents, isoniazid and rifampicin)
  - Ingestion of poisons (mushrooms and herbal concoctions)
  - Contact with chemicals (vinyl chloride)
  - Massive trauma, iatrogenic injury or multiple organ failure.
- Progressive failure occurs in metabolic diseases (Wilson's disease, fatty infiltration, fatty liver of pregnancy and Reye's syndrome), cirrhosis and primary and secondary malignant disease.

Clinical features

- Weakness, lethargy and malaise.
- Fever and jaundice (as a result of unconjugated bilirubinaemia).
- Palmar erythema, spider naevi (upper limbs and trunk) and Dupuytren's contracture.

- Cyanosis, hyperdynamic circulation and raised pulse pressure.
- Flapping tremor, cog-wheel limb rigidity and disorientation leading to coma.
- Features of portal hypertension: caput medusae and ascites.

Investigation

Haematological and biochemical parameters:

➤ Anaemia (normocytic, normochromic), leukocytosis and thrombocytopenia
➤ Raised serum bilirubin (normal 5–17 μmol/L, conjugated fraction <5 μmol/L)
➤ Alkaline phosphatase raised in cholestasis and hepatic infiltrations (normal 35–130 IU/L)
➤ Transaminases raised in hepatocellular disease (aspartate aminotransferase and alanine aminotransferase; normal levels 5–40 IU/L)
➤ Gamma-glutamyl transpeptidase raised in biliary obstruction and alcoholism (normal 10–48 IU/L)
➤ Gamma-globulin raised in chronic hepatitis and cirrhosis (normal 5–15 g/L)
➤ Decreased serum albumin (normal 35–50 g/L)
➤ Abnormal coagulation profile precipitating bleeding diathesis.

Imaging:

➤ Ultrasound, computerized tomography (CT)/ magnetic resonance imaging (MRI) scans reveal the extent of fatty or neoplastic infiltration, cirrhosis or necrosis
➤ Coeliac angiography may define intrinsic liver lesions
➤ Image-guided liver biopsy for histology.

Treatment

➤ Restrict protein and increase carbohydrate intake.
➤ Remove nitrogenous bowel contents by purgation.
➤ Treat the cause and any complication arising.
➤ Liver transplantation for end-stage liver failure.

Viral hepatitis

Definitions

- Viral hepatitis is sufficiently prevalent in all communities to cause diagnostic difficulties with cholecystitis and obstructive jaundice.
- Hepatitis A and E are self-limiting diseases spread by the orofaecal route; hepatitis B, C and D are sexually and parenterally (e.g. blood transfusion, needlestick injury) transmitted and may become chronic with progressive liver damage.
- Viral hepatitis produces acute inflammation of the entire liver with cholestasis and scattered or confluent areas of liver cell necrosis.
- The pre-icteric phase of hepatitis must be distinguished from an acute surgical abdomen and the icteric phase from surgical jaundice.

Clinical features

- Malaise, weakness, anorexia, mild pyrexia and cholestatic jaundice.
- Hepatic pain with a smooth, tender hepatomegaly.

Investigation

➤ Leukopenia, lymphopenia and raised erythrocyte sedimentation rate.
➤ Raised liver enzymes and bilirubin.

Treatment

➤ Symptomatic measures with bed rest and a high carbohydrate and low protein diet.
➤ Drug therapy has little effect in altering the course of the disease (including corticosteroid therapy).

Hepatic encephalopathy

Definitions

- Reversible neuropsychiatric manifestations that are sequelae to progressive liver disease.
- Various neurotransmitter systems are affected to produce clinical signs.

Clinical features

- Apathy, sleep disorders, disturbed consciousness and coma.
- Personality changes with speech and intellectual impairment.
- Flapping tremor and exaggerated deep tendon reflexes.

Treatment

➤ Treat precipitating cause.
➤ Reduce production and absorption of ammonia and other toxins in the gut (by purgation or ion exchange resin).
➤ Modify neurotransmitter balance by drugs (bromocriptine, flumazenil).
➤ Occlusion of an existing portocaval shunt may reverse the encephalopathy.

Cirrhosis

Definitions

- Progressive destruction of liver parenchyma, with fibrosis and nodular regeneration replacing normal liver architecture; a late sequela to chronic liver cell damage.
- Ductal atresia results in primary biliary cirrhosis.
- Predisposing factors:
  - Alcohol abuse
  - Viral hepatitis B and C
  - Cytotoxic agents (chemotherapeutic or industrial)
  - Wilson's disease and haemochromatosis.

Clinical features

- Malaise, lethargy and weakness (insidious onset) with loss of appetite and weight loss.
- Anaemia, oedema and ascites.
- Signs of portal hypertension.
- Hepatomegaly (in early phase of disease, later fibrosis leads to shrinkage of the organ).

Investigation

➤ Liver function may not be compromised until approximately two-thirds of the liver parenchyma is affected and hypoproteinaemia and coagulation defects appear.
➤ Ultrasound, CT/MRI scans delineate the extent of cirrhotic change.
➤ Image-guided core needle biopsy confirms the diagnosis and defines the type of cirrhosis.

Treatment

➤ Eliminate causative factors to halt disease progression.
➤ High carbohydrate and vitamin-enriched diet with salt restriction.
➤ Ascites: oral diuretic therapy (spironolactone 100–200 mg daily or frusemide 20–40 mg daily).
➤ Refractory ascites: paracentesis with replacement of albumin and K^+ or insertion of a peritoneal–jugular shunt.

Complications

● Cirrhosis predisposes to liver malignancy; liver imaging is used to exclude coexisting tumour.

Portal hypertension and gastro-oesophageal varices

Definitions

● Portal hypertension results from obstruction to the venous return from the gut.
● Pre-hepatic causes are splenic or portal venous thrombosis (from portal pyaemia).
● Hepatic causes are cirrhosis (macronodular or micronodular) and hepatocellular carcinoma.
● Post-hepatic causes are hepatic vein or inferior vena caval occlusion (Budd–Chiari syndrome).
● Portal hypertension produces variceal dilatation of the portosystemic venous communications at the gastro-oesophageal and the anorectal watersheds; gastro-oesophageal varices may produce life-threatening haemorrhage.

Clinical features

- Haematemesis.
- History of chronic liver disease.
- Visible abdominal wall varices (caput medusae).
- Rectal bleeding from varicose haemorrhoidal veins.
- Hepatomegaly may be present.

Investigation

➤ Upper endoscopy or barium swallow and meal reveal the varices and exclude other bleeding lesions in the stomach or duodenum.

Treatment

➤ Non-bleeding varices: endoscopic sclerotherapy or banding and prophylactic lowering of venous pressure with oral propranolol 40–80 mg daily.
➤ Acute haemorrhage:
  - Control of airway and ventilation
  - Rapid transfusion of blood or colloid
  - Emergency endoscopic sclerotherapy or banding
  - Vasopressin 20 units i.v. over 15 min or a somatostatin analogue to lower portal venous pressure.
➤ Uncontrolled or recurrent haemorrhage:
  - Balloon tamponade of the bleeding varices by Sengstaken–Blakemore tube
  - Surgical devascularization or oesophageal transection
  - Portosystemic shunt surgery provides long-term palliation by lowering portal venous pressure (may produce hepatic encephalopathy).

Benign liver lesions

Hepatic adenomas

Definitions

- A high incidence in young women with prolonged oral contraceptive use.
- Adenomas may undergo haemorrhagic necrosis with the risk of significant intrahepatic bleeding.
- They are not premalignant.

Treatment

> When situated close to the liver surface, excision is advised.

Focal nodular hyperplasias

Benign derangement of liver architecture with no pre-malignant potential. They are also commoner in young women, the incidence of rupture or bleeding is minimal and they require no treatment.

Simple liver cysts

These are not uncommon and are usually asymptomatic. Large cysts may produce a dragging abdominal pain and may be treated with image-guided aspiration, surgical fenestration or excision.

Haemangiomas

Haemangiomas are benign vascular anomalies in the liver parenchyma and are asymptomatic. There is a risk of haemorrhage from peripherally placed large lesions.

Hydatid cysts

These are parasitic cysts (page 161).

Liver abscesses

Liver abscesses are caused by parasites or anaerobic bacteria (page 149).

Hepatocellular carcinoma

Definitions

- A primary malignancy of the liver, unicentric or multicentric in origin.
- Highest incidence is in West Africa, where it is associated with the ingestion of aflatoxin (a mycotoxin present in mouldy peanuts).
- Portal cirrhosis, viral hepatitis B and C and liver fluke infestation (*Clonorchis sinensis* in South-East Asia) are predisposing factors.
- Late presentation is usual.

Clinical features

- Malaise, anorexia, lethargy, rapid weight loss and weakness.
- Pallor, jaundice and craggy hepatomegaly.
- Features of portal hypertension.
- Dyspnoea from direct extension to the diaphragm.
- Inferior vena caval syndrome from invasion or compression of the vein.
- Haematological spread to lung and bone producing dyspnoea, bone pain or pathological fractures.

Investigation

➤ Liver function tests may show elevated enzyme and bilirubin levels.
➤ Alpha-fetoprotein and carcino-embryonic antigen titres may be elevated.
➤ Ultrasound, contrast-enhanced CT/MRI scan to demonstrate the lesion.
➤ Image-guided needle biopsy for histology.
➤ Coeliac axis angiography delineates the lesion and its vascularity for embolization or perfusion chemotherapy.

Treatment

➤ Segmental resection or hemihepatectomy when tumour is unifocal or localized to one lobe.
➤ Liver transplantation for multifocal lesions in the absence of extrahepatic spread.
➤ Advanced or multicentric tumours may be palliated with tumour embolization, hepatic arterial ligation or perfusion with cytotoxic agents or liver radiotherapy.

Other primary hepatic malignancies

- Sarcomas (angiosarcoma, rhabdomyosarcoma).
- Intrahepatic cholangiocarcinoma.
- Hepatoblastoma (in children).

Secondary tumours of the liver

- These are blood-borne metastatic deposits and are typically multiple.

- They are resistant to chemotherapy (an extension of poor prognostic features of the primary tumour).
- Treated by liver resection when the deposits are limited to one lobe, with good medium-term survival.

Liver trauma

Definitions

- Types:
  - Grade I: minor laceration
  - Grade II: superficial lacerations that continue to bleed
  - Grade III: deeper lacerations with bile duct injury
  - Grade IV: lobar destruction
  - Grade V: hepatic vein or inferior vena cava injury.
- Aetiology:
  - Penetrating trauma
  - High velocity gunshot wounds: major venous injury
  - Severe blunt trauma.

Clinical features

- Features of penetrating or blunt abdominal trauma.
- Bruising or penetrating wound over right lower ribs.
- Concealed haemorrhage.
- Shock.

Investigation

➤ General investigation of the multiply injured patient (page 599).
➤ Laparotomy is usually indicated on clinical grounds.
➤ Abdominal CT shows:
  - Perihepatic haematoma and major lacerations
  - Central intrahepatic haematoma.

Treatment

➤ General management of the multiply injured patient (page 599).
➤ Laparotomy:
  • Lacerations that continue to bleed:
    - Perihepatic packing
    - Remove packs after 48 hours when coagulation has been corrected.

➔

- Major disruption and major venous injury:
  - Perihepatic packing
  - Transfer to hepatobiliary unit for partial liver resection or repair of major veins under caval–atrial bypass.

BILIARY TREE

Definitions

- Approximately 500–1000 mL of bile is secreted by the liver into the biliary tree and consists of bile acids, cholesterol, lecithin and bile pigments.
- The gallbladder concentrates the bile and contracts to empty into the duodenum following a meal and stimulation by cholecystokinin.
- Bile aids fat digestion and absorption and most of the bile is then reabsorbed in the terminal ileum to be re-secreted by the liver (thereby maintaining a constant bile acid pool).

Congenital anomalies

Biliary atresia

Definitions

- Non-canalization of the extrahepatic bile ducts in the newborn; may be associated with cardiac and/or bowel anomalies.

Clinical features

- Deepening jaundice at birth or soon afterwards.
- Pale stools and dark urine.

Investigation

➤ Liver function tests show obstructive jaundice.
➤ Ultrasound/CT scan of the liver reveals associated liver disease (biliary cirrhosis) and the state of the biliary tree.
➤ Radionuclide excretion scan [hepatic iminodiacetic acid (HIDA)] identifies the proximal extent of duct atresia.
➤ Image-guided needle biopsy reveals extent of parenchymal damage.

Treatment

➤ Excision of all biliary tissue with anastomosis of a jejunal Roux loop to the porta hepatis.
➤ Anastomotic stenosis may occur over the years and liver transplantation is considered in selected patients.

Caroli's disease

Definitions

● A rare, inherited non-obstructive cystic dilatation of the intrahepatic ducts.
● Young female adults are predominantly affected.
● Leads to recurrent bacterial cholangitis or stone formation.
● Associated with hepatic fibrosis and cholangiocarcinoma.

Clinical features

● Abdominal pain with febrile episodes.
● Signs of cholangitis.

Investigation

➤ Contrast-enhanced liver CT/MRI scan is diagnostic.
➤ Haematological and biochemical profiles are usually normal unless cholangitis ensues.

Treatment

➤ Biliary drainage in cholangitis [sphincterotomy or stenting by endoscopic retrograde cholangio-pancreatography (ERCP) or percutaneous transhepatic catheterization] under broad-spectrum antibiotic cover.
➤ Surgical drainage (hepaticojejunostomy).
➤ Lobectomy if pathology is confined to one lobe.
➤ Liver transplantation in diffuse disease.

Choledochal cyst

Definitions

● A rare dilatation of the common bile duct that is prevalent in South-East Asia, with a female:male ratio of 3–4:1.

- Common varieties are:
  - Type I: fusiform or cystic dilatation of the common bile duct (65% incidence)
  - Type IV: cystic dilatations of the intrahepatic and/or extrahepatic ducts (30% incidence).
- Choledochal cysts predispose to recurrent cholangitis and cholangiocarcinoma if left untreated.

Clinical features

- Episodes of upper abdominal pain as a result of recurrent pancreatitis.
- Low-grade pyrexia and intermittent jaundice (rigors suggest cholangitis secondary to bile stasis).
- Tender hepatomegaly and, occasionally, a palpable cystic swelling in the upper abdomen.

Investigation

➤ Abdominal X-ray may show a soft tissue mass in the right upper quadrant.
➤ ERCP and abdominal ultrasound, CT or HIDA scan demonstrate the cystic lesion and surrounding anatomy.

Treatment

➤ Excision of dilated extrahepatic bile duct with Roux-en-Y hepaticojejunostomy (anastomosing the Roux loop to the porta hepatis).

Gallbladder and bile ducts

Definitions

- Gallstones (cholesterol, pigment and mixed stones) form in the gallbladder as a result of bile stasis and/or infection, or because of a reduction in the bile acid pool, and cause acute cholecystitis.
- Acalculous cholecystitis occurs in the absence of gallstones in 5–10% of adults and in 30% of children with acute cholecystitis; predisposing causes are severe systemic infections, following major abdominal surgery, trauma or burns, and typhoid and parasitic infections of the gallbladder.

Clinical features

- Acute cholecystitis:
  - Sudden onset of upper abdominal or right upper quadrant pain with nausea and/or vomiting
  - Low-grade pyrexia and mild jaundice
  - Positive Murphy's sign (pain on inspiration when hand depressed under the right costal margin)
  - The gallbladder may be palpable as a tender swelling.

Investigation

➤ Ultrasound scan reveals gallstones, distension and/or inflammatory thickening of the gallbladder wall.

➤ Duct dilatation >10 mm suggests the presence of duct stones.

Treatment

➤ Acute cholecystitis – supportive measures:
  - Bed rest and analgesia (morphine 10 mg or pethidine 50–100 mg 4- to 8-hourly i.m.)
  - Intravenous fluid, electrolyte and antibiotic therapy with cefuroxime 750 mg and metronidazole 500 mg i.v. 8-hourly.

➤ Surgical removal of the diseased gallbladder (by laparotomy or laparoscopically) is performed within 12 hours of the onset of symptoms or following resolution of all symptoms (after 6–16 weeks).

➤ Peroperative cholangiography is performed to identify duct stones that require surgical exploration of the common duct with stone extraction.

Complications

Complications of acute cholecystitis:

- Mucocoele: distension of the gallbladder with mucus as a result of calculus impaction in Hartmann's pouch or cystic duct
- Empyema: abscess formation in the gallbladder caused by stasis and infection
- Gangrene: ischaemic necrosis of the gallbladder wall resulting from inflammation and distension

- Fistulation: inflammatory adhesion of the gallbladder to the duodenum or common hepatic duct may lead to a gallstone eroding into the adjacent viscus.

Gallstones in the bile duct (choledocholithiasis)

Definitions

- Gallstones migrating into or primary duct stones forming in the common bile duct produce obstructive jaundice and/or acute pancreatitis when the stone impacts in the ampulla of Vater.
- Calculus in Hartmann's pouch or cystic duct may produce extrinsic compression of the common hepatic duct and biliary obstruction (Mirizzi syndrome).
- Cholangitis (as a result of infection in stagnant bile) causes inflammation or ulceration of the common bile or hepatic ducts (infecting organisms are *Escherichia coli*, *Klebsiella* spp, *Streptococcus* spp, *Bacteroides* spp and *Clostridium* spp).

Clinical features

- Hepatic pain.
- Progressive jaundice.
- Low-grade pyrexia.
- Tender hepatomegaly.
- Gallbladder is usually not palpable ('Courvoisier's law'; page 472).

Ascending cholangitis:

- Rigors, pain and jaundice
- Tachycardia and hypotension.

Investigation

➤ Raised bilirubin and liver enzymes.
➤ Leukocytosis and raised CRP levels.
➤ Raised platelet count and prothrombin time.
➤ Blood cultures.
➤ Renal function tests.

➜

➤ Ultrasound, CT or HIDA scan or MR cholangiogram reveal the state of the biliary tree and site of obstruction.
➤ ERCP or percutaneous transhepatic cholangiogram; in addition to imaging the biliary tree obtain bile for aerobic and anaerobic blood cultures.

Treatment

➤ Intravenous hydration and electrolyte therapy with 10% dextrose.
➤ Parenteral broad-spectrum antibiotics (ampicillin, ciprofloxacin or a cephalosporin).
➤ Biliary decompression prior to surgery by percutaneous transhepatic catheter drainage or by ERCP with removal of duct stones and sphincterotomy and/or stenting of the bile duct.
➤ Choledochotomy (surgically opening the common bile duct) with exploration of the bile duct and stone extraction is performed with cholecystectomy; an impacted stone at the lower end of the bile duct is bypassed by means of a choledochoduodenostomy; emergency surgical decompression is associated with a mortality of 16–40%.

Complications

● Gallstone ileus:
  – Gallstones or duct stones >2.5 cm in size may erode into the duodenum and cause small bowel obstruction at the terminal ileum.
  – Plain abdominal X-ray shows signs of small bowel obstruction and possibly the obstructing calculus and gas in the biliary tree (indicating a biliary enteric fistula).
  – Surgical relief of obstruction (enterotomy and calculus removal) following optimal rehydration with fluids and electrolytes.

Biliary strictures

Definitions

● Duct injury during cholecystectomy is the commonest cause (incidence of 0.5%).

- Primary sclerosing cholangitis produces multiple strictures of the extrahepatic and intrahepatic ducts as a result of fibrous thickening of the duct wall (is associated with ulcerative colitis).
- Chronic pancreatitis may produce strictures distally, close to the ampulla of Vater.
- Malignant strictures are caused by cholangiocarcinoma.

Clinical features

- Iatrogenic injury: there is increasing postoperative pain, deepening jaundice, abdominal distension and ileus.
- There may be signs of biliary peritonitis.

Investigation

➤ Liver function shows cholestasis (elevated enzymes and bilirubin).

➤ Ultrasound, CT scan or MR cholangiogram may delineate the site of stricture.

➤ ERCP or HIDA scan may, in addition, reveal a bile leak.

Treatment

➤ Management is by joint participation of surgeon, radiologist and endoscopist in a tertiary referral centre.

➤ Strictures are endoscopically dilated or stented and drained.

➤ Surgical repair is undertaken early in order to forestall obliterative cholangitis, adhesion formation and secondary liver changes. Surgical drainage involves anastomosing a Roux loop of small bowel to the proximal hepatic duct or the porta hepatis (Roux-en-Y choledochojejunostomy or hepaticojejunostomy).

➤ Prevention of duct injuries: experienced and competent operating surgeon and team; identification of anatomy of Calot's triangle – common hepatic duct, cystic duct and the cystic artery – (with the aid of peroperative cholangiogram).

➤ Primary sclerosing cholangitis is progressive and high-dose steroid therapy is of short-term benefit; liver transplantation is indicated in the face of deterioration of liver function and poor prognosis.

Carcinoma of the gallbladder

Definitions

- A rare tumour associated with chronic calculous cholecystitis with a female:male ratio 3–4:1.
- Incidental finding on histology for 1% of cholecystectomies for gallstones.
- Papillary adenocarcinoma is the most frequent lesion (others are squamous cell and anaplastic carcinomas).
- The tumour spreads to the porta hepatis, liver, adjacent viscera, and there may be peritoneal seeding by the time the diagnosis is made; the prognosis is poor (<5% 5-year survival).

Clinical features

- Presentation may be similar to cholecystitis.
- Rapidly deepening jaundice, pain and weight loss.
- A mass may rarely be palpable in the right hypochondrium.

Investigation

➤ Liver function shows cholestasis.
➤ Ultrasound and CT scans may show a mass replacing the gallbladder, with enlarged lymph nodes.
➤ Spiral MRI scan or laparoscopy would stage the disease.
➤ ERCP with sampling of the bile and brushings of the bile duct wall may provide cytological evidence of tumour.

Treatment

➤ Radical cholecystectomy with resection of the porta hepatis and part of the overlying liver with Roux loop reconstruction.
➤ Inoperable lesions are palliated by stenting of the proximal common duct and porta hepatis to relieve the jaundice.
➤ Chemoradiotherapy is palliative.
➤ Adenomas of the gallbladder are premalignant and are treated by cholecystectomy.

Carcinoma of the bile duct (cholangiocarcinoma)

Definitions

- Tumours of the biliary tree are adenocarcinomas and may arise intrahepatically or extrahepatically; they are associated with ulcerative colitis, sclerosing cholangitis, choledochal cyst and Caroli's disease (liver fluke infestation with *Clonorchis sinensis* and *Opisthorchis viverrini* is a predisposing factor in the Far East; page 152).
- Gallbladder and bile duct cancers occur in the elderly (>65 years of age).
- Produces complete obstruction of the extrahepatic bile duct with intrahepatic duct dilatation and hepatomegaly, which may progress to liver atrophy or biliary cirrhosis.

Clinical features

- Malaise, anorexia and weight loss.
- Abdominal pain and low-grade pyrexia and jaundice.
- Pale stools, dark urine and pruritus.
- Charcot's triad of symptoms (pain, jaundice and rigors) indicates acute cholangitis secondary to obstruction.
- Courvoisier's 'law' states that in obstructive jaundice, if the gallbladder is palpable, then the obstruction is unlikely to be the result of gallstones; this is because gallstones are associated with gallbladder fibrosis.

Investigation

➤ Ultrasound and CT/MRI scans delineate tumour and associated liver pathology.
➤ Percutaneous transhepatic cholangiogram or ERCP with bile sampling and brush cytology.
➤ MR cholangiogram and digital subtraction angiography assists in the assessment of resectability.

Treatment

➤ Tumours are rarely resectable as a result of hilar/nodal involvement; endoscopic or percutaneous stenting provides satisfactory biliary drainage and palliation.

➤

> Tumours of the lower half of the common bile duct may be resected (pancreatoduodenectomy).
> Early intrahepatic tumours may be treated by lobectomy or hemihepatectomy.

SPLEEN

Definitions

Main functions of the spleen are:

- Destruction of ageing and abnormal red blood cells, foreign protein and microorganisms by the splenic reticulo-endothelial system
- Immunological defence by splenic B- and T-cell lymphocytes produces humoral agents, antibodies, opsonins and interferons.

Splenomegaly

Definitions

- Infective causes: malaria, schistosomiasis, hydatid disease, kala-azar (page 148 Tropical diseases).
- Haematological causes: chronic leukaemia, polycythaemia rubra vera, sickle-cell disease, thalassaemia, hereditary spherocytosis (page 176 Anaemias).
- Liver and autoimmune (collagen) diseases: portal hypertension, Felty's syndrome, Still's disease.
- Tumours: Hodgkin's and non-Hodgkin's lymphomas and metastatic deposits from gastrointestinal primaries.

Clinical features

- Spleen is generally palpable and tender (in tropical splenomegaly syndrome it may become massively enlarged and occupy most of the abdomen).
- Idiopathic thrombocytic purpura: purpuric skin and mucosal patchy rash with mucosal bleeding and positive tourniquet test (splenomegaly is not a constant feature).
- Hereditary spherocytosis: pallor, lassitude, jaundice (haemolytic), pigmented gallstone colic and chronic

leg ulcers (in adults); large palpable spleen with occasional hepatomegaly.
- Acquired autoimmune haemolytic anaemia: triggered by viral infection, drug reaction or connective tissue disease (systemic lupus erythematosus); results in red cell sequestration in spleen with splenomegaly and formation of pigmented gallstones.
- Hereditary haemolytic anaemias:
  - Thalassaemia presents with chronic anaemia, jaundice and splenomegaly
  - Sickle-cell disease presents with anaemia, splenic and/or bone pain from infarcts during sickle-cell crisis.

Treatment
➤ Autoimmune haemolytic anaemias respond to steroid therapy, and relapses to azathioprine or immunoglobulin G transfusion.
➤ Haemolytic crises are treated with blood transfusion.
➤ Splenectomy is reserved for refractory haematological disease (in hypersplenism when all accessory splenic tissue is removed) or neoplastic conditions or for a grossly enlarged tropical spleen; prophylactic anticoagulation is advised because of an increased incidence of venous thromboembolism.

Splenic trauma

Definitions
- Complete rupture, laceration, or capsular haematoma.
- Delayed rupture may occur: usually during the subsequent 2 weeks.
- Aetiology: blunt or penetrating abdominal trauma, or fracture of the lower ribs (left 9, 10, 11).

Clinical features
- Bruising or penetrating injury over left ninth to eleventh ribs.
- General features of abdominal trauma (page 405).
- Tenderness in left upper quadrant.
- Shock: complete rupture.

Investigation

➤ General investigation of the multiply injured patient (page 599).
➤ Plain chest and abdominal radiographs may show rib fractures, with haemothorax/pneumothorax and loss of splenic and psoas outlines.
➤ Laparotomy is usually indicated on clinical grounds.
➤ Abdominal ultrasound or CT: identifies perisplenic and capsular haematoma in stable patients with localized injury.

Treatment

➤ Blood volume replacement.
➤ Splenectomy at laparotomy.
➤ Repair and enveloping spleen in an absorbable mesh bag may be attempted in some centres, especially in children.
➤ Post-splenectomy protection from pneumococcal and *Haemophilus* infection.
➤ Pneumococcal polysaccharide vaccine 0.5 mL i.m. or s.c.
➤ Penicillin V 500 mg b.i.d. orally for life (benzylpenicillin 600 mg t.i.d. when the patient is unable to take oral medication).

PANCREAS

Definitions

● Daily exocrine secretion of 1.5–3.0 L of alkaline fluid is produced by the pancreatic acini, containing enzymes trypsin, chymotrypsin and carboxypeptidase (digest proteins), amylase (digests carbohydrate) and lipase, cholesterol esterase and phospholipase (digest fat). Proteolytic enzymes are secreted as pro-enzymes to prevent autodigestion of the pancreas; pancreatic secretion is stimulated in response to food in the stomach or duodenum by gastrin, cholecystokinin, secretin and acetylcholine.

- Endocrine secretion by the islet cells produces:
  - Insulin (beta cells) regulates uptake, metabolism and storage of glucose (glycogen), free fatty acids and keto-acids (insulin lowers the blood glucose level; insulin insufficiency leads to the mobilization of endogenous metabolites from the liver, adipose tissue and muscle and raises the blood glucose level)
  - Glucagon (alpha cells) raises blood glucose level by stimulating glycogenolysis and glucose release from the liver.

Annular pancreas

Definitions

- Results from prenatal failure of rotation of the ventral pancreatic bud resulting in pancreatic tissue surrounding and thereby narrowing the second and third part of the duodenum (associated with Down's syndrome and other congenital anomalies).

Clinical features

- Vomiting, which may be bile stained, following feeds in the newborn.
- Upper abdominal distension with visible gastric peristalsis.

Investigation

➤ Plain abdominal X-ray may show the 'double-bubble' sign, which is diagnostic.

Treatment

➤ Duodenojejunostomy (side-to-side anastomosis of the duodenum to the jejunum) bypasses the narrowed duodenal segment (avoid dividing the band of constricting pancreatic tissue, which may result in pancreatic fistula).

Acute pancreatitis

Definitions

- An acute inflammation of the pancreas, with raised levels of pancreatic enzymes in the blood and urine, and involvement of other tissues or organs as part of a systemic inflammatory response syndrome.

- Severe acute pancreatitis may result in haemorrhagic necrosis, peripancreatic fluid collections, pseudocyst or abscess formation.
- Multi-organ failure in fulminating disease caused by systemic inflammatory response syndrome.
- Causes: biliary calculi and alcoholism account for 75% of cases; other causes are trauma, systemic infections, autoimmune and metabolic diseases.
- Pancreatic damage is caused by autodigestion by extravasation of its own enzymes.

Clinical features

- Severe upper abdominal pain radiating to the upper back with nausea and vomiting; the patient tends to adopt a flexed position in bed.
- Pyrexia, tachycardia and tachypnoea.
- Diffuse upper abdominal tenderness and guarding.
- Ecchymoses of the body wall (Cullen's sign at the umbilicus, Grey Turner's sign in the flanks).
- Oliguria (in severe pancreatitis).

Investigation

➤ Serum amylase and lipase are elevated.
➤ Leukocytosis $>15 \times 10^9$/L; CRP >210 units/L.
➤ In severe pancreatitis there is derangement of liver, lung and renal function:
  - Glucose >10 mmol/L
  - Pao_2 <60 mmHg
  - Urea >16 mmol/L
  - Calcium <2 mmol/L
  - Albumin <32 g/L
  - Lactate dehydrogenase >600 units/L
  - Aspartate/alanine aminotransferase >100 units/L.
➤ Plain abdominal X-ray may show a 'sentinel loop' of small bowel in the left upper quadrant, moderate distension of the duodenum and the transverse colon.
➤ Ultrasound and CT scan may show pancreatic swelling, fluid collections, define a pseudocyst or areas of necrosis. Biliary calculi may be visualized.

Treatment

➤ The course of the disease is often unpredictable and varies from mild to fulminant; the patient is monitored in a high dependency or intensive care unit for cardiac, respiratory, hepatic or renal dysfunction supported by intravenous fluid therapy, nasogastric decompression and opiate analgesia.

➤ Severe gallstone pancreatitis in the presence of liver dysfunction or cholangitis requires immediate ERCP and sphincterotomy, with duct stone extraction and/or stenting.

➤ Elective cholecystectomy and peroperative cholangiography are performed 6–8 weeks after recovery from the acute attack.

➤ In acute necrotizing pancreatitis there are indications for pancreatic debridement and peritoneal lavage with drainage; occasionally a laparotomy may be required to facilitate drainage and to monitor healing.

Chronic pancreatitis

Definitions

● A persistent inflammation of the pancreas characterized by remissions and relapses with irreversible changes in the gland and its function.

● Affects men more than women (ratio M:F 4:1) with a mean age of onset of 40 years and associated with chronic alcoholism (high level of alcohol and animal protein consumption has also been implicated).

● The pancreas undergoes progressive atrophy and sclerosis, with distortion of the duct and formation of duct stones and proteinaceous material in the ducts causing obstruction.

● Pain may be the predominant symptom and there may be pancreatic insufficiency resulting in steatorrhoea and diabetes.

Investigation

➤ Plain abdominal X-ray: pancreatic calcification may be demonstrable.
➤ ERCP: assesses pancreatic and sphincter function by analysis of pure pancreatic juice and papillary manometry; delineates pancreatic duct pathology and assists planning of surgical drainage.

Treatment

➤ Pain relief with opiates is usually necessary, with steps taken to guard against narcotic habituation.
➤ Pancreatic enzyme supplementation for failing exocrine function and a low fat diet with abstinence from alcohol.
➤ Onset of diabetes mellitus requires insulin therapy.
➤ Surgery for poorly controlled pain in relapsing disease:
  – When the pancreatic duct is grossly dilated, drainage of the duct is carried out by anastomosing a Roux loop of ileum to the distal end of the duct, or longitudinally by filleting the duct (modified Peustow operation)
  – When the disease is confined to the body a distal pancreatectomy or, when involving the head, a pancreatoduodenectomy may provide symptom relief with a good quality of life (surgery is not appropriate in the presence of narcotic and/or alcohol habituation).

Pancreatic pseudocyst

Definitions

● A collection of fluid and tissue debris in the lesser sac as a complication of acute or chronic pancreatitis.
● Presents 3–4 weeks after an episode of acute pancreatitis.

Clinical features

● Nausea, anorexia, epigastric pain and a tender upper abdominal mass.

Investigation

➤ Ultrasound and CT scans define size and position.
➤ Image-guided aspiration enables enzyme estimation and cultures.

Treatment

➤ Indications for drainage: intractable pain or pseudocysts >6 cm in size or persisting for >6 weeks.
➤ Image-guided needle aspiration may resolve small collections.
➤ Internal drainage of pseudocyst into the stomach (cystogastrostomy) or, rarely, into the duodenum or jejunum for large or recurrent cysts.
➤ Distal pancreatectomy for pseudocysts in the tail of the pancreas.

Carcinoma of the pancreas

Definitions

● Ductal adenocarcinoma of the pancreas afflicts the elderly, with an equal incidence in both sexes, and involves the head (70%), the body (15%) and the tail (10%).
● Peri-ampullary tumours arising in the vicinity of the ampulla of Vater present early with obstructive jaundice.
● Tumours of the body are diagnosed late and have usually spread by perineural and lymphatic invasion to the liver, peritoneum and lung.

Clinical features

● Insidious onset with malaise, anorexia, abdominal discomfort or pain and weight loss.
● Jaundice (peri-ampullary tumour or spread to porta hepatis) with a palpable gallbladder ('Courvoisier's law').
● Hepatomegaly (liver metastases).

Investigation

➤ Ultrasound and CT scans identify the pancreatic lesion and regional nodal or liver secondaries.
➤ Hypotonic duodenogram may reveal a widened duodenal curve in tumours of the pancreatic head.
➤ Upper endoscopy (duodenoscopy) may identify peri-ampullary lesions, which may be biopsied.

Treatment

➤ Ampullary tumours (<3 cm) are resected (pancreato-duodenectomy or Whipple's operation) with a 30% 5-year survival.
➤ Larger ampullary and pancreatic head tumours causing obstructive jaundice may either be endoscopically stented or surgically bypassed (cholecystojejunostomy or choledochojejunostomy).
➤ Tumours <3 cm in the body and tail may be resected, with good palliation.
➤ Most pancreatic tumours are well advanced when diagnosed and treatment is directed at symptomatic relief and nutritional support:
  – Pain relief is with morphine or diamorphine 5–10 mg 4- to 6-hourly with fentanyl patches 25 or 50 μg/hour for 'breakthrough' pain
  – Cholestyramine 4–8 g daily for pruritus (caused by jaundice); pancreatic enzyme supplements for loss of exocrine secretion (one to two pancreatin capsules with meals).

Pancreatic endocrine tumours

Insulinomas

Definitions

● These are functional, benign and usually unifocal tumours of the islet cells of the pancreas (beta cells), which affect young adults.

Clinical features

- Bizarre symptoms attributable to hypoglycaemia, range from hunger pains, sweating, dizziness, blurring of vision, uncoordinated limb movements and fits.

Investigation

- Blood glucose of <40 mg/dL with elevated insulin levels of $>6\,\mu$U/mL and C-peptide levels of >0.2 nmol/mL.
- Absence of sulfonylurea in the plasma and raised plasma insulin radioimmunoassay titres are diagnostic.
- Stimulation by insulin secretagogues (tolbutamide test) produces an exaggerated release of insulin.

Treatment

- Excision or enucleation with intra-operative ultrasound localization.
- Diazoxide therapy suppresses insulin production and palliates inoperable lesions.

VIPomas

Definitions

- These tumours arising from vasoactive polypeptide-secreting cells are found mainly in the pancreas; they are usually solitary, and are malignant, metastasizing to the regional lymphatics, kidneys, lungs, stomach or mediastinum.

Clinical features

- Vasoactive polypeptides and amines cause flushing and watery diarrhoea.
- Diagnosis is usually delayed following the onset of symptoms by 2–3 years, by which time patients are usually passing in excess of 3 L of liquid stool daily, with accompanying weakness and dehydration.

Investigation
➤ Hypokalaemia, hypoglycaemia and metabolic acidosis.
➤ Fasting plasma vasoactive intestinal peptide (VIP) levels of >200 pg/mL are diagnostic in the presence of clinical features.
➤ Tumour localization is by CT, MRI and intra-operative ultrasound scanning or mesenteric angiography.
➤ Somatostatin-receptor scintigraphy with radiolabelled octreotide has a high incidence of localizing primary tumours and/or metastases.

Treatment
➤ Correct fluid and electrolyte deficits (severe cases may require >6 L of fluid and >350 mmol of K^+ ions over 24 hours).
➤ Correct hypomagnesaemia and metabolic acidosis.
➤ Symptomatic treatment with somatostatin analogues (octreotide 50–600 µg subcutaneously daily) is effective while awaiting definitive therapy.
➤ Benign VIPomas are curable by pancreatic resection; metastatic tumours may be surgically debulked with good results.
➤ Streptozotocin and 5-fluorouracil therapy produces a modest response.

Glucagonomas

Definitions
● Glucagonomas are rare alpha-cell tumours of the pancreas that secrete various forms of glucagon, the majority occurring in the pancreatic tail; liver metastases are common.
● They may form part of the multiple endocrine neoplasia syndrome (MEN type 1), an inherited disorder consisting of islet tumours of the pancreas (producing gastrin, insulin, glucagons, somatostatin and VIP), pituitary chromaffin adenomas (producing prolactin), thyroid and adrenocortical tumours.

Clinical features

- Cachexia, weight loss and bowel hurry.
- A skin rash that, starting in the groin and perineum and progressing distally, also affects the oral mucosa (necrolytic migratory erythema) is a common feature.
- Psychiatric manifestations may be present.

Investigation

- ➤ Normochromic, normocytic anaemia.
- ➤ Diabetes mellitus with a raised fasting plasma glucagon level (>50 pmol/L).
- ➤ Contrast-enhanced CT scan or selective visceral angiography image the lesion.

Treatment

- ➤ Surgical excision (with intraoperative ultrasound localization) is the treatment of choice for the primary lesion (enucleation or distal pancreatectomy and splenectomy).
- ➤ Tumour embolization for hepatic disease.
- ➤ Octreotide (somatostatin analogue) therapy and chemotherapy (streptozotocin and 5-fluorouracil) produce sustained symptom relief and palliation.

Gastrinomas

Definitions

- An endocrine tumour of the pancreas (less commonly of the duodenum) that targets the stomach by releasing gastrin and causing severe, recurrent peptic ulceration, bleeding and ulcer perforation (the Zollinger–Ellison syndrome).
- The majority of gastrinomas are malignant.

Clinical features

- Gastric acid hypersecretion produces abdominal pain, which may be accompanied by diarrhoea, haematemesis or melaena.

● Signs of acute abdomen in the event of peptic perforation.

Investigation

➤ Fasting serum gastrin assays are elevated with a low gastric pH (<2.5) and a peak acid output higher than 27 mmol H^+.
➤ Tumour localization by CT, abdominal or endoscopic ultrasound scans or by mesenteric angiography.
➤ Somatostatin-receptor scintigraphy with radiolabelled octeotride identifies most gastrinomas.

Treatment

➤ Proton pump inhibition (omeprazole or lansoprazole 60–120 mg in divided daily oral dose) controls gastric hypersecretion.
➤ Total gastrectomy is reserved for failed medical therapy.
➤ Streptozotocin with doxorubicin or 5-fluorouracil chemotherapy gives good remission.
➤ Tumour embolization, interferon or somatostatin (octeotride 50–600 µg subcutaneously daily for 1 week) therapies are palliative (inhibit further tumour growth).

Trauma to the pancreas

Definitions

● Aetiology: severe blunt, crush or penetrating abdominal trauma (lap seatbelt compression).
● Usually occurs in conjunction with multiple organ injuries.
● Most significant if there is main pancreatic duct injury.

Clinical features

● Unexplained systemic inflammatory response, peritonism and ileus from haemoperitoneum and leakage of pancreatic juice.

Investigation

➤ Serum amylase: significantly elevated in 90% of injuries.
➤ Corrected serum Ca^+ may be low.
➤ Abdominal CT may identify oedema, haematoma, or lesser sac collection.
➤ Tends to underestimate severity of injury.
➤ Endoscopic retrograde cholangiopancreatography identifies pancreatic duct injury, but is not often possible in these patients.

Treatment

➤ Resuscitation with volume replacement.
➤ At laparotomy:
    – Drainage of the peripancreatic collection
    – Omental plugging of the damaged area
    – Resection of a damaged tail with the spleen
    – Major duct transection may require drainage into a Roux-en-Y arrangement
    – Establish feeding jejunostomy.

Complications

● Iatrogenic injury of the pancreas may occur in splenectomy, proximal gastric surgery, pancreatic surgery and endoscopic sphincterotomy. It may result in acute pancreatitis or a pancreatic fistula.

ADRENAL GLAND

Adrenal cortex

Definitions

● Glucocorticoids (hydrocortisone/cortisol and its precursor cortisone) are produced by the adrenal cortex and metabolize the conversion of body proteins to carbohydrates (gluconeogenesis).
● Corticotropin-releasing factors (CRF), secreted by the hypothalamus, stimulate adrenocorticotropic hormone

(ACTH) release by the anterior pituitary and circulating ACTH, in turn, stimulates cortisol secretion by the adrenal cortex; circulating cortisol then produces a negative feedback on the hypothalomopituitary axis, inhibiting further CRF/ACTH release.

- Sex hormones (androgens and oestrogens) are also produced, and excessive production as a result of cortical hyperplasia or tumours causes virilism in females and, rarely, feminization in males.
- Haemorrhage into the adrenals in the newborn as a result of trauma at birth or in children and adults as a result of fulminating infections, severe haemorrhage or burns (Waterhouse–Friderichsen syndrome) produces catastrophic adrenal failure.

Addison's disease

Definitions

- Progressive adrenocortical insufficiency caused by lymphocytic infiltration of the gland, usually affecting young adults, or as a result of tuberculosis or amyloidosis.

Clinical features

- Malaise, weakness, postural hypotension and muscle cramps.
- Non-specific abdominal pain, febrile episodes, vomiting, diarrhoea and weight loss.
- Hyperpigmentation of the palm, skin creases and buccal mucosa.

Investigation

➤ Low levels of plasma cortisol and low 24-hour urinary free cortisol level (normal 5–28 mg/24 hours).
➤ ACTH stimulation by Synacthen produces a poor cortisol response, as detected in plasma and urine.

Treatment

➤ Long-term hydrocortisone 20–30 mg daily in divided doses with fludrocortisone 0.1 mg daily (mineralo-corticoid replacement).

Cushing's syndrome

Definitions

- Overproduction of cortisol by the adrenal cortex (female:male ratio of 3:1).
- Pituitary adenomas overproducing ACTH are the commonest form of endogenous hypercorticism (65%); adrenal adenoma/hyperplasia (20%), adrenal carcinoma (5%) and ectopic ACTH production account for others.
- Iatrogenic Cushing's syndrome is caused by long-term cortisone therapy for non-endocrine disease (rheumatoid arthritis) and transplant recipients.

Clinical features

- Moon facies, pursed lips, buffalo hump and 'lemon-on-matchsticks' body contour.
- Thinned and inelastic skin with purple striae.
- Hypertension and congestive cardiac failure.
- Amenorrhoea and impotence.
- Backache (and pathological fractures) resulting from osteoporosis.

Investigation

Raised plasma cortisol levels and loss of diurnal rhythm.

➤ Elevated 24-hour urinary free cortisol level (normal 5–28 mg/24 hours).
➤ Dexamethasone suppression test: normally dexamethasone (a synthetic glucocorticoid) administration suppresses CRF/ACTH and thus cortisol production; no effect is observed in Cushing's syndrome.

- CT surgical localization of adrenal and pituitary tumours.

Treatment

➤ Pituitary tumours: trans-sphenoidal adenectomy or irradiation with yttrium-90 implants.
➤ Adrenal tumours: adrenalectomy.
➤ Adrenal hyperplasia and refractory pituitary disease: bilateral adrenalectomy.

➜

➤ Medical therapy: metyrapone inhibits cortisol production (0.25–6.0 g daily orally tailored to cortisol production) and is given when surgery is contraindicated.

Primary hyperaldosteronism (Conn's syndrome)

Definitions

- Excessive production of aldosterone from a cortical adenoma (Conn's syndrome) or from bilateral cortical hyperplasia resulting in Na^+ retention and K^+ depletion.
- Secondary hyperaldosteronism is associated with cirrhosis and renal artery stenosis with raised plasma levels of renin and angiotensin.

Clinical features

- Polyuria and polydipsia.
- Lethargy, fatigue and muscular weakness.
- Hypertension.

Investigation

➤ Hypokalaemia (<3.5 mmol/L), hypernatraemia and alkalosis with raised plasma aldosterone levels.
➤ CT/magnetic resonance imaging (MRI) localize the lesion and differentiate adenoma from hyperplasia.

Treatment

➤ Adrenalectomy is curative for an adenoma (poor results in bilateral hyperplasia).
➤ Pre-operatively K^+ supplements are given for 4 weeks and hypertension is controlled by calcium channel blockers.
➤ Medical therapy for bilateral cortical hyperplasia with long-term oral spironolactone 100–400 mg or amiloride 10–40 mg daily.

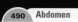

Adrenal medulla

Phaeochromocytoma

Definitions

- Tumours of the sympathetic chain, the majority arising in the adrenal medulla producing mainly noradrenaline with some adrenaline.
- Most are benign, and hormone production (and clinical effects) may be intermittent or continuous.
- Associated with the multiple endocrine neoplasia syndrome (MEN type 2) consisting of parathyroid tumours, medullary carcinoma of the thyroid (producing calcitonin) and phaeochromocytomas.

Clinical features

- Features of catecholamine excess:
  - Paroxysmal hypertension
  - Palpitations, tachycardia/bradycardia with arrhythmias
  - Headaches and vomiting
  - Sweating and tremor
  - Dyspnoea and weakness
  - Pallor or flushing.

Investigation

➤ Raised 24-hour urinary free catecholamines ($>100\,\mu g$), vanillylmandelic acid ($>7\,mg$) and metadrenalines ($>1.3\,mg$).

➤ Plasma noradrenaline and adrenaline levels are raised ($>1000\,\mu g/mL$).

➤ Abdominal ultrasound, CT/MRI scans or ^{131}I meta-iodobenzyl-guanidine (MIBG) scan localizes adrenal and ectopic lesions.

Treatment

➤ Peri-operative alpha and beta blockade with phenoxy-benzamine (20–80 mg) followed by propranolol (120–240 mg) daily to control hypertensive episodes and arrhythmias, respectively, and fluid therapy to

➜

> expand the circulatory volume. Two week preoperative course.
> ➤ Adrenalectomy is curative (except in malignant disease) with long-term surveillance.

Adrenal mass lesion as an incidental finding

Adrenal tumours that are found incidentally on abdominal imaging are usually benign, non-functioning lesions; those <3 cm in size may be kept under surveillance and larger lesions excised to exclude malignancy.

Neurofibroma

Definitions

- Malignant tumour of infants and children arising from the sympathetic chain or the adrenal gland with an incidence of 1 per 10 000 live births.
- Produces catecholamines and vasoactive peptides.
- Metastasizes early, with a poor prognosis.

Clinical features

- Failure to thrive, anaemia and weight loss.
- Abdominal pain and distension with a palpable mass.
- Flushing, sweating, hypertension and irritability (catecholamine effect).
- Watery diarrhoea and hypokalaemia (VIP effect).

Investigation

➤ Raised urinary vanillylmandelic acid and homovanillic acid.
➤ Stippled calcification in the tumour in plain abdominal radiographs.
➤ CT or ^{131}I MIBG scan localize the lesion.

Treatment

➤ Surgical excision in the absence of widespread disease produces long-term remission.

➤

> ➤ Chemoradiotherapy is palliative in advanced disease.
> ➤ Overall survival is 30–35% (the younger the patient, the better the long-term prognosis).

GENITOURINARY SYSTEM AND GENITALIA

KIDNEY AND URETER

Absent kidney

- Congenital absence of one kidney is asymptomatic and may be found incidentally on imaging.
- Complications: renal failure if disease process affects the other kidney, and a blind-ending ureter is present in 50% of cases, which can predispose to urinary tract sepsis.
- Treatment: excision of the redundant ureter may be required for recurrent sepsis.
- Bilateral renal agenesis results in stillbirth – oligo-hydramnios is noted on antenatal ultrasound.

Duplex ureter

Definitions

- Partial or complete congenital ureteric duplication.
- Commonest urinary tract malformation – noted in 1% of post-mortems.
- Usually separate ureters arise from the upper and lower poles of the kidney, later joining so that a single ureter enters the bladder – Y-shaped duplication; but complete duplication can occur; upper pole ureter enters lowermost.
- Abnormal peristalsis and vesico-ureteric reflux may cause hydroureter.

Clinical features

- Usually asymptomatic.
- Recurrent urinary tract sepsis – if abnormal ureteric function.

- Chronic pyelonephritis, with scarring of the affected pole of the kidney.
- Urinary incontinence if ureter enters the urethra below the sphincter.

Investigation
➤ Ultrasound of the urinary tract.
➤ Intravenous urography (IVU).

Treatment
➤ Ureteric re-implantation: may be required if there is incontinence or recurrent sepsis.
➤ Heminephro-ureterectomy: resection of the scarred portion of the kidney and the refluxing ureter – may be required for chronic pyelonephritis.

Horseshoe kidney

- Congenital fusion of the kidneys across the mid-line occurs in 1/1000 cases.
- Asymptomatic: may be found incidentally on abdominal examination or imaging.

Polycystic kidney of the newborn

- Congenital dysplasia results in a lobulated palpable kidney with no collecting system – ultrasound shows a multicystic kidney.
- Treatment: none required; but if there is doubt about the nature of the renal mass, nephrectomy is performed.
- Bilateral cases result in stillbirth – oligohydramnios is noted on antenatal ultrasound.

Adult polycystic kidney

Definitions

- Bilateral cystic destruction of renal parenchyma.
- Cysts also occur in liver, pancreas and spleen.
- Affects adults >40 years of age.
- Aetiology: autosomal dominant inherited condition.

Clinical features

- Loin pain from infection or haemorrhage into a cyst.
- Haematuria.
- Abdominal mass.
- Palpable lobulated kidneys.
- Chronic renal failure (page 496) gradually develops.

Investigation

- Full blood count (FBC) – anaemia.
- Serum potassium, urea and creatinine – elevated in late stages.
- Ultrasound – polycystic kidneys.
- Computerized tomography (CT) – polycystic kidneys; renal failure may limit the use of contrast.

Treatment

- Treatment of chronic renal failure (page 498).
- Treatment of pyonephrosis (page 505).

Infant polycystic kidney

- An autosomal recessive condition that progresses to chronic renal failure and death.
- Treatment: as for chronic renal failure.

Simple renal cysts

- Simple cysts usually arise from the lower pole of the kidney – some renal parenchyma is destroyed, but not sufficient to cause renal failure. They are usually asymptomatic – incidental finding on imaging – and require no treatment. Differentiate from cystic adenocarcinoma.

Acute renal failure

Definitions

- Acute – reversible failure of the kidney to excrete potassium, urea and creatinine, and to regulate body water content.
- May be transient cessation of glomerular filtration, or more established acute tubular damage.

- Aetiology:
  - Pre-renal:
    - Dehydration
    - Postoperative fluid balance problems
    - Shock (page 96) – haemorrhagic/hypovolaemic, cardiogenic, septic/systemic inflammatory response.
  - Renal:
    - Renal artery occlusion – embolism, aortic dissection, surgical
    - Renal ischaemia – shock
    - Toxins – gentamicin, radiological contrast
    - Glomerulonephritis
    - Impaired uric acid metabolism
    - Myoglobinuria – crush syndrome
    - Haemoglobinuria – haemolysis.
  - Post-renal:
    - Ureteric obstruction – stone, invasive pelvic malignancy, retroperitoneal fibrosis
    - Chronic retention
    - Blocked catheter.

Clinical features

- Oliguria – urine output <20 mL/hour for >2 hours for an average adult.
- Anuria – no production of urine.
- Fluid retention and pulmonary oedema – may occur if not pre-renal.
- Manifestations of elevated potassium – electrocardiographic changes; tented T-waves, reduced P-waves, sine-wave pattern; asystolic cardiac arrest.
- Manifestations of underlying cause.

Investigation

➤ Clinical evaluation of fluid balance, circulatory status and other underlying causes.
➤ Serum potassium, urea and creatinine – raised.
➤ Blood gases – metabolic acidosis.
➤ Urinary sodium – <40 mmol/L.
➤ Urine osmolality – <350 mosm/L.
➤ Investigation of underlying cause.

Treatment

➤ Repeated challenges of 250–500 mL colloid – postoperative oliguria.
➤ Management of shock:
  – Replace volume/transfuse – estimation of preload with central venous pressure trends or pulmonary artery wedge pressures
  – Inotropic support
  – Treat sepsis.
➤ Haemofiltration – arterial blood is cleared of water and solutes by the pressure gradient across a semi-permeable membrane, and then returned to the venous circulation.
➤ Haemodialysis – blood from a double lumen tube in a major vein is allowed to exchange solutes with crystalloid, across a semi-permeable membrane.

Chronic renal failure

Definitions

● Chronic – irreversible failure of the kidney to excrete potassium, urea and creatinine, and to regulate body water content.
● Aetiology:
  – Severe or prolonged acute renal failure
  – Hypertension
  – Diabetes
  – Chronic retention
  – Bilateral ureteric obstruction: pelvic tumour, retroperitoneal fibrosis, severe uterine prolapse
  – Vesico-ureteric reflux
  – Renal artery stenosis or occlusion
  – Adult polycystic disease (page 493)
  – Chronic pyelonephritis
  – Vasculitis – polyarteritis nodosa, Wegener's granulomatosis
  – Glomerulonephropathy – systemic lupus erythematosus, Henoch–Schönlein purpura
  – Toxic glomerular damage – gold, penicillamine

- Sarcoidosis
- Amyloidosis – myeloma.

Clinical features

- Asymptomatic: incidental finding – serum biochemistry, or small, scarred kidneys on ultrasound.
- Oliguria and anuria eventually.
- Uraemia – insidious onset of symptoms from accumulation of renally excreted toxins:
  - Fatigue
  - Dyspnoea
  - Ankle swelling
  - Vomiting
  - Pruritus
  - Impotence or amenorrhoea
  - Anaemia from reduced erythropoietin production
  - Pallor and yellow-brown skin discoloration
  - Hypertension
  - Pericardial rub
  - Gastritis and peptic ulceration
  - Rickets – children; and osteomalacia – adults from hypophosphataemia and reduced production of 1,25-dihydroxy cholecalciferol
  - Encephalopathy causing confusion, flapping tremor and, eventually, seizures
  - Death from hyperkalaemia-induced asystole

Investigation

- Clinical evaluation of fluid balance, circulatory status and other underlying causes.
- Serum potassium, urea and creatinine – raised.
- Serum bone alkaline phosphatase – raised.
- FBC – normochromic normocytic anaemia.
- Blood gases – metabolic acidosis.
- Isotope studies:
  - Renogram – demonstrates renal perfusion and extent of non-functioning renal tissue
  - Excretion studies – demonstrate obstructive causes.
- Renal biopsy – can exclude acute renal failure in cases where kidneys are of normal size.
- Investigation of underlying cause.

Treatment

➤ Remove causes.
➤ Avoid further damage:
  – Avoid nephrotoxic drugs and contrast media
  – Maintain hydration if using contrast media or during dehydrating illness
  – Treat hypertension.
➤ Restrict protein intake to 0.6 g/kg per day.
➤ Restrict sodium to 60 mmol/day – others may require sodium supplements.
➤ Restrict fluids in severe cases.
➤ Reduce serum potassium if >5 mmol/L – Resonium-A 15 g in water tds orally; 10 units of insulin in 50 mL of 50% glucose over 10 minutes and repeat if there are ECG changes.
➤ Erythropoietin 100 units/kg per week – for anaemia.

Uraemic syndrome and urea >40 mmol/L on protein restriction:

➤ Peritoneal dialysis:
  – A Tenckhoff catheter is surgically implanted in the peritoneal cavity
  – 2 L of dialysate is run in and out four times a day.
➤ Haemodialysis:
  – An arteriovenous fistula is created in the forearm, which can be cannulated, or a large-bore haemodialysis catheter is placed in the jugular vein
  – Blood is allowed to exchange solutes with crystalloid, across a semi-permeable membrane
  – 4 hours of dialysis are required three times a week.
➤ Renal transplantation – usually a cadaveric kidney (allograft) is implanted in the iliac fossa; the renal vessels are anastomosed to the iliac vessels.

Complications

● Continuous ambulant peritoneal dialysis-related peritonitis.
● Thrombosis of haemodialysis fistula – eventual difficulty in obtaining vascular access.
● Transplant rejection (page 598).

Pelviureteric junction obstruction

Definitions

- Congenital incomplete obstruction can occur at the pelviureteric junction.
- More common on the left side; bilateral in 15% of cases.
- Affects: mainly boys, from infancy to young adult life.
- Aetiology: unknown; but associated abnormal peristaltic function, kinking of the junction, pressure from a separate lower pole renal artery and weak familial tendency.

Clinical features

- Asymptomatic: incidental finding on imaging.
- Chronic loin pain.
- Haematuria.
- Recurrent urinary tract sepsis.

Investigation

➤ Ultrasound: demonstrates enlarged renal pelvis and hydronephrosis.
➤ Intravenous urography: confirms pelvicaliceal dilatation and incomplete obstruction of the pelviureteric junction.
➤ Micturating cystogram: excludes vesico-ureteric reflux.

Treatment

➤ Surveillance: yearly review and ultrasound, with isotope scans to assess loss of functioning renal tissue.
➤ Surgical pyeloureteroplasty: for symptomatic cases, hydronephrosis, stones, recurrent infection or reduced renal function.

Wilms' tumour (nephroblastoma)

- Embryonic tumour presenting at <3 years of age as failure to thrive and an abdominal mass – bilateral cases occur.

- Treatment: radical nephrectomy with adjuvant chemotherapy and radiotherapy.
- Prognosis: up to 90% cure for non-metastatic cases.

Renal cell carcinoma (Grawitz's tumour, hypernephroma)

Definitions

- Clear cell carcinoma, typically of the upper pole.
- Locally invasive, extending into the renal vein, and blood-borne metastases.
- Affects: mainly males >50 years of age.
- Aetiology: cigarette smoking, adult polycystic disease, and hereditary as part of Von Hippel–Lindau syndrome (familial renal, cerebellar, spinal, retinal and pancreatic tumours).

Clinical features

- Painless haematuria.
- Loin pain.
- Abdominal mass.
- Anaemia.
- Polycythaemia – from erythropoietin production.
- Hypertension – from renin production.
- Pyrexia of unknown origin – from pyrogens.
- Left varicocoele – from left testicular vein occlusion.
- Inferior vena cava obstruction.
- Metastatic disease – lungs, liver, bone, brain and subcutaneous tissue.
- Incidental finding on CT or ultrasound, or of metastases on chest X-ray.

Investigation

➤ Urine microscopy and cytology: confirms haematuria and excludes transitional cell tumours.
➤ Chest X-ray: may demonstrate lung metastases – large solitary 'cannonball' metastases may occur.
➤ CT: demonstrates the tumour; identifies renal vein or vena cava involvement, and liver and lung metastases.

Treatment
➤ Radical nephrectomy: extracting tumour from the renal vein and inferior vena cava.
➤ Partial nephrectomy: possible in some cases, but indicated if there is loss of function of the contralateral kidney.
➤ Radiological embolization of the renal artery: useful to control severe haemorrhage prior to surgery.
➤ Solitary lung metastases can be resected.

Pelviureteric carcinoma
● Transitional cell carcinoma can occur in the renal pelvis and ureter.
● Aetiology: as bladder cancer (page 524).
● Treatment: nephro-ureterectomy and cystoscopic surveillance of the bladder.

Renal and ureteric calculi

Definitions
● Upper urinary tract stones form by crystallization when solvent/solute proportions change.
● Stones comprise: calcium oxalate, uric acid, or cystine.
● Aetiology:
  – Dehydration
  – Calcium intake – excessive milk and calcium salts in peptic ulcer disease
  – Calcium metabolism – hyperparathyroidism, renal failure, destructive bone disease
  – Calcium excretion – idiopathic hypercalciuria
  – Oxalate intake – tea, strawberries
  – Oxalate excretion – primary hyperoxaluria
  – Chemotherapy – excessive uric acid production
  – Cystine excretion – homocystinuria.

Clinical features
● Painful haematuria:
  – Dull loin aching for renal stones
  – Severe colicky loin to groin pain for ureteric stones.

- Symptoms settle if the stone is passed into the bladder.
- Stone may be passed per urethram.
- High fever and loin tenderness indicate associated infection.
- Recurrent infection and chronic pyelonephritis – occur with staghorn calculi of the renal pelvis.

Investigation

➤ Urinalysis: shows haematuria.
➤ Plain X-ray of kidneys, ureters and bladder: majority of calculi are radio-opaque, but identification may be difficult.
➤ IVU: delay in the nephrogram, continuous contrast in the ureter down to the calculus – normally only segments of the ureter are seen in any one film; a completely obstructed system may show no excretion.
➤ Ultrasound: when IVU is contraindicated (pregnancy and contrast reaction).
➤ Isotope studies demonstrate the remaining functioning kidney in chronic pyelonephritis.

Treatment

Renal calculi:

➤ Observation – asymptomatic intrarenal calculi
➤ Nephrolithotomy or percutaneous nephrolithotomy – symptomatic intrarenal calculi
➤ Gil–Vernet pyelolithotomy – calculi in major calyces or renal pelvis
➤ Nephrectomy – staghorn calculus and chronic pyelonephritis where there is significant loss of functioning kidney.

Ureteric calculi:

➤ Observe stones <5 mm if there is no sepsis or obstruction – most pass spontaneously
➤ Ureteric stent and extracorporeal shock-wave lithotripsy – larger stones or no progression on observation

➔

> ➤ Ureteroscopy and ultrasound or laser lithotripsy –
>   larger stones or no progression on observation
> ➤ Open or laparoscopic ureterolithotomy – if other
>   techniques are unsuccessful.

Hydronephrosis and hydroureter

Definitions

- Hydronephrosis: dilatation of the renal calyces with loss of parenchyma from urinary outflow obstruction.
- Hydroureter: dilatation of the ureter from urinary outflow obstruction.
- Aetiology:
  - Hydronephrosis:
    - Pelviureteric junction obstruction
    - Long-standing impaction of stone at the renal pelvis
    - Staghorn calculus.
  - Hydronephrosis and hydroureter:
    - Vesico-ureteric reflux
    - Long-standing stone in the ureter or vesico-ureteric junction
    - Chronic retention – causes of bladder outflow obstruction (page 509).

Clinical features

- Chronic loin pain.
- Recurrent urinary tract sepsis.
- Features of underlying conditions.
- Chronic renal failure (page 496).

Investigation

> ➤ Serum potassium, urea and creatinine: assess chronic renal failure.
> ➤ Ultrasound: confirms.
> ➤ IVU: demonstrates the level of obstruction.
> ➤ Isotope renograms: demonstrate degree of parenchymal damage.
> ➤ Investigation of underlying conditions.

Treatment
➤ Treatment of underlying conditions.

Perinephric abscess

Definitions

- A collection of pus in the perinephric space – between the kidney and Gerota's fascia.
- Aetiology:
  - Secondary to infected hydronephrosis
  - Haematogenous spread of infection – rare.

Clinical features

- Loin pain.
- Rigors.
- High, swinging fever.
- Loin swelling and tenderness – may be overlying inflammation.

Investigation
➤ Urine microscopy: pyuria.
➤ Blood, urine and pus cultures: identify the causative microorganism.
➤ Ultrasound: demonstrates a perinephric collection.

Treatment
➤ Percutaneous radiologically guided drainage.
➤ Ceftazidime 1 g tds i.v., then change according to culture.

Tuberculous perinephric abscess

- Presents more insidiously, with loin swelling, which may eventually point to the surface, and general features of tuberculosis (page 142).
- Treatment: percutaneous or surgical drainage, and antituberculous therapy.

Pyonephrosis

- Severe infection of the kidney with pus in an obstructed collecting system – an infected hydronephrosis; causes loin pain and tenderness, rigors and high, swinging pyrexia.
- Ultrasound shows echogenic pus in a dilated pelvi-caliceal system.
- Treatment: urgent drainage by percutaneous radiologically guided nephrostomy, or passage of a ureteric stent; ceftazidime 1 g 8-hourly i.v., then change according to culture.

Tuberculosis of the urinary tract

Definitions

- Tuberculous infection of the urinary tract may involve:
  - Chronic pyelonephritis and renal scarring
  - Ureteric stricture and hydronephrosis
  - Scarring of the ureteric orifice and vesico-ureteric reflux
  - Chronic cystitis
  - Chronic prostatitis and destruction of seminal vesicles
  - Chronic epididymitis and sinus formation through the scrotum.
- Affects: mainly adults aged 20–40 years.
- Aetiology: *Mycobacterium tuberculosis* – haematogenous spread from pulmonary tuberculosis.

Clinical features

- History of previous tuberculosis at another site.
- Frequency, nocturia and dysuria – unresponsive to antibiotic therapy.
- Haematuria.
- Hard, nodular, non-tender epididymal enlargement.
- Nodular enlargement of the prostate.

Investigation

➤ Urine microscopy and culture: 'sterile pyuria'.
➤ Early morning urine specimens × 3 for mycobacterial culture.

→

➤ Heaf or Mantoux tests.
➤ Cystoscopy: ulcerative, nodular scarred areas; and 'golf-hole' ureteric orifice – held wide open by scarring.
➤ Intravenous urography: demonstrates scarred kidneys with 'moth-eaten' calices, ureteric strictures, bladder irregularity and reflux on micturating cystogram.
➤ In chronic epididymitis, excision of the abnormal epididymis for histology – caseous granulomatous chronic epididymitis, may be the only way to establish a diagnosis.

Treatment
➤ Isoniazid 300 mg and rifampicin 450–600 mg daily orally for 6 months; and pyrazinamide 1.5–2.0 g and ethambutol 15 mg/kg daily orally for the first 2 months.

Retroperitoneal fibrosis

- Chronic idiopathic inflammatory fibrosis of the retroperitoneum causes bilateral ureteric obstruction, and may be suspected from CT or MRI findings, which may demonstrate indrawing of the ureters.
- Treatment: prednisolone 20 mg daily, reducing over days to 10 mg daily orally; surgical release of the ureters may be required.

Renal trauma

Definitions

Aetiology:

- Blunt trauma to the loin: falling onto a protruding object, motor vehicle accidents, blow from a blunt weapon
- Penetrating trauma: knife and gunshot wounds
- Deceleration: fall from a height in the upright position.

Types of injury:

- Contusion: blunt trauma
- Laceration of the kidney: severe blunt, penetrating and deceleration trauma
- Perinephric haematoma

- Perinephric urinoma
- Disruption of the renal pedicle: severe blunt, penetrating and deceleration trauma
- Complete avulsion of the renal pedicle: penetrating and deceleration trauma.

Clinical features

Immediate:

- Associated multiple trauma (page 599)
- Bruising and tenderness over the loin
- Haematuria
- Shock from retroperitoneal haemorrhage.

After a few hours:

- Loin swelling and fever from a urinoma – urinary leakage into the retroperitoneum.

Investigation

➤ Urine dipstick: microscopic haematuria.
➤ Renal ultrasound: useful following dipstick haematuria where severe injury is not suspected.
➤ CT with contrast can identify haematoma, urinoma and major disruption.
➤ Intravenous urogram can identify haematoma distorting the kidney, urinary extravasation and major disruption.
➤ Arteriography identifies renal vascular injuries.

Treatment

➤ Management of other injuries and shock (page 599).
➤ Observation: blunt trauma causing contusion and minor laceration, and uncomplicated perinephric haematoma resolve without intervention.
➤ Urgent surgical exploration and repair: disruption of the pedicle, or urinary extravasation; and penetrating trauma.
➤ Nephrectomy: severe disruption and ischaemic damage at exploration; and to control severe haemorrhage from pedicle disruption.

Complications

- Hypertension.
- Hydronephrosis.
- Arteriovenous fistula.

BLADDER AND PROSTATE

Acute urinary retention

Definitions

- Acute complete bladder outflow obstruction.
- Aetiology:
  - Benign prostatic hypertrophy
  - Carcinoma of the prostate
  - Neurological conditions: multiple sclerosis, spina bifida, and spinal cord compression
  - Drugs: therapeutic anticholinergic agents, tricyclic antidepressants, phenothiazines, monoamine oxidase inhibitors, and beta agonists.
- Precipitating factors: surgical operations – groin hernias and pelvic surgery; constipation; cold; alcohol; or diuretics.
- Affects: mainly elderly males.

Clinical features

- Sudden inability to pass urine.
- Dribbling incontinence may occur from overflow.
- Suprapubic pain.
- Previous history of prostatic symptoms.
- Hernia or pelvic surgery within 24 hours or constipation.
- Palpable bladder enlargement.
- Prostatic enlargement may be evident on rectal examination.
- Passage of a catheter releases 500–1000 mL of urine.

Investigation

➤ Serum urea and creatinine: identify associated renal failure.

➜

➤ Serum prostate-specific antigen (PSA) (must be taken prior to catheterization) – see carcinoma of the prostate (page 512).
➤ Renal tract ultrasound with premicturition and postmicturition volumes: identifies associated hydronephrosis and chronic retention.
➤ Investigation of benign prostatic hypertrophy (page 511) or other underlying condition.

Treatment
➤ Urethral catheterization: suprapubic catheterization if unsuccessful.
➤ Prazosin (alpha blocker) 500 µg bd, increasing after 7 days up to 2 mg bd orally – may enhance flow by relaxing smooth muscle.
➤ Trial without catheter after 3 days – catheterize again if retention recurs.
➤ Treatment of benign prostatic hypertrophy or other underlying condition.

Chronic urinary retention

Definitions
● Chronic distension of the bladder from partial outflow obstruction.
● Affects: mainly elderly males.
● Aetiology:
  – Benign prostatic hypertrophy and prostate cancer
  – Neurological conditions: multiple sclerosis, spina bifida and spinal cord compression
  – Cystocoele (page 524).

Clinical features
● May present as acute retention; but >1 L of urine is released on catheterization.
● Obstructive symptoms: hesitancy, weak stream, prolonged voiding, postmicturition dribbling – gradual onset.

- Irritative symptoms: frequency of micturition by day, nocturia, urgency.
- Renal failure.
- Urinary tract infection or epididymitis (page 540).

Investigation

➤ Serum urea and creatinine: identify associated renal failure.
➤ Serum PSA (must be taken prior to catheterization) – see carcinoma of the prostate (page 512).
➤ Renal tract ultrasound with premicturition and post-micturition volumes: identifies associated hydronephrosis and chronic retention.
➤ Investigation of benign prostatic hypertrophy or other underlying condition.

Treatment

➤ Urethral catheterization: suprapubic catheterization if unsuccessful.
➤ Hourly fluid balance: intravenous fluid replacement may be required if large hourly volumes are passed – the diuretic phase of recovery of postrenal renal failure.
➤ Prazosin (alpha blocker) $500\,\mu g$ bd, increasing after 7 days up to $2\,mg$ bd orally – may enhance flow by relaxing smooth muscle.
➤ Trial without catheter after 3 days – catheterize again if retention recurs.
➤ Ultrasound follow-up of residual volume – catheterize again if large residual volumes recur.
➤ Treatment of benign prostatic hypertrophy or other underlying condition.
➤ Intermittent self-catheterization or indwelling catheter with leg bag – for those unfit for other methods.

Complications

- Chronic renal failure, hydronephrosis, hydroureter and bladder diverticula.
- Urinary tract infection and epididymitis.

Benign prostatic hypertrophy

Definitions

- Gradual benign enlargement of the prostate.
- Affects: men >50 years of age.
- Aetiology: glandular and smooth muscle hyperplasia at the transition zone.

Clinical features

- Obstructive symptoms: hesitancy, weak stream, prolonged voiding, postmicturition dribbling – gradual onset.
- Irritative symptoms: frequency of micturition by day, nocturia, urgency.
- Acute retention.
- Chronic retention.
- Haematuria may occur acutely from associated prostatic varices.
- Urinary tract infection.
- Rectal palpation of the prostate reveals smoothly enlarged lateral lobes with/without obliteration of midline sulcus.

Investigation

- ➤ Serum urea and creatinine: identify associated renal failure from chronic retention.
- ➤ Serum PSA – see carcinoma of the prostate (page 512).
- ➤ Renal tract ultrasound with premicturition and postmicturition volumes: identifies associated hydronephrosis and chronic retention.
- ➤ Transrectal ultrasound and biopsies: where carcinoma is suspected.
- ➤ Urodynamics: confirms low flow rate from prostatic obstruction; and distinguishes bladder instability from irritative prostatic symptoms.
- ➤ Cysto-urethroscopy for haematuria: excludes other causes.

Treatment

➤ Observation: mild symptoms.
➤ Prazosin (alpha blocker) 500 μg bd, increasing after 7 days up to 2 mg bd orally – may enhance flow by relaxing smooth muscle.
➤ Finasteride (anti-androgen) 5 mg daily orally, review at 6 months; may reduce prostatic size.
➤ Transurethral resection of the prostate (TURP): for fit patients with intolerable symptoms uncontrolled by medication.
➤ Open prostatectomy: indicated if the gland is very large.
➤ Prostatic stents: short-term benefit for those unfit for TURP.
➤ Microwave therapy: avoids impotence but relief of obstruction is not as good as after surgery.

Complications

● Impotence: occurs with alpha blockers and anti-androgens; and in 30% after TURP.
● Retrograde ejaculation: ejaculation occurs into the bladder rather than per urethram in 70% after TURP.

Carcinoma of the prostate

Definitions

● Adenocarcinoma arises from glands in the peripheral prostate.
● Slow growing, but local invasion of pelvis, and metastases to axial skeleton, lungs and liver.
● Affects: males, usually >50 years of age.
● Common: subclinical disease found in the majority of male post-mortems.
● Aetiology: hereditary in some cases; also high incidence in North American blacks and low incidence after castration.

Clinical features

● Incidental finding on screening PSA measurement, rectal examination, or X-rays – metastatic disease – or histologically after TURP.

- Obstructive symptoms: hesitancy, weak stream, prolonged voiding, postmicturition dribbling – gradual onset.
- Irritative symptoms: frequency of micturition by day, nocturia, urgency.
- Acute retention.
- Chronic retention.
- Haematuria or haematospermia.
- Rectal palpation of the prostate – a hard nodule, or more extensive hard fixed enlargement of the gland.
- Pelvic pain, iliac vein occlusion and renal failure from ureteric obstruction – locally advanced disease.
- Pathological fracture or cord compression – metastatic disease.

Investigation

➤ PSA: used as a screening test yearly in some countries:
  - <4 ng/mL: carcinoma unlikely
  - 4–10 ng/mL: 20–25% carcinoma on histology
  - >10 ng/mL: >50% carcinoma on histology.
➤ Transrectal ultrasound with sextant biopsies: shows structural features and gives histology.
➤ Ultrasound to assess upper tract.
➤ Radio-isotope bone scan: may demonstrate bone metastases if PSA >10 ng/mL.

Treatment

Intracapsular disease – options:

➤ Observation and 3–6 monthly PSA monitoring: this is the best option if life expectancy <10 years
➤ Radical radiotherapy: complications are impotence, diarrhoea and urinary frequency
➤ Radical retropubic or perineal prostatectomy: complications are impotence and incontinence.

Locally invasive disease:

➤ External beam radiotherapy
➤ Hormonal therapy – in metastatic disease.

➜

Metastatic disease:

➤ Hormonal therapy:
  – Orchidectomy
  – Diethylstilboestrol (oestrogen) 1–3 mg daily orally –
    now rarely used because of feminizing side-effects
  – Goserelin (gonadorelin analogue) 3.6 mg monthly
    implant, with cyproterone acetate 100 mg tds orally
    from 3 days before implant for 3 weeks – because
    gonadorelin initially increases testosterone
    production
  – Flutamide (anti-androgen) 50 mg tds orally – if
    resistant to other hormonal therapy.
➤ Prognosis: locally invasive and metastatic disease are
  controlled by hormonal therapy for 12–18 months;
  after relapse survival is <6 months.

Acute cystitis

Definitions

● Bladder infection.
● Affects mainly women – short female urethra.
● Cystitis in males may indicate abnormality of the
  urinary tract: urethral stricture – post-gonococcal
  in young men, or benign prostatic hypertrophy in
  older men.
● Aetiology: *Escherichia coli*, *Staphylococcus saprophyticus*,
  Klebsiella spp, *Proteus mirabilis* or other organisms.

Clinical features

● Burning dysuria.
● Irritative symptoms: frequency of micturition by day,
  nocturia, urgency.

Investigation

➤ Midstream urine specimen.
➤ Dipstick: blood, protein, ketones and white cells.
➤ Microscopy: $>10^5$ bacteria/mm^3.
➤ Culture: identifies pathogen.
➤ Investigation of associated abnormalities.

Treatment
- ➤ Increase fluid intake.
- ➤ Potassium citrate 5% 10 mL tds orally relieves dysuria by increasing the alkalinity of the urine.
- ➤ Appropriate antibiotic: usually trimethoprim 200 mg bd orally for 3 days or ciprofloxacin 250–500 mg orally for 3 days – 7 or more days for diabetics, pregnant women and associated abnormalities.
- ➤ Treat underlying associated conditions.

Recurrent cystitis

- Recurrent infection of the bladder occurs with outflow obstruction – urethral stricture and benign prostatic hypertrophy, bladder diverticulum, neuropathic bladder – and bladder calculus, indwelling catheter or other bladder foreign body.
- Investigation and treatment are those of the associated condition.

Prostatitis

Definitions
- Prostatitis results from ascending infection of the urethra.
- Aetiology: *Escherichia coli*, *Pseudomonas aeruginosa*, *Serratia* spp, *Klebsiella* spp and *Proteus* spp.

Clinical features
- Fever and rigors.
- Low back and perineal pain.
- Urgency, frequency, nocturia and dysuria.
- Acute retention may occur.
- Arthralgia and myalgia.

Investigation
Four-glass test – microscopy and culture of:

- ➤ First 10 mL of voided urine – representative of the urethra

➜

➤ Late midstream urine – representative of the bladder
➤ Secretions obtained from prostatic massage – representative of the prostate
➤ First 10 mL of urine after prostatic massage – representative of the prostate
➤ High colony counts in the last two specimens distinguish prostatitis from other infection.

Treatment

➤ Cefuroxime 750 mg tds i.v. and gentamicin 80 mg bd i.v., adjusting according to levels after four doses – initially in severe infection.
➤ Ciprofloxacin 250 mg bd orally for 28 days, or other antibiotics according to microbiology.

Vesico-ureteric reflux

Definitions

● Loss of valvular function of the ureteric orifice allowing reflux of high-pressure urine.
● Congenital vesico-ureteric reflux affects mainly girls from childhood to young adult life.
● Aetiology:
  – Congenital weakness of the trigone
  – Ectopic ureteric orifice and duplex ureter
  – Post-prostatectomy
  – Postureteric meatotomy
  – Interstitial cystitis – late stage
  – Tuberculosis of the bladder – scarring of ureteric orifice
  – Prune-belly syndrome – abnormal smooth muscle, deficient abdominal wall musculature, undescended testes, talipes equinovarus and hip dislocation.

Clinical features

● Recurrent cystitis.
● Acute pyelonephritis.
● Chronic pyelonephritis.
● Chronic renal failure.

Investigation

➤ Urine microscopy and culture: may identify bacteria without pyuria.
➤ Ultrasound: shows associated hydronephrosis.
➤ IVU – the ureter contains contrast throughout its length: shows associated hydroureter or hydronephrosis.
➤ Micturating cystogram: demonstrates reflux.
➤ Isotope cystogram: radioisotope instilled into the bladder enables reflux to be demonstrated with a gamma camera.
➤ Isotope renogram: demonstrates extent of renal parenchymal damage.

Treatment

Vesico-ureteric reflux with no renal damage:

➤ Trimethoprim 100 mg bd orally for 6 months
➤ Regular voiding every 3 hours to minimize residual urine
➤ Cystograms 6 monthly to assess whether reflux is still occurring
➤ Isotope renogram yearly to detect loss of renal function.

Vesico-ureteric reflux with renal damage:

➤ Surgical reconstruction of the ureteric orifice
➤ Urinary diversion by formation of an ileal conduit – may be required to prevent chronic renal failure if reconstruction is unsuccessful in bilateral cases.

Interstitial cystitis (Hunner's ulcer)

Definitions

● Fibrosis of the bladder wall with ulceration.
● Slow, progressive loss of bladder capacity.
● Aetiology: unknown.
● Affects: middle-aged women.

Clinical features

- Gradually worsening frequency and nocturia.
- Suprapubic pain when the bladder is full – relieved on voiding.

Investigation

➤ Urine microscopy and culture: often normal; sometimes microscopic haematuria.
➤ Ultrasound:
  - Upper tract: usually normal, but there may be hydronephrosis from vesico-ureteric reflux in late cases
  - Bladder: there may be reduced volume.
➤ Micturating cystogram: may demonstrate vesico-ureteric reflux in late cases.
➤ Cystoscopy:
  - Diffuse mucosal oedema and petechiae
  - Small bladder capacity on filling
  - Pain on filling; if so, cystoscopy is performed under local anaesthesia
  - Arcuate splitting and profuse bleeding of the mucosa on distension.

Treatment

➤ Intermittent cystoscopic distension of the bladder.
➤ Prednisolone 20 mg daily orally for up to 3 weeks, reducing to 10 mg daily.
➤ Ileocystoplasty:
  - A vascularized segment of ileum is interposed in the bladder to increase capacity
  - Intermittent self-catheterization may be required to ensure emptying
  - Indicated for severe urinary frequency that is unresponsive to other measures.
➤ Urinary diversion with formation of ileal conduit may be necessary for significant vesico-ureteric reflux and renal parenchymal loss.

Tuberculosis of the bladder

- Tuberculosis of the urinary tract (page 505).

Schistosomiasis (bilharziasis)

Definitions

- Protozoal infection of the lower urinary tract.
- Endemic to India, Africa, the Middle-East, and Central and South America.
- Aetiology: *Schistosoma haematobium* from an intermediate host – the freshwater snail *Bulinus*.
- Lifecycle:
  - Miracidia hatch from ova in fresh water – rivers, lakes, irrigation systems
  - Miracidia penetrate foot of snail and form sporocysts
  - Cercariae from sporocysts rupture from the surface of the snail into fresh water
  - Cercariae penetrate skin of humans standing or bathing in the water
  - Cercariae travel via blood and lymphatics
  - Schistosomules mature in pelvic veins, and lay ova
  - Ova are released into the bladder, and passed in urine which then contaminates fresh water.

Clinical features

- Hyperaemia and itching at the site of skin penetration.
- Malaise and fever.
- Painful haematuria, which may be profuse.
- Frequency and nocturia.
- Loin pain, high fever and rigors indicate ascending infection.
- Secondary infertility from infection of the seminal vesicles.
- Chronic renal failure may eventually result from vesico-ureteric reflux.

Investigation

➤ Urine microscopy: may identify ova and sometimes malignant squamous cells.
➤ FBC: eosinophilia and hypochromic normocytic anaemia.
➤ Serum potassium, urea and creatinine: may identify renal failure.
➤ X-ray of bladder: may show calcification or bladder calculus.

➜

➤ Ultrasound: may demonstrate hydronephrosis in late stages.
➤ IVU: may demonstrate ureteric stenosis and hydronephrosis in late stages.
➤ Cystoscopy: grey tubercles with surrounding hyperaemia, old calcified tubercles, bladder calculus or ulceration – may be squamous carcinoma.

Treatment
➤ Praziquantel 40 mg/kg divided into two doses 6 hours apart for 1 day.
➤ Treatment of vesico-ureteric reflux (page 517).
➤ Ileocystoplasty may be required for a small-volume, scarred bladder.
➤ Total cystectomy with urinary diversion to an ileal conduit for squamous carcinoma.

Complications
● Vesico-ureteric reflux.
● Renal failure from long-standing reflux.
● Small-volume, scarred bladder.
● Squamous carcinoma of the bladder.

Stress incontinence

Definitions
● Leakage of urine when intra-abdominal pressure is raised.
● Affects mainly women; may follow childbirth, or occur with advancing age.
● Pelvic floor muscle weakness allows the bladder neck to descend beyond the external sphincter.

Clinical features
● Involuntary loss of urine on coughing, sneezing or laughing.
● Vaginal examination may demonstrate leakage and bladder neck mobility on coughing.

Investigation

➤ Urodynamics: excludes detrusor instability.
➤ Ultrasound – premicturition and postmicturition: assesses bladder emptying.
➤ Videocystourethrography: radiographic imaging during coughing may demonstrate bladder neck mobility.

Treatment

➤ Physiotherapy: developing pelvic floor muscles by holding a weight in the vagina.
➤ Intravaginal electrical pudendal nerve stimulator: may be successful, but is unpopular.
➤ Burch colposuspension: surgical elevation of the bladder neck by suturing to the ileopectineal ligament – excellent results where other treatment fails.
➤ Stamey bladder neck suspension: cystoscopically guided slinging of the bladder neck to the rectus sheath – a simpler procedure, but with less durable results.
➤ Perurethral collagen or silicone injection may be of benefit if unsuitable for surgery.

Urge incontinence (detrusor instability)

Definitions

● Overwhelming desire to micturate, followed by involuntary voiding.
● Pelvic floor muscle weakness allows the bladder neck to descend beyond the external sphincter.
● Aetiology: idiopathic and neurological conditions: multiple sclerosis, spina bifida, and spinal cord compression.
● Affects: mainly women, but men thought to have irritative prostatic symptoms may in fact have detrusor instability.

Clinical features

● Urgent desire to micturate with involuntary voiding.
● Frequency.

- Nocturia.
- Nocturnal enuresis.

Investigation

➤ Urodynamics: detrusor pressure spikes during bladder filling, then uncontrolled voiding after a high pressure spike.
➤ Ultrasound premicturition and postmicturition: assesses bladder emptying.
➤ Videocystourethrography: excludes stress incontinence.

Treatment

➤ Behavioural therapy: avoiding fluids at certain times; avoiding diuretics – tea, coffee and alcohol.
➤ Oxybutynin (anticholinergic) 5 mg tds
➤ Desmopressin (antidiuretic hormone analogue) 40 µg of nasal spray at bedtime.
➤ Clam cystoplasty: interposition of a segment of bowel into the bladder increases its capacity.
➤ Urinary diversion: formation of an ileal conduit may be necessary in intolerable cases unresponsive to other methods.

Dribbling incontinence

- Continuous leakage of urine results from: chronic retention (page 509), ectopic ureter, and vesicovaginal fistula (page 523).

Colovesical fistula

Definitions

- A fistulous tract between the bladder and colon.
- Aetiology:
  - Sigmoid diverticular disease – the usual cause
  - Colonic cancer
  - Bladder cancer.

Clinical features

- Pneumaturia: gas bubbles in the urine.
- Faecal particles in the urine.
- Persisting urinary sepsis.

Investigation

➤ Barium enema.
➤ Cystography.
➤ Examination under anaesthesia.

Treatment

➤ Surgical resection of the affected segment of bowel and repair of the bladder.

Vesicovaginal fistula

Definitions

- A fistulous tract between the bladder and vagina.
- Aetiology:
  - Iatrogenic: obstetric, radiation or surgical injury
  - Obstructed labour: common in developing countries
  - Cervical cancer.

Clinical features

- Urinary incontinence – constant leakage.

Investigation

➤ Cystography.
➤ Cystoscopy and examination under anaesthesia.

Treatment

➤ Diathermy of the tract and indwelling catheter for 2 weeks – tiny, surgically created fistula.
➤ Resection and layered closure – transvaginal or transvesical.
➤ Urinary diversion with formation of an ileal conduit – bladder or cervical carcinoma.

Cystocoele and urethrocoele

Definitions

- Herniation of the bladder and urethra through the anterior vaginal wall.
- Aetiology: pelvic floor weakness following childbirth.

Clinical features

- Vaginal discomfort.
- Difficulty voiding urine.
- Overflow incontinence.
- Bladder herniation anteriorly on examination with a Sim's speculum.

Investigation

➤ Urodynamic studies identify abnormalities of bladder function.

Treatment

➤ Surgical repair of the pelvic floor if childbearing is complete; further vaginal delivery may damage the repair.
➤ Ring pessary – in those unsuitable for surgery.

Carcinoma of the bladder

Definitions

- Transitional cell carcinoma is the commonest type of bladder cancer; squamous carcinoma, adenocarcinoma and sarcoma are rare.
- Affects: mainly males (M:F 3:1), with peak incidence in the 60- to 70-year age group.
- Aetiology: smoking; occupational exposure to carcinogens (2-naphthylamine, benzidine) in aniline dye, rubber industry and cable making; recurrent or chronic infections; and cyclophosphamide.

Clinical features

- Painless haematuria.
- Urinary frequency.

Investigation

➤ Urinalysis – dipstick or microscopic haematuria.
➤ Urine cytology.
➤ Cystoscopy and biopsy.

TNM classification of bladder cancer

- Tumour:
  - Tis carcinoma-in-situ (CIS) – flat tumour confined to mucosa
  - Ta   papillary tumour confined to the mucosa
  - T1   tumour invades lamina propria
  - T2   tumour invades superficial muscle
  - T3   tumour invades perivesical fat
  - T4   tumour invades adjacent organs.
- Nodes:
  - N0   none
  - N1   single node <2 cm
  - N2   node <2 cm but >5 cm
  - N3   nodes >5 cm.
- Metastases:
  - M1   metastases.

Treatment

➤ BCG (bacille Calmette–Guérin) instillation – CIS.
➤ Transurethral resection of bladder tumour with check cystoscopy at 3 months, then 6-monthly – Ta.
➤ Cystectomy and urinary diversion via an ileal conduit – invasive tumours.
➤ Radiotherapy – invasive tumours.
➤ Chemotherapy (cisplatinum, methotrexate, vinblastine) – metastatic disease.

Prognosis

- Non-invasive tumours (Ta) may be controlled by repeated transurethral resection at check cystoscopy, but some may later become invasive.
- Invasive tumours have a 60% 5-year survival after cystectomy.

Squamous carcinoma of the bladder

Definitions
- A high incidence of squamous cell carcinoma of the bladder in Africa is associated with mucosal epithelial hyperplasia caused by chronic schistosomal bladder infection.

Clinical features
- Painless haematuria (often ignored in areas with endemic schistosomiasis).
- Late presentation with urinary obstruction and/or abdominal or pelvic mass.

Investigation
➤ Cystoscopy and biopsy.

Treatment
➤ Radical or palliative cystectomy with urinary diversion.
➤ Adjuvant radiotherapy.

Bladder trauma

Definitions
- Bladder rupture may be intraperitoneal or extraperitoneal.
- Aetiology:
  - Blunt abdominal trauma to a full bladder – intraperitoneal rupture
  - Penetrating abdominal or perineal trauma
  - Fractured pelvis – extraperitoneal rupture
  - Iatrogenic – electroresection of bladder tumours, injury during pelvic surgery.

Clinical features
- Unable to pass urine – but spontaneous voiding occurs.
- Haematuria.
- Pelvic/lower abdominal pain.

- Palpable mass in lower abdomen: extraperitoneal rupture or pelvic haematoma.
- Peritonitis: intraperitoneal rupture.

Investigation

➤ Cystography: demonstrates extravasation, particularly after emptying out contrast.
➤ CT with bladder contrast: may demonstrate extravasation.

Treatment

➤ Surgical exposure and repair of the bladder with suprapubic cystostomy and urethral catheters for 10 days – cystography before removing catheters.
➤ No surgical repair, but urethral catheter for 2 weeks – small iatrogenic injuries.

PENIS

Hypospadias

- Urethral meatus opens on the ventral side of the penis, proximal to the glans.
- Congenital abnormality occurring in 1/300 males.
- Openings near the glans may pose little problem to urinary or sexual function.

Epispadias

- Urethral meatus opens on the ventral surface of the penis, or in a bifid clitoris.
- Congenital abnormality occurring in 1/120 000 males and in 1/450 000 females.
- Openings near the glans may pose little problem to urinary or sexual function.
- Penoscrotal and perineal locations of urethral openings are associated with the intersex state; investigation of chromosomal and hormonal status is required.
- Treatment: surgical reconstruction before school age.

- Openings on the penile shaft and female hypospadias are associated with abnormal sphincters – causing incontinence.
- Treatment: surgical reconstruction – artificial sphincters – and bladder augmentation for incontinence.

Phimosis

- A narrow prepuce prevents retraction of the foreskin over the glans.
- May cause recurrent balanitis and interfere with micturition.
- Aetiology:
  - Children: congenital narrowing and preputial adhesions, exacerbated by scarring from recurrent balanitis
  - Adults: scarring from recurrent balanitis.
- Treatment: circumcision; observation for children <2 years without recurrent balanitis; preputial dilatation.

Paraphimosis

- Oedema of a retracted foreskin prevents its replacement over the glans.
- Associated with failure to replace the foreskin after urethral catheterization.
- Treatment: reduction by sustained pressure over 5 minutes; if unrelieved, incision of the dorsal foreskin under local anaesthetic and later circumcision.

Balanitis

- Painful inflammation of the glans from infection and retained smegma.
- Phimosis may result in recurrent balanitis; recurrent balanitis may result in scarring, causing phimosis.
- Occurs more often in diabetics: investigate for newly presenting cases.
- Treatment: co-amoxiclav 250/125 mg tds orally for 5 days, clean under foreskin; circumcision may be required for recurrent cases.

Balanitis xerotica obliterans

- White patch of atrophic, chronically inflamed epidermis on the glans or prepuce.
- Affects: middle-aged, diabetic males.
- May be premalignant.
- Treatment: hydrocortisone 1% cream and observe; may require excision if progressing.

Peyronie's disease

- Curvature of the erect penis because of scarring of the tunica albuginea of the corpora.
- Aetiology: unknown; possibly related to trauma in sexual intercourse; associated with Dupuytren's contracture (page 695) in 30%.
- Treatment: surgical correction is possible by excision of the scar, or interposing dermal grafts into the affected segment of the corpora.

Carcinoma of the penis

Definitions

- Squamous cell carcinoma.
- Affects: males, incidence increasing with age.
- Aetiology: poor hygiene; associated with herpes virus infection, human papilloma virus and genital condylomata acuminata; rare in those that have undergone childhood circumcision.

Clinical features

- Slowly enlarging ulcer of the glans.
- Gradual progression to an ulcerative mass involving the whole penis.
- Inguinal lymphadenopathy from associated infection.
- Inguinal and iliac lymph node metastases.
- Distant metastases are uncommon.
- Often presents late.

Investigation

- Surgical biopsy and histology.
- CT/MRI assess local invasion and lymph node involvement.

Treatment

➤ Partial or total resection of the penis.
➤ Radiotherapy: for young patients with small tumours who accept the risk of recurrence or complications, and in those unfit for surgery.
➤ Neoadjuvant radiotherapy or chemotherapy (bleomycin, cisplatin and methotrexate) may downstage the lesion for excision and reconstruction of the penile shaft.
➤ Co-amoxiclav 500/125 mg and metronidazole 400 mg tds orally for 4 weeks – for suspected infective lymph node enlargement.
➤ Bilateral ilio-inguinal node resection – if nodes persist after antibiotics, or clinically appear malignant.

Erythroplasia of Queyrat

● Premalignant, non-invasive, malignant changes appearing as a red marginated lesion of the glans.
● Requires surgical biopsy and histology.
● Treatment: local excision, or laser excision.

Priapism

Definitions

● Persistent erection of the penis.
● Low-flow priapism – occlusion of venous drainage:
  – Sickle-cell disease
  – Leukaemia
  – Hypercoagulable states
  – Antihypertensives – alpha blockers, e.g. prazosin
  – Intracorporeal prostaglandin E_1 injection – treatment of impotence.
● High-flow priapism – arteriovenous fistula:
  – Penile trauma.

Clinical features

Low-flow:

• Thrombotic disorder or corporeal injection
• Painful persisting erection
• Firm, tender penis; but soft glans.

High-flow:

- Penile trauma – hours or days earlier
- Painless persistent erection
- Soft, non-tender penis.

Investigation

➤ Aspirate blood:
  – Dark blood – low-flow priapism
  – Bright blood – high-flow priapism; blood gas analysis confirms arterial blood.
➤ Duplex ultrasound – also distinguishes low-flow and high-flow types.

Treatment

➤ Aspiration of blood from the base of one of the corpora may give immediate relief.

Low-flow priapism:

➤ Creation of fistula between the corpora and the glans, or between the corpus cavernosum and spongiosum
➤ Grayhack procedure – anastomosis of the corpora to the distal end of the mobilized long saphenous vein.

High-flow priapism:

➤ Radiological embolization of the arteriovenous fistula.

Urethral injury

Definitions

Bulbous urethra:

- Blunt perineal trauma – usually falling astride a narrow bar, e.g. bicycle frame, upturned manhole cover
- Penetrating perineal trauma – knife, gunshot or fall onto a sharp object
- Instrumentation – catheter introducer.

Penile urethra:

- Instrumentation – catheter introducer, foreign body insertion.

Membranous urethra:

- Pelvic fracture – particularly if all four pubic rami are fractured; and unstable pelvic fractures
- Penetrating perineal trauma – knife, gunshot, landmine or falling astride onto a hard object.

Clinical features

Bulbous and penile urethra:

- Blood at the external meatus
- Inability to pass urine
- Haematoma or urinoma of the perineum
- 'Butterfly' pattern of perineal bruising – indicates rupture of Buck's fascia.

Membranous urethra:

- Blood at the external meatus
- Inability to pass urine
- Bladder distension
- High, mobile prostate on rectal examination.

Investigation

➤ Urethrocystography: X-rays are taken as contrast is passed through the urethra into the bladder – demonstrates discontinuity of the urethra or extravasation of contrast.
➤ Cysto-urethroscopy.

Treatment

Initial treatment:

➤ Drainage of the bladder by open cystostomy and suprapubic catheter placement – initial management of other injuries
➤ A urethral catheter can be drawn into position from within the bladder (railroading) – if there is complete loss of urethral continuity.

Subsequent treatment – once life-threatening associated injuries have been managed:

➤ Incomplete disruption: allow healing with suprapubic drainage over 2 weeks until urethrography confirms continuity; manage subsequent stricturing

→

➤ Complete disruption: immediate repair – membranous urethral injuries
➤ Delayed primary urethral repair with spatulated anastomosis – for bulbous and penile urethral injuries; suprapubic and urethral catheters remain for 2 weeks until urethrography confirms continuity without stricture.

Urethral strictures

● Arise after healing following urethral injury – including catheterization – or following sexually transmitted infection – typically gonorrhoea.
● Treatment: endoscopic optical urethrotomy; but sometimes open surgical stricturoplasty is required.

SCROTUM AND TESTES

Undescended testis

Definitions

● Testis lies in an abnormal position:
  – Cryptorchidism: along the line of embryological descent from the posterior abdominal wall; usually in the inguinal canal
  – Ectopic: femoral, perineal or pubic.
● Aetiology: abnormal embryonic development of the testis and related structures.
● Affects: 4% male neonates; 1% boys at 1 year.
● Bilateral in one-third of cases.

Clinical features

● Absent testis on routine developmental assessment.
● Distinguish from retractile tests – brought down by squatting or anaesthesia.

Investigation

➤ Clinical diagnosis.
➤ Ultrasound: may identify the location of the testis.
➤ MRI: may identify a deeply located testis if ultrasound fails.

Treatment

➤ Observation if <2 years of age: some may descend.
➤ Orchidopexy at 2 years of age: the inguinal canal is surgically explored, and the testis placed in a superficial scrotal pouch.
➤ Orchidectomy may be considered for an undescended testis identified in an adult because of the risk of malignancy.

Complications

● Infertility – particularly if the testis is not brought down before puberty.
● Torsion.
● Testicular cancer in later life – 10 times the risk; even greater if torsion has occurred.
● Contralateral testicular cancer.

Torsion

Definitions

● Acute rotation of a testis on its pedicle; which may occlude its blood supply.
● Aetiology: abnormal embryonic development of the testis, where the testis has a long pedicle within the tunica vaginalis and lies horizontally – Bell clapper testis.
● Affects: boys aged 10–16 years; but rarely may occur later.

Clinical features

● Sudden severe testicular pain or iliac fossa pain, which may radiate to the loin.
● Vomiting.
● Sometimes previous less severe episodes of pain – intermittent torsion.
● Testis lies high in the scrotum.
● Compare with acute epididymitis.

Investigation

> ➤ Clinical diagnosis: confirmed on surgical exploration.
> ➤ Duplex ultrasound: may assist diagnosis in uncertain cases and identify whether blood supply is compromised.

Treatment

> ➤ Urgent surgical exploration of the testis via the scrotum, and fixation of the repositioned testis; the contralateral testis is also fixed – orchidopexy.
> ➤ Orchidectomy may be required if the testis is black and non-viable; a prosthetic testis may be implanted later if required.

Testicular seminoma

Definitions

- Commonest malignant testicular tumour.
- Solid, lobulated, malignant tumour of germ cell origin.
- Affects: males aged 30–40 years.
- Associations: undescended testis (page 533) and previous testicular tumour.

Clinical features

- Testicular pain or testicular swelling.
- Hard swelling of the body of the testis.
- Large para-aortic nodes may be detectable on abdominal examination – the lymphatic drainage of the testicle is directly to the para-aortic nodes.
- Gynaecomastia may occur.
- Presentation may be from bone or lung metastatic disease.

Investigation

> ➤ Serum beta-human chorionic gonadotrophin: elevated in 25%.
> ➤ Serum placental alkaline phosphatase: elevated in 50%.

➔

➤ CT abdomen and chest: para-aortic and mediastinal nodes; and liver and lung metastases.
➤ Exploration of the testis via an inguinal incision with biopsy and frozen section.
➤ Staging:
   – I   rising tumour markers post-orchidectomy
   – II abdominal nodes
   – III supradiaphragmatic nodes
   – IV lung or liver metastases.

Treatment

➤ Orchidectomy via an inguinal approach.
➤ Radiotherapy to para-aortic nodes – stage I and II.
➤ Combination chemotherapy (e.g. bleomycin, etoposide, cisplatin) – stage II, if nodes >5 cm diameter persist after radiotherapy; and stages III and IV.

Testicular teratoma

Definitions

● Undifferentiated necrotic, haemorrhagic and locally invasive malignant tumour of germ cell origin.
● Metastasizes earlier than seminoma.
● Affects: males aged 20–30 years.
● Associations: undescended testis (page 533) and previous testicular tumour.

Clinical features

● Testicular pain or testicular swelling.
● Hard swelling of the body of the testis.
● Large para-aortic nodes may be detectable on abdominal examination: the lymphatic drainage of the testicle is directly to the para-aortic nodes.
● Gynaecomastia may occur.
● Presentation may be from bone or lung metastatic disease.

Investigation

➤ Serum beta-human chorionic gonadotrophin: elevated in 90%.
➤ Serum alpha-fetoprotein: elevated in 50%.
➤ CT abdomen and chest: para-aortic and mediastinal nodes; and liver and lung metastases.
➤ Exploration of the testis via an inguinal incision with biopsy and frozen section.
➤ Staging:
  – I   rising tumour markers post-orchidectomy
  – II abdominal nodes
  – III supradiaphragmatic nodes
  – IV lung or liver metastases.

Treatment

➤ Orchidectomy via an inguinal approach.
➤ Retroperitoneal lymph node dissection – advocated in some countries.
➤ Surveillance with monthly tumour markers and 3-monthly CT for 1 year, then 2-monthly tumour markers and further CT at the second year.
➤ Combination chemotherapy (e.g. bleomycin, etoposide, cisplatin): stage II, III and IV; relapse on surveillance; and more than two adverse histological findings:
  – Undifferentiated
  – Absence of yolk-sac elements
  – Lymphatic invasion
  – Vascular invasion.
➤ Prognosis:
  – Stage I and no adverse histology: >90% 3 year survival; but 25% relapse in the first year of surveillance and require chemotherapy
  – Other stages and adverse histology: <70% 3 year survival.

Testicular lymphoma

● Uncommon, high grade non-Hodgkin's lymphoma, which may be bilateral, occurring >50 years of age.
● Treatment: orchidectomy and chemotherapy.

Carcinoma of the scrotum

- Sir Percival Pott described carcinoma of the scrotum in London chimney sweeps in 1775 – the first recognized occupational cause of cancer.
- Aetiology: industrial exposure to polycyclic aromatic hydrocarbons – mainly cutting oils in engineering works.
- The condition is now rare thanks to improved conditions and protection, and occupational surveillance.
- Appears as a scrotal ulcer with raised everted edges: the surface may bleed, with spread to inguinal lymph nodes.
- Treatment: radical excision and lymphatic dissection.

Fournier's gangrene

Definitions

- Necrotizing fasciitis around the male genitalia.
- Synergistic infection by aerobic and anaerobic organisms.
- Infection spreads along the dartos fascia of the penis and scrotum and along Colles' fascia of the perineum.
- Aetiology: *Escherichia coli*, *Klebsiella* spp, *Bacteroides* spp, *Fusobacterium* spp, *Clostridium* spp, *Streptococcus* spp.
- Associated:
  - Urethral trauma – catheter introducer or other instrumentation
  - Diabetes
  - Urethral stricture from sexually transmitted infection
  - Peri-anal infection
  - Inguinoscrotal and penile surgery.

Clinical features

- Rapidly spreading:
  - Cellulitis
  - Crepitus – from surgical emphysema
  - Gangrene.
- Severe septic state.

Investigation

➤ Clinical diagnosis.
➤ Gas in tissue planes on incidental plain X-ray.
➤ Swab and tissue microscopy and culture – obtained during debridement.
➤ Histology of tissue confirms necrotizing fasciitis.

Treatment

➤ Urgent debridement of all affected tissue – the testes can often be preserved.
➤ Repeated review under anaesthesia and further debridement every 24 hours until the process has abated.
➤ Benzylpenicillin 1.2 g 8-hourly i.v., metronidazole 500 mg 8-hourly i.v., gentamicin 80 mg 12-hourly i.v. – adjust according to levels after four doses.
➤ Further antibiotics according to cultures and microbiological advice.
➤ Plastic reconstruction and skin grafts – after all infection has settled.
➤ Re-implantation of testes in lower abdominal wall – after all infection has settled.

Filariasis (page 158)

Definitions

● Nematode infection of lymphatics.
● Endemic to the West Indies, South Pacific islands, China and Japan.
● Aetiology: *Wuchereria bancrofti*, introduced by mosquito bites.

Clinical features

● Fever and malaise.
● Lymphangitis and lymphadenitis.
● Epididymo-orchitis and scrotal inflammation.
● Hydrocoele.
● Elephantiasis: massive enlargement of the scrotum or limbs may occur in advanced cases.
● Chylous urine: fat in the urine, giving it a milky colour.

Investigation

➤ Urine specimen: on standing, separates into:
- – Fatty layer – upper layer
- – Blood-stained – middle layer
- – Clear – lower layer.
➤ FBC: eosinophilia.
➤ Blood film: microfilariae may be identified (the blood should be taken at night).
➤ Lymphangiography: demonstrates major lymphatic occlusion.
➤ Isotope lymphoscintigraphy: demonstrates major lymphatic occlusion.

Treatment

➤ Diethylcarbamazine 1 mg/kg increasing over 3 days to 6 mg/kg orally for 3 weeks.
➤ Irrigation of renal pelvis with 2% silver nitrate seals off lymphatics – for severe chyluria.
➤ Surgical excision of excess scrotal tissue.

Epididymal cyst and spermatocoele

● Multilocular epididymal swellings may arise as retention cysts of the vasa efferentia, which after puberty may be termed spermatocoeles.
● Treatment is by excision, but surgery may impair fertility.

Acute epididymitis

● Occurs in young adult males with non-specific urethritis from sexually transmitted *Chlamydia trachomatis* infection, and in elderly males with bladder outflow obstruction – benign prostatic hypertrophy (page 511) – from organisms causing urinary tract infection.
● Treatment: rest, analgesia and scrotal support; doxycycline 100 mg bd orally for 7 days if chlamydial infection is likely; or ciprofloxacin 250 mg bd orally for bladder outflow obstruction. Treat underlying prostatic

hypertrophy – vasectomy may be required to prevent recurrent infections.

Chronic epididymitis

- Recurrent infections result in hard, irregular epididymal swelling; genitourinary tuberculosis (page 505) must be excluded.

Orchitis

- Inflammation of the testis causing testicular pain, swelling, scrotal inflammation; occurs with epididymitis or infectious disease – mumps, Coxsackie virus and dengue fever.
- Urinalysis may show red and white cells, or may be normal; ultrasound shows hyperaemia of the testis – excluding torsion (page 534), and a small hydrocoele.
- Treatment: rest, analgesia and scrotal support; doxycycline 100 mg bd for 7 days if chlamydial infection is likely, or ciprofloxacin 250 mg bd for bladder outflow obstruction. Treat underlying prostatic hypertrophy – vasectomy may be required to prevent recurrent infections.

Hydrocoele

- A fluid collection in the tunica vaginalis can occur secondary to testicular trauma, infection or malignancy, or as idiopathic hydrocoele in elderly males.
- Treatment of idiopathic hydrocoele: excision of the tunica vaginalis – Jaboulay's procedure – or radial plication of the tunica vaginalis from within the sac – Lord's procedure. In those unfit for surgery, repeated aspiration is possible.

Varicocoele

- Tortuous, dilatation and elongation of the pampiniform plexus of veins results in a scrotal swelling resembling a 'bag of worms', which empties on elevation.

- Typically affects young men – associated with primary infertility; varicocoele occurs more commonly on the left side.
- Sudden onset of left-sided varicocoele in an older man may occur with left renal cell carcinoma (page 500).
- Treatment: ligation of the plexus of veins through an inguinal approach, or excision through a scrotal approach.

Haematocoele and testicular trauma

- Blood may collect in the tunica vaginalis after scrotal trauma. Treatment is with analgesia and scrotal support.
- Associated rupture of the testes may be identified on ultrasound. Treatment is by surgical exploration and repair of the tunica albuginea.

SEXUALLY TRANSMITTED DISEASE

Gonorrhoea

- *Neisseria gonorrhoeae* acquired from unprotected sexual intercourse results in urethral discharge and burning dysuria after 3–10 days.
- Confirmed by urethral swabs and culture.
- Treatment: ciprofloxacin 100 mg single dose orally. Trace and treat contacts.
- Urethral strictures may develop later causing bladder outflow obstruction.
- Treatment: endoscopic optical urethrotomy.

Non-specific urethritis

- *Chlamydia trachomatis* acquired from unprotected sexual intercourse may result in urethral discharge, urethral itching and burning dysuria after 1–5 weeks; but other cases are asymptomatic.
- Affects: young men.
- Confirmed by urethral swabs and culture.
- Treatment: doxycycline 100 mg bd orally for 7 days. Trace and treat contacts.

Pelvic inflammatory disease

Definitions

- Ascending subacute infection of the vagina, cervix, endometrium and fallopian tubes.
- Aetiology: infection introduced by unprotected sexual intercourse – *Chlamydia trachomatis*, *Neisseria gonorrhoeae* – or possibly poor toilet hygiene – aerobic streptococci, *Escherichia coli*, *Bacteroides* spp and *Peptostreptococcus* spp.
- Affects: young women.

Clinical features

- Often unrecognized minor symptoms.
- Lower abdominal pain, which may radiate to the inside of the thigh.
- Purulent cervical and vaginal discharge.
- Acute salpingitis: a more acute presentation of pain, high fever, lower abdominal tenderness and guarding; and adnexal tenderness on vaginal examination – appendicitis may be suspected.

Investigation

➤ Swabs:
  - Endocervix: *Chlamydia trachomatis*
  - High vaginal: *Neisseria gonorrhoeae* and others.
➤ Erythrocyte sedimentation rate (ESR)/C-reactive protein (CRP)/white cell count are all raised in acute infection.
➤ Urinary beta-human chorionic gonadotrophin: excludes ectopic pregnancy.
➤ Transvaginal ultrasound: may identify a pelvic abscess, or identify ovarian disease.
➤ Laparoscopy: salpingitis and purulent pelvic fluid; and excludes appendicitis.

Treatment

➤ Doxycycline 100 mg bd orally for 7 days and metronidazole 400 mg bd orally for 14 days – start treatment on clinical suspicion.
➤ Appendicectomy may be required if there is doubt about its appearance at laparoscopy.

➜

> ➤ Surgery may be required to drain a tubo-ovarian abscess.
> ➤ Contact tracing for sexually transmitted disease.

Complications

- Infertility – from tubal damage.
- Fitz–Hugh–Curtis syndrome – perihepatitis results in adhesions between the liver and the diaphragm, causing chronic right upper quadrant pain.

Herpes

- Herpes simplex virus type II acquired from unprotected sexual intercourse may result in multiple vesicular lesions with surrounding erythema after 2–7 days, with tender inguinal lymphadenopathy.
- Confirmed by swabs and viral culture.
- Treatment: aciclovir 200 mg 5 times daily orally for 10 days.
- Herpes simplex virus type II infection in women is associated with cervical carcinoma.

Genital warts

- Papilloma virus infection acquired by unprotected sexual intercourse may cause multiple warts around the penis and anus.
- Treatment: podophyllum 15% paint applied weekly, then washed off after 6 hours; cryotherapy, diathermy, surgical excision.
- Papilloma virus cannot be eradicated. Patients must abstain from unprotected sexual intercourse.

VASCULAR

ARTERIES

Atherosclerotic disease

Definitions

- Chronic occlusive disease of elastic arteries.

- Commonest cause of death or major morbidity in the Western world.
- Pathology: multifactorial, degenerative process of arterial intima and media; results in arterial narrowing, thrombosis and occlusion.
- Aetiology – risk factors:
  - Cigarette smoking
  - Hyperlipidaemia
  - Hypertension
  - Diabetes mellitus
  - Obesity*
  - Sedentary lifestyle*
  - 'Type A' personality – aggressive, high stress, high achievement*

*More for coronary disease than for peripheral arterial disease.

Clinical features

- Initially asymptomatic.
- Possible manifestations:
  - Coronary arteries (page 364) – angina, myocardial infarction, arrhythmia, sudden death
  - Carotid arteries (page 546) – transient ischaemic attack (TIA), stroke
  - Upper limb arteries (page 560) – usually not significantly affected
  - Mesenteric arteries (page 569) – mesenteric angina (rare), or infarction
  - Renal arteries (page 569) – hypertension, renal failure
  - Lower limb arteries (page 552) – claudication, rest pain, ulceration, gangrene.

Investigation

Risk factor assessment:

➤ Serum cholesterol >5 mmol/L
➤ Blood pressure: diastolic >110 mmHg, systolic >160 mmHg
➤ Serum blood glucose: random >11 mmol/L, fasting >7 mmol/L
➤ Thrombophilia screening (page 567) – only if clinical suspicion of prothrombotic disorder.

Treatment

➤ Stop smoking: support groups, nicotine replacement gum or patches.
➤ Aspirin 75 mg daily.
➤ Atorvastatin 10 mg daily – if serum cholesterol >5 mmol/L.
➤ Treat hypertension by progressive use of additional antihypertensive agents until control is achieved:
  – Bendroflumethiazide 2.5 mg mane (diuretic)
  – Atenolol 50 mg daily (beta-adrenoceptor blocker)
  – Captopril 12.5 mg bd (angiotensin-converting enzyme inhibitor) or amlodipine 5 mg daily (calcium-channel blocker)
  – Doxazosin 1 mg (alpha-adrenoceptor blocker)
  – Requirement for four antihypertensive agents may indicate underlying renal artery stenosis.
➤ Treat diabetes and monitor control with BM-Test of capillary blood, dipstick testing of urine glucose, and serum HBA1C measurement.

Complications

Prognosis for atherosclerotic disease and risk factor management:

• 30% 5-year mortality from myocardial infarction or stroke for a claudicant without risk factor management
• Stopping smoking – 50% reduction in subsequent repeat myocardial infarction
• Serum cholesterol reduction by statins – 42% reduction in cardiovascular death for patients under 70 years.

Carotid artery disease

Definitions

• Atherosclerotic disease affects the carotid bifurcation.
• Often asymptomatic; more likely to cause symptoms if:
  – Severe stenosis
  – Ulcerated plaque.
• Asymptomatic disease becomes symptomatic by:
  – Embolism of plaque debris and thrombus to intracranial vessels or central retinal artery

– Thrombosis may cause complete internal carotid artery occlusion.

Clinical features

Transient or permanent 'carotid territory' neurological deficit:

- Contralateral hemiparesis
- Contralateral sensory loss
- Contralateral facial weakness
- Dropping objects
- Difficulty with writing
- Catching toe when walking
- Speech deficit:
  - Aphasia – absence of speech
  - Expressive dysphasia – know what they want to say, but cannot say it
  - Sensory dysphasia – incoherent speech.

Types of neurological deficit:

- Transient ischaemic attacks (TIA) – sudden onset of 'carotid territory symptoms', which usually resolve over a few minutes but may last up to 24 hours
- Prolonged, reversible, ischaemic neurological deficit – resolves after 24 hours
- Stroke – sudden onset of 'carotid territory' symptoms, or collapse and unconsciousness in severe cases, with progression over hours; sometimes some recovery over days, but permanent residual neurological deficit
- Amaurosis fugax – ipsilateral visual loss, which resolves over minutes; a curtain appears to fall across the field of one eye
- Permanent loss of vision to one eye – central retinal artery occlusion.

Investigation

➤ Duplex ultrasound of carotid arteries – determines degree of carotid stenosis by physiological means: calculated from velocity changes; formula varies between institutions.

➡

➤ Carotid and vertebral angiography:
  – Demonstrates anatomic nature of carotid atherosclerotic disease
  – Identifies intracranial vessel involvement
  – Distinguishes tight stenosis from carotid occlusion where there are doubts on duplex
  – Determines degree of stenosis by anatomic means: formula varies between institutions.
➤ Cerebral computerized tomography (CT) >48 hours after symptoms: identifies areas of new and old cerebral infarction; supportive evidence that symptoms are of cerebrovascular origin.
➤ Echocardiography and 24 hour ECG monitoring – look for cardiac sources of embolism – and associated paroxysmal arrhythmias.

Treatment
➤ Treatment of atherosclerotic disease risk factors (page 546).
➤ Aspirin 75 mg daily.
➤ Carotid endarterectomy – surgical removal of carotid atheroma – indications:
  – Severe (70–99%) carotid stenosis with carotid-territory symptoms within the past 6 months
  – Moderate (50–70%) carotid stenosis with carotid-territory symptoms in the past 6 months – depending on local variations in practice
  – Significant (50–99%) asymptomatic stenosis – as part of a trial; or carotid endarterectomy/medical treatment according to local practice.

Complications
Complications of carotid endarterectomy:

* Stroke 2% – can be fatal
* Hypoglossal nerve palsy – deviation of tongue to side of injury.

Carotid stenting
● Carotid atheroma may be dilated and excluded by angioplasty and deployment of a covered stent.

- Largely an experimental procedure, with unacceptably high stroke rate, but certain centres are obtaining good results.

Carotid dissection

Definitions

- A subintimal false passage for blood flow may form in the carotid artery.
- Aetiology:
  - Hypertension
  - Hyperextension (whiplash injury) of the neck.

Clinical features

- Sudden onset of ipsilateral frontoparietal headache and Horner's syndrome (page 267).
- TIA or stroke.

Investigation

➤ Duplex ultrasound.
➤ Magnetic resonance angiography (MRA) in doubtful cases.
➤ Carotid and vertebral angiography – occasionally required.

Treatment

➤ Anticoagulation with heparin, then warfarin for 6 months.
➤ Continue anticoagulation if there are any further symptoms.

Vertebrobasilar artery disease

- Transient or permanent neurological deficit including: vertigo, balance and gait problems, involvement of cranial nerve nuclei – including bulbar palsy (page 215) – and, in severe cases, changes in consciousness.
- Treatment is medical: atherosclerotic risk factor management and aspirin 75 mg daily; treatment of any concomitant carotid artery disease.

Subclavian steal

- An uncommon cause of TIA in proximal subclavian artery stenosis or occlusion.
- Arm exercise results in reversal of blood flow in the ipsilateral vertebral artery, 'stealing' blood from the cerebral circulation.
- Arm 'claudication' is relatively rare because of excellent anastomoses around the scapula – upper limb circulation is less affected by atherosclerotic disease.

Carotid body tumour (chemodectoma)

Definitions

- Carotid body tumour.
- Usually benign, but may eventually compress or invade adjacent structures.
- Associations:
  - High altitude dwellers
  - Autosomal dominant tendency in 10% – more common in bilateral cases.
- Affects those in the 40- to 50-year age group.

Clinical features

- Hard, regular, painless mass at the carotid bifurcation.
- Transmitted pulsation – may be expansile.
- Some horizontal mobility; no vertical mobility.
- Cranial nerve palsy in 10% of VIII, IX, X, XI or XII.

Investigation

➤ Duplex ultrasound: splaying of the carotid bifurcation.
➤ Angiography: splaying of the carotid bifurcation, a blush of fine vessels in the tumour, feeding vessels from external carotid or vertebral arteries.
➤ CT: demonstrates extent of tumour.
➤ Gadolinium-enhanced magnetic resonance imaging: shows extent of tumour and screens for contralateral tumour; can identify tumour <5 mm diameter.
➤ Laryngoscopy/pharyngoscopy: recurrent laryngeal nerve palsy; excludes local invasion.

Treatment
- ➤ Conservative: for the elderly or unfit.
- ➤ Surgical excision: complicated by stroke and recurrent laryngeal nerve palsy:
- • Shamblin classification:
  - – I: Small, easily resectable
  - – II: Large, adherent to vessels
  - – III: Tumour surrounding vessels or nerves.
- ➤ Radiotherapy – subsequent contralateral tumours – avoids bilateral complications.

Prognosis:
- ➤ Slow-growing tumour
- ➤ Most patients are cured by surgery
- ➤ Local recurrence and metastases are rare.

Subclavian aneurysm
- Usually occurs as post-stenotic dilatation of the subclavian artery associated with thoracic outlet compression syndrome (TOCS, page 562), but may occur with giant cell arteritis or, rarely, in isolation.
- Typically presents with micro-embolic phenomena – splinter haemorrhages of the nail beds, Raynaud's phenomenon, and sometimes digital ischaemia and gangrene.
- Investigation: duplex ultrasound and angiography.
- Treatment: treatment of any source of arterial compression (page 562), and resection of the aneurysm with end-to-end anastomosis, or interposition graft of the subclavian artery.

Carotid aneurysm
- Rare aneurysms, which may present as pulsatile neck swellings, or with stroke from thrombosis, dissection or embolism.
- Investigation: duplex ultrasound.
- Treatment: resection and interposition vein graft.

Prominent innominate artery
- Elongation and tortuosity of the innominate artery, often with shortening of the neck from spondylosis,

may result in a prominent, visible, arterial pulsation in the right side of the neck.

- Made more prominent by hypertension and wasting of sternocleidomastoid muscle.
- Typically seen in elderly women, and often initially misdiagnosed as a carotid artery aneurysm.
- Investigation: duplex ultrasound.
- Treatment: reassurance.

Chronic lower limb ischaemia

Definitions

- Atherosclerotic disease affects the lower limb arteries.
- Fontaine's grading of severity by symptoms:
  - I   Asymptomatic
  - II   Claudication
  - III Rest pain
  - IV Ulceration and gangrene.

Clinical features

- Intermittent claudication:
  - Cramp-like leg pain induced by walking a certain distance; relieved by rest; recurs on walking a similar distance
  - Calf claudication – superficial femoral artery disease
  - Thigh and calf claudication – external iliac disease
  - Buttock, thigh and calf claudication – common iliac or aortic disease.
- Rest pain:
  - Severe pain at rest, usually in the toes and forefoot
  - Exacerbated by elevation of the leg – keeps the patient awake at night
  - Relieved by dependency – hanging the affected foot out of the bed at night, or sleeping in a chair.

Signs of lower limb ischaemia depend on severity:

- None – in mild cases
- Absent dorsalis pedis, posterior tibial, popliteal or femoral pulses – indicating level of major occlusive disease
- Cool, pale foot

- Delayed capillary refilling of the toes – after blanching by pressure, colour normally returns within <1 second; refilling in an ischaemic foot is delayed. Compare affected/unaffected sides
- Trophic changes to foot and lower leg: thin, dry, hairless, cracked skin; brittle nails
- Buerger's sign: pallor of the foot and collapse of superficial veins may be induced by elevating a severely ischaemic leg; reactive hyperaemia then results in red/purple discoloration on dependency, developing over 2 minutes.

Investigation

➤ Ankle–brachial pressure index, measured using a hand-held Doppler probe and expressed as a ratio:
  - Claudication: usually 1.0–0.6 at rest, falling by >0.15 after exercise
  - Rest pain, ulceration or gangrene: usually <0.6 at rest, often lower.
➤ Angiography: to plan intervention.
➤ Duplex ultrasound: to plan intervention in patients where angiography is contra-indicated, e.g. in renal failure, contrast reactions, poor angiographic access – iliac occlusive disease.
➤ MRA: to plan intervention in patients where angiography is contra-indicated, e.g. renal failure, contrast reactions, poor angiographic access; iliac occlusive disease.

Treatment

Treatment of atherosclerotic disease risk factors:

➤ Claudication:
  - Structured exercise programme
  - Angioplasty or bypass surgery in severe cases.
➤ Rest pain, ulceration:
  - Angioplasty or bypass surgery – long saphenous vein is preferable to synthetic graft.

Complications

- Angioplasty may occasionally result in more extensive occlusion and precipitate acute limb-threatening ischaemia.

- Bypass surgery may fail:
  - Immediately: usually technical problems with the bypass
  - <2 years: graft stenosis from neo-intimal hyperplasia
  - 2 years: progression of atherosclerotic disease.
- Approximate 5-year graft patency:
  - 90%: synthetic (Dacron) aortobifemoral
  - >70%: synthetic/saphenous vein from femoral artery to above-knee popliteal artery
  - <70%: saphenous vein from femoral to below-knee popliteal artery
  - <50%: synthetic (ePTFE, polytetrafluoroethylene) with distal vein cuff from femoral to below-knee popliteal artery.
- Synthetic graft infection necessitates removal of the graft with a high incidence of amputation – 5% overall incidence, but more common in revascularization for ulcers.

Leriche's syndrome

- Impotence and bilateral buttock claudication resulting from chronic aortic occlusion.
- Treatment: aortobifemoral synthetic (Dacron) bypass.

Acute lower limb ischaemia

Definitions

- Sudden impairment of the arterial circulation to the leg.
- Aetiology:
  - Embolism
  - Thrombosis of atheromatous narrowing
  - Thrombosis of vascular graft
  - Trauma.
- Embolism – arterial occlusion by migration of thrombus from:
  - Left atrial appendage – in atrial fibrillation
  - Mitral valve disease – after childhood rheumatic fever
  - Aortic atheroma.
- Aortic occlusion and 'saddle embolism' – see below.

Clinical features

- Sudden onset in leg of:
  - Pain
  - Pallor
  - Pulselessness
  - 'Perishing cold'
  - Paraesthesia and anaesthesia*
  - Paralysis.*
- Non-salvageable leg:
  - Anaesthesia and paralysis of increasing duration
    >4 hours
  - Mottled purple colour that does not blanch on
    pressure
  - Pain on squeezing the calf
  - Wet gangrene
  - Muscle rigidity.

*Features indicating very severe ischaemia, requiring
urgent intervention.

Investigation

➤ Clinical diagnosis.
➤ Angiography: to plan intervention, if available and if
   time permits.

Treatment

Embolus most likely:

➤ Surgical embolectomy – usually by exploration of
   femoral artery, but sometimes popliteal artery:
  - Fogarty balloon catheter is used to retrieve embolus
  - On-table angiography guides the procedure
  - Direct intra-arterial administration of 20 mg tissue
    plasminogen activator (TPA) may be used for
    thrombolysis of small vessels.

Thrombosis of previous atheroma or old graft most likely:

➤ Radiological aspiration of thrombus; thrombolysis with
   TPA; and angioplasty of underlying disease
➤ Emergency surgical bypass may be required for
   thrombosis of pre-existing atheroma not responsive to

➤

interventional radiology, or where interventional radiology is not immediately available.

Thrombosis of recent (<2 weeks) graft most likely:

➤ Surgical exploration and revision of the graft
➤ Flow through vein grafts must be restored within hours or the vein will become non-viable.

Non-viable leg:

➤ Trans-tibial (below-knee) amputation, if calf viable; palpable femoral pulse
➤ Trans-femoral (above-knee) amputation, if calf non-viable; absent femoral pulse.

Acute aortic occlusion/saddle embolism

- A large arterial embolism impacting at the aortic bifurcation may cause:
  - Acute severe bilateral leg ischaemia and pain
  - Mottled blue/purple skin colour to the level of the buttocks and lower abdominal wall
  - Shock
  - Myocardial infarction – cardiac strain from increased peripheral resistance.
- Clinical diagnosis, requires urgent embolectomy via both femoral arteries.
- High risk of bilateral leg gangrene requiring above-knee amputation, and high mortality.
- Contrast with relatively mild changes in chronic aortic occlusion – Leriche's syndrome (page 554).

Micro-embolism and 'trash-foot'

- Micro-embolism of platelet aggregates that do not occlude major arteries, may cause patchy purple mottling of the toes, 'trash-foot', or sometimes small, black areas of infarction of the tips of the toes or nail bed.
- Aetiology:
  - Aortic cross-clamping
  - Aortic balloon pump
  - Aortic atheroma and aortic aneurysm

- Popliteal aneurysm
- Mitral valve disease – after childhood rheumatic fever
- Acute and subacute bacterial endocarditis.
- 'Trash-foot' after aortic surgery often does not require any intervention.
- Revascularization is not required – in severe cases consider iloprost (prostacycline) infusion.
- Treat sources of embolism.
- Anticoagulation with heparin and warfarin, if embolic source cannot be eliminated.
- Severe cases may require debridement or limited amputation.

Buerger's disease

Definitions

- Clinical syndrome from occlusion of small and medium arteries and veins in the lower limb, and sometimes upper limb.
- Pathology: obliterative thrombo-angitis – vessels are occluded by thrombus filled with inflammatory cells.
- Aetiology: unknown.
- Associations:
  - Racial – originally described in Ashkenazi Jews, but also affects Oriental, Indian and African races
  - Heavy cigarette smoking.
- Males are affected almost exclusively.

Clinical features

- Foot rest pain.
- Dry ulceration/digital gangrene.
- Raynaud's phenomenon affecting the fingers (page 565).
- Typically palpable femoral and popliteal pulses, but absent distal pulses.

Investigation

➤ Angiography: normal arteries proximal to the popliteal, then sudden occlusions of crural vessels, with characteristic 'corkscrew' collaterals and segmental reconstitution of the vessels.

Treatment

➤ Stop smoking: essential to hold the progression of the disease.
➤ Aspirin 75 mg daily or other antiplatelet agents.
➤ Epoprostanol (prostacyclin) infusions: benefit is uncertain; available in some centres.
➤ Amputations: as required according to extent of gangrene.

Diabetic foot

Definitions

● A multifactorial process leading to necrosis or gangrene of the foot.
● Aetiology:
  – Atherosclerotic disease: early onset and more extensive
  – Microvascular occlusive disease
  – Impaired resistance to infection
  – Neuropathy: increased likelihood of ulceration from repeat trauma
  – Pressure necrosis: exacerbated by neuropathy.

Clinical features

● Diabetic neuropathy:
  – Autonomic: foot appears warm and pink in spite of severe ischaemia
  – Motor: claw foot and hammer toes accentuate bony prominences, encouraging pressure necrosis
  – Sensory: reduced sensation of the sole allows minor injury to go unnoticed.
● Spectrum of severity:
  – Infected nail bed or toe tips
  – Ulcers over/under bony prominences: metatarsal heads, heels, malleoli
  – Distal gangrene
  – Fascia and tendon destruction, and osteomyelitis – often more extensive than surface appearances suggest.

Investigation
➤ Investigation of diabetes.
➤ X-rays: to identify underlying osteomyelitis.
➤ Investigation of atherosclerotic disease risk factors (page 545).
➤ Investigation of chronic lower limb ischaemia (page 545).
➤ Doppler pressure measurements may be less reliable: calcified calf vessels are less compressible by the sphygmomanometer cuff.

Treatment
➤ Treatment of diabetes.
➤ Neuropathic ulcer without severe ischaemia:
  • 'Walking plaster' with 'rocker bottom' protects and redistributes weight to allow healing.
➤ Evidence of ischaemia:
  • Treatment of chronic lower limb ischaemia (page 552).
➤ Extensive deep necrosis:
  • Debridement
  • Amputation: where there is osteomyelitis, extensive deep necrosis or gangrene
  • In the absence of chronic lower limb ischaemia, other patterns of amputation may be possible:
    – Toe amputations: for isolated severe infection or gangrene of a toe
    – Ray amputations: transmetatarsal amputation of an individual toe, with V-shaped extension over the metatarsal
    – Transmetatarsal forefoot amputation: for extensive forefoot ischaemia.

Popliteal artery entrapment
● The popliteal artery may be compressed against the femoral condyle by a congenitally abnormal gastrocnemius or popliteus muscle.
● Typical presentation is calf claudication in a young man, although, rarely, thrombosis may cause acute lower limb ischaemia (page 554).

- Duplex ultrasound/angiography/MRA shows lateral displacement of the popliteal artery, which is compressed by passive foot dorsiflexion or active plantarflexion.
- Treatment: surgical division of the medial head of the gastrocnemius; vein bypass graft for occlusion.

Cystic adventitial disease of the popliteal artery

- A rare condition, where mucinous degeneration results in an adventitial cyst that narrows the popliteal artery.
- May cause claudication, or precipitate acute lower limb ischaemia (page 554).
- Duplex and MRA demonstrates the cyst, whereas angiography shows a characteristic 'hourglass' stenosis.
- Treatment: surgical resection and repair; angioplasty is contra-indicated because of distal embolism of the cyst contents.

Popliteal aneurysm

- Aneurysmal dilatation of the popliteal artery to >2 cm diameter may occur in isolation, but is often bilateral and occurs in 40% of patients with abdominal aortic aneurysm.
- Affects males over 50 years of age, with various presentations:
  - Acute lower limb ischaemia: from thrombosis of the aneurysm
  - Micro-embolism to the toes
  - Incidental finding of an expansile pulsation behind the knee.
- Saphenous vein bypass with ligation of the aneurysm is indicated for asymptomatic aneurysm >2.5 cm diameter and symptomatic cases.
- Acute limb ischaemia may require emergency bypass with distal embolectomy or thrombolysis.

Acute upper limb ischaemia

Definitions

- Sudden impairment of the arterial circulation to the arm.

- Aetiology:
  - Embolism: most likely
  - Thrombosis of subclavian/axillary artery stenosis from compression or radiotherapy: relatively rare
  - Atheroma does not usually cause significant upper limb ischaemia
  - Trauma.

Clinical features

- Sudden onset in arm of:
  - Pain – at rest or on arm claudication
  - Pallor
  - Pulselessness
  - 'Perishing cold'
  - Paraesthesia and anaesthesia
  - Paralysis
  - Features indicating very severe ischaemia, requiring intervention as soon as possible.

Investigation

➤ Clinical diagnosis.
➤ Angiography: to plan intervention.

Treatment

Embolus most likely:

➤ Surgical embolectomy:
  - Usually by exploration of brachial artery, but rarely the axillary artery
  - Fogarty balloon catheter is used to retrieve embolus
  - On-table angiography guides the procedure
  - Direct intra-arterial administration of 20 mg TPA may be used for thrombolysis of occluded small vessels.

Thrombosis of subclavian or axillary stenosis most likely:

➤ Radiological thrombolysis with TPA and angioplasty of underlying disease
➤ Emergency surgical bypass may be required for severe cases unresponsive to radiological intervention

➔

> ➤ Conservative treatment with full anticoagulation for less severe cases unresponsive to or unsuitable for intervention – heparin 5000 units loading dose, then 1000 units/hour until warfarin stabilized; warfarin 10 mg, 10 mg, 5 mg, then 2–3 mg daily to achieve international normalized ratio (INR) 2–3.

Thoracic outlet compression syndrome (TOCS)

Definitions

- Syndrome resulting from compression of the brachial plexus, or the subclavian vein or artery against the first rib and Sibson's fascia.
- Aetiology: cervical rib, fibrous bands, long C7 transverse process, scalene muscle hypertrophy.
- Affects: young adults, more common in swimmers.

Clinical features

- Pain, paraesthesia and numbness over the neck, shoulder, arm and hand – exacerbated by exercise of the arm, particularly work with the arm raised, or carrying heavy bags.
- If the upper brachial plexus is compressed, symptoms affect the lateral and radial aspects of the arm and hand.
- If the lower brachial plexus is compressed, symptoms affect the medial and ulnar aspects of the arm and hand.
- Raynaud's phenomenon.
- Venous compression may result in heaviness, swelling and cyanosis of the arm, or, rarely, axillary vein thrombosis.
- Arterial compression (rare) may result in arm pain and cyanosis on exertion, post-stenotic aneurysmal dilatation of the subclavian artery or micro-embolic phenomena to the hand.

Clinical tests (unreliable):

- Roos' test: clenching and opening the fists repeatedly for up to 2 minutes in the 'hands-up' position induces the symptoms

- Allen's test: 90% abduction and external rotation of the shoulder with the head turned to the opposite side induces the symptoms.

Investigation
➤ Thoracic outlet X-ray: to identify cervical ribs.
➤ Nerve conduction studies: to exclude other nerve compression.
➤ Duplex ultrasound: to identify subclavian artery or vein abnormalities, particularly in conjunction with the clinical test manoeuvres above.
➤ Venography or angiography: may be required if arterio-venous abnormalities are suspected.
➤ MRI: to identify bands.

Treatment
➤ Physiotherapy: neck and shoulder girdle exercises.
➤ Transaxillary first rib resection.
➤ Supraclavicular cervical rib resection: also allows access for treatment of subclavian arteriovenous abnormalities.
➤ Surgical resection of scalenus anterior muscle: for upper brachial plexus compression.

Complications
- Subclavian artery stenosis and aneurysm.
- Subclavian–axillary vein stenosis or occlusion.
- Phrenic nerve and vascular injury during surgery.

Vasculitic disorders

Takayasu's arteriopathy

Definitions
- Obliterative condition of major aortic branches and pulmonary arteries.
- Pathology: giant cell arteritis.
- Aetiology: unknown.
- Affects mainly women, 10–30 years of age, usually oriental.

Clinical features

Acute phase:

- Malaise, fever, weight loss, arthralgia.

Chronic phase:

- Claudication: may affect upper limb
- Cerebrovascular symptoms (page 547) (may present to an ophthalmologist)
- Absent pulses: particularly upper limb
- Bruits
- Hypertension: blood pressure inequality between the arms
- Cardiac murmurs.

Investigation

➤ Erythrocyte sedimentation rate (ESR)/C-reactive protein (CRP): elevated in acute phase.
➤ Angiography: for symptomatic limbs.

Treatment

➤ Treatment of hypertension (page 547).
➤ Prednisolone 40 mg daily until clinical remission, then 7.5 mg daily for 2 years – where obliterative disease is progressing, with raised ESR/CRP.
➤ Surgical bypass: for established symptomatic occlusive disease.

Temporal arteritis

Definitions

- Obliterative condition of cranial branches of the aorta, typically temporal arteries.
- Pathology: giant cell arteritis.
- Aetiology: unknown.
- Affects mainly women >50 years of age.

Clinical features

- Headache: temporal region.
- Tenderness: over superficial temporal artery.
- Jaw claudication.

- Amaurosis fugax: a warning sign of impending blindness.
- Sudden blindness: from occlusion of the ophthalmic or posterior ciliary artery.

Investigation

➤ ESR >100 mm/hour.
➤ Temporal artery biopsy: negative result does not rule out temporal arteritis, particularly if steroid treatment has been started.
➤ Duplex ultrasound: used in some centres to identify abnormal temporal artery flow.

Treatment

➤ Prednisolone 40 mg daily until clinical remission, then 7.5 mg daily for 2 years. Urgent treatment is given on clinical suspicion, because of the risk of blindness; for ophthalmic symptoms use prednisolone 60 mg daily initially.

Raynaud's phenomenon, syndrome and disease

- Raynaud's phenomenon is caused by exposure to cold, which induces characteristic changes in fingers or toes: pallor, then cyanosis, then red hyperaemia; sometimes with severe pain.
- Cause: Raynaud's disease; and vasospasm in vasculitic and rheumatological disorders.
- Raynaud's syndrome: includes everyone with Raynaud's phenomenon.
- Raynaud's disease: painful Raynaud's phenomenon, mainly affecting the hands, with no associated vasculitic or rheumatological disorder; occurs in young women.
- Treatment: avoid sudden cold exposure; heated gloves; nifedipine 5 mg tds, naftidrofuryl 100 mg tds, inositol nicotinate 1 g tds, prazosin 500 μg bd.

Vasculitis

Definitions

- Complex multisystem conditions including:
  - Polyarteritis nodosa

- Wegener's granulomatosis
- Connective tissue disorders: systemic lupus erythematosus (SLE), systemic sclerosis/scleroderma
- Rheumatoid disease
- Other non-specific forms.
- Pathology: inflammation of small blood vessels causing ischaemic tissue damage.
- Aetiology: unknown, autoimmune.

Clinical features

- Polyarteritis nodosa:
  - Affects mainly men; age >40 years
  - Malaise, fever, weight loss, abdominal pain
  - Progressive chronic renal failure
  - Acute bowel infarction, perforation or haemorrhage
  - Mononeuritis multiplex.
- Wegener's granulomatosis:
  - Granulomatous occlusion of upper respiratory tract – chronic sinusitis (page 278)
  - Lung fibrosis
  - Progressive chronic renal failure
  - Discoid granulomatous skin ulcers
- Cutaneous vasculitis:
  - Usually affects lower leg
  - Raised purpuric areas progress to ulceration
  - Features of connective tissue disorders.

Investigation

➤ Full blood count: anaemia.
➤ ESR/CRP: raised.
➤ Autoantibody screen.
➤ Antineutrophil cytoplasmic antibody: polyarteritis nodosa, Wegener's granulomatosis.
➤ Rheumatoid factor: rheumatoid disease, some cases of SLE, and other non-specific forms.
➤ Antinuclear antibodies: SLE.
➤ Angiography: saccular aneurysms and small vessel occlusions – polyarteritis nodosa
➤ Histology of arterial biopsy or affected areas of skin: vasculitis.

Treatment
> Prednisolone 40 mg orally daily, reducing to the minimum dose required to suppress disease activity, usually 10 mg.
> Other forms of immunosuppression in severe cases.

Scleroderma
- A collagen disease with associated vasculitis, resulting in occlusion of small arteries.
- Mainly affects young women as: Raynaud's phenomenon; then thickened skin over the fingers and brittle nails; and eventually painful fingertip necrosis, with withering, and sometimes gangrene and auto-amputation of the fingertips.
- Systemic sclerosis results in a similar process affecting small vessels of the heart, lungs and gastrointestinal tract, and may result in oesophageal stenosis.

Vibration white finger
- Occurring in those operating certain vibrating machinery; severity relates to length of exposure; symptoms, including Raynaud's phenomenon, may develop up to 20 years later.
- Characteristic pattern of finger involvement for each machine.
- Prevention: modern machinery is designed to reduce vibration.
- Treatment: avoid vibrating machinery; otherwise treat as Raynaud's; recognized as a condition for industrial compensation and disablement in some countries (e.g. UK).

Thrombophilia (hypercoagulable states/prothrombotic disorders)

Definitions
- Conditions predisposing to thrombosis.
- Pathology:
  - Antithrombin III deficiency
  - Leiden V mutation

– Protein S or C deficiency
– Activated protein C resistance
– Abnormal fibrinolysis
– Antiphospholipid syndrome – associated with SLE.
- Aetiology: autoimmune conditions, hereditary conditions and genetic mutations.

Clinical features

- Recurrent miscarriages.
- Recurrent deep venous thrombosis.
- Early onset of occlusive arterial disease.
- Recurrent vascular graft occlusion.

Investigation

➤ Serum assays of antithrombin III, protein S/C, Leiden factor V, lupus anticoagulant and anticardiolipin antibody.

Treatment

Acute thrombosis:

➤ Heparin 5000 units i.v., then 1000 units/hour – adjusted to maintain activated partial thromboplastin time (APTT) ratio 2–3 until warfarin therapy is stable
➤ Warfarin daily dose 10 mg, 10 mg, 5 mg; then adjusted to achieve INR 3–4.

Long term:

➤ Warfarin daily dose to achieve INR 3–4
➤ Management of SLE.

Complications

- Skin necrosis is a rare complication of warfarin therapy, associated with protein C deficiency.

Visceral arteries

Acute intestinal ischaemia

Definitions

- Aetiology: acute embolic occlusion of the superior mesenteric artery or major branches.

- Embolic sources: as for acute lower limb ischaemia.
- Thrombosis in terminal illness.

Clinical features

- Central constant abdominal pain.
- Diarrhoea: dark blood-stained stool.
- Gradually developing signs of sepsis.
- Peritonitis develops hours later.

Investigation

➤ White cell count: $>20 \times 10^9/L$, often $>30 \times 10^9/L$.
➤ Serum amylase: may be slightly raised ($>200\,IU$).
➤ Mesenteric angiography.

Treatment

➤ Laparotomy: superior mesenteric embolectomy; resection of areas of non-viable bowel.
➤ 'Second look' laparotomy at 24 hours for further resection of non-viable bowel.

Complications

- Most cases are recognized late and are fatal.

Chronic mesenteric ischaemia

- Atherosclerotic disease affecting the coeliac and mesenteric arteries may rarely produce chronic symptoms: food fear, weight loss, diarrhoea, and vague abdominal pains after eating – mesenteric angina.
- Surgical bypass of the occlusion may be required.

Renal artery stenosis

Definitions

- Aetiology:
  - Atherosclerotic disease – of the aorta, causing osteal stenosis
  - Fibromuscular dysplasia – a rare condition where intima/media thickening produces a smooth focal renal artery stenosis; occasionally seen in carotid and other medium-sized arteries.

Clinical features

- Asymptomatic: majority.
- Hypertension: from excessive renin release; may occur even if only one kidney is affected; typically patients are on multiple antihypertensive medications.
- Renal failure: may be precipitated by angiotensin-converting enzyme inhibitors – block efferent arteriolar contraction and exacerbate renal hypoperfusion.
- Flash pulmonary oedema: sudden severe pulmonary oedema, requiring intensive care.

Investigation

➤ Ultrasound: demonstrates atrophy of the poorly perfused kidney; length <8 cm indicates that intervention will not be successful.
➤ Angiography: demonstrates nature of stenoses.
➤ Captopril renography: radio-isotope renal excretion studies demonstrate marked reduction in excretion after captopril administration.

Treatment

➤ Treatment of hypertension (page 546).
➤ Treatment of atherosclerotic disease (page 546).
➤ Angioplasty and stents: particularly for fibromuscular dysplasia.
➤ Surgical revascularization by aortic atherectomy, patch angioplasty or bypass grafts.

Aortic aneurysm

Definitions

- Slow, progressive, fusiform dilatation of the aorta (>1.5 times the normal size).
- Typically affects the infrarenal (abdominal) aorta; often with extension to iliac arteries.
- Thoracic and thoraco-abdominal aortic aneurysms are less common.
- Eventually rupture may occur (see below); the larger the aneurysm, the greater the risk.
- Affects mainly males >60 years of age.

- Aetiology: unknown.
- Associations: familial tendency (father, brothers), atherosclerotic disease, and hypertension; increased incidence in Marfan's and Ehlers–Danlos syndromes.

Clinical features

- Asymptomatic: often incidental finding on examination or investigation for other conditions; or identified by screening programmes.
- Associated popliteal aneurysms (page 560).
- Back pain, left loin pain, or epigastric pain: may indicate enlargement or rupture.
- Epigastric swelling with expansile pulsation.
- May present with rupture (see below).

Investigation

➤ Investigation of associated atherosclerotic disease (page 545).
➤ Ultrasound scan: identifies abdominal aortic aneurysm and quantifies size: typically as maximum antero-posterior diameter.
➤ Chest X-ray: may identify associated thoracic aortic aneurysm.
➤ CT for more detailed information: relation to renal arteries, iliac involvement.
➤ Crawford classification of thoraco-abdominal aneurysms:
    I   Majority of descending thoracic aorta and proximal abdominal aorta
    II Majority of descending thoracic aorta and majority of abdominal aorta
    III Distal descending aorta and majority of abdominal aorta
    IV Majority of abdominal aorta, but including visceral origins.

Treatment

Asymptomatic infrarenal aneurysm <5.5 cm A–P diameter:

➤ Surveillance: 6-monthly ultrasound scan.

➔

Symptomatic infrarenal aneurysm, and asymptomatic
infrarenal aneurysm >5.5 cm anteroposterior diameter:

➤ Surgical synthetic graft replacement of the abdominal
aorta – major procedure.

Unfit for surgery – usually with cardiorespiratory disease:

➤ Atherosclerotic risk factor management – particularly
hypertension
➤ Early discussion of outcome in the event of rupture.

Thoraco-abdominal aneurysms:

➤ Graft replacement is possible, but more complex –
decision to operate depends on expertise of centre.

Complications

Complications of surgical synthetic graft replacement of
the abdominal aorta:

- Death >5%: myocardial infarction; peri-operative,
multisystem organ failure; later in intensive care
- Renal failure: may stabilize, but rarely dialysis is required
- Distal embolism: range from trash-foot (page 556) to
acute lower limb ischaemia (page 554) with risk of
limb loss
- Graft infection (page 576): may present weeks or
months later, mortality >50%.

Thoraco-abdominal aneurysm surgery:

- Spinal stroke: paraplegia occurs in >10% of thoraco-
abdominal aneurysm surgery – spinal cord ischaemia
results when the aortic clamp is placed above the arteria
radicularis magna, a posterior aortic or upper lumbar
vessel supplying the spinal cord
- Surgical mortality of up to 35%.

Endoluminal repair of abdominal
aortic aneurysm

● Method of aneurysm repair where a stent–graft system
is passed via the femoral and iliac arteries, to exclude
the aneurysm from within.

- Theoretic advantages:
  - Smaller incisions
  - Lesser magnitude of procedure.
- Practical disadvantages:
  - Inferior anatomic repair
  - Unknown longevity
  - Increased risk of limb and visceral ischaemia
  - Mortality no less than for open surgery.
- Some centres produce excellent results but results of randomized trials are awaited.

Ruptured abdominal aortic aneurysm

Definitions

- The larger the anteroposterior diameter of an aortic aneurysm, the greater the risk of rupture:
  - <5.5 cm: <5% per year
  - 5.5–6.0 cm: 5–10% per year
  - 6 cm: up to 30% per year.

Clinical features

Intraperitoneal rupture:

- Sudden death.

Retroperitoneal rupture:

- Usually progression over hours:
  - Sudden severe back, left loin, left iliac fossa or central abdominal pain
  - Tender left-sided abdominal mass – may not be pulsatile
  - Shock
  - Death.

Treatment

Shock or resuscitated from shock:

➤ Immediate surgical synthetic graft replacement of the abdominal aorta.

Symptomatic but stable:

➤ Immediate CT: confirm diagnosis, and assess aneurysm
➤ Urgent surgical synthetic graft replacement of the abdominal aorta.

Complications

Outcome of ruptured abdominal aortic aneurysm:

* 90% mortality before reaching hospital
* 50% peri-operative mortality
* In shocked patients and those aged >80 years survival is unlikely.

Mycotic/inflammatory aortic aneurysm

- Aortic aneurysm with associated inflammation: has a very thick wall, adherent to adjacent structures.
- Aetiology: unknown; sometimes salmonella, tuberculosis or other infection.
- May present with fever, malaise and abdominal pain.
- Surgery is more complex, with high risk of complications – particularly graft infection (page 576).

Aortic dissection (dissecting aortic aneurysm)

Definitions

- A subintimal false passage for blood flow may form in the aorta.
- If the diameter of dissected aorta is abnormal, it is termed a dissecting aneurysm.
- May obstruct flow to major aortic branches by isolating their origins.
- Aetiology: most commonly intimal tear associated with hypertension, but also abnormal aortic media in inherited disorders.
- Association: Marfan's and Ehlers–Danlos syndromes.
- Affects: 50–70 year age group.

Clinical features

Acute cases:

* Sudden onset central chest pain radiating to the back
* Symptoms and signs from separation of the major aortic branches:
  - Stroke
  - Myocardial infarction

- Acute upper or lower limb ischaemia
- Acute visceral ischaemia.
- Collapse in severe cases
- Aortic regurgitation murmur – early diastolic murmur in aortic area
- Asymmetry of pulses
- Different blood pressure readings between the arms (>15 mmHg)
- May rupture leading to death.

Chronic cases:

- May be asymptomatic.

Investigation

➤ Chest X-ray: shows widened mediastinum.
➤ Transoesophageal echocardiography: demonstrates relation to aortic root.
➤ CT aortogram: diagnoses and demonstrates extent of dissection.
➤ Aortography: demonstrates relation to aortic root, and major arterial branches.
➤ DeBakey classification:
  I   Tear in ascending aorta back to aortic valve, forward to-arch-descending aorta (type A)
  II Tear in ascending aorta back to aortic valve (type A)
  III Tear at left subclavian origin forward descending aorta (type B).

Treatment

➤ Control of hypertension: most uncomplicated dissection may be managed this way.
➤ Fenestration by intervention during aortography: major arterial branches may be opened up by deliberately making a hole in the dissection flap with a radiologically guided wire.
➤ Surgical graft replacement of the aortic root, with aortic valve replacement, and aortic arch: for fitter patients with type A dissections.
➤ May be amenable to stenting.
➤ Prognosis: type A 80% mortality without surgery; 25% mortality for surgery in those who are fit enough.

False aneurysm of the femoral artery

Definitions

- A cavity containing haematoma, with active communication to the arterial lumen, with walls of compressed surrounding tissues.
- Aetiology: arterial puncture for coronary angiography; accidental puncture in intravenous drug abuse; other arterial trauma.
- Some may thrombose over days, and resolve over weeks; others enlarge and rupture.

Clinical features

- Expansile groin mass, surrounding bruising, evidence of recent arterial puncture.

Investigation

➤ Duplex ultrasound: confirms diagnosis, assesses size, locates site of arterial leak.

Treatment

➤ Compression of the site of arterial leak for half an hour using the Duplex probe.
➤ Thrombin injection.
➤ Surgical exploration and suturing of the arterial puncture site.

Vascular graft infection

Definitions

- Infection complicates 5% of synthetic (PTFE or Dacron) grafts.
- Pathology: typically *Staphylococcus*, *Streptococcus*, *Pseudomonas*.
- Aetiology: contamination of graft during implantation from patient's own skin or perineum, or any other source of micro-organisms in the operative environment, e.g. bowel injury; spread of infection from leg ulcers; haematogenous spread of micro-organisms from any site of entry.

Clinical features

Presentation days or weeks after surgery: usually virulent organisms, e.g. *Pseudomonas*, *Streptococcus*, *Staphylococcus aureus*, methicillin-resistant *Staph. aureus*:

- Inflammation and suppuration of groin or popliteal incisions
- Failure to recover after aortic surgery, with general weakness, anaemia, back pain, pyrexial illness, and sometimes ileus.

Presentation weeks or months after surgery: usually less virulent organisms, e.g. *Staph. epidermidis*:

- Chronic thickening of groin or popliteal wound, with lymphocoele and sinus formation
- Risk of dramatic wound haemorrhage from anastomotic breakdown
- Late general deterioration after aortic surgery, with general weakness, anaemia, back pain, pyrexial illness
- Crescendo upper gastrointestinal haemorrhages, with final large fatal haemorrhage – aortoduodenal fistula in aortic graft infection.

Investigation

➤ Microbiology of any wound discharge/ulcer.
➤ Blood cultures: in systemic sepsis.
➤ Duplex ultrasound: may identify peri-graft fluid collection or anastomotic false aneurysm for peripheral grafts.
➤ Angiography: determines anatomy for further surgery.
➤ CT: may identify peri-graft collection (with gas–fluid level) for aortic grafts, may demonstrate abnormal tissues adherent to upper anastomosis suggestive of aortoduodenal fistula.
➤ Oesophagogastroduodenoscopy: excludes peptic ulcer or other cause of upper gastrointestinal haemorrhage in suspected aortoduodenal fistula; the aortoduodenal fistula is rarely visualized.
➤ Radiolabelled white cell scan: may support suspected aortic graft infection where other methods fail.

Treatment

➤ Extra-anatomic graft (via a route away from the site of infection), using vein – best option, non-synthetic cryopreserved homografts, or rifampicin-impregnated coated Dacron; excision of the infected graft.

➤ In aortic grafts axillobifemoral bypass is required, with oversewing of the aortic stump after graft excision.

➤ Graft removal without immediate limb revascularization is a good option where collateral circulation is adequate.

➤ Amputation may be an option where there are no good alternative routes for revascularization.

➤ Palliation with long-term antibiotics may be an option for infected aortic grafts in patients unfit for further major surgery.

Complications

● 50% mortality for infected aortic grafts.
● High risk of limb loss for infected peripheral grafts.

Vascular injury

Definitions

● Aetiology:
  – Gunshot, knife or other penetrating injuries – may sever an artery or vein
  – Crush injury – intimal tearing and occlusion by thrombosis
  – Fractures – laceration by bone fragments, crushing or kinking by associated angular deformity
  – Iatrogenic – arterial puncture – for angiography, leading to false aneurysm formation (page 576); major abdominal vessel laceration – in laparoscopic surgery.

Clinical features

● Haemorrhage: external via the wound, or concealed, e.g. into the abdomen.
● Ischaemia: features of acute ischaemia of the affected area, e.g. acute limb ischaemia (page 554).

- Pulsatile haematoma or false aneurysm.
- Arteriovenous fistula.

Investigation

Haemorrhage:

➤ No investigation, immediate surgical exploration.

Ischaemia:

➤ Angiography: to determine the location and nature of injury (NB muscle ischaemia produces renal damage on revascularization after 4–6 hours; beyond 12 hours irreversible damage and amputation rather than revascularization should be considered).

Treatment

➤ Surgical exploration via the site of injury, and to key areas above and below where control of the vessels is possible.
➤ Direct repair if local injury, with vein patch if narrowing of the vessel is likely.
➤ Excision of damaged region, with anastomosis of the ends or vein bypass graft.
➤ Shunts to temporarily restore circulation while other significant injuries are treated.
➤ Venous injuries may be ligated without reconstruction if there is good collateral venous drainage; except in total limb re-implantation where venous repair must be undertaken prior to arterial repair.

Compartment syndrome after limb ischaemia

- Muscle oedema after limb revascularization may compress smaller vessels and nerves within the compartments of the lower leg or arm, to produce further ischaemic damage.
- Fasciotomy should be performed immediately after a limb has been revascularized for prolonged acute severe ischaemia (duration >4 hours, but there are no absolute criteria), or after severe limb trauma.

- Failure to decompress the limb will result in a tensely swollen, paralysed, anaesthetic, ischaemic limb, with subsequent need for debridement of necrotic tissue or even limb loss. If the limb recovers, muscle contractures will develop, and there will be permanent loss of sensation and movement, e.g. foot drop, Volkmann's contracture of the wrist/arm (page 685).

Carotid injury

- Usually penetrating trauma from bullet or knife wounds.
- Considered according to zones:
  - I: from 1 cm above the manubrium sterni downwards
  - II: from zone I to the angle of the mandible
  - III: from the angle of the mandible upwards.
- In general, angiography is always performed to assess zone I and III injuries, whereas zone II injuries may be surgically explored without angiography.
- Internal and common carotid artery injuries are repaired: shunts may be used to temporarily restore circulation, whereas the external carotid artery and jugular vein may be ligated.

VEINS AND LYMPHATICS

Varicose veins

Definitions

- Dilated, tortuous, elongated superficial leg veins.
- Women more often affected.
- Pathology: often associated with valvular incompetence at communication of superficial and deep veins.
- Aetiology:
  - Heredity
  - Female sex hormones
  - Pregnancy.
- May be secondary to:
  - Deep venous thrombosis, occlusion or injury
  - Pelvic mass compressing iliac veins.

Clinical features

- Aching legs – particularly on standing for long periods.
- Past history of: pregnancy, deep vein thrombosis (leg fracture or immobilization in plaster).
- Dilated, tortuous, elongated superficial leg veins.
- Thread veins and venous flares.
- There may be associated changes of chronic venous insufficiency (page 585).
- Groin cough-impulse: indicates saphenofemoral incompetence.
- Trendelenburg tests:
  - Elevation of the leg to empty the veins, application of a tourniquet, then observing filling of veins on standing
  - Rapid filling indicates incompetent communications below the level of tourniquet application, e.g. if varicosities do not fill rapidly (within 20 seconds) on standing with a high-thigh tourniquet, the saphenofemoral junction is likely to be the only site of incompetence.

Investigation

➤ Doppler probe (hand-held Doppler, continuous wave Doppler):
  - A long signal after squeezing and releasing the calf indicates reflux in the examined vein
  - Can identify saphenofemoral reflux and 'popliteal fossa' reflux, but cannot distinguish short saphenopopliteal reflux from popliteal vein reflux.
➤ Duplex ultrasound:
  - Confirms sites of incompetence
  - Distinguishes saphenopopliteal from popliteal reflux
  - Locates the short saphenopopliteal junction.

Treatment

➤ Class 2 compression stocking: relieves aching and protects against changes of chronic venous insufficiency.
➤ Varicose vein surgery: varicosities are avulsed via tiny stab incisions, and the incompetent junction and its

→

tributaries are ligated; the long saphenous vein is stripped out to just below the knee.
➤ Injection sclerotherapy: sodium tetradecyl sulphate 3%, with immediate application of a compression stocking or elastic bandage – associated major venous incompetence must be treated surgically first.
➤ Photodermal therapy and laser coagulation of thread veins and flares – associated major venous incompetence must be treated surgically first.

Complications

Varicose veins:

* Chronic venous insufficiency and ulceration (see below)
* Bleeding – fragile superficial varicosities are easily torn, and may bleed profusely
* Thrombophlebitis.

Injection sclerotherapy:

* Skin ulceration – from extravasation of sclerosant
* Brown skin pigmentation
* Recurrence – particularly if major venous incompetence is untreated.

Varicose vein surgery:

* Recurrence
* Sural nerve injury (page 772) – may be injured during short saphenous surgery
* Saphenous nerve injury (page 773) – may be injured if the long saphenous vein is stripped below the knee
* Deep vein thrombosis – in women taking oral contraceptives.

Thrombophlebitis

Definitions

* Thrombosis and inflammation result in painful, tender, hard discoloured superficial veins – associated with varicose veins of the legs.
* Palpable thrombosis of the main long saphenous trunk in the thigh may be associated with deep venous thrombosis.

- Thrombophlebitis migrans: repeated episodes of thrombophlebitis affecting different areas – associated with advanced malignancy.

Investigation
➤ Duplex ultrasound – if deep venous thrombosis is suspected.

Treatment
➤ Rest, elevation of the leg, anti-inflammatory agents, e.g. ibuprofen 400 mg tds, compression stocking – if tenderness has settled.
➤ Ligation of the saphenofemoral junction: sometimes required if extensive thrombosis of the main long saphenous trunk extends to the deep veins.

Deep vein thrombosis (venous thromboembolism)

Definitions
- Thrombosis begins in deep calf vein tributaries.
- May propagate into and occlude popliteal, femoral and iliac veins.
- Aetiology – Virchow's triad:
  - Stasis: immobility – surgery, treatment of long bone fractures, serious illness or a long-haul flight; pregnancy
  - Blood viscosity/coagulability: dehydration, carcinomatosis, thrombophilias; hormones of pregnancy, combined oral contraceptive, hormone replacement therapy
  - Disruption of integrity of normal vein wall: venous injury; impairment of normal endothelial function by many unexplained factors.

Clinical features
- Sudden onset of pain and swelling:
  - Calf: popliteal vein thrombosis
  - Calf and thigh: iliofemoral vein thrombosis.
- Pitting oedema of calf/thigh.
- Increased skin temperature over calf/thigh.

- Superficial venous dilatation over the leg.
- Cyanosis/pallor: see phlegmasia (page 585).
- Homan's sign: calf pain on passive foot dorsiflexion

Investigation

➤ Duplex ultrasound.
➤ Compression tests with B-mode ultrasound: major venous thrombosis can be observed as a non-compressible venous segment using non-Duplex ultrasound machine.
➤ Venography.
➤ Serum D-dimer >0.3 mg/L: sensitive, but not specific – may be elevated for other reasons.

Treatment

Prevention – in successive combination:

➤ Thrombo-embolic deterrent stockings: for all hospitalized patients, except those with limb ischaemia or reperfusion states
➤ Heparin 5000 units subcutaneous bd (or low molecular weight alternatives): for patients who are non-ambulant; older patients or those with risk factors undergoing intermediate surgery; all patients undergoing major surgery; or those with a history of previous deep venous thrombosis or pulmonary embolism
➤ Intermittent intra-operative pneumatic calf compression: patients with risk factors undergoing major surgery; all patients undergoing prolonged surgery.

Treatment:

➤ Heparin i.v. 5000 unit bolus, then 1000 units/hour adjusted to maintain activated partial thromboplastin time ratio 2–3: continued until oral anticoagulation is stabilized
➤ Warfarin orally daily: 10 mg, 5 mg, 5 mg, then dose adjustment to maintain international normalized ratio around 2

→

> ➤ Duration of warfarin therapy:
>   – 3–6 months – idiopathic thrombosis
>   – Indefinite – persisting causal factor.
> ➤ Vena cava filter (a metal-wire trap inserted radio-logically): to trap free-floating thrombus and recurrent pulmonary embolism
> ➤ Deep venous thrombosis in pregnancy: heparin is continued throughout the pregnancy, and warfarin started only after delivery.

Complications

- Pulmonary embolism.
- Varicose veins.
- Chronic venous insufficiency.

Phlegmasia alba dolens

- Pallor of a massively swollen leg in iliofemoral venous thrombosis – may progress to phlegmasia caerulea dolens.

Phlegmasia caerulea dolens

- Blue discoloration of a massively swollen leg in ilio-femoral venous thrombosis: perfusion of the leg has been compromised, which may lead to gangrene.
- Hand-held Doppler: absence of arterial signals at the ankle.
- Requires urgent angiography and arterial/venous thrombolysis, or surgical arterial/venous thrombectomy.

Chronic venous insufficiency

Definitions

- A state of characteristic changes resulting from long-standing venous valvular dysfunction and persisting high venous pressures in the leg.
- Aetiology:
  - Varicose veins – but not all varicose veins lead to this
  - Deep venous thrombosis

– Venous injury
– Long-term leg dependency, e.g. wheelchair users
– Calf muscle pump dysfunction, e.g. contractures/
  fractures preventing ankle dorsiflexion.

Clinical features

- Dark red/purple skin pigmentation in the gaiter area:
  from haemosiderin deposition.
- Lipodermatosclerosis: waxy skin texture with
  indentation of the gaiter area from subcutaneous
  fibrosis.
- Varicose eczema: flaking skin, with vesicle formation.
- Ulceration: typically superficial, irregular, moist ulcers
  above the malleoli, with a flat edge and granulating
  base.

Investigation

➤ History and findings are diagnostic.
➤ Duplex ultrasound: confirms patency of deep veins and
  identifies sites of superficial or deep reflux.

Treatment

➤ Treatment of varicose veins (page 581).
➤ Moisturizing creams and steroid creams for eczema.
➤ Class 2 (18–24 mmHg) compression stocking, usually
  below-knee – but not used if co-existing arterial
  disease with resting ankle pressure <100 mmHg.

Complications

- Perforating vein reflux may be identified on duplex in
  these cases – significance and effects of treatment are
  still debated.

Leg ulcers

Definitions

- Aetiology:
  – Chronic lower limb arterial disease
  – Chronic venous insufficiency

- Diabetic neuropathy
- Vasculitis – rheumatological disease
- Other: infection, trauma, cutaneous malignancy, sickle-cell disease, pressure necrosis, various tropical diseases.
- Marjolin's ulcer: malignant change (squamous cell carcinoma) may develop at the edge of a chronic ulcer.

Clinical features

Arterial:

- Location: toe joints/tips, heel, malleoli, anterior shin
- Appearance: dry, circular – but may slough with infection, punched-out edge.

Venous:

- Location: above malleoli
- Appearance: moist, irregular, flat edge.

Diabetic neuropathic:

- Location: under metatarsal heads and as in arterial
- Appearance: moist, sloughy; often associated with extensive underlying plantar space infection or necrosis of fascia and tendon.

Vasculitic:

- Location: any
- Appearance: variable, but there may be rapid progression of skin discoloration and necrosis; punched-out edge.

Investigation

➤ Investigation of: arterial disease (page 553), chronic venous insufficiency (page 585), diabetes (page 558), vasculitis (page 565).
➤ Investigation of specific causes of ulceration if suspected.
➤ X-rays: to look for osteomyelitis, particularly in diabetes.
➤ Biopsy and histology: for suspected Marjolin's ulcer, vasculitis or primary malignancy.

Treatment

Arterial ulcers:

➤ Treat arterial disease: angioplasty or bypass surgery (page 553).

Venous ulcers:

➤ Four-layer bandage (Charing Cross bandage): graduated compression from forefoot to upper calf with: wool/crepe/Elset/Coban layers; replaced weekly or sooner if soiled
➤ Surgery to treat origin of underlying venous reflux.

Diabetic ulcers:

➤ Treat diabetes
➤ Protective shoes.

Severe diabetic foot necrosis:

➤ Debridement of dead tissue
➤ Appropriate antibiotics for infection
➤ Plaster boot with window over the ulcer.

General management of ulcers:

➤ Debridement of any dead tissue: hydrocolloid gel dressing or surgical debridement
➤ Split skin grafting: for large ulcers, where underlying cause has been treated and infection eliminated.

Severe ulcers with untreatable underlying cause:

➤ Amputation may sometimes be required.

Complications

● Leg ulcers may have a combination of causes, e.g. diabetic neuropathy and arterial; arterial and venous.
● Long-standing ulceration may undergo malignant change: Marjolin's ulcer – raised, everted edges.

Lymphoedema

Definitions

● Oedema from absence, dysfunction or occlusion of lymphatics.

- Aetiology:
  - Primary:
    - Congenital abnormality of lymphatics occurring at birth (congenitalia), at puberty (praecox) or later (tarda), and may be familial (Milroy's disease).
  - Secondary:
    - Malignant infiltration of lymphatics: iliac and para-aortic nodes in prostatic or other pelvic carcinoma; inguinal region in melanoma; axilla in breast carcinoma or after axillary radiotherapy
    - Infection: filarial parasitic organisms.

Clinical features

General features:

- Limb swelling that, once established, does not pit on digital pressure.

Late features:

- Prominent skin creases with hyperkeratotic skin changes
- Papillomatosis.

Age of onset:

- At or soon after birth
- Post-puberty: minor infection precipitating lymphoedema where there is previously asymptomatic congenital abnormality
- Older age groups: often malignant involvement of pelvic, inguinal or axillary nodes.

Features of specific types:

- Tropical area: filariasis
- Giant scrotal swelling: filariasis
- Lymphoedema of the arm: carcinoma of the breast or after axillary radiotherapy.

Investigation

➤ Lymphoscintigraphy: the progress of radiolabelled colloid injected into the first foot web-space is followed with a gamma camera – distinguishes lymphoedema from other causes of leg swelling.

Treatment

➤ Massaging fluid out of the limb: sequential compression devices.
➤ Compression hosiery: Class 3 (25–35 mmHg).
➤ Surgical reduction of limb girth with/without skin grafting: in severe cases with secondary changes.

Vascular malformations

Definitions

● Anomalous vascular structures: capillary, venous, arterial or lymphatic.
● Aetiology: abnormal embryonic vasculogenesis.

Clinical features

Low-flow:

• Capillary: flat 'port-wine stain'; or the prominent, rapidly enlarging 'strawberry naevus' in neonates/children
• Venous: painful large prominent veins, with overlying eczema, prone to thrombosis; empty on elevation or pressure/fill on dependency or release of pressure; may be apparent in childhood, or enlarge after puberty
• Lymphatic: large, soft, transilluminable, 'fluid-filled' swelling; 'cystic hygroma' in neonates; may become apparent in later life from secondary infection.

High-flow:

• Arteriovenous malformations:
  – Pulsatile swelling with visible dilated veins
  – 'Thrill' on palpation
  – Bruit or hum on auscultation
  – Hyperhidrosis of overlying skin
  – Stunted or increased growth of an involved limb
  – High-output cardiac failure may lead to death in large arteriovenous fistulae.
• Post-traumatic arteriovenous fistulae: occur at any age and at any site following penetrating trauma, or associated with fractures.

Investigation

➤ Duplex ultrasound: distinguishes low-high-flow types, and may identify the vessels of origin.
➤ MRI: excellent for demonstrating the extent of deep/complex malformations.
➤ Angiography: useful for identifying the source of a high-flow malformation.
➤ Biopsy: best performed as a surgical procedure under anaesthesia. May rarely be necessary if angiosarcoma is suspected.

Treatment

Port-wine stain:

➤ Laser treatment if available, otherwise leave untreated.

Strawberry naevus:

➤ Spontaneous regression as puberty approaches; may be excised if cosmetically unacceptable or interfering with vision.

Venous malformation:

➤ Injection sclerotherapy under general anaesthesia: 3% sodium tetradecyl sulphate with compression for several weeks
➤ Surgical excision: small malformations
➤ Surgical compartmentalization: underrunning with sutures.

Lymphatic malformation (cystic hygroma):

➤ Injection sclerotherapy under general anaesthesia: 3% sodium tetradecyl sulphate with compression for several weeks
➤ Surgical excision.

Arteriovenous malformation:

➤ Radiological embolization of the major feeding artery with metal coils/alcohol/tissue glue
➤ Radiologically placed covered stents: to close off large arteriovenous fistulae
➤ Surgical skeletalization of arteries, excision of focal malformation, and vascular reconstruction.

TRANSPLANTATION

Principles of transplantation

General principles

- Effective treatment for organ failure incompatible with life.
- Organs or tissue for transplantation may be obtained from living or cadaveric donors.
- The immune response to transplants from unrelated individuals is similar to that for pathogens, but transplants stimulate a far stronger immune response, resulting in antibody-mediated damage to the graft.
- Transplantation is achieved at the expense of immunosuppression, and when donor and recipient are unrelated, acute rejection is assumed and a baseline immunosuppressive regimen is used.
- Immunosuppressive treatment reduces the frequency of rejection but leads to an increased incidence of common and opportunistic infections.
- Donor prerequisites are freedom from diabetes mellitus, hypertension, renal disease, general sepsis, malignancy (except primary brain tumours), organ-specific disease and transmissible infection.
- Recipient organ failure risks are age >65 years, diabetes mellitus and cardiorespiratory disease.

Criteria and procedure for donation

- Living (related or emotionally attached) donors may donate one kidney, a lung or a liver lobe without adverse effect.
- Brainstem-dead (heart beating) donors may donate multiple organs and are maintained on a ventilator with cardiovascular support.
- Asystolic (non-heart-beating) donors are those who have arrested suddenly with unsuccessful resuscitation and may donate corneas, heart valves, bone and skin up to 24 hours following cardiac arrest; kidneys may be harvested soon after cardiac arrest.

- Warm ischaemia is avoided by perfusing donor organ with cold perfusate immediately on interruption of blood flow.
- Donor organ is packed in sterile plastic bags and stored on ice for transport.

Criteria for brainstem death in donor (page 100)

- Absent pupillary response to light.
- Absent corneal reflexes.
- Absent motor response to pain.
- Absent gag and cough reflex.
- Absent spontaneous respiration following induction of hypercapnoea ($P_{CO_2} > 60$ mmHg).

Permission for organ donation must be obtained from the relatives, following counselling by a senior clinician caring for the patient.

Donor and recipient screening

- Full blood count and haematocrit.
- Urea, electrolytes and creatinine.
- Liver function tests and fasting blood glucose.
- Hepatitis B and C antibody titres and HIV screen.
- Chest radiography and electrocardiogram.
- A mixed lymphocyte culture compatibility (non-essential for cadaveric donors).
- Major histocompatibility antigen matching. These are involved in allograft rejection, are found in chromosome 6 and are of two classes: class I antigens – HLA-A, HLA-B and HLA-C; class II antigens – HLA-DR, HLA-DP and HLA-DQ. Graft survival is based on matching HLA-DR, HLA-B and HLA-A in order of priority; the better the match, the less the chance of rejection.
- For avascular grafts (cornea and cartilage) tissue matching is usually not required.

Management of the organ donor

- Physiological effects of brainstem ischaemia and death (increased sympathetic outflow followed by loss of

sympathetic tone) are:
- Cardiac arrhythmia and ischaemia
- Pulmonary oedema
- Hypotension
- Hypothermia
- Electrolyte imbalance, hyperglycaemia and diabetes insipidus.
- These require cardiovascular and respiratory support, electrolyte and endocrine regulation and thermoregulation.

The donor organ may be transplanted:

- Into the site of the diseased organ following its removal (liver, lungs, heart and small bowel)
- Adjacent to the diseased organ (pancreas)
- Distal to the retained diseased organ (kidney, in the pelvis).

Renal transplantation

Definitions

- Indications: end-stage chronic renal failure; the majority of patients are on dialysis awaiting donor organ.
- Contra-indications: chronic bladder dysfunction may cause graft damage (self-catheterization or urinary diversion is required prior to transplantation); severe atherosclerotic disease affecting ileofemoral arteries.
- Recipients may require dialysis pre-operatively to optimize blood chemistry, and postoperatively until donor kidney starts functioning.

Liver transplantation

Definitions

- Indications: cholestasis (biliary cirrhosis, primary sclerosing cholangitis), alcoholic cirrhosis, viral cirrhosis (hepatitis B/C) and hepatocellular carcinoma (without extrahepatic spread).
- Contra-indications: extrahepatic malignancy, sepsis, mesenteric venous thrombosis.
- Liver and heart grafts are less immunogenic than kidney grafts and tissue matching is not necessary,

but ABO blood group antigen compatibility is required.

Complications

- Reperfusion syndrome: inflammatory mediators and cold perfusion solution in the donor liver are washed out into the recipient circulation, producing hypotension and cardiac irregularities.
- Bleeding/coagulopathy: sequelae to extensive surgery and blood loss, with loss of hepatic synthetic function; require transfusion of blood and clotting factors.
- Nutritional deficits: may require nutritional support parenterally/enterally.

Complications of transplantation

Complication	Clinical	Investigations	Management
Renal			
Anastomotic haemorrhage	Oliguria BP and CVP fall	Ultrasound scan	Re-exploration
Graft/vessel thrombosis/stenosis	Renal failure Anaemia Hypertension	Ultrasound scan Angiography Isotope scan	Revascularization
Ureteric stenosis/ obstruction/ lymphocoele	Progressive renal failure Oliguria Anuria	Ultrasound scan Isotope scan Renography IVU	Re-exploration ±stenting
Liver			
Haemorrhage	Oliguria BP and CVP fall	Ultrasound scan	
Hepatic/portal vessel thrombosis	Liver failure Anaemia	Duplex Ultrasound scan	Revascularization
Biliary leak	Peritonitis	Cholangiogram	Drainage Repair
Biliary stricture	Jaundice Progressive liver failure Bleeding	Ultrasound scan Liver function	Re-exploration or stenting

(Continued)

(Continued)

Complication	Clinical	Investigations	Management
Coagulopathy	Convulsions	Coagulation screen	Transfuse clotting factors
Neuropathy	Arrhythmias	ECG	
Reperfusion syndrome	Hypotension	U&E	

BP, blood pressure; CVP, central venous pressure; ECG, electrocardiograph; IVU, intravenous urography; U&E, urea and electrolytes.

Heart/lung transplantation

Definitions

- Indications: end-stage heart/lung disease.

Complications

- Cardiopulmonary bypass and anticoagulation.
- Abnormalities of heart rhythm, rate and output caused by conduction disruption and denervation of the transplanted heart; temporary pacing is required to ensure adequate ventricular filling.

Other transplants

- Pancreas (diabetes mellitus, chronic recurrent pancreatitis).
- Small bowel (short bowel syndrome).
- Bone (skeletal reconstruction).
- Cornea.
- Skin (grafting after burn injury).
- Bone marrow (marrow aplasia, treatment of haematological cancers).

Complications of transplantation

Surgical complications

- Majority of grafts function immediately.
- Primary non-function is a result of donor organ pathology or long ischaemic period.
- Delayed primary function is seen in 25% of kidney recipients.

- Acute anastomotic arterial/venous thrombosis or stenosis require revascularization.
- Urinary tract complications in renal transplants, acute ureteric leak, obstruction or stenosis require surgical repair.
- Soon after visceral transplants, recipients are vulnerable to intra-abdominal complications (bowel ischaemia, obstruction or perforation, peptic ulceration, pancreatitis or cholecystitis), which may be masked by immunosuppression.

Immunosuppression

- All transplant recipients require immunosuppression for life.
- Triple drug regimen used: prednisolone (oral 20–40 mg daily), azathioprine (oral 1–4 mg/kg daily) and cyclosporin (oral 2–6 mg/kg daily) or FK506.
- Other agents: antilymphocytic serum and monoclonal antibodies.
- The initial high doses are tapered down to maintenance levels.

Monitoring of transplant function

- Renal: urine output, serum creatinine, radio-isotope scan.
- Liver: function tests.
- Lung: blood gases, chest radiology.
- Heart: electrocardiogram and echocardiogram.
- All transplants: ultrasound or CT scan; angiography.
- Progressive transplant failure: fine-needle biopsy to determine type of rejection.
- Long-term steroid therapy can give rise to Cushing's syndrome, with classic skin and fat changes, poor wound healing, osteoporosis, diabetes mellitus and psychoses.

Infection in transplant patients

Definitions

- Immunosuppressed patients are very susceptible to all forms of infection. Opportunistic infections are:
  - Cytomegalovirus

- *Pneumocystis carinii* (pneumonia)
- Papilloma virus (skin warts).

Clinical features

- Symptoms: fever and malaise (exclude onset of rejection).

Investigation

➤ Wound, urine, sputum (bronchial washings), bile and blood cultures for bacterial, viral and fungal infections.

Treatment

➤ Immediate 'best guess' antibiotic therapy, to be modified as per sensitivity testing; if infection is severe or difficult to control, reduce or stop immunosuppressive therapy.

Complications

Graft rejection:

- Hyperacute rejection is a rapid reaction of pre-existing antibodies to antigens in the graft within hours of surgery; this causes fibrin deposition in the intima and vascular occlusion; immediate removal of the transplant is usually indicated
- Acute rejection is caused by graft invasion by host T-lymphocyte and/or plasma cell infiltration following recognition of the graft as foreign, and leads to eventual graft failure occurring within 14 days of surgery. It responds well to high doses of steroids and standard immunosuppressive drugs and/or antilymphocytic/ antithymocytic globulin therapy. [Dose monitored by T-lymphocyte count in plasma; monoclonal murine antibodies (OKT3) may be used against T-cells and T3 antigens.]
- Chronic rejection is a slow deterioration of graft function over a period of years and is caused by a chronic fibrosis of the graft and its vasculature and is irreversible.

Malignancy in transplant recipients:

- Malignancy is associated with long-term immuno-suppression
- Primary cancers develop in 5% of recipients, namely, squamous skin cancer, Kaposi's sarcoma, non-Hodgkin's lymphoma and colon cancer
- Treatment is by standard anticancer therapy
- Reduce immunosuppression if tumour response is poor
- In metastatic disease consider stopping immuno-suppression.

MANAGEMENT OF THE MULTIPLY INJURED PATIENT

The management of trauma requires a structured approach, prioritizing life-threatening problems while not overlooking any other injuries. The Advanced Trauma Life Support (ATLS) system, developed by the American College of Surgeons and franchised to many centres worldwide, is an excellent example of such an approach, which instructs, examines and awards credentials to clinicians in these measures.

Initial assessment and resuscitation

Definitions

- Motor vehicle accidents – except low speed.
- Fall from significant height.
- Multiple sites of injury.
- Penetrating trauma to neck, thorax or abdomen (knife wounds).
- Ballistic trauma (bullet or bomb blast).
- Burns >15% or facial burns.
- Initial survey: assessment and treatment of immediately life-threatening problems.
- Priority:
  - **A**irway and cervical spine
  - **B**reathing
  - **C**irculation
  - **D**isability – neurological assessment
  - **E**xposure and environment.

Clinical features

Airway (mouth, oral cavity, nose and pharynx)

- Unobstructed:
  - Normal respiration
  - Talking normally.
- Obstructed:
  - Respiratory distress or stridor
  - Vomit, blood or other fluid in mouth
  - Severe facial injury/burns
  - Apnoea.

Cervical spine

- Suspected injury in all major trauma
- More likely if:
  - Injuries above clavicular level
  - Motor vehicle accidents with extreme deceleration and deformation of the vehicle
  - Motorcycle accidents
  - High falls
  - Blast injuries.

Breathing

- Open chest wound (page 361)
- Tension pneumothorax (page 361):
  - Respiratory distress
  - Shock
  - Tracheal deviation away from the affected side
  - Decreased chest movement with respiration
  - Resonance on percussion
  - No breath sounds on auscultation.
- Flail chest (page 362).
- Massive haemothorax:
  - Shock
  - Less movement with respiration
  - Dullness on percussion
  - No breath sounds on auscultation.
- Cardiac tamponade (page 362)

Circulation

- Shock:
  - Heart rate >100 bpm

- Pale, cool, clammy periphery
- Capillary refilling time >2 seconds
- Visible blood at the scene of the trauma
- Visible bleeding from a wound
- Conscious level impaired.
- Concealed haemorrhage:
  - Shock and impaired breathing – thorax
  - Shock and abdominal findings (page 405) – abdomen
  - Retroperitoneal haematoma
  - Haematoma around fractures.

Disability

- Glasgow Coma Scale (page 226)
- ATLS system:
  - Alert
  - Voice response
  - Pain response
  - Unconscious.

Investigation

➤ Monitor:
  - Electrocardiograph (ECG)
  - Oxygen saturation.
➤ Venous blood samples:
  - FBC
  - Cross-match blood
  - Serum biochemistry.
➤ Arterial blood gas analysis.
➤ Trauma series of X-rays:
  - Lateral cervical spine
  - Chest
  - Pelvis.

Treatment

Airway

- Remove debris, dentures; use suction.
- Chin lift or jaw thrust manoeuvres: prevents obstruction by tongue.
- Needle cricothyroidotomy: if acute, unrelieved upper airway obstruction.

- Guedel airway: if no gag reflex.
- Nasopharyngeal airway: if no basilar skull fracture suspected.
- 100% oxygen: by mask with reservoir bag.
- Endotracheal or nasotracheal intubation, indications:
  - Protection from aspiration
  - Airway obstruction or impending obstruction
  - Apnoea
  - Severe head injury
  - Need for artificial ventilation (see below).
- Surgical cricothyroidotomy: if upper airway injury prevents endotracheal intubation.

Cervical spine

- In-line traction.
- Rigid cervical collar.
- Side blocks and straps across head and chin.

Breathing

- Tension pneumothorax:
  - Cannula placed through the second intercostal space, midclavicular line
  - Chest drain.
- Open chest wound:
  - Asherman seal: a flutter valve allowing air exit but not entry
  - Chest drain away from the site of injury.
- Haemothorax:
  - Intravenous access and fluid (see circulation)
  - Chest drain >28Ch.
- Artificial ventilation (endotracheal/nasotracheal intubation) indications:
  - Respiratory distress
  - Pao_2 <9 kPa on 100% oxygen
  - Severe head injury – hyperventilation for raised intracranial pressure (page 229).

Circulation

- Pressure applied to sites of visible haemorrhage.
- Two large-bore peripheral intravenous cannulae inserted.

- Rapid infusion of 2 L of warmed Hartmann's solution.
- Pericardiocentesis: for cardiac tamponade (page 362).
- Thoracotomy: for life-threatening intrathoracic haemorrhage.
- Laparotomy: for intra-abdominal haemorrhage.

Disability

- Restore oxygen delivery to the brain: management of airway, breathing and circulation.

Exposure and environment

- Remove/cut away all clothing to allow complete examination.
- Prevent heat loss: space-blanket/warming blanket, use warmed fluids.
- Cover burns with polythene film.

Second assessment and further management

Definitions

- History.
- Examination.
- Investigation results from initial survey.
- Management plan.
- Components of initial survey are re-applied at any time if there is sudden deterioration.

Clinical features

History

- Events resulting in the trauma: time and nature.
- Past medical history.
- Medication.
- Allergies.
- Last meal: time, nature, drugs and alcohol.

Examination

- Head and face:
  - Laceration, haematoma, depressed/open fracture

- – 'Panda eyes' or cerebrospinal fluid (CSF) rhinorrhoea – anterior fossa basilar fracture (page 219)
  - – CSF otorrhoea – middle fossa skull base fracture.
- Neurology:
  - – Glasgow Coma Scale – conscious level
  - – Pupil size and reaction to light
  - – Hemiplegia – localizing sign of intracranial haematoma (page 226)
  - – Paraplegia – indicates thoracolumbar spinal injury (page 745)
  - – Quadriplegia – indicates cervical spinal injury.
- Neck:
  - – Tenderness and deformity of the line of spinous processes – fracture dislocations of the cervical spine (page 749).
- Thorax (page 360):
  - – Deformity, asymmetry of movement, bruising from: seat-belt or steering-wheel; penetrating/open wounds; air entry – auscultation, resonance – percussion.
- Abdomen (page 405):
  - – Distension, bruising, penetrating wounds, evisceration
  - – Palpation, tenderness, masses.
- Pelvis:
  - – Pressure to the iliac crests laterally and anteroposteriorly – mobility in severe pelvic fracture (page 699).
- Genitalia:
  - – Blood at urethral meatus – may indicate urethral injury (page 531)
  - – Haematuria – indicates significant renal tract injury
  - – Dipstick haematuria – indicates renal tract injury.
- 'Log-roll' – examination of the back:
  - – Patient is rolled while maintaining a constant alignment of the spine.
- Spine:
  - – Loss of alignment or a step in the spinous processes
  - – indicates spine fracture/dislocation (page 749).
- Limbs:
  - – Bruising, haematoma, deformity, lacerations and penetrating wounds – suggest fractures

– Distal ischaemia or profuse bleeding – suggests arterial injury (page 578)
– Distal anaesthesia – suggests nerve injury (page 759).
- Rectal examination:
    – Irregular bony fragments – major pelvic fracture
    – Disruption or laceration of the anus, rectum or perineum
    – High mobile prostate – complete rupture of the membranous urethra (page 531).

Investigation

According to suspicion of injury and local availability:

➤ Head computerized tomography (CT): severe head injury
➤ Facial X-rays or CT: facial fractures
➤ Cervical spine X-rays (anteroposterior, lateral, oblique) or CT: suspected cervical spine fracture
➤ ECG: ischaemic changes suggest cardiac contusion
➤ Thoracic spiral contrast CT: suspected great vessel injury
➤ Diagnostic peritoneal lavage: blunt abdominal injury
➤ Abdominal contrast CT: stable abdominal injury and retroperitoneal injury
➤ Pelvic X-rays/CT: pelvic fracture
➤ Limb X-rays: limb fractures
➤ Urethrogram: suspected urethral injury
➤ Spinal CT/magnetic resonance imaging (MRI): spine and spinal cord injury.

BALLISTIC TRAUMA

Gunshot wounds

Definitions

- Produce a track of damaged tissue; debris (e.g. clothing, dirt) is drawn into the track.

- Types:
  - Low velocity projectiles: pistol bullets, shotgun pellet wounds
  - High velocity projectiles: rifle bullets, explosive fragments (see also blast injury and antipersonnel mines, page 609).
- 'Cavitation': bullets rotate as they fly, 'tumbling', producing a wider volume of damaged tissue.
- 'Temporary cavitation': high velocity projectiles produce a 'shock-wave' dissipating energy over a wide volume of tissue.
- Soft-tipped bullets are designed to fragment/deform to increase tissue damage (dum-dum).
- Subsequent infection of contaminated wounds by:
  - *Clostridium perfringens*: gas gangrene
  - *Clostridium tetani*
  - *Streptococcus pyogenes*
  - *Staphylococcus aureus*
  - Gram-negative organisms.

Clinical features

- Limb trauma:
  - Small entry wound and sometimes no exit wound: low velocity projectiles
  - Large exit wound: high velocity projectile
  - Muscle, tendon, nerve and vascular injury.
- Abdominal penetrating trauma (page 405).
- Thoracic penetrating trauma (page 360).
- Fatal disruption of major liver and lung veins: high velocity projectile.
- General features of wound infection after 1–3 days:
  - Pain, fever and inflammation.
- Gas gangrene after 1–3 days:
  - Severe toxaemia
  - Sweet smell from wound
  - Surgical emphysema
  - Blistering.
- Tetanus after 1–3 days:
  - Limb tingling and spasm
  - Trismus – 'lock-jaw'
  - Neck rigidity

– Pyrexia
– Difficulty in micturition.

Investigation

➤ General investigation of the multiply injured (page 599).
➤ Investigation of thoracic trauma (page 360).
➤ Investigation of abdominal trauma (page 405).
➤ X-rays show:
  – Location of bullet/fragments
  – Associated fractures.
➤ CT for abdominal, thoracic, spinal and head injuries may show:
  – Location of bullet/fragments
  – Nature of injuries.

Treatment

➤ General management of the multiply injured.
➤ Benzylpenicillin 3 g (5 mega-units) i.v. qds 24 hours, then penicillin V 500 mg qds orally for 5 days.
➤ Tetanus antiserum 500 IU i.m. and tetanus toxoid 0.5 mL i.m.
➤ Thoracotomy for penetrating thoracic trauma.
➤ Laparotomy for penetrating abdominal trauma.
➤ Observe limb wounds with minimal disruption:
  – Entry and exit wounds less than 1 cm diameter
  – No gross haematoma or other evidence of internal disruption
  – No fragmentation of bullet/shrapnel on X-ray.
➤ Surgically explore more extensive wounds:
  – Excise wound edge
  – Incise over wound tracks: excise dead tissue and remove debris
  – Extend wounds to allow excision of retracted divided muscle ends
  – Ligate bleeding vessels
  – Surgical exploration and repair of major vessel injury
  – Tag tendon and nerve ends with non-absorbable sutures
  – Irrigate wound well with saline

→

> - Apply dry dressings
> - Do not change dressings for 5 days unless there is evidence of wound sepsis
> - Do not close wounds
> - Immobilize large wounds and fractures.
- ➤ Immediate amputation in:
  - Severe limb disruption
  - Crushed limb
  - Ischaemia or tourniquet >6 hours.
- ➤ Further surgical exploration if sepsis develops over the following days.
- ➤ Delayed primary closure, nerve and tendon repair, and split skin grafts of non-infected wounds at 5 days.
- ➤ Reconstructive procedures after wound healing, e.g.:
  - Tendon transfer to restore function
  - Nerve grafts.

Blast injury

Definitions

Explosions cause injury by:

- Blast and shock waves
- Generation of heat
- Shrapnel – high velocity projectiles:
  - From the casing of the device
  - Deliberately included ball-bearings and nails
- Glass and other debris carried by the blast
- Falling masonry.

Clinical features

- Traumatic amputations for severe limb disruption.
- Crush injuries.
- Penetrating abdominal and chest trauma.
- Head injury.
- Spinal injury.
- Flash burns: superficial burns to all exposed areas.
- Pulmonary contusion: immediate respiratory failure.

- Adult respiratory distress syndrome: decreased pulmonary compliance and progressive respiratory failure after 48 hours.
- Tympanic membrane rupture: conductive deafness (page 244).
- Olfactory nerve injury: loss of smell and taste.

Treatment
➤ General investigation and management of the multiply injured patient (page 599).
➤ Head injury (page 226).
➤ Spinal injury (page 749).
➤ Abdominal trauma (page 405).
➤ Thoracic trauma (page 360).
➤ Limb injury (page 618).
➤ Burns (page 610).

Anti-personnel mines

Definitions
- Small explosive devices concealed in the ground, triggered by foot pressure or trip-wires.
- Produce traumatic amputation of the foot, with contaminated material being blasted into the fascial compartments of the leg and body.
- Some types fire into the air before exploding, causing shrapnel injuries.

Clinical features
- Traumatic amputation of the foot or lower limb.
- Blast and shrapnel injuries to other limbs and perineum.

Investigation
➤ General investigation of the multiply injured patient (page 599).
➤ X-rays identify metallic debris.
➤ Surgical exploration of limb wounds.

Treatment

- ➤ General management of the multiply injured patient (page 599).
- ➤ Benzylpenicillin 3 g (5 mega-units) i.v. qds 24 hours, then penicillin V 500 mg qds orally for 5 days.
- ➤ Tetanus antiserum 500 IU i.m. and tetanus toxoid 0.5 mL i.m.
- ➤ Immediate amputation of severely disrupted limbs – do not close wound.
- ➤ Surgically explore other wounds:
    - Excise damaged tissue
    - Ligate bleeding vessels
    - Irrigate wound well with saline
    - Apply dry dressings
    - Do not change dressings for 5 days unless there is evidence of wound sepsis
    - Do not close wounds
    - Immobilize associated fractures.
- ➤ Later re-fashioning of amputations – suitable for prosthetic limb fitting.

BURNS

Definitions

Depth of thermal injury

- First-degree burn:
    - Superficial
    - Heal by regeneration of epithelium
    - No scarring
    - Aetiology: sunburn, flashburns.
- Second-degree burn:
    - Dermal injury
    - Heal from preserved epithelium in skin appendages
    - Relatively little scarring
    - Aetiology: hot liquids and steam; fire and explosion; chemicals, e.g. phosphorus, phenol, hydrofluoric acid; and electrical burns.
- Third-degree burn:
    - All skin layers destroyed

- Heal by granulation, contraction and in-growth of surrounding epithelium
- Severe scarring
- Aetiology: more severe exposure to hot liquids and steam; fire and explosion; chemicals, e.g. phosphorus, phenol, hydrofluoric acid; and electrical burns.

Clinical features

Assessment of depth of burn

- First-degree burn:
  - Red: blanches on pressure
  - Painful to pinprick
  - May blister after 24 hours.
- Second-degree burn:
  - Pink: blanches less on pressure
  - Painful to pinprick
  - Blisters after a few hours.
- Third-degree burn:
  - Creamy or discoloured base: does not blanch
  - Painless to pinprick
  - Does not blister.

Assessment of total body surface area burnt

- Standard burn charts.
- Estimation by 'rule of nine':
  - Head and neck: 9%
  - Trunk – front: 18%
  - Trunk – back: 18%
  - Arm – each: 9%
  - Leg – each: 18%
  - Genitalia: 1%.

Other injuries associated with burns

- Thermal injury to the respiratory tract:
  - Facial burns/soot in nostrils
  - Hoarseness/stridor
  - Wheezing
  - Drooling of saliva
  - Dysphagia.
- Carbon monoxide poisoning:
  - Depressed conscious level
  - Cherry-red mucous membranes.

- General multiple injuries.
- Haemoglobinuria/myoglobinuria: treacle-coloured urine.
- Multisystem organ failure may complicate severe cases.

Investigation

➤ General investigation of the multiply injured patient (page 599).
➤ Clinical assessment of body surface area burnt (see above).
➤ Peak expiratory flow measurement: reduced in airway injury.
➤ Carboxyhaemoglobin concentration at 1 hour: nomogram allows estimation of exposure to carbon monoxide.
➤ Arterial blood gas analysis – repeated as required for assessing:
  - Thermal injury to the respiratory tract
  - Carbon monoxide poisoning
  - Cyanide poisoning: severe metabolic acidosis, high lactate, increased anion gap.
➤ Chest X-ray:
  - Associated chest injuries
  - Features of adult respiratory distress syndrome (page 67) after 48 hours.
➤ ECG: cardiac arrhythmia or ischaemia in electrocution.
➤ Urine analysis for haemoglobin and myoglobin.

Treatment

Early management of severe burns

➤ General management of the multiply injured patient (page 599).
➤ Intubation and ventilation for:
  - Severe facial burns
  - Thermal injury to the respiratory tract
  - Carbon monoxide and cyanide poisoning.
➤ Analgesia: 50% nitrous oxide/50% oxygen by face mask if conscious and no facial burns, morphine 5–10 mg i.v. and ondansetron 4 mg i.v.
➤ Tetanus antiserum 500 IU i.m. and tetanus toxoid 0.5 mL i.m.

➜

➤ Intravenous fluid replacement: if >15% burns in an adult, or >10% burns in a child calculate according to the Muir/Barclay formula.

$$\text{Volume (mL)} = \frac{\% \text{ body surface area of burn} \times \text{weight (kg)}}{2}$$

➤ To be given over each of the following periods: 4, 4, 4, 4, 6, 12 hours post-burn
  – N/saline: first 500 mL
  – Colloid: subsequent volumes
  – Blood: if >10% burn area
  – Larger volumes may be required with haemoglobinuria/ myoglobinuria: keep urine output >1 mL/kg per hour.
➤ Cover burns with 'Clingfilm' or other dry dressings.
➤ Prevent hypothermia.
➤ Escharotomy: longitudinal incision of full-thickness circumferential burns:
  – Chest: allows adequate ventilation
  – Limb: prevents tourniquet effect.
➤ Nutritional support: nasogastric feeding is required in severe cases.
➤ Intensive support for multisystem organ failure.

Transfer to burns unit considered

➤ Total body surface area of burn >15% adult or >10% child.
➤ Thermal injury to the respiratory tract.
➤ Burns of the face, hands or perineum.
➤ Circumferential burns of the limbs or chest.

Prognosis

Survival is unlikely with >70% burns.

Subsequent management of severe burns

➤ First-degree burn:
  – Dressings: Vaseline gauze and wool for 48 hours, then hydrocolloid.
➤ Second-degree burn:
  – Dressings: antibacterial silver sulfadiazine cream, Vaseline gauze and wool daily.

➔

> ➤ Third-degree burn:
>   - Excision of burn (tangential excision of non-viable tissue) and application of meshed split skin grafts
>   - Elastic supports and splints for 18 months to reduce hypertrophic scarring
>   - Plastic surgery to improve form and function may be required years later.

PAEDIATRIC TRAUMA

Differences from management of the multiply injured adult

Airway

- Anatomic differences make maintenance and intubation more difficult.
- Uncuffed endotracheal tubes are used until puberty.
- Endotracheal tube diameter = (age in years/4) + 4.
- Needle cricothyroidotomy is used where intubation is impossible.
- Cricothyroidotomy is avoided: causes stenosis.

Breathing

- Ventilation using a mask requires a 30 cmH$_2$O blow-off valve to avoid barotrauma and gastric dilatation.
- Orogastric tubes avoid gastric distension during ventilation.

Circulation

- Greater circulatory reserve: vital signs are less affected by significant blood loss.
- Normal heart rate is higher and systolic blood pressure lower in children <12 years of age.
- Intra-osseous needle passed into the medullary cavity of the upper tibia may be required for vascular access <6 years of age.
- Initial resuscitation fluid volume = 20 mL/kg.

Disability

Modified Glasgow Coma Scale:

- Verbal response:
  - Appropriate words or follow object: 5
  - Cries, will not settle: 4
  - Irritable: 3
  - Agitated: 2
  - Silent: 1.
- Eyes: as adult (page 261)
- Motor: as adult (page 227).

Exposure and environment

- Greater heat loss from high surface area to weight ratio: use of overhead heaters and warming blankets.

Head injury

- More vulnerable to acceleration/deceleration forces producing intracranial haematoma.
- Acute subdural haematoma:
  - May occur without skull fracture
  - Often bilateral
  - Associated with underlying brain injury.
- Extradural haematoma:
  - Usually occurs with skull fracture
  - Often unilateral
  - Lucid interval may not occur in children
  - Vomiting and epileptic fits are more common.

Spinal cord injury

- Spinal cord injury is less likely.
- X-rays may do not identify up to 50% of serious spinal injuries.
- Unstable cervical spine injury may be ligamentous: identified by manipulation under fluoroscopic control.

Thoracic trauma

- Second intercostal space chest drains should be placed more laterally than in an adult to avoid the great vessels.
- Flail chest, myocardial contusion and aortic rupture are less common.

Abdominal blunt trauma

- Clinical assessment is more difficult: serial ultrasound may be useful.

Skeletal injuries

- Radiological and fracture-type differences: growing bone with epiphyses.

Burns

- Total body surface area burnt requires use of specialized paediatric charts.
- Estimation differs: the head area is larger:
  - Head: 19%
  - Trunk – front: 18%
  - Trunk – back: 18%
  - Arm – each: 9%
  - Leg – each: 13%

Non-accidental injury

- Suggestive features:
  - Delayed presentation
  - Repeated presentation
  - History of trauma inconsistent with findings
  - Abnormal child–parent interaction
  - Suspicious injuries: cigarette burns, bites
  - Internal organ injury without history of significant trauma
  - Retinal haemorrhage
  - Multiple subdural haemorrhage
  - Long bone fractures in non-ambulant children
  - Perineal injury.

TRAUMA IN PREGNANCY

Differences from management of the multiply injured non-pregnant adult

General principles – treating the mother effectively is the best treatment for the fetus also.

Airway

- Increased risk of vomiting and aspiration: establish nasogastric drainage.

Breathing

- Respiratory alkalosis is normal in later pregnancy: acidosis may be less apparent from blood gas analysis.

Circulation

- Greater circulatory reserve: vital signs are less affected by significant blood loss.
- Normal heart rate is higher and systolic blood pressure lower in pregnancy.
- The patient's body should be tilted to the left with a wedge to relieve pressure on the vena cava and enhance venous return.

Abdominal trauma

- Peritoneal lavage (if required) should be performed through a supra-umbilical incision.

Assessment of the fetus

Adverse findings are:

- Absence of fetal movements
- Fetal distress on cardiotocography:
  - Bradycardia <110 bpm
  - Inadequate accelerations to uterine contraction
  - Late decelerations to uterine contraction.

Complications of blunt abdominal trauma:

- Fetal distress
- Premature labour
- Abortion/stillbirth death
- Vaginal bleeding
- Placental abruption: vaginal bleeding, shock, increasing fundal height, fetal distress.

Delivery by caesarean section may be considered for a suitably developed fetus if:

- Necessary for treatment of maternal injuries
- Penetrating abdominal injury

- Uterine rupture
- Placental abruption
- Fetal distress
- Burns >50%
- Maternal death.

ORTHOPAEDICS

BONES AND FRACTURES

Fractures

Definitions

A break in the continuity of bone, which may be:

- Oblique: direct force or bending
- Transverse: tension force
- Spiral: twisting
- Butterfly fragment: bending and compression
- Comminuted (many small fragments): severe crushing force
- Closed: no break in surrounding soft tissue
- Compound (open): break in surrounding soft tissues.

Gustilo's classification of compound fractures:

- Type I: puncture from within by a bone spike
- Type II: external wound <1 cm long
- Type III: extensive skin and soft tissue damage.

Clinical features

Local features

- Swelling.
- Bruising.
- Deformity.
- Tenderness.
- Abnormal movement.
- Crepitus.

Associated features

- Vascular injury.
- Nerve injury.

- Joint dislocation.
- Compartment syndrome: mainly lower leg and forearm.

General features of major long bone and pelvic fractures

- Shock from blood loss:
  - Humerus 1–3 units
  - Tibia 1–3 units
  - Femur 2–6 units
  - Pelvis 2–10 units.
- Associated chest, abdominal, head and spinal injuries.

Investigation

➤ X-rays – principles:
  - Two views at right-angles: fracture may not be apparent on a single view
  - Include the joints above and below: associated joint dislocation
  - Both limbs for comparison: especially in children, where epiphyses make interpretation difficult
  - Repeat X-rays at 2 weeks: for suspected fractures of carpus or scaphoid.
➤ Computerized tomography (CT): demonstrates extent of fracture of spine or tibial condyles.
➤ Magnetic resonance imaging (MRI): identifies associated spinal cord compression in spinal fractures.

Treatment

Principles:

➤ Reduction of fracture
➤ Hold reduced position while union occurs
➤ Allow movement of joints to preserve function.

Closed reduction:

➤ Minimally displaced fractures
➤ Method:
  - Traction in line with the bone
  - Reversal of original direction of force

Open (operative) reduction:

➤ When closed reduction fails
➤ If internal fixation is required.

➜

Methods of holding reduction:

➤ Continuous traction: skin or skeletal
➤ Cast:
  – Plaster of Paris or lightweight, waterproof synthetic material
  – Splitting the cast along its length allows for swelling when applied to fractures in the first 48 hours
  – To avoid rotational instability in long bone fractures the cast must extend proximal to the joint above the fracture.
➤ Functional brace: cast extends above and below a joint with hinges to allow movement of the joint
➤ Internal fixation: operative fixation of the bone fragments using:
  – K (Kirschner) wire: a stiff wire with sharpened ends; driven into bone using a compressed airgun
  – Dynamic compression plate: a metal plate fixed across the fracture site with screws
  – AO (Arbeitsgemeinschaft für Osteosynthesefragen) nail: a metal rod driven into the medullary cavity of long bones; may have screws inserted under radiological guidance to prevent rotational instability of the bone fragments.
➤ External fixation: an external framework fixed to the bone with threaded pins.

Treatment of open fractures:

➤ Benzylpenicillin 1.2 g i.v. tds and flucloxacillin 500 mg i.v. qds, or other broad-spectrum antibiotics: until satisfied that major wound sepsis is controlled
➤ Tetanus toxoid 0.5 mL booster if previously immunized; tetanus immunoglobulin (HTIG) 250 units if no previous immunization, then three doses of tetanus toxoid 0.5 mL at monthly intervals
➤ Surgical debridement, repeated as required
➤ Stabilize fracture with split cast or external fixator
➤ Antiseptic-soaked dressings to wound.

Impacted fracture

● Fragments are jammed together making the fracture line indistinct.

Greenstick fracture

- Fractures in long bones of children in which only one cortex is broken.

Epiphyseal fractures

- Fractures through the epiphysis of a growing bone.
- May result in premature fusion and subsequent deformity.
- Salter–Harris radiological classification:
    - I Complete separation of epiphysis
    - II Separation of epiphysis with a triangular fragment of metaphysis
    - III Vertical fracture from the articular surface to the metaphysis
    - IV Vertical fracture from the articular surface continuing through the metaphysis
    - V Crushing of the epiphysis.
- Premature fusion most likely in types III–V.
- MRI is useful in assessment.
- Treatment follows general principles: perfect reduction reduces subsequent deformity in types II and IV.
- Surgical fat interposition may prevent premature epiphyseal fusion.
- Established deformity may require corrective osteotomy.

Pathological fractures

Definitions

- Fracture secondary to underlying bone disease.
- Aetiology:
    - Children: osteogenesis imperfecta, rickets
    - Young adults: bone cysts, benign tumours, primary malignant tumours
    - Older adults: metastatic tumour, myeloma
    - Elderly: osteoporosis, Paget's disease.

Clinical features

- Site of fracture:
    - Long bone shafts
    - Vertebral bodies.

- Generalized features of underlying condition.
- Cord compression may complicate vertebral collapse.

Investigation

➤ X-rays: may show abnormal surrounding bone.
➤ Investigations of underlying conditions.
➤ Biopsy for histology: during open reduction/ fixation.

Treatment

➤ Internal fixation of long bone fractures.
➤ Radiotherapy to underlying malignant tumour.
➤ Emergency surgical decompression of cord compression.
➤ Treatment of underlying conditions.

Complications of fractures

Compartment syndrome

Definitions

- Increased pressure in a fascial compartment of a limb causing ischaemic tissue damage.
- Aetiology: traumatic soft tissue swelling, reperfusion after ischaemia.
- Typically complicates fractures of elbow, forearm and proximal tibia.
- Internal fixation and infection may contribute.

Clinical features

- Painful, swollen limb.
- Pain on passive hyperextension of the fingers or toes.
- Features of acute limb ischaemia (page 554).

Investigation

➤ Intracompartment pressure measurement: >40 mmHg.

Treatment

Pressure <40 mmHg:

➤ Observation.

Pressure >40 mmHg, or if no measurement equipment available:

➤ Fasciotomies
➤ Debridement of necrotic muscle
➤ Delayed closure or split skin grafts to cover defects.

Arterial injury (page 578)

Nerve injury (page 759)

Adult respiratory distress syndrome
(page 67)

Fat embolism

Definitions

- Embolism of fat globules to the lung.
- Occurs in most adult long bone fractures but symptomatic fat embolism is rare.

Clinical features

Progressively at approximately 72 hours after injury:

- Pyrexia.
- Tachycardia.
- Breathlessness.
- Confusion.
- Petechiae on thorax and conjunctival folds.
- Respiratory failure.
- Coma.

Investigation

➤ Blood gas analysis: hypoxaemic respiratory failure.

Treatment

➤ Oxygen.
➤ Intensive monitoring.
➤ Ventilatory support (page 90).
➤ Cardiovascular support (page 91).
➤ Heparin 5000 units i.v. bolus; then heparin 1000 units i.v. per hour to maintain activated partial thromboplastin time (APTT) ratio of 2 to 3 times normal.

Delayed union

Definitions

● A delay in the natural repair process of bone:
  – Union is the point at which the bone fragments are held together by the repair process, but the fracture is still visible on X-ray
  – Consolidation is the point at which the repair process is complete.
● Causes of delayed union:
  – Inadequate blood supply: bone separated from surrounding muscle
  – Infection: open fractures
  – Inadequate splintage
  – Excessive traction.

Clinical features

● Tender fracture site.
● Pain on stressing bone.
● Angulation may occur on stressing bone.

Investigation

➤ X-ray:
  – Fracture remains visible
  – Callus deficient.

Treatment

➤ Conservative.
➤ Adjust plaster/traction.
➤ Internal fixation and bone grafting if delayed >6 months.

Non-union

Definitions

- Failure of the natural repair process of bone.
- Causes:
  - Inadequate blood supply: bone separated from surrounding muscle
  - Infection: open fractures
  - Soft tissue interposition between the fragments
  - Inadequate splintage
  - Excessive traction.

Clinical features

- Painless angulation on stressing bone.

Investigation

➤ X-ray:
  - Fracture remains visible
  - Sclerosis or atrophy of bone ends.

Treatment

➤ Conservative.
➤ Functional bracing.
➤ Internal fixation and bone grafting.

Malunion

Definitions

- Fragments unite in an unacceptable position.

Clinical features

- Deformity.

Investigation

➤ X-ray during the first 3 weeks of healing to identify incipient malunion:
  - Angulation >15°
  - Rotational deformity
  - Shortening of leg >2.5 cm.

Treatment

Incipient malunion:

➤ Remanipulation
➤ Angulation near bone ends in children corrects with growth.

Established malunion:

➤ Osteotomy and fixation.

Osteomyelitis (page 628)

Deep venous thrombosis (page 583)

Reflex sympathetic dystrophy (Sudek's atrophy)

Definitions

● A post-traumatic syndrome.
● May affect: hand, foot, knee, hip or shoulder.
● Aetiology: unknown.

Clinical features

Early:

• Persistent pain
• Slight swelling
• Mild inflammation
• Stiffness of adjacent joints.

Late:

• Smooth shiny skin
• Hair loss
• Brittle nails
• Loss of movement.

Investigation

➤ X-rays: patchy osteoporosis.

Treatment

➤ Ibuprofen 400 mg tds orally.
➤ Physiotherapy.
➤ Sympathectomy.

Prognosis:

➤ Usually subsides over 1–2 years.
➤ May be irreversible.

Myositis ossificans

Definitions

● Ossification in muscles after injury.
● Aetiology: unknown.

Clinical features

● Pain.
● Soft tissue tenderness.
● Palpable bony mass at 8 weeks.

Investigation

➤ X-ray: normal initially, fluffy calcification in muscle at 2 weeks.
➤ Bone scan: increased metabolic activity.

Treatment

➤ Rest until pain subsides.
➤ Then mobilize.
➤ Excise bony mass when movements have returned.
➤ Indometacin 25 mg bd orally may reduce recurrence.

Post-traumatic osteoarthritis (page 648)

Bone necrosis in sickle-cell disease

● Sickle-cell disease (page 177) results in ischaemia and infarction of bone.

- Repeated attacks of severe pain lasting for hours or days.
- Typically affects tubular bones of hands and feet: ischaemic damage eventually results in digits of unequal length.
- Salmonella osteomyelitis may develop in infarcted bone.
- Femoral head necrosis resembles Perthes' disease.
- Treatment is rest and pethidine 0.5–2.0 mg/kg 3-hourly as required; blood transfusion may be required in severe cases.
- Surgical treatment is usually excluded because of the risks of anaesthesia.

Acute osteomyelitis

Definitions

- Usually affects children.
- Adult cases in diabetes, immunosuppression, drug addiction.
- Aetiology: haematogenous spread of infection to metaphysis of bone.
- Pathogens:
  - *Staphylococcus aureus*
  - *Streptococcus pyogenes*
  - *Streptococcus pneumoniae*
  - Gram-negative organisms: rare
  - *Haemophilus influenzae*: children <4 years
  - Salmonella: sickle-cell disease.

Clinical features

- Severe pain: limb held still.
- Malaise.
- Fever.
- Local inflammation.
- Commonest site:
  - Proximal femur: children
  - Thoracolumbar spine: adults.

Investigation

➤ X-ray:
  - Displacement of fat planes: early
  - Peri-osteal new bone formation: 2 weeks

➔

- Patchy rarefaction of the metaphysis: late
- Osteoporosis with apparent adjacent increased density.
➤ Bone scan: increased activity.
➤ MRI: identifies pus in atypical cases.
➤ Aspiration of pus: Gram stain and culture.
➤ White cell count (WCC)/erythrocyte sedimentation rate (ESR)/C-reactive protein (CRP): elevated.
➤ Antistaphylococcal antibodies: elevated.

Treatment

➤ Pain relief.
➤ Rehydration.
➤ Splintage.
➤ Antibiotics – adult:
  - Flucloxacillin 1 g qds i.v. and fusidic acid 1 g tds i.v. until systemic sepsis and severe local inflammation settle
  - Flucloxacillin 500 mg orally qds and fusidic acid 500 mg qds orally for 6 weeks.
➤ Antibiotics – child 5 years of age and over:
  - Flucloxacillin 500 mg qds i.v. and fusidic acid 500 mg tds i.v. until systemic sepsis and severe local inflammation settle
  - Flucloxacillin 250 mg orally qds and fusidic acid 250 mg tds orally for 6 weeks.
➤ Antibiotics – child <5 years of age:
  - Amoxicillin 100 mg/kg divided tds i.v. until systemic sepsis and severe local inflammation settle
  - Amoxicillin 250 mg tds orally for 6 weeks.
➤ Surgical drainage of pus.

Prognosis:

➤ Most cases resolve.

Complications

- Suppurative arthritis.
- Metastatic infection.
- Altered bone growth.
- Chronic osteomyelitis.

Chronic osteomyelitis

Definitions

- Aetiology: acute osteomyelitis, open fractures, bone and joint prosthesis.
- Pathogens:
  - As acute osteomyelitis
  - *Staphylococcus epidermidis*: infection associated with prosthetic joints.

Clinical features

- Chronic draining sinuses.
- Relapsing inflammation and systemic sepsis.
- Pathological fracture.

Investigation

➤ X-ray:
  - Patchy bone resorption
  - Surrounding sclerosis
  - Sequestrum: may resemble bone tumour.
➤ Sinogram: may demonstrate communication to bone.
➤ Bone scan: increased activity.
➤ MRI: assess extent prior to surgery.
➤ Culture from sinus discharge.
➤ WCC/ESR/CRP: elevated.
➤ Antistaphylococcal titres: elevated.

Treatment

➤ Palliation:
  - Appropriate antibiotics
  - Dressings/appliances to contain sinus discharge.
➤ Surgery:
  - Debridement of devitalized tissues
  - Removal of prostheses
  - Instillation of antibiotics via tubes for 6 weeks.
➤ Papineau technique:
  - Cavity packed with bone graft/antibiotic/fibrin sealant
  - Closure: coverage with muscle.

Prognosis:

➤ Palliative rather than curative.

Brodie's abscess

Definitions

- A subacute form of haematogenous osteomyelitis, resulting in a granulating infected cavity in cancellous bone.
- Sites: distal femur, proximal tibia, cuboidal bones.
- Affects: children or adolescents.

Clinical features

- Pain near a joint for months.

Investigation

- ➤ X-ray demonstrates round 2 cm diameter cavity with sclerotic halo.
- ➤ ESR/CRP: elevated (WCC often normal).
- ➤ Biopsy: distinguishes from osteoid osteoma.

Treatment

- ➤ Immobilization.
- ➤ Appropriate antibiotics for 6 weeks.
- ➤ Surgical curettage.

Osteoporosis

Definitions

- Diminution of mass of fully mineralized bone.
- Aetiology:
  - Primary:
    - Age-related changes
    - Post-menopausal.

  - Secondary:
    - Idiopathic
    - Endocrine: Cushing's, hyperparathyroidism, gonadal insufficiency, thyrotoxicosis
    - Drug induced: steroids, alcohol, heparin
    - Nutritional: scurvy, malnutrition, malabsorption
    - Malignancy

- Renal failure
- Rheumatoid, ankylosing spondylitis, tuberculosis
- Immobility/lack of weight bearing: bed-bound, astronauts/cosmonauts.

Clinical features

Primary:

- Back pain
- Increased thoracic kyphosis
- Pathological fracture: Colles', neck of femur.

Secondary:

- Features of underlying condition
- Pathological fracture.

Investigation

➤ X-rays: wedging of vertebrae.
➤ Investigation of underlying conditions.
➤ Investigation of pathological fracture.

Treatment

Postmenopausal:

➤ Calcium 1 g/ergocalciferol (vitamin D_2) 20 µg tablets daily
➤ Physical activity
➤ Hormone replacement therapy, e.g. 625 µg oestrogen/150 µg norgestrel calendar pack
➤ Calcitonin 100 units daily s.c. or alendronic acid (bisphosphonate) 10 mg daily orally
➤ Treatment of pathological fractures.

Secondary:

➤ Treatment of underlying condition
➤ Treatment of pathological fractures.

Scurvy

- May cause subperiosteal haematoma, pathological fracture and epiphyseal separation in infants.

- X-ray demonstrates rings of calcification around the ossific centres.

Paget's disease of the bone

Definitions

- Enlargement and thickening of bone.
- Affects: pelvis, tibia, femur, skull, spine and clavicle.
- Pathology: increased osteoclastic/osteoblastic activity.
- Epidemiology:
  - Age >50 years
  - Affects men and women equally
  - North America, Britain, Germany
- Aetiology: possibly slow viral infection.

Clinical features

- Mainly asymptomatic: incidental finding on X-rays.
- Pain.
- Bowed tibia and femur.
- Enlarged skull.
- Flattened skull base: apparent short neck.
- Kyphosis.
- Cranial nerve compression: impaired vision, facial palsy, trigeminal neuralgia, deafness.
- Cerebrovascular insufficiency.
- Spinal claudication.
- Pathological fracture.
- High-output cardiac failure.

Investigation

➤ X-rays:
  - Flame-shaped region of osteolysis along the shaft of a bone
  - Circumscribed patch of skull osteolysis
  - Thick sclerotic bone with coarse trabeculation later.
➤ Serum alkaline phosphatase and hydroxyproline: elevated.
➤ Serum calcium: elevated if immobilized.

Treatment

Asymptomatic:

➤ No treatment necessary.

Symptomatic:

➤ Calcitonin 50 units three times a week up to 100 units daily by subcutaneous injection
➤ Alendronic acid 10 mg daily
➤ Treatment of pathological fractures.

Rickets and osteomalacia

Definitions

- Manifestations of inadequate bone mineralization:
  - Rickets: regions of endochondral growth are affected in children
  - Osteomalacia: generalized demineralization in adults.
- Aetiology:
  - Deficiency of calcium or vitamin D
  - X-linked impaired renal tubular phosphate reabsorption: commonest cause in developed countries
  - Abnormalities of vitamin D metabolic pathway
  - Renal failure and secondary hyperparathyroidism
  - Drug-induced liver impairment: anticonvulsants or rifampicin.

Clinical features

Rickets

Infant:

- Tetany
- Failure to thrive.

Children:

- Deformity of skull
- Thickening of knees, ankles, wrists
- Enlargement of costochondral junctions (rickety rosary)
- Lateral indentation of the chest
- Spinal curvature
- Bowing of long bones.

Osteomalacia

- Bone pain.
- Backache.
- Muscle weakness.
- Vertebral collapse: kyphosis.
- Pathological fractures.

Investigation

➤ X-rays in cases of rickets show:
   – Thick, wide growth plate
   – Cupping of metaphysis
   – Bowing of diaphysis.
➤ X-rays of osteomalacia show:
   – Thin transverse band of rarefaction across the shaft
     of a long bone or scapula (Looser's zone)
   – Biconcave vertebrae
   – Lateral indentation of acetabula.
➤ Serum calcium and phosphate: reduced.
➤ Serum alkaline phosphatase: elevated.
➤ Urinary calcium: elevated.
➤ Serum 25-hydroxycholecalciferol: reduced in vitamin D
   deficiency.
➤ Bone biopsy: diagnostic in radiologically uncertain cases.

Treatment

Deficiency:

➤ Calcium 500 mg/ergocalciferol 10 μg tablets daily orally.

Metabolic and renal:

➤ Calciferol 1 mg daily orally: malabsorption and liver
   disease
➤ Alfacalcidol 1 μg daily orally: renal failure
➤ Withdraw drugs causing liver impairment
➤ Treat renal failure.

Marble bone disease

Definitions

- Aetiology: inherited – autosomal dominant and recessive
  forms.

Clinical features

Autosomal dominant:

- Presents in adolescence
- Incidental finding on X-ray
- Pathological fracture
- Cranial nerve palsy
- Prone to mandibular infection after dental extraction.

Autosomal recessive:

- Presents at birth
- Pancytopenia, haemolysis, splenomegaly
- Optic and facial nerve palsy
- Haemorrhage and infection.

Investigation

➤ X-rays: extremely dense bones.

Treatment

➤ Autosomal dominant: no treatment necessary.
➤ Autosomal recessive: fatal in early childhood.

Primary hyperparathyroidism and Von Recklinghausen's disease of bone

- Primary hyperparathyroidism (page 318) may result in bone erosion, and replacement of marrow space with granulations and fibrous tissue.
- X-rays: subperiosteal erosions of phalanges, clavicle and proximal humerus.
- Treatment of primary hyperparathyroidism (page 318).

Dwarfism

Achondroplasia

- Autosomal dominant inheritance but most cases are sporadic.
- Proximal segments of limbs are disproportionately short.
- Splayed fingers (trident hands).

- Lordotic spine.
- Spinal stenosis and cord compression.
- Treatment: leg lengthening procedures, and spinal surgery for cord compression.

Spondyloepiphyseal dysplasia

- Autosomal dominant (severe) and X-linked recessive (mild) disorders.
- Shortening of limbs, trunk and neck.
- Corrective osteotomies after skeletal maturity.
- Atlanto-axial fusion may be required to stabilize the neck.

Multiple epiphyseal dysplasia

- Range of severity: but less severe than achondroplasia.
- Distortion of long bone ends: reduced limb length.
- Corrective osteotomies after skeletal maturity and treatment of secondary arthritis

Mucopolysaccharidoses

- Defective enzymes for degrading proteoglycans.
- Syndromes: Hurler's, Hunter's, Morquio–Brailsford.
- Features:
  - Shortening of limbs, trunk and neck
  - Coarse facies
  - Hepatosplenomegaly
  - Mental retardation.
- Corrective osteotomies after skeletal maturity.
- Atlanto-axial fusion may be required to stabilize the neck.

Osteogenesis imperfecta

Definitions

- Generalized connective tissue disorder.
- Autosomal dominant and autosomal recessive types.
- Variable severity.

Clinical features

- Fractures following minor trauma: may result in deformity.
- Blue sclerae.
- Thin dentine: crumbling teeth.

- Fractures become much less common after adolescence.
- Severe forms result in stillbirth.

Investigation

➤ X-rays:
  - Osteopenia: thin cortices
  - Multiple old fractures.

Treatment

➤ Avoid injury: prevent fractures.
➤ Normal fracture management.
➤ Correction of deformities: osteotomies and fixation.

Fibrous dysplasia

Definitions

- Developmental disorder.
- Bone is replaced by fibrous tissue.
- May be localized or generalized.
- Extensive cases become evident in childhood or adolescence.

Clinical features

- Asymptomatic if a single small area is affected.
- Pain.
- Deformity.
- Pathological fracture.
- Café-au-lait patches on the skin and precocious puberty in girls: Albright's syndrome.

Investigation

➤ X-rays:
  - Cystic lucent areas of metaphysis or shaft
  - Shepherd's crook deformity of femur.

Treatment

➤ No treatment for asymptomatic disease.
➤ Curettage and bone grafting of painful regions.
➤ Surgical correction of deformities.

Bone tumours: benign

Solitary bone cyst

Definitions
- Cyst of long bone metaphysis.
- Common location: proximal humerus or femur.
- Affects: children.

Clinical features
- Pathological fracture.
- Incidental finding on X-ray.

Investigation
➤ X-ray: radiolucent area of metaphysis.

Treatment
Asymptomatic non-enlarging cyst:

➤ Observation.

Enlarging cyst:

➤ Aspiration and steroid injection.

Pathological fracture:

➤ Curettage, bone grafting and internal fixation.

Osteochondroma

Definitions
- Cartilage-capped exostosis at physeal plate.
- Common location: end of long bone or ileum.
- Aetiology: developmental abnormality.
- Affects: teenagers.

Clinical features
- Lump over metaphysis or iliac crest.
- Enlarges with bone growth.
- Stops enlarging at end of bone growth.
- Sometimes painful.

Investigation

> ➤ X-ray: bony exostosis surrounded by clouds of calcified cartilage.

Treatment

Asymptomatic lump:

> ➤ No treatment.

Enlarging lump in an adult:

> ➤ Treat as chondrosarcoma.

Enchondroma

Definitions

- Persisting island of cartilage in a metaphysis of hand or foot long bones.
- Malignant change may eventually occur in 2%.

Clinical features

- Incidental finding on X-ray.

Investigation

> ➤ X-ray: central radiolucent area with flecks of calcification at junction of metaphysis and diaphysis.

Treatment

Asymptomatic:

> ➤ No treatment.

Enlarging tumour:

> ➤ Curettage and bone grafting: high recurrence rate.

Osteoid osteoma

Definitions

- Small tumour.
- Common location: skull, or metaphysis of femur or tibia.
- Affects: males >30 years.

Clinical features

- Severe pain.
- Limp if in femur or tibia.
- Muscle wasting

Investigation

➤ X-ray: lucent nidus surrounded by sclerosis.

Treatment

➤ Surgical excision with X-ray localization.
➤ Internal fixation if weakening after excision.
➤ Laser coagulation may be used as an alternative in some centres.

Aneurysmal bone cyst

Definitions

- Spontaneous haemorrhagic lesion.
- Common location: long bone metaphyses.
- Affects: young adults.

Clinical features

- Pain.
- Sometimes visible swelling over bone.

Investigation

➤ X-ray: eccentric lucent area of metaphysis.

Treatment

➤ Curettage and bone grafting.
➤ May recur several times.

Giant cell tumour

Definitions

- Soft tumour of mature bone, which extends up to the articular surface.

- Pathology: multinucleate giant cells; may be malignant – giant cell sarcoma.
- Common location: distal femur, proximal tibia, proximal humerus, distal radius.
- Affects: young adults.

Clinical features

- Pain over end of long bone.
- Pathological fracture.
- Palpable swelling.

Investigation

➤ X-ray: eccentric lucent area extending to subchondral bone plate.
➤ MRI/CT: staging procedures.
➤ Arthroscopy: identifies whether articular surface has been broached.
➤ Biopsy: frozen section at time of operative treatment.

Treatment

Surgery based on histology of frozen section biopsy:

➤ Curettage and bone grafting: benign
➤ Excision and prosthetic replacement: aggressive tumours
➤ Postoperative radiotherapy: aggressive tumours where complete resection is difficult
➤ Radical resection or amputation: sarcoma.

Bone tumours: malignant

Multiple myeloma

Definitions

- Plasma cell bone marrow tumour.
- Affects: age 45–65 years.

Clinical features

- Weakness.
- Malaise.

- Anaemia.
- Bone pain.
- Pathological fracture.

Investigation

➤ X-rays:
  - Sometimes no change
  - Multiple punched-out defects, typically of skull
  - Pathological fracture.
➤ Urinalysis: Bence-Jones protein.
➤ Serum protein electrophoresis: identifies abnormal immunoglobulin band.
➤ Bone marrow aspirate and biopsy: histopathology.

Treatment

➤ Melphalan 150 μg/kg for 4 days, repeated at 6-week intervals until remission.
➤ Radiotherapy of bone metastatic deposits.
➤ Internal fixation of pathological fractures.
➤ Fatal over 36 months.

Osteosarcoma

Definitions

- Highly malignant bone tumour arising within bone, spreading out to surrounding tissues.
- Common location: long bone metaphyses – particularly at the knee.
- Affects: children and adolescents.

Clinical features

- Gradual onset of pain: becomes severe.
- Later a mass develops with inflamed overlying soft tissues.
- Pathological fracture is rare.

Investigation

➤ X-ray:
  - Hazy osteolytic and dense osteoblastic areas
  - Breach of cortex

➔

- 'Sunburst': streaks of new bone formation into adjacent tissue
- Codman's triangle: peri-osteal elevation by new bone formation.
➤ MRI/CT: local and metastatic staging.
➤ Biopsy (such that the track will be excised by subsequent surgery).

Treatment

➤ Amputation through or above the proximal joint.
➤ Limb-sparing operations: if patient accepts higher risk of recurrence.
➤ Chemotherapy pre-operatively and postoperatively improves survival.
➤ Radiotherapy: controls inoperable sites.
➤ Surgical resection of small pulmonary metastases.

Complications

- Poor prognosis.
- 50% long-term (10-year) survival after resection and chemotherapy.

Parosteal osteosarcoma

Definitions

- Low-grade osteosarcoma at the surface of long bones.
- Common location: distal femur or proximal tibia.
- Affects: young adults.

Clinical features

- Slowly enlarging mass.

Investigation

➤ X-ray: dense mass on the surface of the bone, but no erosion of the cortex.
➤ CT/MRI: local and metastatic staging.

Treatment

➤ As osteosarcoma.

Complications

- >90% long term survival after resection and chemotherapy.

Chondrosarcoma

Definitions

- Malignant tumour of cartilaginous origin:
  - Primary: arise in metaphysis of long bone
  - Secondary: malignant change in cartilage cap of exostosis – usually pelvis and scapula.
- Affects: men aged 30–40 years.

Clinical features

- Dull ache.
- Slow-growing lump.

Investigation

➤ X-rays:
  - Primary: lucent area with calcific flecks
  - Secondary: cloud of calcification.
➤ MRI/CT: local and metastatic staging.

Treatment

➤ Wide excision and prosthetic replacement.
➤ Amputation if complete excision is impossible.

Complications

- Slow-growing tumours: metastasize late.

Fibrosarcoma

Definitions

- Fibrosarcoma may rarely occur in bone.
- Common location: previously abnormal bone: infarct, fibrous dysplasia, post-irradiation.
- Affects: adults.

Clinical features

- Pain or swelling.
- Pathological fracture.

Investigation
➤ X-ray: non-specific bone destruction.
➤ Biopsy.

Treatment
➤ Wide excision and prosthetic replacement: low grade.
➤ Amputation or radiotherapy: high grade.

Giant cell sarcoma

Definitions
● Giant cell tumours may be malignant sarcomas.

Clinical features
● As giant cell tumour (see above).

Investigation
➤ As giant cell tumour (see above).

Treatment
➤ Radical resection or amputation.

Ewing's tumour

Definitions
● Tumour arising from endothelial cells of bone marrow.
● Common location: diaphysis of tibia, fibula or clavicle.
● Affects: age 10–20 years.

Clinical features
● Painful swelling.
● Inflammation.

Investigation
➤ X-ray:
  – May be similar to osteosarcoma, but at the diaphysis
  – 'Onion-peel' appearance of layers of new bone formation.

➜

> MRI/CT: local and metastatic staging.
> Biopsy.

Treatment
> Pre-operative chemotherapy.
> Amputation.
> Radiotherapy.

Complications
- Poor prognosis.
- 50% 5-year survival after combination therapy.

Secondary neoplasia

Definitions
- Commonest bone tumour age >50 years.
- Primary tumour:
  - Breast
  - Bronchus
  - Thyroid
  - Kidney
  - Prostate
  - Bladder
  - Gastrointestinal tract.

Clinical features
- Incidental finding on X-ray.
- Pain.
- Pathological fracture.
- Acute cord compression.

Investigation
> X-ray: osteolytic areas (rarely sclerotic from prostatic carcinoma).
> Bone scan: increased uptake.
> Tumour markers: rise during follow-up may be indicative.

Treatment

➤ Radiotherapy.
➤ Hormonal therapy: carcinoma of breast and prostate.
➤ Internal fixation of pathological fractures.
➤ Surgical decompression of cord compression.

JOINTS AND MUSCLES

Osteoarthritis

Definitions

● Chronic progressive destructive joint disorder.
● Pathology:
   – Disintegration of articular cartilage
   – Osteophyte formation: new cartilage and bone formation at joint margins
   – Capsular fibrosis.
● Aetiology: genetic, pre-existing joint abnormalities, wear and tear.
● Common location: hip, knee or interphalangeal joints.
● Affects: mainly >50 years of age.

Clinical features

● Insidious onset: remission and relapse over months.
● Affected joints may show:
   – Stiffness after inactivity
   – Swelling: intermittent or continuous
   – Deformity
   – Bouchard's nodes: proximal interphalangeal joints
   – Loss of function: difficulty climbing stairs, reduced walking distance
   – Reduced range of movement
   – Crepitus.

Investigation

➤ X-rays:
   – Asymmetric narrowing of joint space
   – Sclerosis of subchondral bone
   – Cysts close to joint surface
   – Osteophytes at joint margin.

Treatment

Early cases:

➤ Paracetamol up to 1 g orally qds, or co-codamol 2 tablets qds: avoid long-term use of non-steroidal anti-inflammatory drugs
➤ Physiotherapy
➤ Reduce load:
  – Walking stick
  – Weight loss
  – Osteotomy.

Late cases:

➤ Arthrodesis
➤ Prosthetic joint replacement.

Complications

- Baker's cyst: posterior capsular herniation of the knee joint.
- Locking of the knee joint: from cartilage/bone loose bodies.
- Rotator cuff syndrome.
- Spinal stenosis (page 746).
- Spondylolisthesis (page 747).

Rheumatoid arthritis

Definitions

- Chronic inflammatory disease affecting joints.
- Pathology:
  – Synovitis and tenosynovitis
  – Destruction of articular cartilage and tendon rupture
  – Deformity and joint instability.
- Aetiology: unknown, human leukocyte antigen (HLA)-DR4 association.
- Common location: fingers, wrist, knee, shoulder, cervical spine, extensor tendons of wrist and flexor tendons of fingers.
- Affects: mainly women >30 years of age.

Clinical features

Articular manifestations

Polyarthritis spreading through affected joints:

* Pain
* Swelling
* Stiffness after inactivity
* Loss of function
* Deformity in late stages:
  - Ulnar deviation of fingers
  - Swan-neck deformity of fingers
  - Boutonnière deformity (page 697)
  - Heberden's nodes: distal interphalangeal joints
  - Radial and volar deviation of wrist
  - Valgus knees
  - Valgus feet
  - Claw toes.

Extra-articular manifestations

* Subcutaneous nodules behind elbows or in tendons.
* Muscle wasting.
* Lymphadenopathy.
* Scleritis.
* Nerve entrapment syndromes.
* Skin ulceration.
* Peripheral sensory neuropathy.

Investigation

➤ X-rays:
  - Peri-articular osteoporosis
  - Marginal bony erosion
  - Narrowing of joint space.
* Late stages:
  - Destruction and deformity
  - Subluxation of atlanto-axial and mid-cervical vertebrae on flexion/extension views.
➤ Full blood count (FBC): normocytic, hypochromic anaemia.
➤ Erythrocyte sedimentation rate (ESR)/C-reactive protein (CRP): elevated.

➜

➤ Rheumatoid factor: positive in 80%.
➤ Antinuclear factor: positive in 30%.
➤ Synovial biopsy via arthroscope.

Treatment

Acute exacerbation:

➤ Rest
➤ Naproxen 500 mg bd orally, or other non-steroidal anti-inflammatory drugs
➤ Prednisolone up to 20 mg orally daily; reduced rapidly to 5 mg maintenance dose.

Long-term suppression of the disease process – 'second-line therapy':

➤ Sodium aurothiomalate ('gold') 50 mg i.m. weekly after 10 mg test dose; continued until disease process is halted
➤ Penicillamine 125 mg daily orally for 1 month: alternative to 'gold'; also hydroxychloroquine, methotrexate.

Localized treatment of affected joints:

➤ Intra-articular injection of steroid
➤ Synovectomy
➤ Splints
➤ Physiotherapy.

Late stages:

➤ Prosthetic joint replacement
➤ Arthrodesis.

Systemic lupus erythematosus

Definitions

● Commonest connective tissue disorder, causing damage to small joints and multiple other systems.
● Pathology: widespread vasculitis and antinuclear autoantibodies.

- Affects: women aged 20–40 years, mainly Afro-Caribbean and Polynesian.
- Aetiology: unknown; hereditary component – affects 5% of first-degree relatives.

Clinical features

- Chronic relapsing condition, ranging from arthritis to multisystem disease.
- Joints: arthritis of small joints, rarely, femoral head necrosis.
- Skin: photosensitivity, butterfly facial rash, purpura, urticaria.
- Lungs: pleurisy, effusions, fibrosis.
- Heart: pericarditis, endocarditis, aortic valvular disease.
- Kidneys: glomerulonephritis progressing to nephrotic syndrome and renal failure.
- Nervous system: psychiatric disturbances, epilepsy, cranial and peripheral nerve palsy.
- Eyes: retinal hard exudates and haemorrhages, Sjögren's syndrome.
- Gastrointestinal: abdominal pain.
- Blood: anaemia, leukopenia, thrombocytopenia.
- Raynaud's phenomenon (page 565).
- Myopathy.

Investigation

➤ ESR/CRP: indicate level of disease activity.
➤ Serum antinuclear antibodies: positive in almost all cases, double-stranded DNA binding occurs in 50% of cases and is specific for systemic lupus erythematosus (SLE).
➤ Serum rheumatoid factor: positive in 50%.
➤ Serum complement levels: reduced in active disease.
➤ Renal biopsy: membranous glomerulonephritis.

Treatment

➤ Prednisolone 30 mg daily orally, reducing over 6 weeks: for acute exacerbations.
➤ Prednisolone 5 mg daily orally long term: maintenance therapy.

Polymyalgia rheumatica

Definitions

- A condition causing aching shoulders and hips.
- Pathology: vasculitis.
- Aetiology: unknown.
- Affects: mainly women aged 60–70 years

Clinical features

- Sudden onset.
- Myalgia, weakness and tenderness around shoulder and pelvic girdles.

Investigation

➤ ESR: >100 mm/hour, returns to normal with treatment.
➤ No specific test.

Treatment

➤ Prednisolone 15 mg daily orally, reducing over 2 years to 1 mg daily.

Ankylosing spondylitis

Definitions

- Chronic inflammatory condition resulting in ankylosis of joints: bony bridges form across joints.
- Aetiology: unknown, association HLA-B27.
- Common location: spine and sacro-iliac joints.
- Affects males aged 15–25 years.

Clinical features

- Backache and stiffness at intervals over years.
- Tenderness at tendo Achilles insertion.
- Eventually deformity develops:
  - Loss of lumbar lordosis
  - Increased thoracic kyphosis
  - Compensatory stance with hips and knees flexed
  - Diminished spinal movements

  – Decreased chest expansion
  – Shoulder, hip and knee involvement in one-third of cases.

Extra-articular manifestations:

- Prostatitis
- Uveitis
- Conjunctivitis
- Aortic valve disease
- Carditis
- Pulmonary fibrosis.

Investigation

➤ X-rays:
  – Erosion and fuzziness of sacroiliac joints
  – Sclerosis of joints
  – Squaring of vertebrae
  – Bony ankylosis: bamboo spine.
➤ ESR/CRP: elevated in active phases.
➤ HLA-B27: in 90%.

Treatment

➤ Spinal extension exercises.
➤ Naproxen 500 mg bd orally: or other non-steroidal anti-inflammatory drugs.
➤ Osteotomy of spine: rarely indicated.
➤ Prosthetic joint replacement: for rare hip involvement.

Psoriatic arthropathy

Definitions

- Psoriasis is a skin disease, associated with arthritis in 10%.
- Aetiology: unknown, but HLA-B27 associated.
- Affects: adults of any age.

Clinical features

- Scaled plaques over the extensor surfaces.
- Pitting of nails and onycholysis: separation of distal portion of nail from vascular bed.

- Arthritis of distal interphalangeal joints of hands: pain and stiffness.
- Sacroiliitis: buttock pain.

Investigation

➤ Serum rheumatoid factor: negative.
➤ X-rays: arthritic changes of small joints and sacroiliitis.
➤ No specific tests.

Treatment

Skin:

➤ Coal tar topically tds
➤ Dithranol ointment 0.1% applied only to plaques daily, washed off after 30 minutes; increase to 1% after 1 week if no skin irritation
➤ Photochemotherapy: psoralen with ultraviolet-A radiation.

Arthritis:

➤ Ibuprofen 400 mg tds daily orally.

Severe resistant skin disease and arthritis:

➤ Azathioprine up to 3 mg/kg daily orally for up to 3 months: danger of neutropenia; blood count must be monitored
➤ Methotrexate up to 2.5 mg/kg daily orally: danger of neutropenia; blood count must be monitored.

Gout

Definitions

- Acute arthritis resulting from abnormal uric acid metabolism.
- Pathology: sodium urate crystal deposition in joints, soft tissues, urinary tract.
- Aetiology:
  - Increased production of uric acid: idiopathic, inborn errors of metabolism; myeloproliferative disorders, e.g. polycythemia rubra vera; lymphoproliferative disorders, e.g. leukaemia, carcinomatosis, severe psoriasis

    – Impaired excretion of uric acid: chronic renal failure, drugs, e.g. thiazides and aspirin, hypertension, lead toxicity, primary hyperparathyroidism, hypothyroidism, alcohol, starvation, glucose-6-phosphatase deficiency.
- Affects: mainly males >40 years of age.

Clinical features

- Acute severe painful arthritis of the small joints: characteristically affecting the metatarsophalangeal joint of the great toe.
- Tophi: white crystal deposits in the ear lobes and around joints.

Investigation

➤ Synovial fluid aspiration: characteristic birefringent crystals.
➤ Serum uric acid: often raised but may be normal.

Treatment

Acute gout:

➤ Indometacin 50 mg tds orally
➤ Colchicine 500 μg 3-hourly orally until pain is relieved; stop if vomiting or diarrhoea occur.

Prophylaxis:

➤ Allopurinol 100–300 mg daily orally.

Reiter's syndrome

Definitions

- Syndrome of arthritis, urethritis and conjunctivitis.
- Aetiology: unknown.
- Associated:
  - HLA-B27
  - Non-specific urethritis
  - Gastrointestinal infection: *Shigella* spp, *Salmonella* spp, *Yersinia* spp, *Campylobacter* spp.
- Affects: mainly young adult males.

Clinical features

- Urethral discharge and dysuria.
- Features of associated gastrointestinal infections: vomiting, diarrhoea and blood in stool.
- Asymmetric arthritis of joints of the lower limbs: 2 weeks after urethral or enteric symptoms.
- Mild bilateral conjunctivitis.
- Keratoderma blennorrhagicum: intense scaling of the soles of the feet and shedding of the toenails: occurs in 10%.

Investigation

- ➤ ESR: raised acutely.
- ➤ Rheumatoid factor: negative.
- ➤ Urethral swabs: negative.
- ➤ Stool culture: for enteric infections may show *Shigella* spp, *Salmonella* spp, *Yersinia* spp, *Campylobacter* spp.

Treatment

- ➤ Indometacin 50 mg tds daily orally.
- ➤ Aspiration of joints and injection of prednisolone 40 mg and lidocaine 10 mg.
- ➤ Prognosis: recurrent arthritis of the knee is common.

Still's disease

Definitions

- Commonest form of juvenile chronic arthritis; other types are rheumatoid arthritis and ankylosing spondylitis.
- Aetiology: unknown.
- Affects: children 2–5 years of age; but also some 10–15 years of age.

Clinical features

- Episodic pattern; features may include:
  - High fever and erythematous patches on trunk and limbs
  - Arthritis

- Lymphadenopathy
- Splenomegaly
- Pericarditis.
- Arthritis may be:
  - Mild generalized arthralgia
  - Hips, knees and ankles
  - Rheumatoid pattern of involvement.

Investigation

➤ FBC: may be anaemic.
➤ ESR: raised.
➤ Rheumatoid factor: negative. A positive result indicates juvenile rheumatoid arthritis.

Treatment

➤ Ibuprofen 50 mg (aged 1–2 years) tds orally; 100 mg (aged 3–7 years) tds orally; 200 mg (aged 8–12 years) tds orally.

Severe arthritis unresponsive to above:

➤ Sodium aurothiomalate 1 mg/kg weekly deep intramuscular injection for up to 5 years; but discontinue if no response after 2 months
➤ Penicillamine 15 mg/kg daily orally for up to 6 months.

Complications

- Danger of haematological disorders and nephritis with sodium aurothiomalate and penicillamine: regularly monitor FBC and test urine for proteinuria.

Septic arthritis

Definitions

- Joint infection.
- Aetiology:
  - Penetrating wound
  - Osteomyelitis
  - Bacteraemia.
- Bacteriology: *Staphylococcus aureus*, *Haemophilus influenzae*, *Neisseria gonorrhoeae*; less commonly: *Streptococcus pyogenes*, *Escherichia coli*, *Proteus* spp.

Clinical features

Infant:

* Septicaemia
* Refusal to feed
* Warm, tender, immobile joint: may not be too apparent.

Child:

* Acutely painful, immobile large joint: usually the hip
* Redness, warmth and swelling around the joint
* Septicaemia
* Primary source of infection may be present, e.g. boil, septic toe, otitis.

Adult:

* Painful, red, warm swollen superficial joint: usually the knee, wrist or ankle
* Primary source of infection may be present, e.g. gonococcal infection or drug abuse.

Investigation

➤ Joint aspiration: urgent Gram stain and culture.
➤ Blood cultures.
➤ X-ray: joint effusion, associated osteomyelitis.

Treatment

➤ Bed rest.
➤ Splintage: e.g. split plaster for knee, skin traction for hip.
➤ Antibiotics:
   * Infants and children <4 years of age (*Haemophilus influenzae*):
     – Cefuroxime 240 mg/kg daily, divided tds i.v.
   * Children >4 years of age and adults:
     – Flucloxacillin 250 mg–1 g qds and fucidin 6 mg/kg up to 500 mg tds daily i.v.; orally once systemic sepsis has subsided: for 6 weeks.

Complications

* Deformity and shortening of limb: damage to epiphyses in children.

- Osteoarthritis.
- Bony ankylosis: destruction of articular cartilage.

Tuberculous arthritis

Definitions

- Tuberculous infection of a joint.
- Pathology: chronic granulomatous inflammation with caseous necrosis destroying articular cartilage and adjacent bone.
- Aetiology: spread of infection from pulmonary tuberculosis (5% of cases): tertiary disease.
- Bacteriology: *Mycobacterium tuberculosis*.
- Affects: mainly children and young adults; from Asia and other developing regions.

Clinical features

- History of tuberculous infection or contacts.
- Intermittent fever and weight loss.
- Swollen, immobile joint: with severe pain at night when surrounding muscles relax.
- Chronic discharging sinus communicating with the joint.
- Muscle wasting.
- Deformity and shortening of the limb after months.

Investigation

➤ X-ray:
  – Narrowing of joint space and peri-articular osteoporosis
  – Enlargement of epiphyses in children
  – Cystic lesions in subarticular bone
  – Gross disruption and subluxation.
➤ Mantoux or Heaf test: positive.
➤ Synovial fluid aspiration: cultures positive in 20%.

Treatment

➤ Bed rest.
➤ Splintage: e.g. split plaster for knee, skin traction for hip.

➔

➤ Pyrazinamide 1.5–2.0 g daily for 2 months; and isoniazid 300 mg, rifampicin 450–600 mg, ethambutol 15 mg/kg daily for 6 months.
➤ Arthrodesis: for painful destroyed joint.
➤ Joint replacement: only if disease has been inactive for years.

Complications

● Chronic infection.
● Osteoarthritis and fibrous ankylosis.
● Deformity and shortening of limb: destruction of surrounding tissues and epiphyseal damage in children.

Haemophilic arthropathy

Definitions

● Recurrent intra-articular bleeding in haemophilia.
● Pathology: chronic synovitis and destruction of articular cartilage.
● Aetiology: haemophilia A (page 34) and haemophilia B – Christmas disease (page 34).
● Affects: male children: intra-articular haemorrhage from when the child begins to walk; joint degeneration develops later, but before 15 years of age.

Clinical features

● Acute intra-articular haemorrhage:
  – Sudden onset of painful, boggy swelling, with severe limitation of movement
  – Affects knees, ankles, elbows, shoulders and hips
  – Less commonly haemorrhage into muscle can occur
  – Gradually resolves over 2 weeks.
● Joint degeneration:
  – Gradual loss of range of movement
  – Muscle wasting
  – Instability.

Investigation

➤ Investigation of haemophilias (page 34).
➤ X-ray – stages:
  - I: Soft tissue swelling
  - II: Osteoporosis and epiphyseal overgrowth
  - III: Narrowing of joint space
  - IV: Severe narrowing of joint space and disorganization
  - V: Joint disintegration.

Treatment

Acute intra-articular haemorrhage:

➤ Factor VIII or IX concentrate intravenous infusion
➤ Pethidine 0.5–2.0 mg/kg 3-hourly as required
➤ Splintage: for 48 hours
➤ Aspiration: only if high suspicion of infection.

Joint degeneration:

➤ Physiotherapy: to prevent contractures
➤ Intermittent splintage: to prevent contractures
➤ Tendon lengthening and osteotomy may occasionally be used to correct deformity
➤ Arthrodesis: may occasionally be required for painful joint destruction.

Charcot's joint

- Severely deformed and unstable joint, resulting from abnormal stress and injury associated with neuropathy.
- Aetiology: tabes dorsalis, syringomyelia, meningo-myelocoele (page 773), diabetic neuropathy (page 773), lepromatous neuropathy.
- Treatment: stabilization with a brace or calliper.

Cerebral palsy

Definitions

- Abnormal mental and physical development from non-progressive brain damage; occurring in uterine development, at birth or in the neonatal period.

- Types:
  - Spastic paresis: hemiplegic, diplegic, or tetraplegic
  - Ataxia
  - Athetoid: follows kernicterus
  - Aetiology: hypoxia, birth trauma, prematurity, maternal toxaemia, prolonged febrile convulsions or coma, hypoglycaemia, kernicterus, cerebral haemorrhage or infarction
  - Affects: 2/1000 live births.

Clinical features

Gradually becomes apparent over the first year of life with delay in normal developmental milestones:

- Grasp, withdrawal, sucking reflexes: neonatal period
- Hold up head: 3 months
- Sitting: 6 months
- Walking: 1 year.

After 1 year features upper motor neuron spastic paresis:

- Scissors stance: stands assisted with legs crossed
- Equinus feet
- Abnormal posture aggravated by movement
- Flexion contractures and scoliosis begin to develop
- Facial contortions
- Involvement of tongue and speech muscles: difficulty with developing speech
- Athetosis: writhing movements of the limbs
- Ataxia: a rare pattern of intention tremor and incoordination of the trunk and limbs
- Associated mental retardation: range from mild to severe deficit.

Treatment

➤ Physiotherapy.
➤ Splints: to prevent fixed deformity, e.g. equinus, and limit dynamic spastic contractions.
➤ Division of tendons to release flexion contractures.
➤ Tendon transfers to augment weak muscles.
➤ Osteotomy or arthrodesis to improve the position of fixed deformities.

Multiple sclerosis

Definitions

- Chronic relapsing neurological disorder, which may cause paralysis.
- Pathology: multiple areas of demyelination of the brain and spinal cord:
  - Optic nerves
  - Brainstem and cerebellar connections
  - Cervical cord
  - Periventricular region.
- Affects: 1/50 000; more frequent in females than males; onset between 20 and 35 years of age.
- Aetiology: unknown; increased incidence in first-degree relatives; HLA-A3/B7/DR2 association.

Clinical features

- Relapsing and remitting (80%), or chronic progressive (20%) symptoms.
- Features depend on sites of demyelination:
  - Retrobulbar neuritis: blurring of vision in one eye, progressing over days to visual loss, which recovers over the period of a month
  - Brainstem demyelination: diplopia, vertigo, facial numbness, dysphagia; recovers over weeks
  - Cord demyelination: spastic paraparesis – difficulty in walking, urinary retention or incontinence, constipation, impotence
  - Late stages: spastic tetraparesis, ataxia, optic atrophy, nystagmus, pseudobulbar palsy, incontinence, dementia, pressure necrosis. Death results from uraemia or bronchopneumonia.

Investigation

➤ MRI: multiple plaques in periventricular region and brainstem.
➤ Visually evoked response: cerebral electrical responses to optic stimulation by light – delayed responses indicate optic neuropathy.
➤ Syphilis serology: negative.

➜

➤ CSF: elevated total protein with >15%
immunoglobulin G (IgG), oligoclonal IgG on
electrophoresis, increased mononuclear cells >5/mm³.

Treatment

➤ Prednisolone up to 1 g daily i.v. for 4 days: in acute
exacerbations.
➤ Abdominal pressure/intermittent self-catheterization:
for difficulty in micturition; oxybutynin 5 mg tds orally,
for bladder instability.
➤ Laxatives, enemas: for constipation.
➤ Papaverine injections: for impotence.
➤ Propranolol 40 mg daily orally: for tremor.
➤ Cinnarizine 30 mg tds orally: for unsteadiness.
➤ Baclofen 5–30 mg tds orally, or by intrathecal infusion
pump: for spasticity.
➤ Neurosurgical division of reflex pathways.
➤ Electric wheelchair, home adaptations and devices to
assist with daily activities.
➤ Pressure area care: inflatable mattresses, fleece pads,
regular inspection of pressure points.

Motor neuron disease

Definitions

● Chronic progressive condition leading to paralysis and
muscle wasting.
● Pathology: progressive degeneration of upper and lower
motor neurons of the spinal cord, cranial nerves and
cortex.
● Aetiology: unknown, associated gene identified on
chromosome 21.
● Affects: 6/100 000, mainly middle-aged males.

Clinical features

Progressive muscular atrophy:

● Muscle wasting, weakness and fasciculation
● Begins in the small muscles of one hand, spreading to
the arm and then contralaterally

- Reflexes may be lost or exaggerated: variable involvement of anterior horn cells or corticospinal neurons.

Amyotrophic lateral sclerosis:

- Paraparesis or tetraparesis: involvement of lateral corticospinal tracts
- Muscle wasting, weakness and fasciculation
- Reflexes exaggerated
- Bulbar palsy (page 215).

Investigation
➤ No specific tests.
➤ Exclusion of other conditions.

Treatment
➤ Riluzole 50 mg bd orally may slow disease progression.
➤ Adaptation of home for disabilities.
➤ Electric wheelchair.
➤ Computerized communication devices.
➤ Feeding gastrostomy.
➤ Mechanical ventilation.

Prognosis:

➤ Relentless progression to death from broncho-pneumonia over a 3 year period.

Poliomyelitis

Definitions

- Viral infection that causes paralysis by damaging anterior horn cells of spinal cord.
- Aetiology/pathology: polio virus – an RNA virus spread by the faecal–oral route.
- Affects: mainly children in developing countries.
- Epidemics occurred worldwide before vaccination programmes were introduced.

Clinical features

- Asymptomatic infection 95%.
- Fever, sore throat, myalgia 4–5%.

- Paralytic polio <1%:
  - Meningitis: fever, headache, neck stiffness, vomiting
  - Myalgia
  - Painful muscle spasm on passive stretching
  - Asymmetric paralysis develops after 2 days: lower limbs most often affected in children <5 years of age
  - Dysphagia: bulbar palsy (page 215)
  - Respiratory muscle paralysis.

Investigation

➤ Clinical diagnosis: lack of sensory loss and asymmetric pattern distinguish from Guillain–Barré.
➤ Viral culture.

Treatment

Acute stage:

➤ Isolation: infective for 4 weeks from onset
➤ Rest
➤ Physiotherapy: passive stretching to prevent contractures
➤ Artificial ventilation: for respiratory paralysis.

Rehabilitation (gradual partial recovery over first 6 months):

➤ Physiotherapy
➤ Splintage to prevent fixed deformity.

Residual paralysis (>6 months):

➤ Quadriceps weakness: calliper to hold the knee straight
➤ Unbalanced paralysis of flexors/extensors: splintage, tendon transfers or arthrodesis.

Complications

- Residual paralysis: typically a weak, wasted lower leg.
- Flail joint from balanced paralysis of flexors/extensors: calliper or arthrodesis.
- Limb shortening: lack of muscle activity impairs growth; employ built-up shoe; limb-lengthening procedures or epiphyseal plate stapling of normal limb.
- Cool, blue limb from vasomotor dysfunction: may require sympathectomy.

Myasthenia gravis

Definitions

- Episodic condition causing muscular weakness.
- Pathology: defective neuromuscular transmission; autoimmune destruction of postsynaptic acetylcholine receptors.
- Aetiology: unknown.
- Associations: thymic hyperplasia and thymoma, HLA-B8/DR3; and autoimmune thyrotoxicosis, diabetes mellitus, rheumatoid arthritis, SLE, pernicious anaemia.
- Affects: women more than men, typically aged around 30 years.

Clinical features

- Relapsing and remitting skeletal muscle weakness: most pronounced at the end of the day and exacerbated by exercise.
- Diplopia and ptosis at the end of the day: early features.
- Weakness of mastication and facial muscles, dysarthria, dysphagia, dysphonia.
- Weakness of neck and shoulder girdle.
- Proximal limb muscle wasting but brisk reflexes: in later stages.

Investigation

- ➤ Tensilon test: test dose of edrophonium (anticholinesterase) 1 mg i.v., then 5 mg i.v.: improves the weakness for a few minutes.
- ➤ Serum acetylcholine receptor antibodies: titres raised in 90%.
- ➤ Thoracic CT: identifies thymic enlargement.

Treatment

- ➤ Pyridostigmine (anticholinesterase) 30–120 mg up to qds orally as required.
- ➤ Propantheline 15 mg tds orally: may be required to counteract abdominal cramps induced by pyridostigmine.

Polymyositis and dermatomyositis

Definitions

- Inflammatory disease of muscle and skin.
- Aetiology: unknown.
- Associated: viral infection (rubella, influenza, Coxsackie), HLA-DR3, autoimmune rheumatic diseases (rheumatoid, SLE, systemic sclerosis), malignancy.
- Affects: children; also adults >60 years of age.

Clinical features

- Insidious onset of malaise, weight loss and fever.
- Progressive proximal muscle weakness and tenderness:
  - Difficulty rising from a chair or from a squatting position
  - Difficulty walking up stairs
  - Difficulty raising the arms above the head.
- Dysphagia.
- Respiratory muscle weakness: in severe cases.
- Heliotrope (purple) discoloration of eyelids and peri-orbital oedema.
- Purple vasculitic patches over extensor surfaces.
- Ulcerative vasculitis

Investigation

- ESR: often raised.
- Serum creatinine phosphokinase: often raised.
- Serum anti-Jo1 antibodies: positive in 30%.
- Rheumatoid factor: positive in 50%.
- Electromyelography – characteristic combination:
  - Fibrillation at rest
  - Short duration potentials on voluntary contraction
  - Salvos on nerve stimulation.
- Muscle biopsy: inflammation; degeneration, abnormal regeneration and necrosis of fibres.
- Investigations for associated malignancy: most likely in males >50 years of age.

Treatment
➤ Prednisolone 60 mg initially (adult cases), reducing to 10 mg daily orally: often required for years.
➤ Cyclophosphamide 1 mg/kg daily orally: for severe disease unresponsive to steroids.
➤ Physiotherapy and splints: rehabilitation.

Pyomyositis and other types of myositis

- Local bacterial infection: *Clostridium welchii* (temperate countries), *Staphylococcus aureus* (tropical countries) (page 143).
- Systemic viral infections: adenovirus, rhinovirus, influenza, Coxsackie.
- Systemic parasitic infections: cysticercosis, trichinosis, toxoplasmosis, trypanosomiasis.
- Systemic inflammatory disorders: sarcoidosis, poly-arteritis nodosa, Wegener's granulomatosis, eosinophilic polymyositis.

Muscle tears

- Sharp pain during muscular exertion: bruising develops later; treatment is by analgesia and gradual reintroduction of activity.
- Intramuscular haemorrhage may occur with haemophilic arthropathy (page 34).
- Tenosynovitis: inflammation of tendon sheaths occurs in rheumatoid arthritis (page 649) and DeQuervain's disease (page 691).

Duchenne's muscular dystrophy

Definitions

- Progressive muscle weakness from absence of the muscle protein dystrophin.
- Aetiology: X-linked recessive inherited disorder of protein synthesis; may also arise by spontaneous mutation.
- Affects: 1/3000 males; begins in infancy.

Clinical features

- Proximal muscle weakness usually becomes apparent by 3 years of age:
  - Difficulty in running
  - Difficulty in rising from the floor; using the hands to climb up the legs – Gower's sign.
- Hypertrophy of the calf, and sometimes of the deltoid muscles.
- Progressive weakness: confined to wheelchair by 10 years of age.
- Cardiomyopathy and respiratory muscle weakness: death by 20 years of age.

Investigation

➤ Serum creatinine phosphokinase: elevated up to 200 times the normal level.
➤ Muscle biopsy and histology: variation in fibre size; fibre necrosis, regeneration and replacement by fat; absence of dystrophin – immunochemical stains.

Treatment

➤ Adaptations and wheelchair.
➤ Prevention:
  - Genetic detection of carriers
  - Genetic counselling
  - Selective abortion of males.
➤ Prognosis: progression from disability to death by 20 years of age.

Becker's muscular dystrophy

- Less severe weakness develops between 5 and 25 years of age with no cardiac involvement.

Dystrophia myotonica

- Progressive distal muscle and facial weakness from defective membrane conductance developing at 20–50 years of age.
- Myotonia is the characteristic feature: continued muscle contraction after cessation of voluntary contraction.

- Part of an autosomal dominant inherited syndrome comprising: frontal baldness, cataracts, mild intellectual impairment, cardiomyopathy, hypogonadism, glucose intolerance.
- Treatment: procainamide 250 mg tds orally or phenytoin 300 mg daily orally; adaptation for disabilities.
- Prognosis: death by middle age.

Myotonia congenitalia (Thomsen's disease)

- Less severe form of autosomal dominant inherited myotonia occurring in childhood: the condition improves with increasing age.

Tendon injury

- Tendons may be transected by knives or other sharp instruments, or rupture under excessive strain, e.g. mallet finger (page 696), ruptured tendo Achilles (page 725).
- Penetrating injury to flexor surfaces of the palm or wrist may result in flexor tendon and sensory nerve injury, with subsequent contractures that may severely impair hand function.
- These flexor injuries are best treated by early surgical exploration and repair by experienced hand surgeons or plastic surgeons: extensile plastic exposures may be required to retrieve the divided ends of the tendons, which tend to retract, and tendon grafts may be required.
- After surgery, the arm and hand are splinted in supportive slabs in a position to relax the repair, often with elastic bands attached to the fingers ('lively splint') to avoid contracture but allow gentle flexion exercise.

Repetitive strain injury

- Pain in the dorsum of the forearm during repetitive hand movements, e.g. keyboard operators.
- Rest from the activity for 4 weeks; physiotherapy with ultrasound; elastic support.

Arthrogryphoses

- Congenital disorders where there is restricted movement and deformity from soft tissue contractures, which may result from nerve or muscle pathology.
- Treatment: manipulation and splintage; rebalancing joints by tendon transfers, and osteotomies.

Rhabdomyosarcoma

Definitions

- Malignant tumour of skeletal muscle.
- Aetiology: unknown.
- Affects: two age groups:
  - Aged 2–6 years: head, neck and genitourinary tract
  - Aged 14–18 years: extremities, trunk, head, neck and genitourinary tract.

Clinical features

- Aching, rapidly enlarging hard lump: typically in muscles around hip and shoulder joints.
- Fixed by tensing affected muscle.

Investigation

➤ CT/MRI of affected region: poorly demarcated mass in muscle, spreading along fascial planes.
➤ CT of thorax and abdomen: staging for lymph nodes and metastases.
➤ Biopsy and histology: confirms diagnosis and gives histological type and grade.

Treatment

➤ Radical resection.
➤ Amputation of affected limb: if tumour has spread beyond the fascial sheath, or in cases of recurrent tumour.
➤ Radiotherapy and chemotherapy: for head, neck and prostatic tumours; and as adjuvant treatment after resection of limb tumours.
➤ Prognosis: up to three-quarters of cases are cured.

UPPER LIMB

SHOULDER JOINT AND PECTORAL GIRDLE

Painful arc syndrome

Definitions

- Chronic tendinitis with impingement under the coraco-acromial arch.
- Aetiology: overuse, subacromial bursitis, partial rupture of supraspinatus tendon, acromial osteophytes, arthritis.

Clinical features

Young adults:

- Shoulder pain after vigorous activity
- Tenderness over acromion
- Painful arc of active abduction 60–120.

Older adults:

- Recurrent pain after activity: worse at night
- Painful arc of active abduction 60–120
- Crepitation over the shoulder on passive movement
- Complete tear of supraspinatus: active shoulder abduction is lost.

Investigation

➤ X-rays:
  - Normal in early stages
  - Osteophytes
  - Thinning of acromion
  - Calcification of supraspinatus.
➤ Arthrography: demonstrates supraspinatus tear.
➤ Ultrasound: demonstrates supraspinatus tear.
➤ Magnetic resonance imaging (MRI): demonstrates supraspinatus tear.

Treatment

➤ Modify activities to avoid symptoms.
➤ Physiotherapy.
➤ Ibuprofen 400 mg t.i.d. orally.
➤ Prednisolone 40 mg subacromial injection weekly as required.
➤ Surgical excision of coraco-acromial arch for symptoms lasting >6 months.

Acute calcific tendinitis

Definitions

● Deposition of hydroxyapatite crystals just medial to insertion of supraspinatus tendon.
● Affects: young adults.

Clinical features

● Shoulder pain becomes severe over hours: subsides over a few days.

Investigation

➤ X-ray: opacity just above the greater tuberosity.

Treatment

➤ Rest in a sling.
➤ Indometacin 50 mg t.i.d. orally.
➤ Prednisolone 40 mg and bupivacaine 0.5% subacromial injection weekly as required.
➤ Surgical evacuation of crystals for persisting symptoms.

Biceps tendon rupture

Proximal tendon:

• Accompanies rotator cuff syndrome in patients aged >50 years
• Sudden snap when lifting
• Prominent lump in lower arm on elbow flexion
• No disability: elbow flexion from brachialis

- No treatment necessary in majority of cases
- Surgical reattachment in young, fit patients as part of rotator cuff surgery.

Distal tendon:

- Rare disabling injury requiring surgical repair

Frozen shoulder

Definitions

- Tendinitis progressing to capsulitis.
- Aetiology: unknown.
- Affects: patients aged 40–60 years.

Clinical features

- Minor trauma precedes onset.
- Gradually worsening shoulder pain.
- Pain subsides as shoulder stiffness develops over 6–12 months.

Investigation

➤ X-rays: sometimes decreased humeral bone density.

Treatment

➤ Ibuprofen 400 mg t.i.d. orally.
➤ Physiotherapy: active exercises.
➤ Prednisolone 40 mg subacromial injection repeated weekly as required.
➤ Manipulation under anaesthesia.

Surgical management of arthritis of the shoulder

- Indication: severe pain not controlled by analgesics.

Osteoarthritis

- Prosthetic shoulder replacement: relieves pain but gives a limited range of movement.
- Arthrodesis at: 50° abduction, 25° flexion, internally rotated.

Rheumatoid arthritis

- Prednisolone 40 mg subacromial injection repeated weekly as required.
- Synovectomy.
- Shoulder replacement: little improvement in mobility.
- Arthrodesis.

Milwaukee shoulder

- A term describing extensive destructive osteoarthritis.

Sprengel's deformity

Definitions

- Congenital elevation of the scapula.
- Usually unilateral.
- Bilateral cases occur in Klippel–Feil syndrome:
  - Bilateral high scapulae
  - Abnormal cervical spine: short neck
  - Failure of occipital bone fusion
  - Associated kyphosis or scoliosis.

Clinical features

- Painless limitation of abduction.

Investigation

➤ X-rays may show:
  - Fusion of vertebrae
  - Bony bridge between the scapula and cervical spine.

Winging of scapula

- Injury of long thoracic nerve of Bell.

Fractured clavicle

Definitions

- Fracture usually between medial and middle one-third: sometimes the outer one-third.
- Aetiology: a fall on the outstretched hand.

Clinical features

- Arm is held close to chest to limit pain.
- Lump over clavicle.
- Outer one-third fractures produce greater deformity and subsequent weakness.

Investigation

➤ X-rays.

Treatment

➤ Sling for 3 weeks: middle one-third fractures.
➤ Open reduction and internal fixation: outer one-third fractures.

Acromioclavicular dislocation

- A fall on the shoulder may cause subluxation (partial displacement) or complete dislocation of the acromioclavicular joint.
- A 'step' is visible over the joint.
- Subluxation requires no treatment.
- Dislocation is reduced by direct pressure and held by internal fixation.

Sternoclavicular dislocation

- Rare injury from a fall on the shoulder.
- Treatment: reduction and use of a sling for 6 weeks.

Fractured scapula

- Types:
    - Body of scapula: severe direct force
    - Neck of scapula: fall on the shoulder
    - Glenoid: accompanies shoulder dislocation.
    - Arm is held close to chest to limit pain.
    - Body fractures are stable: rest in a sling.
    - Neck and glenoid fractures: internal fixation.

Fractured proximal humerus

Definitions
- Aetiology: moderate trauma from a fall on the outstretched hand, with osteoporosis.
- Affects: postmenopausal women.

Clinical features
- Large bruise on upper arm.
- Associated shoulder dislocation.
- Associated vascular and radial nerve injury.

Investigation
➤ X-rays.

Treatment
Undisplaced fractures:

➤ Sling until pain subsides.

Displaced fractures:

➤ Manipulation and Velpeau chest bandage: circumferential bandaging of the thorax and affected shoulder, with the arm held against the chest and the elbow flexed.

Three part fractures:

➤ Open reduction and internal fixation.

Complex multipart fractures:

➤ Shoulder replacement: movement remains severely limited.

Dislocations of the shoulder

Anterior shoulder dislocation

Definitions
- Common injury.
- Aetiology: fall on outstretched hand.

Clinical features

- Severe shoulder pain: relieved by supporting arm with opposite hand.
- Flattened shoulder outline.
- Bulge of humeral head below clavicle.
- Associated axillary nerve injury: anaesthesia over distal attachment of the deltoid and wasting of the deltoid.
- Associated fracture of the greater tuberosity.

Investigation

➤ X-ray:
   - Overlapping humeral head and glenoid fossa on anteroposterior view
   - Associated fracture.

Treatment

➤ Reduction:
   - Traction in slight abduction, with counter-traction from a sling under the axilla
   - Kocher's manoeuvre: traction from the flexed elbow in lateral shoulder rotation, then adduction with medial shoulder rotation
   - Hippocratic method: traction via the extended arm with counter-traction from a foot placed in the axilla.
➤ Sling or 'collar and cuff' for 3 weeks.

Prognosis:

➤ Recurrent dislocation in half of those aged under 25 years
➤ Axillary nerve injury usually recovers over weeks.

Posterior shoulder dislocation

Definitions

- Rare injury.
- Aetiology: forced internal rotation, often from epileptic fit or electric shock.

Clinical features

- Arm locked in medial rotation.

Investigation

➤ X-ray:
  - 'Light bulb' appearance of humeral head
  - Often missed on anteroposterior view.

Treatment

➤ Reduction: traction in slight abduction then external rotation.
➤ Sling or 'collar and cuff' for 3 weeks.

Irreducible and late presentation:

➤ Open reduction and capsular repair.

Irreducible and late presentation in elderly:

➤ Mobilize without reduction.

Recurrent shoulder dislocation

Definitions

- Usually anterior dislocation.
- Aetiology:
  - Capsular/humeral head injury from acute dislocation
  - Bankart lesion: detachment of labrum from glenoid
  - Hill–Sachs lesion: compression fracture of humeral head.
- Affects: young men.

Clinical features

- Previous acute dislocation.
- Occurs after further but progressively lesser injury.
- Apprehension sign: sensing pending dislocation on abduction, external rotation and extension.

Investigation

➤ X-rays: Hill–Sachs lesion.
➤ MRI: Bankart/Hill–Sachs lesions.

Treatment

➤ Capsular repair and reinforcement operations:
  - Bankart: reattachment of the capsule
  - Putti–Platt: overlapping the capsule and subscapularis
  - Bristow: the coracoid process is transferred and fixed to the anterior scapular neck.

ARM

Cubitus valgus

Definitions

- Abnormally exaggerated valgus carrying angle of elbow.
- Aetiology: non-union of lateral condylar fracture of the humerus.

Clinical features

- Previous elbow fracture.
- Deviation of forearm in supination >15° away from the body.
- Late-onset ulnar nerve palsy.

Investigation

➤ Nerve conduction studies: ulnar nerve palsy.

Treatment

➤ No treatment for deformity.
➤ Ulnar nerve may be surgically transposed anterior to the medial epicondyle: for symptoms of developing palsy.

Cubitus varus ('gun-stock' deformity)

Definitions

- Abnormal varus carrying angle of forearm.
- Aetiology: malunion of supracondylar fracture.

Clinical features

- Deviation of forearm in supination towards the body.

Treatment

➤ Wedge osteotomy of lower humerus for significant deformity.

Tennis elbow

Definitions

- Chronic tendinitis over lateral epicondyle of humerus.
- Aetiology: overuse injury, common in tennis players.

Clinical features

- Pain over lateral epicondyle on movement.
- Tenderness over lateral epicondyle.
- Pain on passive stretching of wrist extensors.

Investigation

➤ X-rays: sometimes calcification at common extensor origin.

Treatment

➤ Avoid activities that cause pain if possible.
➤ Prednisolone 40 mg injection around the tendon insertion.
➤ Physiotherapy.
➤ Forced elbow extension under anaesthesia.
➤ Surgically detach common extensor origin in severe persistent cases.

Golfer's elbow

- Tendinitis over medial epicondyle of humerus: as for tennis elbow except that it is the common flexor origin that is affected.

Pitcher's elbow

- Overuse injury in baseball pitchers results in hypertrophy of the lower humerus, which no longer fits into the olecranon.

Olecranon bursitis

- Pressure/friction over the olecranon or gout may cause inflammation of the olecranon bursa: treatment is with flucloxacillin 500 mg qds for 10 days; fluid may need aspiration; bursa may be excised in chronic cases.

Supracondylar fracture of the humerus

Definitions

- Transverse fracture just above the condyles.
- Usually affects children.
- Caused by a fall onto outstretched hand.

Clinical features

- Painful, swollen elbow.
- S-shaped deformity.

Investigation

➤ X-ray.
  - Distal fragment usually displaced posteriorly.
  - Fat-pad sign: a black triangle in front of the intra-articular portion of the humerus helps to identify undisplaced fractures.

Treatment

Undisplaced fracture:
➤ Sling for 3 weeks.

Displaced fracture:
➤ Reduction under general anaesthesia
➤ Collar and cuff for 3 weeks
➤ Sling for a further 3 weeks.

Irreducible fracture, brachial artery or median nerve entrapment:
➤ Open reduction and internal fixation.

Complications

- Brachial artery injury.

- Volkmann's contracture: clawing of the hand, resulting from ischaemic contracture of forearm muscle due to brachial artery entrapment.
- Median nerve injury.
- Myositis ossificans.
- Malunion.

Bicondylar fractures

Definitions

- Fracture splitting humeral condyles apart.
- Aetiology: fall on the point of the elbow.
- Occurs in adults >50 years: rare.

Clinical features

- Severe soft tissue swelling and tenderness.

Investigation

➤ X-rays: T- or Y-shaped fracture between the humeral condyles.

Treatment

Undisplaced fracture:

➤ Plaster slab.

Moderately displaced fracture:

➤ Open reduction and internal fixation.

Severely comminuted fractures:

➤ Collar and cuff/hinged brace for 8 weeks.

Fracture separation of lateral condylar epiphysis

Definitions

- Avulsion of epiphysis.
- Aetiology: fall on the hand with elbow in varus.
- Affects children <16 years of age.

Clinical features

- Pain over lateral epicondyle on passive flexion of wrist.

Investigation

➤ X-rays: may show grossly displaced and capsized epiphysis.

Treatment

Undisplaced fracture:

➤ Plaster backslab for 2 weeks.

Displaced fracture:

➤ Open reduction and internal fixation.

Complications

- Non-union/malunion: valgus deformity.
- Recurrent elbow dislocation.

Fracture separation of medial condylar epiphysis

Definitions

- Avulsion of epiphysis.
- Associated elbow dislocation: epicondyle is drawn into joint.
- Affects: children <16 years of age.

Clinical features

- Deformity.
- Associated dislocation of elbow.

Investigation

➤ X-ray: epicondyle appears as loose body in joint.

Treatment

➤ Manipulation: may free trapped epicondyle.
➤ Open reduction and internal fixation.

Fracture separation of entire distal humeral epiphysis

- Treated as a supracondylar fracture.

Fractured capitulum

- Aetiology: fall onto the outstretched hand in adults.
- Treatment:
  - Undisplaced fracture: splintage for 2 weeks
  - Displaced fracture: open reduction and internal fixation.

Fractured head of radius

Definitions

- Aetiology: fall onto outstretched hand.
- Usually affects adults.

Clinical features

- Painful forearm rotation.
- Tender head of radius.

Investigation

➤ X-ray: may show vertical split, single or multiple fragments.

Treatment

Undisplaced fracture:

➤ Collar and cuff for 3 weeks.

Single fragment:

➤ K-wire fixation.

Multiple fragments:

➤ Excise radial head.

Fractured neck of radius

- Occurs in children: reduction required if deformity >20.

Fractured olecranon

Definitions

- Aetiology:
  - Fall onto the olecranon, usually in the elderly: comminuted fracture
  - Fall onto the hand during triceps contraction: transverse fracture.

Clinical features

- Unable to extend arm against gravity: transverse fracture.

Investigation

➤ X-ray.

Treatment

Comminuted fracture in the elderly:

➤ Sling for 1 week.

Transverse fracture with no separation on flexion:

➤ Plaster cast at 60° for 3 weeks.

Displaced fracture:

➤ Open reduction and internal fixation.

Dislocation of elbow

Definitions

- Usually posterior dislocation of ulna at the elbow.
- Aetiology: fall onto outstretched hand in elbow extension.

Clinical features

- S-shaped deformity of the arm.
- Associated vascular and nerve injury: as supracondylar fracture.

Investigation

➤ X-ray.

Treatment

➤ Reduction under anaesthesia.
➤ Collar and cuff for 3 weeks.

Pulled elbow

- The head of the radius slips out of the annular ligament on sudden jerking of the arm, causing a painful, hanging arm in a 3- to 4-year-old.
- The radial head of the child is cylindrical, rather than the conical shape in an adult, and is more liable to dislocate from the annular ligament.
- Reduced by forceful supination and flexion.

Fracture of the forearm

Definitions

Types:

- Spiral fracture: twisting injury
- Transverse fracture: angulation injury
- Greenstick fracture of one or both of the radius and ulna: children.

Associated dislocations:

- Monteggia: proximal one-third ulnar fracture and radial head dislocation.
- Galeazzi: lower one-third radius fracture and inferior radioulnar dislocation.

Clinical features

- Range from little deformity to gross angulation.
- Galleazzi is the commoner fracture–dislocation.
- Associated compartment syndrome.

Investigation

➤ X-ray.

Treatment

Isolated ulnar fracture and angulated fractures in children:

➤ Brace.

Isolated radial fracture:

➤ Reduction and plaster cast including elbow and wrist.

Angulated fractures and fracture–dislocations:

➤ Open reduction and internal fixation.

Carpal tunnel syndrome

Definitions

- Compression of the median nerve in the carpal tunnel.
- Aetiology: unknown.
- Associations: rheumatoid arthritis, pregnancy, menopause and myxoedema.

Clinical features

- Mostly affects women 40–50 years of age.
- Pain and paraesthesiae in the distribution of the median nerve in the hand.
- Symptoms wake the patient at night.
- Symptoms may be induced by:
  - 'Phalen's test': holding wrist palmar-flexed for 1 minute
  - Compressing the arm with a sphygmomanometer cuff for 1 minute
  - 'Tinel's sign': percussing over the median nerve in the carpal tunnel.
- Wasting of thenar muscles.
- Weakness of thumb abduction.

Investigation

➤ Nerve conduction studies: slowing of conduction across the wrist.

Treatment

➤ Division of the anterior carpal ligament.
➤ Splintage during pregnancy.

De Quervain's disease

Definitions

- Thickening and inflammation of the tendon sheath of extensor pollicis brevis and adductor pollicis longus.
- Aetiology: unknown.
- Mainly affects women aged 40–50 years.

Clinical features

- Symptoms may be induced by a change in activity, e.g. pruning.
- Pain on the radial side of the wrist.
- Thickening of tendon sheath.
- Tenderness over radial styloid.
- Pain on thumb abduction against resistance, and on passive adduction.

Investigation

➤ X-ray: excludes malunited scaphoid fracture and arthritis.

Treatment

➤ Prednisolone 40 mg injection into the tendon sheath, repeated as often as weekly if required.
➤ Plaster splintage.

Resistant cases:

➤ Division of the tendon sheath.

Ganglion of wrist (see page 203)

Keinbock's disease

Definitions

- Avascular necrosis of the lunate.
- Aetiology: unknown; possibly injury.
- Affects young adults.

Clinical features

- Aching wrist and decreased grip strength.

Investigation

➤ X-ray – progressive pattern:
  – No change
  – Increased density
  – Collapse
  – Osteoarthritis.

Treatment

➤ Splintage of the wrist.
➤ Radial osteotomy to alter stress distribution.
➤ Excision of the lunate: replacement with silicone prosthesis.

Colles' fracture

Definitions

● Transverse fracture of the radius just above the wrist with dorsal and lateral displacement and angulation.
● Aetiology: fall onto outstretched hand in the elderly.
● Association: osteoporosis.

Clinical features

● Wrist pain and tenderness.
● 'Dinner-fork' deformity of the wrist viewed laterally and pronated.

Investigation

➤ X-ray – radial fragment:
  – Displaced and angulated dorsally
  – Displaced and angulated laterally
  – Impacted.

Treatment

➤ Reduction: traction in wrist flexion, ulnar deviation and pronation.
➤ Plaster dorsal slab for 6 weeks: may need repeat reduction after 1 week.
➤ Internal or external fixation: if unstable in plaster.

Smith's fracture

Definitions

- Transverse fracture of the radius just above the wrist with palmar angulation.
- Aetiology: fall onto the back of the hand.

Clinical features

- Wrist pain and tenderness.
- No dinner-fork deformity.

Investigation

➤ X-ray: opposite deformity to Colles'.

Treatment

➤ Reduction: traction and extension.
➤ Plaster volar slab to include elbow at 90.
➤ Surgery: fixation often required – usually unstable in plaster.

Scaphoid fracture

Definitions

- Aetiology: fall onto dorsiflexed hand.
- Affects adolescents and young adults.

Clinical features

- Localized tenderness in the anatomical snuffbox.

Investigation

➤ X-rays – anteroposterior, lateral and oblique:
  - Often only visible on oblique view initially
  - May become apparent after a few weeks
  - Associated fracture of scaphoid tubercle.

Treatment

Undisplaced fracture and after surgery:

➤ Scaphoid plaster for 6 weeks.

➔

Displaced fracture:

➤ Open reduction and internal fixation.

If still tender at 6 weeks:

➤ Scaphoid plaster for a further 6 weeks.

Complications

- Avascular necrosis of proximal fragment:
  - Persistent pain and non-union
  - X-ray shows high-density scaphoid at 3 months
  - May need excision and bone grafting.

Carpal dislocation

- Tearing of carpal ligaments allows dislocation but the lunate usually remains attached to the radius (perilunar dislocation): requires reduction and plaster slab.

HAND

Congenital abnormalities

- **Syndactyly:** webbing between fingers – can be surgically corrected if required.
- **Polydactyly:** accessory digits; the commonest hand malformation – can be amputated.
- **Macrodactyly:** giant finger – no treatment.
- **Radial club hand:** severe radial deviation of the wrist, with absent thumb and lower radius – improved by manipulation, splintage, and sometimes surgery.
- **Ulnar club hand:** severe ulnar deviation of the wrist, with absent fingers on the ulnar side of the hand and ulna – improved by surgery.
- **Madelung's deformity:** lower radius curves forward leaving a prominent lower ulna – severe deformity requires excision of lower ulna.

Dupuytren's contracture

Definitions

- Nodular hypertrophy and contracture of superficial palmar fascia.
- Affects middle-aged men.
- Aetiology: autosomal dominant inheritance.
- Associations: alcoholic cirrhosis, epilepsy, AIDS, diabetes and tuberculosis.

Clinical features

- Nodular thickening of the palm.
- Flexion deformities of little and ring fingers.
- Similar disease process affects:
  - Sole of the foot
  - Corpus cavernosum (Peyronie's disease).

Investigation

➤ Clinical diagnosis.

Treatment

➤ Excision of thickened fascia in severe cases.
➤ Splintage for 6 weeks after surgery.
➤ Amputation of a finger for severe persisting or disabling deformity.

Trigger finger

Definitions

- A nodule in a flexor tendon becomes trapped at a stenosis of the tendon sheath, or at its entrance.
- Commonly affects: ring and middle fingers.
- Aetiology: trauma, overuse-injury, rheumatoid arthritis.

Clinical features

- Affected finger:
  - Clicks on flexion
  - Remains flexed when others are extended
  - Extends with a sudden snap after further effort
  - Tender nodule over flexor tendon sheath.

Treatment

➤ Prednisolone 40 mg injection into the tendon sheath.
➤ Surgical incision of tendon sheath.

Mallet finger

Definitions

● Rupture of extensor tendon to a terminal phalanx.
● Aetiology: forced flexion injury during active extension.

Clinical features

● Terminal phalanx:
  – Remains in a flexed position
  – Cannot be actively extended
  – Can be passively extended.

Investigation

➤ X-ray may show avulsion fracture at base of terminal phalanx.

Treatment

Acute injury:

➤ Mallet splint for 6 weeks.

Old injury with little deformity:

➤ No treatment.

Old injury with marked deformity:

➤ Tendon reconstruction.

Mallet thumb

● Extensor pollicis longus tendon rupture; occurs with Colles' fracture (page 692) or rheumatoid arthritis. Treatment involves surgical transfer of the tendon from the index finger.

Boutonnière deformity

- Splitting of the intermediate part of the extensor digitorum tendon occurs in rheumatoid arthritis, allowing the proximal phalanx to protrude.
- Surgical correction is possible by transferring the lateral slip of the tendon to the middle phalanx.

Gamekeeper's thumb

- Ruptured ulnar collateral ligament of the carpometacarpal joint of the thumb, from a hyperadduction injury (now more commonly seen in skiers) – surgical repair.

Rheumatoid arthritis (page 649)

Bennet's fracture–dislocation

Definitions

- Oblique fracture of the base of the first metacarpal extending into the joint.
- Aetiology: caused by punching.

Clinical features

- Short, swollen thumb.

Investigation

➤ X-ray: triangular fragment of first metacarpal base remains attached to the trapezium.

Treatment

➤ Reduction: traction along the line of the thumb.
➤ Plaster cast for 4 weeks.
➤ Internal fixation if unstable in plaster.

Fractured base of thumb

- Reduction and plaster for 3 weeks.

Metacarpal fractures

Definitions

- Aetiology: caused by punching.

Clinical features

- Rotational deformity of finger: displaced spiral shaft fracture.
- Dorsal hump of the hand: angulated transverse shaft fracture.
- Flattening of knuckle: metacarpal neck fracture.

Investigation

➤ X-ray.

Treatment

➤ Crepe bandage: undisplaced spiral shaft fractures.
➤ Plaster slab for 10 days: undisplaced metacarpal neck fractures.
➤ Reduction and plaster slab for 3 weeks: angulated shaft and base fractures.
➤ Reduction and K-wire fixation: angulated/rotated shaft and neck fractures.
➤ Reduction of fifth metacarpal neck fractures is unnecessary for deformity <20°.

Phalangeal fractures

- Neighbour strapping for 3 weeks; reduction and internal fixation for severely displaced/rotated fractures.

Carpometacarpal dislocations

- Reduction and K-wire fixation.

Metacarpophalangeal dislocations

- Reduction and strapping in flexion.

Interphalangeal dislocations

- Reduction and neighbour strapping for a few days.

Deep infection of the hand

Definitions
- Relatively trivial puncture wound.
- Pathology: *Staphylococcus*.

Clinical features
- Grossly swollen, red hand.
- Ascending lymphangitis.

Investigation
➤ X-ray: soft tissue swelling; identifies osteomyelitis or septic arthritis.

Treatment
➤ Rest and elevation.
➤ Benzylpenicillin 1.2 g tds i.v. and flucloxacillin 1 g qds i.v.
➤ Surgical drainage of synovial sheaths, and deep palmar and thenar spaces.

Paronychia
- Abscess under the nail fold: surgical drainage by excising part of the nail.
- Rest in cross-arm sling until inflammation subsides.

Whitlow
- Abscess in finger pulp: surgical drainage by direct incision.

LOWER LIMB

PELVIS, HIP JOINT AND THIGH

Pelvic fractures

Definitions

Fractures of the pelvic ring

- Types:
  - 'Open book': anteroposterior compression

- Buckled fractures through the pubic rami: lateral compression
- Vertical split through sacroiliac region and pubic rami: vertical shear.
- Aetiology:
  - Severe compression: motor vehicle accidents
  - Vertical shear: fall from a great height onto one leg.

Fractures of the pelvic bones not involving the pelvic ring

- Aetiology:
  - Fall from a great height onto the ischium or ilium
  - Avulsion of sartorius or rectus femoris tendons in athletes
  - Stress fractures of the pubic rami in osteoporosis.

Clinical features

Stable fractures – fractures not involving the pelvic ring

- Pain on walking.
- Not shocked.
- No visceral injury.

Unstable fractures – fractures of the pelvic ring

- Unable to stand.
- Shocked: iliac vein injury.
- Visceral injury.
- Urethral injury:
  - Blood at the meatus
  - Unable to pass urine.
- Pain on attempting to move the ilium.
- Associated sciatic nerve injury.

Investigation

➤ X-ray: more than one fracture or associated sacroiliac disruption in fractures of the pelvic ring.
➤ Computerized tomography (CT): better assessment of the nature and extent of injury.

Treatment

General management:

➤ As for multiple injury (page 599).

➜

Fractures:

➤ Stable fractures: bed rest for 4–6 weeks
➤ Open-book fractures <2.5 cm: bed rest and sling/elastic girdle for 6 weeks
➤ Open-book fractures >2.5 cm: reduction and external fixation, and bed rest for 6 weeks
➤ Other unstable fractures with minimum displacement: bed rest for 6 weeks
➤ Other unstable fractures with displacement: reduction and external fixation, and bed rest for 6 weeks
➤ Complex unstable fractures: open reduction and internal fixation.

Shock:

➤ Transfuse
➤ Treat sources of intra-abdominal bleeding
➤ Leave retroperitoneal haematoma undisturbed: radiological embolization of pelvic vessels if continued haemorrhage
➤ Stabilize pelvis urgently: external fixator.

Urethral injury (page 531).
Rectal injury:

➤ End colostomy
➤ Anorectal reconstruction: once other injuries are healed
➤ Reversal of colostomy.

Acetabular fractures

Definitions

● Complex fractures involving anterior/posterior rims and the roof are commonest.
● Other fractures involve:
  – Anterior rim
  – Posterior rim: associated with posterior dislocation of the hip
  – Separation of iliac from pubic/ischial parts.
● Aetiology: severe force driving the head of the femur into the acetabulum.

Clinical features

- Often severe generalized injuries.
- Limb lies in internal rotation.
- Associated sciatic nerve injury: particularly with posterior rim fractures and posterior hip dislocation.

Investigation

➤ X-ray.
➤ CT.

Treatment

General management:

➤ Multiple injury (page 599).
➤ Traction.

Fracture:

➤ Minimal weight-bearing with crutches for 6 weeks: for fractures where there is little damage to the weight-bearing acetabular surface
➤ Surgery – most cases:
  - Open reduction and internal fixation
  - Minimal weight-bearing initially
  - Full recovery may take up to a year.

Complications

- Iliofemoral venous thrombosis.
- Sciatic nerve injury.
- Heterotopic bone formation.
- Avascular necrosis of femoral head.
- Osteoarthritis.

Protrusio acetabuli (Otto pelvis)

- A deep acetabulum, with protrusion into the pelvis; may lead to osteoarthritis.
- Aetiology: familial, osteomalacia, Paget's disease, long-standing rheumatoid arthritis.
- Often asymptomatic: incidental finding on X-ray, or as osteoarthritis in later life.
- Treatment of osteoarthritis (page 648).

Congenital dislocation of the hip

Definitions

- Pathology: acetabular and proximal femoral dysplasia.
- Aetiology: polygenic inheritance, high maternal hormones, breech position, swaddling with legs together.
- Affects: up to 20/1000 live births.

Clinical features

Neonate:

- Ortolani's test:
  - Abduction of the hips in 90° flexion is impeded
  - Pressure on greater trochanters reduces the hips with a clunk
  - Further movement is then possible.
- Barlow's test:
  - Attempt to lever the hips in and out during abduction.

Late features:

- Asymmetry
- Clicking hip
- Difficulty in applying napkin.

Investigation

➤ Ultrasound: the hip joints of neonates are not visible on X-ray.
➤ X-ray – after 6 months:
  - Von Rosen's lines: at 45° abduction lines drawn through the femoral shafts should point to the acetabula
  - Perkin's lines – femoral head epiphysis should lie: below a horizontal line drawn through the triradiate cartilages; medial to vertical lines drawn from the outer acetabular edge.

Treatment

3–6 months:

➤ Double napkins for 6 weeks
➤ Abduction splintage for 6 months: if unstable at 6 weeks

➜

> ➤ Splint types:
>   – Von Rosen's malleable splint: holding the thighs to the waist
>   – Pavlik harness: holding the lower legs to the thorax.

6–18 months:

➤ Traction in a vertical frame: to reduce dislocation slowly
➤ Plaster spica at 60° flexion/40° adduction/20° internal rotation for 6 months
➤ Surgery: open reduction if traction unsuccessful.

18 months to 10 years:

➤ Traction: to loosen tissues
➤ Surgery: open reduction and de-rotation osteotomy
➤ Plaster spica for 3 months.

>10 years (>6 years in bilateral cases):

➤ No treatment: attempted reduction may cause avascular necrosis of the femoral head.

Complications

● Avascular necrosis of femoral head: may later result in coxa vara (page 705), flattening of the femoral head, and shortening of the leg, with subsequent osteoarthritis.

Subluxation of the hips

Definitions

● Aetiology: congenital acetabular dysplasia, damage to the acetabular epiphysis or maldevelopment of the femoral head.

Clinical features

● Limited hip abduction: infants.
● Limping and hip pain after strenuous activity: children.
● Osteoarthritis: adults.

Investigation

➤ X-ray.
➤ Exclusion of other causes.

Treatment

Infant:

➤ As congenital dislocation.

Children:

➤ Femoral varus osteotomy.

Adults:

➤ As osteoarthritis.

Intoe gait

- Causes:
  - Anteversion of femoral neck
  - Torsion of tibia
  - Adductus metatarsus (forefoot).
- Affects children.
- Spontaneous correction with growth.
- Corrective osteotomy if condition persists past 8 years of age.

Coxa vara

Femoral neck-shaft angle $<120°$ (normally 160° at birth; 125° in adults).

- Infant:
  - Aetiology: congenital shortening and bowing of the leg when walking begins
  - Treatment: corrective osteotomy.
- Child:
  - Aetiology: Perthes' disease, rickets, fracture through a solitary bone cyst, slipped epiphysis
  - Treatment of the underlying condition.
- Adult:
  - Osteomalacia, osteoporosis, malunion of trochanteric fracture
  - Treatment: underlying condition.

Irritable hip

- Transient synovitis causing hip pain and limited movement for 1–2 weeks: affects mainly boys aged 6–12 years.
- Exclude: Perthes' disease, tuberculosis, juvenile arthritis, slipped epiphysis.
- Treatment: bed rest and traction.

Perthes' disease

Definitions

- Avascular necrosis of the femoral head: remodelling results in abnormal shape.
- Aetiology: post-traumatic joint effusion compressing lateral epiphyseal vessels.
- Affect: boys aged 4–8 years.

Clinical features

- Pain and limping recurring over weeks.
- Limitation of abduction in flexion and internal rotation.

Investigation

➤ X-ray:
  – Widening of joint space in early stage
  – Flattening and lateral displacement of epiphysis in late stage.
➤ Features used to determine Caterall's groups:
  1 Progressive uncovering of epiphysis
  2 Calcification of cartilage lateral to epiphysis
  3 Radiolucent edge of epiphysis: Gage's sign
  4 Severe metaphyseal resorption.

Treatment

➤ Bed rest and traction while the hip is irritable.
➤ Observation: group 1; and patients <7 years of age in groups 2 and 3.
➤ Containment: patients >7 years of age in groups 2 and 3; and group 4.
- Containment:
  – Abduction splint for 1 year
  – Femoral varus osteotomy
  – Pelvic innominate osteotomy.

Slipped upper femoral epiphysis

Definitions

- Posterior displacement of the upper femoral epiphysis.
- Results in premature fusion and remodelling.
- Aetiology: hormonal imbalance and trauma.
- Affects: mainly boys aged 14–16 years; overweight or tall and thin.

Clinical features

- Trauma may precede onset of symptoms.
- Series of minor episodes of hip pain and limping.
- Externally rotated leg with true shortening.
- Limited flexion, abduction and medial rotation.

Investigation

➤ X-ray:
  - Epiphyseal plate is wide
  - Trethowan's sign: femoral head lies below the line of the lateral aspect of the femoral neck
  - Angle of epiphyseal base to femoral neck <90°.

Treatment

Slip <1/3 epiphyseal width and <20° tilt:

➤ Internal fixation.

Slip 1/3–2/3 epiphyseal width and 20–40° tilt:

➤ Internal fixation
➤ Osteotomy if significant deformity after a few years.

Slip >2/3 epiphyseal width and >40° tilt:

➤ Open reduction, subepiphyseal osteotomy and internal fixation.

Complications

- Avascular necrosis/articular chondrolysis: up to 10% of cases requiring reduction.
- Coxa vara.
- Slipping of opposite hip.

Septic arthritis of the hip

Definitions

- Pathology: staphylococcal, streptococcal or *Haemophilus influenzae* infection.
- Aetiology: haematogenous spread, or extension of osteomyelitis.
- Affects: usually those aged <2 years.

Clinical features

- General malaise, fever and pain: difficult to localize.
- Restricted hip movement.

Investigation

➤ Ultrasound: joint effusion.
➤ Aspiration: microbiology.

Treatment

➤ Clindamycin 40 mg/kg daily (divided tds) for 6 weeks.
➤ Traction.

Tuberculosis

Definitions

- Tuberculous infection of the hip joint resulting in ankylosis.
- Aetiology: spread from other site of tuberculous infection.

Clinical features

- Insidious onset.
- Aching and limping.
- Flexed abducted medially rotated hip.
- True and apparent shortening of leg.
- Muscle wasting.

Investigation

➤ X-ray:
  – Destruction of femoral head or acetabular roof
  – Subluxation of hip
  – Calcified ankylosis: late severe cases.
➤ Investigation of tuberculosis (page 142).

Treatment

- ➤ Pyrazinamide 1.5–2.0 g daily for 2 months; and isoniazid 300 mg, rifampicin 450–600 mg, ethambutol 15 mg/kg daily for 6 months.
- ➤ Traction: while hip is symptomatic.
- ➤ Arthrodesis: for painful destroyed joint.
- ➤ Joint replacement: only if disease has been inactive for years.

Rheumatoid arthritis (page 649)

Osteoarthritis

Indications for surgery:

- Progressive pain
- Severe restriction of activity
- Significant deformity
- Joint destruction demonstrated on X-ray.

Types of surgery:

- Prosthetic joint replacement: age >60 years
- Intertrochanteric osteotomy: younger adults with preservation of cartilage
- Pelvic osteotomy: adolescents with acetabular dysplasia
- Arthrodesis: young adults with severe destruction.

Osteonecrosis of the femoral head

Definitions

- Aetiology: idiopathic, iatrogenic – steroids, alcohol abuse, Perthes', sickle-cell disease, Gaucher's disease, septic arthritis and trauma.
- Affects: men aged 20–50 years – idiopathic cases.

Clinical features

- Pain and limping.
- Shortening of leg and muscle wasting.
- Hip rotates externally on passive flexion.
- Internal rotation possible only in extension.

Investigation

➤ X-ray:
  – Segmental sclerosis
  – Subchondral fracture
  – Collapse of femoral head: late stage.

Treatment

No femoral head destruction:

➤ Reduction and fixation: traumatic
➤ Decompression: non-traumatic.

Femoral head destruction:

➤ Osteotomy and grafting: young patients
➤ Joint replacement: older patients.

Collapse of femoral head and osteoarthritis:

➤ Joint replacement.

Bursitis

● Trochanteric bursitis: lateral thigh pain.
● Iliopsoas bursitis: groin pain, tenderness and limited hip movement.
● Occurs with hip implants, gout, rheumatoid arthritis or infection.
● Treatment: rest, non-steroidal anti-inflammatory drugs, injection of steroid and local anaesthetic; and treatment of any underlying cause.

The snapping hip

● Thickened band of gluteus maximus aponeurosis slips over the greater trochanter, causing the hip apparently to 'jump out of place' when walking: affects young women.
● Of importance only in that other causes of the symptom must be excluded.

Complications of total hip replacement

Chronic infection

- Presents with recurrent pain and sometimes a wound sinus.
- Affects 1% of hip replacements: more common in rheumatoid arthritis or psoriasis.
- X-ray: lucent area around implant; erythrocyte sedimentation rate/C-reactive protein are raised.
- Requires removal of the prosthesis and replacement with uncemented type after 4 weeks; alternatively a fibrous union can be allowed to develop at which some movement can occur – girdlestone pseudarthrosis.

Aseptic loosening

- Presents with recurrent pain and X-ray shows lucent area around the implant: requires replacement of prosthesis.

Acute dislocation

- Requires reduction and stabilization with a spica: if recurrent, prosthesis may have to be replaced.

Heterotopic bone formation

- Causes pain and stiffness: non-steroidal anti-inflammatory drugs may reduce incidence.

Fractured neck of femur

Definitions

- Fall on the greater trochanter or external rotation injury from catching the toe.
- Aetiology: osteoporosis.

Clinical features

- Usually affects elderly women.
- Unable to walk; may be able to walk if impacted fracture.
- Shortened and externally rotated leg.

Investigation

➤ X-ray:
  • Femoral neck fracture – Garden's classification:
    – Incomplete impacted fracture
    – Complete undisplaced fracture
    – Moderately displaced fracture
    – Severely displaced fracture.
  • Intertrochanteric fracture.

Treatment

Femoral neck fracture:

➤ Closed reduction and fixation (cannulated screws)
➤ Open reduction and fixation: failed closed reduction and age <70 years
➤ Hemi-arthroplasty (Austin–Moore): failed closed reduction and age >70 years
➤ Total hip replacement: associated acetabular damage, Paget's or metastatic bone disease.

Intertrochanteric fracture:

➤ Internal fixation (dynamic hip screw).

Complications

● Non-union.
● Avascular necrosis of femoral head.
● Osteoarthritis.
● Coxa vara.

Subtrochanteric fracture

● As fractured neck of femur, but also occurs in young patients after severe trauma.
● Most require reduction and internal fixation; severely comminuted fractures require skeletal traction.

Dislocation of the hip

Definitions

● Aetiology:
  – Posterior dislocation: motor vehicle accident where the knee impacts on the dashboard

   – Anterior dislocation (rare): air crashes or weight
     falling onto the back of a bending worker
   – Central dislocation: fall onto the greater trochanter.

Clinical features

Posterior dislocation:

- Leg is shortened, adducted, internally rotated and
  flexed
- Associated long bone fracture
- Associated sciatic nerve injury.

Anterior dislocation:

- Leg is abducted, externally rotated and flexed
- There is no shortening: rectus femoris tendon prevents
  head displacing upwards.

Central dislocation:

- Leg in normal position: no movement possible.

Investigation

➤ X-ray:
   • Posterior dislocation:
     – Femoral head appears above the acetabulum
     – Acetabular roof and posterior rim may be
       broken off.
   • Anterior dislocation:
     – Femoral head appears prominent over the lower
       acetabulum.
   • Central dislocation:
     – Femoral head displaced medially via fractured
       acetabulum.
➤ CT: assesses fractured acetabulum.

Treatment

➤ Closed reduction and traction for 3 weeks (6 weeks for
   central dislocation).
➤ Open reduction: if closed reduction fails.
➤ Joint washout to remove intra-articular fragments.
➤ Internal fixation: of large acetabular fragments.

KNEE

Genu varum (bow leg)

- Distance between knees >6 cm with the heels together.
- Not abnormal in babies.
- Aetiology: variant of normal development; Blount's disease – abnormal growth of posteromedial proximal tibial epiphysis; osteoarthritis, Paget's, epiphyseal injury, vitamin C and D deficiency.
- Surgery: only if significant deformity at age >10 years – staple lateral epiphysis or tibial osteotomy.

Genu valgum (knock knee)

- Distance between malleoli >8 cm with the knees touching.
- Not abnormal <4 years of age.
- Aetiology: variant of normal development, rheumatoid arthritis, epiphyseal injury, vitamin C and D deficiency.
- Surgery: only if significant deformity at age >10 years – staple medial epiphysis or supracondylar osteotomy.

Genu recurvatum

- Hyperextension of the knee from ligamentous laxity.
- Aetiology: congenital – intrauterine position, Ricket's, polio, Charcot's disease.
- No treatment: hyperextension is necessary for stability.
- Calliper: if poor quadriceps power.
- Surgical fixation of patella to the tibial plateau in severe cases.

Meniscal injury

Definitions

- Usually a split along the length of the medial meniscus.
- 'Bucket handle' tear: remains attached at each end.
- Aetiology: twisting strain when weight is taken through the flexed knee, e.g. footballers.
- Affects: usually young men, but can occur with minimal injury in middle age because of fibrosis.
- Lateral meniscus is less often affected.

Clinical features

- Severe pain on medial side of knee: onset on sports field.
- Occasionally knee is locked in flexion.
- Swelling of knee after hours or the following day.
- Recovers with rest.
- Recurrent giving way, pain and swelling.
- McMurray's test: the flexed knee is extended while being rotated, producing sudden locking and snapping free.
- Appley's grinding test: with the patient prone the 90° flexed knee is compressed and rotated, reproducing the pain.

Investigation

➤ X-ray: often normal, may show loose bodies.
➤ Magnetic resonance imaging (MRI): demonstrates tear.
➤ Arthroscopy: allows diagnosis and treatment.

Treatment

If knee is not locked:

➤ Plaster backslab for 3 weeks.

If knee is locked or recurrent symptoms:

➤ Arthroscopy and removal or repair of torn fragment
➤ Open meniscectomy is sometimes required.

Complications

- Associated ligamentous injuries lead to instability and osteoarthritis.

Knee ligament injury

Definitions

- Medial collateral and anterior cruciate ligaments are most commonly injured.
- Aetiology: twisting and valgus/varus force to the flexed knee – sports injury or motor accident.

Clinical features

- Pain and immediate swelling of the knee.
- Severely limited movement.
- Tender over torn ligament.

Examination under anaesthesia:

- Lateral force allows angulation in slight flexion: collateral tear
- Lateral force allows angulation in full extension: collateral and cruciate tear
- Antero-posterior laxity at 90° flexion (drawer test): posterior cruciate tear

Investigation

➤ X-ray:
 – Ligament may have been avulsed with a fragment of bone
 – Stress films may show joint space opening up.
➤ Arthroscopy: contra-indicated in clinically severe injury.

Treatment

Partial tears:

➤ Functional brace
➤ Exercise programme 6 weeks.

Complete tear of medial collateral ligament:

➤ Cast-brace 6 weeks.

Complete tear of anterior cruciate ligament:

➤ Surgical repair within 14 days
➤ Above-knee plaster cast for 6 weeks.

Combined complete tears:

➤ Cast brace 6 weeks
➤ Late surgical anterior cruciate ligament reconstruction.

Unfit for surgery:

➤ Plaster cylinder for 8 weeks.

Chronic ligamentous instability

Definitions
- May result after healing of acute ligamentous injury.

Clinical features
- Feeling that the knee will give way.
- Knee gives way on pivoting to affected side.
- Lateral or anteroposterior instability demonstrable without anaesthesia.

Investigation
➤ X-ray.
➤ MRI.
➤ Arthroscopy.

Treatment
➤ Exercise programme for 6 months.
➤ Surgical repair of ligaments and capsule; may involve graft of patellar tendon or synthetic material, or tendon transfers.

Osteochondritis dissecans

Definitions
- A condition resulting in loose bodies in the knee.
- Pathology: separation of avascular fragments of bone and cartilage.
- Aetiology: repeated minor trauma causing avascular necrosis of subchondral bone.
- Common location: lower or lateral part of medial femoral condyle.
- Affects: men aged 15–20 years.

Clinical features
- Intermittent aching or swelling of the knee.
- Giving way.
- Locking.

Investigation

➤ X-ray:
  – Line of demarcation around a lesion
  – Loose body.
➤ MRI.
➤ Arthroscopy.

Treatment

Early lesion:

➤ Avoid strenuous activity for 6–12 months.

Unstable lesion or loose body:

➤ Arthroscopy and removal of loose bodies; fixation of larger fragments
➤ Plaster cast for 6 weeks after surgery.

Other loose bodies in the knee joint and locking of the knee

● Loose bodies (joint mice) result from trauma and degenerative conditions.
● May cause sudden locking.
● Many are visible on X-ray.
● May require arthroscopic removal.

Chondromalacia patellae

Definitions

● Overuse injury resulting in softening of the articular surface of the patella.
● Aetiology: malalignment or abnormal shape of patellofemoral surfaces predispose.
● Affects: teenage girls or athletic adults.

Clinical features

● Pain below the patella aggravated by climbing stairs.
● Malalignment of the patella may be apparent.
● Pain on pressing patella against femur.
● Effusion.
● Quadriceps wasting.

Investigation
➤ X-rays: skyline views may show tilting or subluxation.
➤ Computerized tomography (CT): reliably demonstrates malposition.

Treatment
➤ Avoid stressful activities.
➤ Physiotherapy.

If persistent incapacitating symptoms or correctable abnormality:

➤ Surgery:
  – Lateral release of patella
  – Realignment of patella
  – Patellectomy is sometimes required.

Patellar tendinitis ('jumper's knee')
● Pain and tenderness from overuse of quadriceps: spontaneous recovery with alteration of activity.

Osgood–Schlatter's disease
● Painful swelling of the tibial tubercle in adolescents – a traction injury to the apophysis: spontaneous recovery with alteration of activity.

Prepatellar bursitis (housemaid's knee)
● Now occurs more often in carpet layers: treated by bandaging, avoiding kneeling and sometimes aspiration.

Infrapatellar bursitis (clergyman's knee)
● Similar to prepatellar bursitis.

Bursitis anserina (breast-stroker's knee)
● A painless lump behind the medial head of the gastrocnemius that resolves spontaneously.

Semimembranosus bursitis

- A painless lump behind the knee.

Baker's cyst

- Synovial herniation producing a fluctuant swelling behind the knee; rupture causes acute painful calf swelling, which may be confused with deep vein thrombosis.

Patellar dislocation

Definitions

- Aetiology: lateral force to the patella with the knee flexed.

Clinical features

- Knee gives way: patient falls to the ground.
- Deformity: medial condyle is prominent but patella actually lies laterally.
- No active or passive knee movement possible.
- Medial bruising indicates quadriceps tear.

Investigation

➤ X-ray: laterally displaced patella.

Treatment

➤ Reduction: push the patella back into place – anaesthesia not always required.
➤ Repair of quadriceps tear prevents recurrent dislocation.

Recurrent dislocation of the patella

- Results from quadriceps tear in acute dislocation, or ligamentous laxity, patellofemoral abnormalities and genu valgus.
- Requires surgical realignment of the patella.

Meniscal cysts

- Repeated trauma results in firm swellings at the joint line anterior to the collateral ligaments.
- Treated by arthroscopic removal of the damaged portion of meniscus from which they arise.

Treatment of rheumatoid arthritis of the knee

- Treatment of the generalized condition.
- Arthroscopic synovectomy: for synovitis not controlled by drugs.
- Supracondylar osteotomy: for marked valgus deformity.
- Prosthetic joint replacement: for extensive joint destruction.

Treatment of osteoarthritis of the knee

- Analgesics.
- Elastic support.
- Prednisolone 40 mg intra-articular injection; repeated weekly if required.
- Arthroscopic washout: removal of degenerate material gives transient improvement.
- Patellectomy: for disease confined to patellofemoral joint.
- Tibial osteotomy: for young patients with medial compartment disease.
- Prosthetic joint replacement: older patients with severe joint destruction.
- Arthrodesis: severe disease where there is a contra-indication to arthroplasty.

Rupture of rectus femoris muscle

- Affects elderly patients and those on steroid therapy.
- Forced knee extension against resistance.
- Torn muscle forms a lump in the thigh but extensor function is usually preserved.
- No treatment required.

Patellar fractures

Definitions

- Aetiology:
  - Stellate fracture: direct force
  - Transverse fracture: forced knee extension against resistance.

Clinical features

- Pain and swelling over the patella.
- Loss of active knee extension: quadriceps mechanism is disrupted.

Investigation

➤ X-ray: stellate or transverse fracture.
➤ Beware incidental finding of a bipartite patella: here a smooth line separates the superolateral part.

Treatment

➤ Aspirate haemarthrosis.
➤ Plaster backslab for 4 weeks: remove intermittently and mobilize as soon as pain allows.
➤ Patellectomy: for displaced stellate fractures.
➤ Tension band wires; wires are tightened across K-wires passed through the fragments – for transverse fractures.

Ligamentum patellae rupture

- Forced knee extension against resistance in young adults may result in rupture of the patellar ligament.
- Only limited active knee extension is possible: CT/ultrasound confirms.
- Treatment: surgical repair.

Femoral shaft fractures

Definitions

- Aetiology:
  - Spiral fracture: severe torsional force
  - Transverse fractures: severe direct force, e.g. motorcycle accidents.
  - Affects: usually young adults.

Clinical features

- Thigh is swollen and bruised.
- Leg is short and externally rotated.
- Leg may have angular deformity.

Possible causes:

- Shock
- Fat embolism
- Associated pelvic fractures.

Investigation

➤ X-ray.

Treatment

➤ As for multiple injury (page 599): general management.
➤ Splintage for transportation to hospital.

Adults:

➤ Skeletal traction (page 620): achieves initial reduction and stabilization
➤ Closed medullary nailing (page 620): method of choice for closed fractures
➤ External fixation (page 620): the method of choice for compound fractures
➤ Continued skeletal traction for 12 weeks: where operative facilities are not available.

Children:

➤ Balanced skin traction: for 2 weeks in infants, up to 6 weeks in teenagers.

Supracondylar fracture of the femur

- Occurs in young adults with severe direct force, and in osteoporosis with lesser injury.
- Requires internal fixation, and non-weight bearing for 12 weeks.

Fracture of a femoral condyle

- Occurs when the tibia is driven at the femur after a fall onto the feet from a significant height.
- Requires internal fixation.

Fracture of the tibial plateau

Definitions

- Aetiology:
  - Severe varus or valgus force with axial loading
  - Sometimes from car bumper impact with a pedestrian.
- Types:
  1 Fracture of lateral tibial condyle
  2 Comminuted fracture of lateral tibial condyle
  3 Comminuted fracture of lateral tibial condyle with depressed articular surface
  4 Fracture of medial tibial condyle
  5 Fracture of both condyles
  6 Associated subcondylar fracture.

Clinical features

- Haemarthrosis.
- Unable to move knee.
- Knee may be unstable.

Investigation

➤ X-rays: anteroposterior, lateral, oblique and sometimes stress views under anaesthesia.

Treatment of fracture types

➤ Types as above:
  1 Internal fixation
  2&3 Elevation and internal fixation (aspiration, traction and cast brace in osteoporosis)
  4 Aspiration, traction and cast brace
  5&6 Aspiration, traction and cast brace; internal fixation of complex injuries in young adults.

LEG AND ANKLE

Ruptured Achilles tendon

Definitions
- Aetiology: stress injury following degeneration of the tendon.
- Affects: usually age >40 years.

Clinical features
- Sudden pain just above the heel when running or jumping.
- Gap noted 5 cm above the insertion of the tendon.
- Simmonds' test: calf squeezed with the patient prone – foot remains still if the tendon is ruptured.

Investigation
➤ Clinical diagnosis.

Treatment
➤ Plaster cast with foot in equinus for 8 weeks.
➤ Surgical repair: if tendon ends do not approximate on passive plantar flexion.

Tears of the soleus muscle
- Similar injury to ruptured Achilles tendon with pain and tenderness halfway up the calf: requires physiotherapy and heel-raise.

Achilles peritendinitis
- Local irritation around the tendon occurring in athletes, joggers, long-distance walkers.
- Treatment: ice-packs, rest, ultrasound, heel-raise; Prednisolone 40 mg/lidocaine 10 mg injection – but may precipitate tendon rupture.

Calcaneal knob

- Prominence of the calcaneum in girls causes painful blistering: requires open-backed shoes or padding.

Sever's disease (osteochondritis of the calcaneum)

Definitions

- Aetiology: traction injury to the apophysis of the calcaneum.
- Affects: boys, at about 10 years of age.

Clinical features

- Pain and tenderness at the tendon insertion.

Investigation

➤ X-ray: fragmentation of the apophysis.

Treatment

➤ Restriction of activity for a few weeks.
➤ Heel-raise.

Tuberculosis of the ankle joint

- Painful swelling of the ankle joint, sinus formation and calf muscle wasting.
- Treatment: non-weight bearing in a calliper, and a course of antituberculous chemotherapy (page 143).
- Arthrodesis is often required later for painful ankle stiffness.

Fracture of the shaft of the tibia and fibula

Definitions

- Aetiology:
  - Spiral fracture of both bones at different levels: rotational force
  - Transverse or oblique fractures at the same level: angulating force.

Clinical features

- Deformity: tented skin may necrose.
- Bruising and swelling.
- Foot externally rotated.
- Often compound.
- Associated vascular and neurological injury.

Investigation

➤ X-ray.

Treatment

Undisplaced fracture:

➤ Plaster cast from thigh to metatarsal heads for 8 weeks
➤ Admit and elevate for 2 days: swelling may require splitting of the cast
➤ Functional brace after 4 weeks for transverse fractures.

Displaced transverse fractures:

➤ Reduction and closed intramedullary nailing.

Displaced long oblique and spiral fractures:

➤ Reduction and external fixation.

Metaphyseal fractures:

➤ Internal fixation.

Compound fractures:

➤ General principles of management of compound fractures (page 618)
➤ External fixation.

Complications

- Compartment syndrome.
- Osteomyelitis.
- Malunion.
- Delayed union.
- Non-union.
- Volkmann's contracture.
- Chronic venous insufficiency.
- Peroneal and tibial nerve injury.

Isolated fracture of the shaft of the fibula

- Results from direct force.
- Splinted by the intact tibia: requires only analgesia.

Isolated fracture of the shaft of the tibia

- Occurs in children.
- Treatment: reduction and plaster cast for 12 weeks.

Stress fracture of the tibia

Definitions

- Transverse tibial fracture occurring in the absence of severe injury.
- Aetiology: repeated athletic stress.
- Affects: soldiers, dancers and runners.

Clinical features

- Pain in the shin.

Investigation

➤ X-ray:
  - Initially no abnormality
  - New bone formation and transverse cortical defect: after 4 weeks
  - May be confused with osteosarcoma.

Treatment

➤ Restriction of stressful activity.
➤ Resolves over an 8-week period.

Shin splints

- Unexplained pain and tenderness in the posteromedial border of the lower tibia after vigorous activity in children.

Sprained ankle

Definitions

- Partial tear of the collateral ligaments of the ankle: usually lateral.
- Aetiology: forced ankle inversion from stumbling.

Clinical features

- Swelling of the ankle.
- Bruising may appear up to 2 days later.
- Tenderness over lateral aspect of joint.

Examination under anaesthesia:

- Excessive inversion: complete tear.

Investigation

➤ X-rays (stress films under anaesthesia): talar tilting >10° indicates complete tear.

Treatment

Partial tear:

➤ Crepe bandage
➤ Walk normally as soon as possible
➤ Physiotherapy and ultrasound.

Complete tear:

➤ Plaster cast knee to toe with foot plantargrade for 6 weeks, then brace and physiotherapy
➤ Surgical repair: may be an advantage where the ankle is subjected to great stress, e.g. dancers, athletes.

Rupture of the medial (deltoid) ligament

- Associated with fracture of the distal fibula or tibiofibular ligament injury.
- X-ray: widening of the joint space.
- Treatment: reduction and internal fixation.

Pott's fracture

Definitions

- Types:
    - Fracture below the tibiofibular syndesmosis
    - Oblique fibular fracture from the joint line
    - Fibular fracture above the syndesmosis with rupture of the interosseous membrane and widening of the mortise
    - Maisonneuve fracture: type C with high (hence possibly overlooked) fibular fracture
    - Pilon fracture: a posterior triangular fragment of tibial articular surface.
- Aetiology:
    - Twisting injury – forced external rotation with abduction or adduction: most fractures
    - Severe axial force – talus driven directly into the articular surface of the lower tibia: pilon fracture.

Clinical features

- Swelling of the ankle.
- Deformity.

Investigation

➤ X-rays: anteroposterior, lateral, oblique and mortise views.

Treatment

Undisplaced fractures and fractures below the tibiofibular joint:

➤ Reduction and plaster cast for 6–12 weeks.

Displaced fractures and fracture dislocations:

➤ Open reduction and internal fixation
➤ Elevation and splintage for 2 weeks.

Fracture-separation of the distal tibial and fibular epiphyses (Salter–Harris fractures)

- Ankle fractures in children: undisplaced – reduction and plaster cast for 3 weeks; displaced – open reduction and internal fixation.

- Asymmetric growth or shortening may result from premature epiphyseal fusion.

Fractures of the talus

Definitions

- Rare.
- Aetiology: falling from great height or motor accident – considerable force required.

Types of injury:

- Fractures: head, neck, body or lateral process
- Dislocations: midtarsal, subtalar or total dislocation
- Fracture dislocation.

Clinical features

- Swelling of the foot.
- Deformity.

Investigation

➤ X-rays: anteroposterior, lateral and oblique views.

Treatment

Undisplaced fractures:

➤ Below-knee plaster cast for up to 8 weeks.

Displaced fractures and fracture dislocations:

➤ Urgent reduction: to avoid skin necrosis and avascular necrosis of the talus
➤ Internal fixation of large fragments
➤ Below-knee plaster cast for 8 weeks.

Complications

- Avascular necrosis of talus: no attached muscle to maintain its blood supply.

Recurrent dislocation of the peroneal tendons

- The patient can demonstrate the tendons moving over the fibula on dorsiflexion and eversion: may require surgical reattachment of the retinaculum.

FOOT

Talipes equinovarus (clubfoot)

Definitions

- Congenital deformity where the foot and ankle turn inwards.
- Bilateral in one-third of cases.
- Aetiology: polygenic inheritance.
- Associated with spina bifida.

Clinical features

- Noticed on routine neonatal examination.
- Talipes deformity:
  - Inverted heel: talus points downwards
  - Foot twisted so that the sole faces posteromedially
  - Forefoot adducted and laterally rotated.
- Foot cannot be dorsiflexed to touch the leg: in a normal neonate this is possible.

Investigation

➤ X-ray: to assess progress of treatment.

Treatment

➤ Splinting from 3 days of age: replaced every week until correction is achieved.
➤ Surgical soft tissue release for resistant cases from 8 weeks of age; this may be delayed until walking begins – the larger foot facilitates surgery.

Postural equinovarus

- A normal baby has an equinus foot but in this case it can be dorsiflexed so that the toes touch the leg: no treatment is required.

Pes cavus

Definitions

- Higher than normal foot arch.
- Usually bilateral.
- Aetiology:
  - Idiopathic
  - Neurological disorders: peroneal muscular atrophy, Friedreich's ataxia.

Clinical features

- Noticed at age 8–10 years.
- High instep.
- Clawed toes: mobile initially, later fixed.
- Callosities under metatarsal heads.

Investigation

➤ X-rays – in the standing position:
  - Calcaneal pith >30°.
  - Meary's angle (the axis of the talus compared to the axis of the first metatarsal) >0°.

Treatment

➤ No treatment if asymptomatic.
➤ Specially made shoes to prevent callosities.
➤ Arch supports.
➤ Corrective surgery for severe cases:
  - Steindler's operation: release of tissues from plantar surface of the calcaneum
  - Robert Jones tendon transfer
  - Calcaneal osteotomy.

Pes planus (flat foot)

Definitions

- Absence of normal foot arch.
- Aetiology: ligamentous laxity, obesity, other deformities of the leg, paralytic and wasting disorders, arthritis.

Clinical features

- Children: noticed by parents.
- Adults: asymptomatic or foot strain.
- Prominent navicular.
- Loss of arch: medial border of foot in contact with the ground.
- Valgus heels.
- Abnormal shoe wear.

Investigation

➤ X-ray/computerized tomography: only for planning surgery.

Treatment

Small children:

➤ No treatment needed.

Older children/adults:

➤ No treatment if asymptomatic
➤ Heel cups or arch support.

Underlying disorder and symptomatic:

➤ Physiotherapy: tendon stretching exercises
➤ Surgery – a variety of procedures involving: tendon advancements; fusion of midtarsal and tarso-metatarsal joints; excision of prominent bone at the navicular.

Fractured calcaneum

Definitions

- Aetiology: fall from a great height onto the heels.
- Associated: injuries of skull base, spine, pelvis or hip.
- Types:
  - Extra-articular
  - Intra-articular
  - Fracture dislocations.

Clinical features

- Painful, swollen foot.
- Bruise over the sole.

- Broad, squat heel.
- Ankle movement is possible.

Investigation
➤ X-rays: lateral, oblique and axial.

Treatment
➤ Admission, elevation and ice packs to reduce swelling.

Extra-articular fractures and undisplaced intra-articular fractures:

➤ Below-knee cast: non-weight bearing 4 weeks, then partial weight bearing 4 weeks.

Displaced intra-articular fractures:

➤ Open reduction and internal fixation
➤ Non-weight bearing for 8 weeks.

Treatment of tarsal injuries

- Sprains: bandaging.
- Undisplaced fractures: elevation then plaster cast for 6 weeks.
- Displaced fractures: open reduction and internal fixation.
- Fracture–dislocations: closed reduction and K-wire fixation and plaster cast for 6 weeks.
- Tarso-metatarsal (Lisfranc's) dislocation: closed reduction and plaster cast for 6 weeks, no treatment if discovered >4 weeks after injury.

Kohler's disease

- Osteochondritis of the navicular causes painful limping in a child aged <5 years: settles with strapping for a few weeks.

Tarsal tunnel syndrome

- Pain and sensory disturbance in the medial forefoot from compression of the posterior tibial nerve in the tarsal tunnel beneath the flexor retinaculum: sometimes requires surgical decompression.

Morton's metatarsalgia

- Entrapment of a digital nerve and subsequent neuroma formation results in pain in the forefoot radiating to the toes: affects women aged 40–50 years.
- Requires protective padding or surgical excision if unresolved.

Freiberg's disease

- Osteochondritis of the second metatarsal head in young women, forming a tender bony lump: X-ray confirms diagnosis.
- Sometimes requires synovectomy and partial excision of the metatarsal head.

Stress fracture of the metatarsal (march fracture)

- Overuse injury of the foot of a young adult: initially no change on X-ray until callous appears.
- No treatment required.

Hallux valgus and 'bunions'

Definitions

- Excessive lateral angulation of the big toe away from the axis of the metatarsal.
- Usually affects women aged >50 years.
- Usually bilateral.
- Aetiology: familial predisposition, loss of muscle tone in elderly, wearing tight shoes, rheumatoid arthritis.
- Associated: varus splaying of first metatarsal.

Clinical features

- There may be pain from shoe pressure.
- Valgus deformity.
- Bunion: thickening and inflammation of bursa over the first metatarsal head.

Investigation

➤ X-rays – taken when standing:
   - Intermetatarsal angle >9°
   - Metatarsophalangeal angle >15°
   - May be osteoarthritis of first metatarsophalangeal joint.

Treatment

<25 years:

➤ Mitchell's osteotomy: excision of the prominent area of the metatarsal head, which is used as a bone graft in a corrective osteotomy at the metatarsal base.

25–50 years:

➤ Reconstructive exostectomy and capsulorrhaphy.

>50 years:

➤ Keller's operation: excision of the metatarsophalangeal joint
➤ Arthrodesis is an alternative.

Hallux rigidus

● Stiffness of the first metatarsophalangeal joint from osteoarthritis, trauma, osteochondritis or gout; causes pain on walking.
● May require rocker-soled shoes, and, in severe cases, osteotomy, joint replacement or arthrodesis.

Hammer toe

● Proximal interphalangeal joint fixed in flexion, distal interphalangeal and metatarsophalangeal joints are extended.
● Causes pain and callosities over dorsal surface of toes.
● May require excision of the proximal interphalangeal joint.

Claw toes

- Flexion of interphalangeal joints, extension of metatarsophalangeal joints.
- Aetiology: usually no cause, but occurs in peroneal muscular atrophy, poliomyelitis and rheumatoid arthritis.
- Presents with metatarsalgia: pain beneath the metatarsal heads.
- Treatment includes: supportive metatarsal bar, osteotomy, joint excision, arthrodesis or amputation.

Ainhum (page 168)

Gout

- Severe inflammation of the first metatarsophalangeal joint: raised uric acid level.
- Indometacin 100 mg bd orally prevents recurrence – in acute gout allopurinol 100 mg daily od orally.

Toenail disorders

Ingrowing toenail

- The nail burrows into the lateral groove, causing inflammation.
- Requires trimming of the nail or raising the edge with a pledget of cotton wool. For persisting problems: excision of the edge of the nail and a wedge of soft tissue, with phenol ablation of the nail bed; or removal of the nail and its germinal matrix (Zadik's operation).

Onychogryphosis

- Hard, thick, curved nail: may result from fungal infection.
- Requires trimming, or sometimes avulsion of the nail; with or without removal of the nail bed.

Subungual exostosis

- Bony outgrowth pushes the nail up.
- Requires excision.

Subungual malignant melanoma

● As malignant melanoma (page 201).

Plantar fasciitis (policeman's heel)

Definitions

● Unexplained condition characterized by heel pain.
● Affects: mainly men aged 30–60 years.
● Aetiology: local trauma.
● Associated with: gonorrhoea, Reiter's disease and ankylosing spondylitis.

Clinical features

● Heel pain.
● Tenderness of the attachment of the long plantar ligament.

Investigation

➤ X-ray: may show bony spur projecting forwards from the calcaneal tuberosity.

Treatment

➤ Ibuprofen 400 mg qds orally.

Severe cases:

➤ Protective cast
➤ Prednisolone 40 mg/lidocaine 10 mg injection.

Diabetic foot (page 558)

Malignant melanoma of the foot

See Malignant melanoma (page 201).

Madura foot (Mycetoma; page 145)

● Tropical chronic infection of the foot from actino-mycosis species, introduced by puncture of the foot by acacia thorns.

- Hard subcutaneous chronic foot swelling, with draining sinuses and eventually bone destruction.
- Investigation: microscopy and culture of discharge.
- Treatment: dapsone 50–100 mg daily.

SPINE

Spina bifida

Definitions

- Congenital condition, which, in severe form, results in exposure of the lower spinal canal, paraplegia and lower limb deformities.
- Types:
  - Spina bifida cystica: severe form with protrusion of cord tissues
  - Spina bifida occulta: mild form without protrusion.
- Aetiology: embryonic failure of fusion of developing posterior vertebral arches.
- Association: possibly folic acid deficiency, and drugs affecting folic acid metabolism.
- Incidence:
  - Spinal bifida cystica 3/1000 live births
  - Spinal bifida occulta 5% of lumbar spine X-rays.

Clinical features

Spinal bifida cystica:

- Saccular lesion over lumbosacral spine:
  - Meningocoele: sac contains only cerebrospinal fluid
  - Meningomyelocoele: sac contains spinal cord or nerve roots
  - 'Open' defects are exposed; 'closed' defects are covered by skin.
- Hydrocephalus
- Paralysis: may deteriorate over a few days
- Extent of paralysis:
  - One-third complete lower motor neuron paralysis below the level of the lesion

- One-third complete paralysis at the level of the lesion, but cord function below
- One-third incomplete paralysis.

Spina bifida occulta:

- Incidental finding on X-ray
- Lumbosacral dimple or tuft of hair
- Cauda equina syndrome may develop at any time:
  - Weakness, numbness and trophic changes in one or both legs
  - Urinary retention.

Investigation

➤ X-ray.
➤ Myelography.
➤ Computerized tomography (CT).
➤ Magnetic resonance imaging (MRI).

Treatment

Spina bifida cystica:

➤ Skin closure: within 48 hours
➤ Treatment of hydrocephalus (page 221): within few days
➤ Correction of deformities:
  - Stretching and strapping: first 12 months
  - Surgical correction: after several months.
➤ Urinary tract monitoring: appliances or diversion may be required
➤ Avoid pressure necrosis of denervated skin.

Scoliosis

Definitions

- Apparent lateral curvature of the spine.
- Types: postural or structural.
- Aetiology:
  - Postural: compensatory curvature from extraspinal disease, e.g. short leg or hip contracture
  - Structural: idiopathic, osteopathic, neuropathic or connective tissue disorder.

- Idiopathic scoliosis:
  - Incidence: 3/1000, affects mainly girls
  - Onset: adolescent (commonest), juvenile or infantile.
- Osteopathic scoliosis:
  - Congenital anomalies: hemivertebrae, wedge vertebrae, fused vertebrae or absent/fused ribs
  - Acquired deformity: rickets or osteogenesis imperfecta.

Clinical features

Postural scoliosis:

- Curve disappears on sitting
- True or apparent leg shortening.

Adolescent idiopathic scoliosis:

- Thoracic curves are convex to the right
- Lumbar curves are convex to the left
- Risk factors for progressive deterioration:
  - Younger age
  - Marked curvature.

Investigation

Adolescent idiopathic scoliosis:

➤ X-rays:
  - Cobb's angle: the degree of deformity, measured between the upper and lowermost vertebrae of the curve
  - Risser's sign: ossification of the iliac crests indicates skeletal maturity; progression is then unlikely.

Osteopathic scoliosis: exclude spinal cord involvement:

➤ Myelography
➤ CT
➤ MRI.

Treatment

Adolescent idiopathic scoliosis:

➤ Observation: measure degree of deformity every 4 months
➤ Support brace: for progressive deformity with >20° Cobb angle:
  - Milwaukee brace: fits under chin and occiput
  - Boston brace: fits under arms.

➔

➤ No further intervention: if skeletal maturity reached with <30° Cobb angle
➤ Surgery: correction and arthrodesis of the curve with Harrington or Cotrel–Dubousset fixation for:
  – Progression in spite of other treatment
  – Cosmetically unacceptable severe curvature.

Osteopathic scoliosis:

➤ Surgery: early posterior fusion.

Scheuermann's kyphosis

Definitions

● Abnormal dorsal curvature of the spine in young women.
● Aetiology:
  – Growth disorder resulting in wedge-shaped vertebrae
  – Unknown.
● Affects: teenagers, mainly girls.

Clinical features

● Backache.
● Progressively round-shouldered appearance.
● Smooth thoracic kyphosis: cannot be corrected by postural change.
● Compensatory lumbar lordosis

Investigation

➤ X-ray:
  – Irregular, fragmented vertebral end-plates
  – Schmorl's nodes: translucent defects of subchondral bone
  – Degree of deformity measured as for scoliosis.

Treatment

➤ Exercises and postural training: for deformity <40°.
➤ Brace: for deformity >40° in a child who is still growing.
➤ Surgical correction and arthrodesis for:
  – Deformity >60° with skeletal maturity
  – Severely painful deformity
  – Impending spastic paresis.

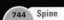

Kyphosis in the elderly

- Osteoporotic wedging of vertebrae and narrowing of disc spaces results in increasing stoop, typically in elderly women.
- Compensatory lumbar lordosis causes lumbosacral pain.

Acute disc rupture

Definitions

- Extrusion of the disc nucleus into the spinal canal or intervertebral foramen.
- Types:
  - Central rupture: cauda equina compression
  - Posterolateral rupture: nerve root compression.
- Aetiology: stress from flexion and compression: greatest at L4/5 and L5/S1; but may occur at higher levels, including thoracic and cervical discs.
- Affects: fit adults.

Clinical features

General symptoms and signs:

- Occurs while lifting and stooping
- Severe lower back pain
- Unable to straighten up
- Sciatica: develops after 1–2 days
- Paraesthesia of the foot
- Scoliosis concave to side of disc herniation
- Sensory loss L5 or S1 dermatome
- Motor weakness and reflex changes at knee (L3–4) or ankle (S1); loss of dorsiflexion of the great toe (L5).

Central disc prolapse:

- Urinary retention
- Sensory loss over sacrum.

Investigation

➤ X-ray: exclude bone disease, but narrowing of disc space is not essential.
➤ Myelogram.
➤ CT.
➤ MRI.

Treatment

➤ Rest:
  - Confine to bed with knees flexed
  - Pelvic traction
  - Analgesics and local warmth.
➤ Reduction:
  - Traction for 2 weeks reduces 90% of cases
  - Epidural injection of Prednisolone 40 mg/lidocaine 10 mg.
➤ Surgery: partial laminectomy, microdiscectomy or percutaneous discectomy. Indications for surgery are:
  - Cauda equina compression not resolving within 6 hours
  - Neurological deterioration during treatment
  - Persisting neurological symptoms after 3 weeks.
➤ Rehabilitation and physiotherapy: how to move with least strain.

Spondylosis

Definitions

● Desiccation of intervertebral discs with disc flattening, chronic herniation and displacement of facet joints.
● Aetiology: normal ageing.
● Affects: age >40 years.

Clinical features

● Lumbar spondylosis.
● Intermittent, recurrent backache.
● Induced by working, standing or sitting for long periods.
● Sciatica.
● 'Locking' and 'giving way'.
● Signs of disc prolapse or spinal stenosis.

Investigation

➤ X-ray:
  - Loss of disc space
  - Sclerosis of vertebral bodies
  - Bony spurs
  - Facet joint malalignment on oblique views
➤ MRI.

Treatment

➤ Physiotherapy.
➤ Corsets.
➤ Facet injection: prednisolone 40 mg/lidocaine 10 mg under X-ray guidance.
➤ Modify activities.
➤ Ibuprofen 400 mg tds orally.
➤ Spinal fusion: persisting symptoms and proven facet joint instability.

Prognosis:

➤ Up to 20% failure of fusion.
➤ Instability may develop at other sites.

Spinal stenosis

Definitions

● Narrowing of the spinal canal from hypertrophy at the posterior disc margin.
● Aetiology: spondylosis and osteoarthritis.
● Affects: males >50 years of age.

Clinical features

● Spinal claudication:
  – Aching and paraesthesiae of one or both legs and thighs on walking
  – Relieved by sitting.

Investigation

➤ X-ray: spondylosis, spondylolisthesis or osteoarthritis.
➤ MRI.

Treatment

➤ Conservative for tolerable symptoms.
➤ Laminectomy to relieve pressure for limiting symptoms.

Spondylolisthesis

Definitions

- Forward shift of the spine relative to that below.
- Aetiology: spondylosis, facet degeneration, congenital anomalies.

Clinical features

- Step noticed by mother: children.
- Backache: young adults.
- Incidental finding on X-ray: patients with spondylosis.
- Cord/cauda equina compression: rarely in early onset cases.

Investigation

➤ X-ray: forward shift of L4 on L5, or L5 on S1.

Treatment

➤ Conservative.
➤ Surgery for:
  - Severe symptoms
  - Progressive slip >50%
  - Neurological compression.

Prognosis:

➤ Early onset cases – congenital in origin: high risk of neurological compression
➤ Adult cases: low risk of progression.

Ankylosing spondylitis (page 653)

Coccydynia

- Pain from the region of the coccyx in the absence of identifiable pathology.
- May require prednisolone 40 mg/lidocaine 10 mg injection, and sometimes excision of the coccyx.

Pyogenic spondylitis and discitis

Definitions

- Infection of disc or vertebrae causes local destruction and abscess formation.
- Aetiology:
  - Haematogenous spread of infection from urinary tract to vertebrae
  - Iatrogenic from instrumentation: of disc space.

Clinical features

- Immunocompromised patient, e.g. drug addict.
- Recent instrumentation of spine or source of sepsis.
- Back pain.
- Occasionally nerve root compression

Investigation

➤ Erythrocyte sedimentation rate (ESR)/C-reactive protein (CRP)/white cell count (WCC): elevated.
➤ Antistaphylococcal antibodies: may be high titre.
➤ X-ray: bone destruction and narrow disc space.
➤ Bone scan: increased activity.

Treatment

➤ Bed rest until symptoms settle.
➤ Intravenous antibiotics for 6 weeks.
➤ Spinal brace for 6 weeks.
➤ Evacuation of an abscess.

Spinal tuberculosis (Pott's disease of the spine)

Definitions

- Tuberculous infection of the spine: commonest site of skeletal tuberculosis.
- Aetiology: haematogenous spread of *Mycobacterium tuberculosis* from pulmonary or other primary site.
- Affects: mainly children.

- Pathological process:
  - Infection begins in the vertebral body adjacent to the disc
  - Bone destruction and caseation spread to adjacent vertebrae
  - Vertebral bodies collapse
  - Vertebrae fuse in angulated arrangement.

Clinical features

- Long history of ill health, primary tuberculosis.
- Backache.
- Angular kyphosis.
- Loin or groin abscess in active disease.
- Reduced spinal movements.
- Pott's paraplegia:
  - Pressure from an abscess: early
  - Pressure from deformity: late.

Investigation

- ➤ Mantoux: positive.
- ➤ ESR/CRP: elevated.
- ➤ Needle biopsy: histology and microbiology.

Treatment

- ➤ Isoniazid 300 mg daily, rifampicin 450–600 mg daily, pyrazinamide 1.5–2.0 g daily orally for 6 months; and in addition ethambutol 15 mg/kg daily orally for the first 2 months.
- ➤ Bed rest.
- ➤ Surgery:
  - Drainage of abscess
  - Decompression: for paraplegia
  - Correction of deformity: for severe kyphosis.

SPINAL INJURIES

Cervical spine

Definitions

- Aetiology: any severe head or supraclavicular trauma.

Clinical features
- Neck pain.
- Deformity.
- Limb neurological signs.

Investigation
➤ X-ray: lateral view (must include C1–C7 and T1):
  - Loss of lordosis
  - Loss of smooth line of front/back of vertebral bodies, lateral masses and base of spinous processes
  - Trachea displaced: haematoma
  - Distance from odontoid to arch of atlas >3 mm (4.5 mm in children)
  - Forward shift of <1/2 vertebral body depth indicates unilateral facet dislocation
  - Forward shift of >1/2 vertebral body depth indicates bilateral facet dislocation.
➤ X-ray – anteroposterior view:
  - Loss of lateral outline
  - Odontoid and C1 lateral mass fracture: open-mouth view.
➤ CT: if doubtful X-ray or cord compression.
➤ MRI: if doubtful X-ray or cord compression.

Treatment
➤ Halo body cast: a metal ring encircling the skull vault is screwed to the cranium and attached by metal rods to a cast surrounding the thorax for 12 weeks.
➤ Surgical decompression and operative fixation for cord compression.

Whiplash injury

Definitions
- Soft tissue hyperextension injury of the neck.
- Aetiology: motor accidents – front-to-back impact.

Clinical features
- Painful, stiff neck.
- Concussion-like symptoms.

Investigation

➤ X-ray.
➤ MRI.

Treatment

➤ Soft collar.
➤ Ibuprofen 400 mg tds orally.
➤ Physiotherapy.

Prognosis:

➤ Most recover over 6 weeks
➤ Some have symptoms for years.

Fracture of the atlas (C1)

Definitions

● Aetiology: severe force to the top of the head.

Clinical features

● General features of spinal injury.

Investigation

➤ X-ray: spreading of lateral masses indicates instability.
➤ CT/MRI.

Treatment

Undisplaced – stable:

➤ Soft collar.

Displaced – unstable:

➤ Halo body cast: 6 weeks.

Fracture of the pedicle of the axis (C2): hangman's fracture

● Aetiology: motor accidents and hanging (hanging usually involves fracture–dislocations at more than one level).
● Treatment: halo body cast: 12 weeks.

Hyperextension injury C3–T1

- Stable injury.
- X-ray: lateral film in hyperextension shows a gap between the anterior aspects of two vertebral bodies.
- Treatment: collar for 6 weeks.

Wedge compression C3–T1

- Stable injury.
- Treatment: collar for 6 weeks.

Burst fractures

- Stable injury.
- Risk of cord compression from fragments.
- Treatment: plaster collar for 6 weeks, hard collar until X-ray demonstrates fusion.
- Halo body cast if CT finds fragments encroaching on spinal canal.

Comminuted body fractures

- Aetiology: axial compression and flexion: diving injury.
- Unstable: cord injury likely.
- Treatment: halo traction for 8 weeks; halo body brace for a further 8 weeks.
- Surgical decompression and spinal fusion:
  - To speed mobilization
  - If fragment is impinging on cord.

Subluxations C3–T1

- Aetiology: flexion injury of posterior ligament.
- X-ray: increased gap between the vertebral spines.
- Treatment: collar for 6 weeks.

Dislocation/fracture–dislocation C3–T1

Definitions

- Aetiology: flexion–rotation injury.

Clinical features

- Cord injury likely.

Investigation

➤ Investigation of spinal injury (page 750).

Treatment

Initial:

➤ Reduction: 10–15 kg halo traction
➤ Open reduction.

Subsequent:

➤ Traction reduced to 5 kg for a further 6 weeks
➤ Collar for 6 weeks.

Or:

➤ Halo body cast for 12 weeks.

Or:

➤ Posterior fusion
➤ Cervical brace for 6 weeks.

Unilateral facet dislocation

- Stable flexion–rotation injury.
- X-ray: vertebral body displaced < 1/2 depth of body.
- Treatment: halo traction for 3 weeks, collar for further 6 weeks, or open reduction and internal fixation.

Thoracic spine

Definitions

- Stable: because of ribcage.

Clinical features

- Cord compression: although stable, the spinal canal is narrow.

Investigation

➤ X-ray:
  – Wedge fractures
  – Fracture–dislocations.
➤ CT: if cord compression.

Treatment

Paraplegia complete with no improvement in 48 hours:

➤ Bed rest for 6 weeks
➤ Physiotherapy.

Paraplegia partial:

➤ Surgical decompression and internal fixation.

Thoracolumbar

Definitions

● Aetiology: severe trauma: axial, rotational, flexion, extension.

Clinical features

● Back pain.
● Cord injury.
● Bruising.
● Gap in spinous processes: unstable injury.

Investigation

➤ X-ray.
➤ CT: assessment of unstable injury and cord injury.
➤ MRI.

Treatment

➤ Initial in-line immobilization.
➤ Log-rolling.
➤ Rigid neck collar.
➤ Later injury-specific treatment.

Transverse process fracture

● No treatment required.

Pars interarticularis fracture

● Results from athletic extension strain: avoid athletic activity during healing.

Wedge compression fracture

- Stable flexion injury.
- Treatment: bed rest, physiotherapy, corset.
- Surgical correction and internal fixation for loss of vertebral height >50%

Burst fracture

- Unstable severe axial compression injury: often with cord compression.

Treatment if no impingement on cord:

- Plaster jacket for 6 weeks
- Polythene jacket for further 12 weeks.

Treatment if cord compression or impingement on cord:

- Surgical decompression and internal fixation.

Jack-knife injury

- Unstable flexion and distraction injury: lap seat-belt injury.
- X-ray: horizontal fracture of pedicles and opening-up of posterior disc space.
- Treatment: plaster jacket for 6 weeks.

Fracture–dislocations

Definitions

- Flexion–compression–rotation injury.
- Thoracolumbar junction commonest site.

Clinical features

- Low spinal cord or cauda equina compression likely.

Investigation

➤ X-ray:
  - Fractures through body, pedicle, articular process or laminae
  - Subluxation or dislocation.
➤ CT: assess cord injury.
➤ MRI.

Treatment

Paraplegia:

➤ Traction for 6 weeks
➤ Physiotherapy
➤ Spinal brace.

Or:

➤ Surgery: internal fixation.

No paraplegia:

➤ Traction: initial stabilization and reduction
➤ Surgery: urgent open reduction and internal fixation.

Types of neurological injury

Neurapraxia

● Flaccid motor paralysis, visceral paralysis and sensory loss.
● No compressing injury.
● Complete recovery over hours

Cord transection

● Flaccid motor paralysis, visceral paralysis and sensory loss.
● Reflex activity recovers after a few hours.
● Paralysis becomes spastic after a few days.

Root transection

● Flaccid motor paralysis and sensory loss.
● Some recovery is possible.

Level of neurological injury

● Vertebrae C1–C5: fatal respiratory paralysis.
● Vertebrae C5: tetraparesis.
● Vertebrae below C5: progressive sparing of upper limbs.
● Vertebrae T1–T10: paralysis of lower limbs and viscera.
● Vertebrae T10–L1: cord and nerve root lesions affecting the lower limbs.
● Vertebrae below L1: nerve root lesions affecting the legs.

Management of paraplegia and tetraplegia

- Spinal injury unit: specialized care.
- Prevention of pressure necrosis.
- Intermittent catheterization/bladder training/later urological intervention.
- Bowel training, laxatives, enemas.
- Physiotherapy.
- Callipers: to prevent contractures.
- Tenotomies: to release contractures.

Tumours of the spine

Osteoblastoma

- Benign.
- Backache in young adults.
- X-ray: osteolytic lesion with surrounding sclerosis.
- Surgical excision and bone grafting.

Haemangioma

- Benign.
- Backache in the middle-aged patient or incidental finding on X-ray.
- X-ray: coarse vertical trabeculation – 'corduroy appearance'.
- Usually no treatment required.
- Radiological embolization and surgical excision with bone grafting: for severe symptoms.

Non-Hodgkin's lymphoma

- Malignant.
- Backache in adults 30–40 years of age.
- X-ray:
  - Mottled area
  - Pathological fracture.
- Chemotherapy.
- Surgical excision and bone grafting.
- Radiotherapy: palliation.

Chordoma

- Rare tumour from notochord remnant.
- Slow-growing mass of sacrum, and backache in young adults.
- X-ray: lucent area in sacrum.
- Wide excision.

Metastases

Definitions

- Elderly.
- Primary tumour:
  - Breast
  - Bronchus
  - Thyroid
  - Kidney
  - Prostate
  - Bladder
  - Gastrointestinal tract.

Clinical features

- Backache.

Investigation

➤ X-ray:
  - Osteolytic lesions: 'moth-eaten' cortex
  - Osteosclerotic lesions: prostatic carcinoma, some breast.
➤ Bone scan: more sensitive than X-ray.
➤ Other investigations: relative to assessment of primary tumours.

Treatment

➤ Palliation: bisphosphonate (sodium pamidronate, sodium clodronate) by slow i.v. infusion 300 mg daily for up to 7–10 days, or sodium clodronate orally 800 mg daily.
➤ Radiotherapy.
➤ Terminal care.

Non-organic back pain

- Pain and tenderness of bizarre distribution.
- Pain on passive rotation of the trunk.
- Variable limitation of straight leg raising.
- Non-dermatomal distribution of limb sensory loss.
- Excessive reactions to examination, e.g. hyperventilation.

PERIPHERAL NERVES

PERIPHERAL NERVE INJURIES

Nerve injury – general principles

Definitions

- Neuropraxia:
  - Anatomically intact but non-functioning nerve
  - Aetiology: minor compression injury.
- Axonotmesis:
  - Damaged nerve fibres with intact sheath
  - Aetiology: prolonged compression or traction.
- Neurotmesis:
  - Complete division
  - Aetiology: severe traction, penetrating trauma, accidental surgical division.

Clinical features

- Weakness.
- Flaccidity.
- Hyporeflexia.
- Sensory loss.
- Trick movements: use of unaffected muscle groups to overcome disability.
- Dry, red skin 7 days post injury: loss of autonomic supply only in neurotmesis.

Investigation

➤ Urgent surgical exploration of new injuries.
➤ Nerve conduction studies in established cases.

Treatment

Neuropraxia:

➤ No treatment; but surgical exploration for diagnosis.

Axonotmesis:

➤ No treatment; but surgical exploration for diagnosis.

Neurotmesis:

➤ Surgical repair
➤ Tendon transfer.

Complications

Neuropraxia:

• Spontaneous recovery over 90 minutes.

Axonotmesis:

• Spontaneous regeneration at 1 mm per day: tapping over the course of the nerve induces paraesthesia when the level of regeneration is reached (Tinel's test).

Neurotmesis:

• Complete recovery is unlikely, but more success with:
  – Immediate repair, or repair as soon as possible
  – Direct repair with minimum deficiency
  – More distal nerve injury
  – Pure motor or sensory nerves
  – Nerve injuries in children.

Accessory nerve

Definitions

● Aetiology: surgical injury during lymph node biopsy.

Clinical features

● Weakness of elevation of scapula: loss of 'shoulder shrugging'.
● Weakness of turning the head towards the side of the injury.
● Trapezius wasting.

Investigation

➤ Clinical diagnosis.

Treatment

➤ Surgical repair if recognized at time of injury.
➤ Physiotherapy.

Cervical sympathetic chain (Horner's syndrome)

Definitions

● Aetiology:
  – Congenital
  – Idiopathic
  – Cervical sympathectomy
  – Brainstem vascular/demyelinating disease
  – Aneurysm of aortic arch, subclavian artery or carotid bifurcation
  – Carotid artery dissection
  – Cervical malignancy: lymph nodes, thyroid, chemodectoma, apical bronchus, skull base.

Clinical features

Ipsilateral:
● Meiosis: pupillary constriction
● Ptosis: drooping eyelid
● Vasodilatation and anhidrosis of the face.

Treatment

➤ No treatment, except in case of severe ptosis.

Brachial plexus injury

Definitions

● Usually affects upper plexus C5 and C6.
● Aetiology: severe traction injury to the arm – typically from motorcycle accidents, where the head and shoulders are stretched in opposite directions.
● Associated: severe shoulder injury.

Clinical features

Upper plexus injury:

- Paralysis of:
  - Shoulder abductors and external rotators
  - Elbow flexors
  - Forearm supinators.
- Sensory loss: outer arm and forearm.

Lower plexus injury (rare):

- Paralysis of:
  - Wrist and finger flexors
  - Intrinsic hand muscles.
  - Sensory loss: ulnar forearm and hand.

Features suggesting root injury:

- Severe pain
- Scapular muscle and diaphragmatic paralysis
- Horner's syndrome
- Vascular injury
- Cervical spine fracture
- Spinal cord dysfunction.

Investigation

Identification of level of injury:

➤ Intradermal injection of histamine: persisting flare in anaesthetic skin indicates root avulsion
➤ Nerve conduction studies
➤ Computerized tomography
➤ Magnetic resonance imaging.

Treatment

➤ Exploration and repair: replace defective segment with sural nerve grafts.
➤ Surgical transfer of tendons from non-paralysed muscles to restore finger extension.
➤ Shoulder arthrodesis allows some arm abduction by the scapular muscles.
➤ Amputation of a useless flail limb: rarely indicated.

Erb's and Klumpke's palsy

Definitions

Erb's palsy:

- Root lesion C5 and C6.

Klumpke's palsy:

- Root lesion C8 and T1
- Aetiology: traction during forceps or breech delivery:
  - Downwards traction on upper limb: Erb's palsy
  - Upwards traction on upper limb: Klumpke's palsy.

Clinical features

Erb's palsy:

- Arm held in 'waiter's tip' position:
  - Elbow extended
  - Internally rotated
  - Pronated.

Klumpke's palsy:

- Paralysis of fingers: claw hand
- Associated sensory loss and Horner's syndrome.

Investigation

➤ Clinical diagnosis.

Treatment

Erb's palsy:

➤ Splint arm in abduction, external rotation and supination
➤ Physiotherapy: passive movement of joints
➤ Sural nerve grafts and surgical correction of deformities: if no recovery over 3 months.

Klumpke's palsy:

➤ Physiotherapy: passive movement of joints.

Complications

- Erb's palsy: recovery in three-quarters of cases.
- Klumpke's palsy: recovery unlikely.

Long thoracic nerve of Bell

Definitions

- Injury causes paralysis of serratus anterior muscle.
- Aetiology:
  - Shoulder and neck injuries
  - Iatrogenic: radical mastectomy and axillary surgery.

Clinical features

- Winging of the scapula: accentuated by pushing against a wall.

Investigation

➤ Clinical diagnosis.

Treatment

Indirect injury:

➤ Spontaneous recovery.

Iatrogenic injury or no recovery after 1 year:

➤ Surgical stabilization of scapula sometimes required.

Suprascapular nerve

Definitions

- Aetiology:
  - Traumatic – fractures of the scapula
  - Non-traumatic: nerve entrapment.

Clinical features

- Weak shoulder abduction and external rotation.
- Supraspinatus wasting.

Investigation

➤ Nerve conduction studies.

Treatment

Traumatic:

➤ No treatment required: usually neuropraxia.

Non-traumatic:

➤ Surgery: decompression for entrapment.

Complications

● Usually spontaneous recovery over a 3-month period.

Musculocutaneous nerve

Definitions

● Aetiology: lacerations of the upper arm, and shoulder surgery.

Clinical features

● Paralysis of biceps, brachialis and coracobrachialis muscles: weakness of elbow flexion.

Investigation

➤ Clinical diagnosis.

Treatment

➤ Immediate repair if recognized at time of injury.
➤ Surgical reconstruction if no recovery after 6 months.

Thoracodorsal nerve

Definitions

● Paralysis of latissimus dorsi muscle.
● Aetiology: iatrogenic – radical mastectomy and axillary surgery.

Clinical features

● Weakness of forced adduction of the shoulder.

Investigation

➤ Clinical diagnosis.

Treatment

➤ Usually no treatment necessary or physiotherapy.

Axillary nerve

Definitions

- Aetiology:
  - Shoulder dislocation
  - Humeral neck fracture
  - Iatrogenic: axillary incisions.

Clinical features

- Weakness of shoulder abduction.
- Numbness over distal attachment of deltoid.

Investigation

➤ Clinical diagnosis.

Treatment

Shoulder dislocation or humeral neck fracture:

➤ Spontaneous recovery after shoulder reduction.

Iatrogenic or no recovery after 3 months:

➤ Surgical repair.

Radial nerve

Definitions

Aetiology:

- Very high injury:
  - Drunken stupor with the arm dangling over the back of a chair
  - Walking with axillary crutches.

- High injury:
  - Fractures of the humeral shaft
  - Iatrogenic: prolonged tourniquet pressure
  - Penetrating wounds.
- Low injury:
  - Fracture–dislocation at elbow.

Clinical features

With ascending level of injury, loss of:

- Extension of metacarpophalangeal joints of hand
- Thumb abduction and interphalangeal extension
- Radial extensor muscles: wrist drop
- Sensation over anatomical snuffbox
- Elbow extension.

Investigation

➤ Nerve conduction studies.

Treatment

Closed injury:

➤ Spontaneous recovery.

Open injury or no recovery after 6 weeks:

➤ Surgical exploration and grafting as soon as possible
➤ Supinator decompression of posterior interosseous nerve
➤ Lively splint: provides support but allows use of the hand.

Ulnar nerve

Definitions

Aetiology:

- High injury:
  - Elbow fractures and dislocations
  - Entrapment in the medial epicondylar cubital tunnel: occurs in severe valgus deformity and osteoarthritis

- Compression at the medial epicondyle: occurs in the anaesthetized patient.
- Low injury:
  - Penetrating injury
  - Entrapment in the pisohamate tunnel: occurs in cyclists
  - Compression: by a deep carpal ganglion.

Clinical features

High injury (in addition to features of low injury):

- Paralysis of ulnar half of flexor digitorum profundus: hand is less clawed than it is in low injury.

Low injury:

- Loss of:
  - Intrinsic muscle function to the hand: claw hand
  - Finger abduction (partial)
  - Thumb adduction.
- Froment's sign:
  - Attempting to grip paper between thumbs and index
  - Excessive flexion of interphalangeal joint of the thumb: from compensation by flexor pollicis longus.
- Combined low injury of median and ulnar nerves produces maximum clawing.

Investigation
➤ Nerve conduction studies.

Treatment
Entrapment:

➤ Anterior transposition at the elbow.

Open injury:

➤ Urgent surgical exploration and repair: anterior transposition allows for loss of length.

Late presentation:

➤ Zancolli's operation: shortening of the volar capsule of the metacarpophalangeal joints.

Median nerve

Definitions

Aetiology:

- High injury:
  - Penetrating injury
  - Elbow dislocation.
- Low injury:
  - Penetrating injury
  - Entrapment:
    - Carpal tunnel syndrome (page 690)
    - Carpal dislocation: myxoedema, pregnancy, rheumatoid arthritis.

Clinical features

- Night pain: carpal tunnel syndrome.
- Thenar wasting.
- With ascending level of injury, loss of:
  - Thumb abduction
  - Sensation over radial three and a half digits
  - Flexion of fourth and fifth fingers, with pointing of index finger
  - Wrist flexion and pronation.

Investigation

➤ Nerve conduction studies.

Treatment

Carpal tunnel syndrome:

➤ Division of the flexor retinaculum.

Open injury:

➤ Urgent surgical exploration and repair.

Late presentation or lack of recovery:

➤ Tendon transfers: division of tendons from unaffected muscles and reattachment to those of paralysed muscles.

Femoral nerve

Definitions

- Aetiology:
  - Spontaneous haemorrhage into psoas muscle when anticoagulated
  - Penetrating injury
  - Iatrogenic: surgery to the thigh or groin.

Clinical features

- Weak knee extension.
- Sensory loss over anterior thigh

Investigation

➤ Clinical diagnosis.

Treatment

➤ Correct abnormal clotting.
➤ Conservative management of psoas haematoma.
➤ Evacuate thigh haematoma.
➤ Surgical repair, with or without grafting.

Late presentation:

➤ Tendon transfer: hamstring to quadriceps.

Lateral cutaneous nerve of thigh (meralgia paraesthetica)

- Entrapment within lateral fibres of inguinal ligament causing paraesthesia of lateral thigh.
- Treatment: surgical decompression.

Sciatic nerve

Definitions

- Aetiology:
  - Penetrating injury
  - Hip dislocation and pelvic fractures
  - Iatrogenic: hip replacement surgery.

Clinical features

- Paralysis of all muscles below the knee: foot drop.
- Paralysis of hamstrings in high injury.
- Sensory loss below the knee, except medial leg.

Investigation

➤ Nerve conduction studies.

Treatment

➤ Surgical repair.
➤ Foot drop splint.

Late presentation:

➤ Tendon transfer: tibialis posterior to front of foot.

Tibial nerve

Definitions

- Aetiology:
  - Penetrating injury
  - Compound tibial fractures.

Clinical features

Proximal:

- Paralysis of ankle plantar flexion
- Sensory loss over the sole and calf.

Distal:

- Paralysis of intrinsic muscles of the foot: claw foot
- Sensory loss over the sole.

Investigation

➤ Nerve conduction studies.

Treatment

➤ Surgical repair.
➤ Splint to prevent excessive dorsiflexion.

Peroneal nerves

Definitions

Aetiology:

- Common peroneal nerve:
  - Fractures of the lateral tibial condyle and proximal fibula (bumper fracture)
  - Iatrogenic: correction of valgus deformity.
- Superficial peroneal nerve:
  - Lateral compartment syndrome.
- Deep peroneal nerve:
  - Anterior compartment syndrome
  - Iatrogenic: ankle surgery.

Clinical features

Common peroneal nerve:

- Foot drop
- Sensory loss over dorsum of foot and anterior/lateral leg.

Superficial peroneal nerve:

- Weak foot eversion
- Sensory loss over dorsum of foot/lateral leg.

Deep peroneal nerve:

- Weak foot dorsiflexion
- Sensory loss over the first web space.

Investigation

➤ Nerve conduction studies.

Treatment

➤ Surgical repair or walking brace.
➤ Reduction and fixation of fractures.

Compartment syndrome:

➤ Fasciotomy.

Sural nerve

- Aetiology: accidental division in short saphenous varicose vein surgery.

- Loss of sensation over the back of leg, and lateral aspect of ankle joint, heel, foot and fifth toe.
- Sural communicating nerve – loss of sensation strip along midcalf.

Saphenous nerve

- Aetiology: damage during stripping of the long saphenous vein, particularly if continued down to the ankle.
- Loss of sensation over the medial border of the leg and foot, as far as the ball of the big toe.

NEUROPATHY

Definitions

- A disorder of peripheral nerves, which may be sensory, motor, autonomic or mixed, and is usually symmetrical.

Aetiology of peripheral neuropathy

Metabolic	Diabetes (page 14)
	Chronic renal failure
	Liver failure
	Hypothyroidism
Drugs	Isoniazid
	Phenytoin
	Vincristine
	Nitrofurantoin
Vitamin deficiency	B_1 (alcoholism)
	B_{12}
Malignancy	Carcinomatosis
	Myeloma
Inflammatory	Guillain–Barré syndrome
	Systemic lupus erythematosus
	Polyarteritis nodosa
Infective	Leprosy (page 140)
Genetic	Charcot–Marie–Tooth
	Friedreich's ataxia
Post intensive care	(page 88)

Clinical features

- Diabetic neuropathy (page 558).
- Malignant neuropathy: 'glove' or 'stocking' sensory loss with proximal muscle wasting.
- Alcoholic neuropathy: numbness, paraesthesia, and pain affecting the feet.
- Guillain–Barré: progressive proximal weakness, bulbar palsy and respiratory failure 1–4 weeks after respiratory or gastrointestinal infection.
- Lepromatous neuropathy (page 140).
- Charcot–Marie–Tooth.
- Friedreich's ataxia.

Investigation

➤ General investigation for underlying causes: full blood count, erythrocyte sedimentation rate, B_1, B_{12}, folate, urea, electrolytes, creatinine, liver function, blood glucose, thyroid-stimulating hormone, serum electrophoresis, venereal disease research laboratory test, autoantibodies (rheumatoid factor, double-stranded DNA, antinuclear factor, extractable nuclear antigens).

➤ Specific investigation of underlying causes.

➤ Nerve conduction studies.

Treatment

➤ Treat diabetes.

➤ Stop drugs.

➤ Replace dietary deficiencies:
  - Alcoholism: intravenous Pabrinex 1 pair of ampoules daily for up to 7 days, then long-term thiamine (B_1) 50–100 mg tds orally
  - Isoniazid prophylaxis: pyridoxine hydrochloride (B_6) 10 mg daily
  - B_{12} deficiency: hydroxocobalamin 1 mg i.m. on alternate days until no further improvement is seen, reducing to every 2 months.

➤ Treat malignancy.

➤ Treat inflammatory conditions with immuno-suppressants, e.g. steroid.

➤

➤ Treat leprosy (page 141).
➤ Physiotherapy helps to maintain general function and allows adaptation.
➤ Amitriptyline 10–25 mg nocte or gabapentin 300 mg nocte increasing to 300 mg tds: for neuropathic pain.

Mononeuritis multiplex

● Serial or concurrent multifocal peripheral neuropathy associated with diabetes, rheumatoid arthritis, polyarteritis and leprosy.

Charcot–Marie–Tooth

● An autosomal dominant condition presenting in two forms:
  - Type I: difficulty in walking during childhood, with pes cavus or talipes equinovarus, kyphoscoliosis, and severe wasting mainly affecting the legs ('Champagne bottle' appearance)
  - Type II: lesser weakness and wasting, mainly of the legs, with onset in the teenage years.

Friedreich's ataxia

● An autosomal recessive condition, with onset at 8–16 years, causing ataxia, nystagmus, dysarthria, spasticity, diabetes mellitus, optic atrophy and cardiac abnormalities.

6

Personal development

PERSONAL DEVELOPMENT

Your surgical development involves the acquisition of appropriate surgical knowledge and clinical skills. The aim is to become surgically competent.

Education

- In the UK, the General Medical Council, universities and Royal Colleges, and the recently established Postgraduate Medical Education Training Board (PMETB) set educational standards, including moral and ethical codes. Medical examinations test competence and the acquisition of these standards.
- Medical students are usually attached to a surgical firm, with one or more consultants in charge of their teaching, and there may also be a tutor.
- The medical student should be aware of the clinical skills that are expected of them on qualification, which must be practised and perfected during their training.
- Surgical trainees should be allocated a consultant as their educational supervisor and develop a learning partnership. The aims of the partnership are discussed, documented and signed as an educational contract at the commencement of an appointment.
- The contract, and its subsequent assessment, forms part of the trainee's training portfolio.
- Students and trainees have a personal responsibility to acquire the necessary knowledge and clinical skills to enter into, and progress within, the medical profession.
- Of prime importance are motivation and the desire to succeed.
- The key features of higher education are critical thinking, scepticism and debate. Time must be allowed to think, reflect, deliberate and analyse clinical activity, in order to evaluate outcome and identify the lessons to be learned.
- Teachers and trainees must foster these characteristics.
- Institutions should provide a supportive learning environment, relevant learning material and clear direction so that the learner knows where he or she is going, and maintains enthusiasm and interest.

- Self-directed learning must continue throughout postgraduate education and subsequent professional development.

Knowledge base

- Medical knowledge is continually changing and under-graduate and postgraduate curricula have to match this progress. Textbooks supply core knowledge, but this information may be 2–4 years out of date. Information is therefore supplemented by lectures, tutorials, ward teaching and journal reading. Clinical-based teaching is an important source of surgical knowledge.
- Individuals learn at a different pace and with different styles. Computer literacy is essential for information retrieval. Access may be through a personal computer with internet access or via a medical library, using the skill, advice and direction that they provide.
- Information is never lacking but learning is best based on need and built on an existing knowledge base.
- Critical appraisal is possible once alternative information is available and, from this, an evidence-based practice can be developed.
- The trainee is expected to read current journals, and is exposed to postgraduate training sessions, external courses and conferences.
- The educational supervisor can help the trainee select appropriate information sources and ensure the level of knowledge equates to educational needs.
- All educators should ensure that students and trainees understand and apply appropriately the information they are gathering, through regular tutorials and feedback sessions.

Clinical skills

- Clinical activities are a prime **educational resource** and student and trainee are responsible for maximizing this experience in the wards, outpatient departments, operating theatres and all other clinical areas.

- **Diagnosis** is based on taking a history, examining a patient and requesting appropriate investigations. These measures also allow **assessment** of a patient's condition, i.e. the severity of their presenting problem and any co-morbidity.

- **Management** includes assessment and treatment; the latter may be surgical or non-surgical and may have to commence before a definitive diagnosis is made.

- All aspects of management should be fully and legibly **documented** in the patient's notes. These entries should be routine, consistent in their format, relevant and informative.

- Student notes provide a learning resource and are important in training; storing and retrieval must take into account the legal requirement of confidentiality.

- Medical students and trainees benefit from a **wide exposure** to all areas of clinical practice. There may be only limited experience of a specialty, but this can provide an understanding of the principles of management in each discipline, allowing appropriate advice and referral of patients if required in the future; it may also influence the choice of specialty.

- A trainee's involvement in management planning increases their confidence and teaches them to deliver relevant and appropriate care. Important skills to acquire are task prioritization and the delivery of sound judgement in routine and emergency situations; hand-overs must encompass all salient features of management.

- **Teamwork** is an essential part of good healthcare and this often means working with colleagues from different disciplines; teams should comprise an appropriate skill mix. Good communication within the team is essential to ensure optimal patient care.

- With seniority comes increasing responsibility and autonomy, together with the need for appropriate delegation. These factors progress into peer respect and professional leadership.

- It is the clinician's moral duty to treat in an ethical manner, and to the highest level of his or her practical skill.

Communication

- Communication skills are essential for obtaining information from a patient, obtaining their consent for investigation and treatment, talking to their relatives and associates, in discussing cases with other members of the profession, and in teaching.
- History taking involves concentrated listening, understanding and empathy.
- Whereas questions follow a routine format, there is no such thing as a routine patient: all must be treated as individuals, respecting the privileged doctor–patient relationship. Much personal information is divulged, and confidentiality must be assured and respected by the management team.
- Questions must be relevant, appropriate and tailored to the patient's level of understanding, and take into account their educational, social and cultural background. Linguistic barriers may be overcome by gestures and diagrams, but may require the help of an interpreter.
- Questions should be delivered in a non-controversial and non-judgemental style. Personal views of a patient's socioeconomic status, disability, age, gender, sexuality, colour, race, culture, creed or belief must not interfere with clinical decisions.
- Effective communication between medical professionals requires good general knowledge of anatomy and basic medical sciences, so that the nature and location of findings are accurately and succinctly described.

Assessment

- Assessment of students and trainees has to ensure that they are fit to practise as a doctor and a surgeon, respectively.
- The assessment may be continuous throughout a course, or by qualifying examinations.
- It is essential that students and trainees have regular appraisals during their course of study and that this is included in their educational contract. These should

include constructive criticism and counselling on progress, to ensure that they are aware of, and progress towards, the required standard.

- Throughout their course of study, students and trainees should be encouraged to undertake self-assessment, and comparison with the views of others provides the necessary insight on progress.
- The main aim of teacher and learner in the medical field is to ensure competence in both medical knowledge and clinical skills, with these merging to provide optimal patient care.
- Assessment of operative competence includes preoperative and postoperative care, knowledge of relevant procedures and, most importantly, technical skills. It may also include a 'triggered' assessment, the success of which influences progress.

Teaching

- Involvement in teaching, whether to one's peers, to juniors or to other health professionals, is an effective and reliable means of learning, ensuring that one's knowledge is current and withstands close questioning.
- The atmosphere of teaching sessions should, where possible, be informal enough to allow exploration of learning methods, encouraging critical and lateral thinking, fostering creativity and responsiveness.
- Setting problems and challenges encourages the critical debate that is the hallmark of higher educational activities.

Research

- All educational activities identify unanswered questions across the field of medicine and these questions form the basis for research initiatives.
- With more intense searching, answers are often to be found.
- The search for both questions and answers that forms the basis of all research is to be encouraged in every-one, but if time is to be put aside for this discipline

it should be undertaken in an institution with specific interest in the question being investigated, and where adequate funding, supervision and guidance are guaranteed.
- Research in basic sciences, which is laboratory based, forms the foundation from which most clinical research originates.
- Research on patients requires approval from an ethical committee and laws on data protection govern identifiable data.
- Clinical research must be valuable and be of benefit to the population being studied; this benefit must far outweigh any risks.
- The patient must be fully informed of the details of the research and give written consent. There must be no coercion in their involvement, and they must understand that they can at any time, and without prejudice to their care, withdraw from the study.
- The experimental design, usually a randomized controlled trial, must be appropriate, and have a reasonable chance of a meaningful outcome within a specified timeframe.
- Throughout the research period the patient's individual rights must be respected.
- Negative findings are almost as valuable as positive results, and direct future studies.
- Regrettably negative findings do not always surface and much time, effort and finance can be wasted following well-trodden but poorly publicized pathways. The researcher thus has a moral obligation to publicize fully all his or her findings.

Health service

- Students and trainees should understand the health service in which they practise.
- Finance has a profound influence on staff remuneration and training and on the provision of healthcare.
- Every health service has finite resources, but observation will indicate whether funds are being used wisely and appropriately.

- Medical practitioners have a responsibility continually to develop and improve health care for their community and are the advocate for their patients, both individually and collectively, to ensure optimal use of resources.
- In the last few years there has been a proliferation of governing bodies in the UK NHS of which medical students and trainees should be aware.
  - The **National Institute of Clinical Excellence (NICE)** was established in 1999 to provide authoritative, robust and reliable guidance on current 'best practice' to patients. Its expert panel includes patients and lay members. NICE provides technical appraisal, clinical guidance on selected problems, and information on the efficiency and effectiveness of new interventional procedures; these include surgical appliances and techniques.
  - The **British Association of Surgical Oncology (BASO)** was established in 1980 and issues guidelines for the diagnosis and treatment of site-specific cancers.
  - The **Commission for Health Improvement (CHI)** was launched in 2000 to review the performance of Health Trusts every 4 years. It checks that clinical guidelines are being adhered to, identifying failures and inequality of standards in the NHS.
  - The **National Clinical Assessment Authority (NCAA)** offers support to the employers of doctors whose performance is giving cause for concern. Its aim is to facilitate local resolution of any problem and it may recommend a period of retraining for the individual concerned.
  - The **National Patient Safety Organization (NPSA)** was established in 2001 to provide a national reporting system for adverse events and near-misses, to allow initiation of preventive measures throughout the NHS.
- The recent implementation of the **European Working Time Directive** into the UK, has imposed restrictions on the working practice of trainees. Adequate training should be fitted into the working week, it should

constitute one-third of the total working time, and at least 50% of the working week should have training opportunities.

- The educational programme should also consist of didactic teaching; there should be one session a week of time protected from other responsibilities, and time should be allowed for attending educational courses.

INDEX

a wave, 382
abdomen
  burst, 74
  hernias, 392–4
  sarcomas, 453–4
  wall developmental
    abnormalities, 390–1
abdominal surgery
  infections, 73
  postoperative problems,
    68–70
abdominal trauma, 405–9
  aetiology, 405
  blast injury, 608
  clinical features, 406
  colon, 408
  duodenum, 408
  gunshot wounds, 606
  investigations, 406–7
  multiply injured, 604
  paediatric, 616
  pregnancy, 617
  rectum, 409
  small bowel, 408
  stomach, 407
  treatment, 407
abducent nerve and nucleus
  palsy, 211
abortion, septic, 411
accessory auricles, 237
accessory nerve
  iatrogenic injury, 760
  palsy, 214–15
acetabulum
  congenital dislocation of hip,
    703
  fractures, 701–2
  Otto pelvis, 702
  subluxation of hip, 704–5
  see also hip
acetaminophen (paracetamol),
    44–5, 107
acetylcholine receptor antibodies, 668
achalasia of the cardia, 414
Achilles tendon
  peritendinitis, 725
  ruptured, 672, 725
achondroplasia, 636–7
acid reflux (gastro-oesophageal
  reflux disease), 417–19

acid–base balance, 29, 62–4, 93
acne, 193, 282
acoustic neuroma, 213, 225,
  244–5
acquired immunodeficiency
  syndrome (AIDS), see HIV
  and AIDS
acromegaly (gigantism), 225
acromioclavicular dislocation,
  678
actinomycosis, 144, 739
activated partial thromboplastin
  time (APTT), 33
acute abdomen, 395–405
  acute mesenteric adenitis,
    402–3
  appendicitis, 402–3
  bowel obstruction, 398–400
  congenital atresias, 395–6
  intestinal ischaemia, 568
  intra-abdominal abscess, 405
  intussusception, 400–1
  malrotation, 396–7
  Meckel's diverticulum, 397–8
  meconium ileus, 398
  neonatal volvulus, 396–7
  peritonitis, 69–70, 403–5
  pseudo-obstruction, 400
  volvulus of bowel, 401–2
acute coronary syndrome, 366
acute haemolytic transfusion
  reaction, 39
acute phase proteins, 115
Addison's disease, 487
adenoidal hypertrophy, 286
adhesive otitis, 243
admission to hospital, 8
adrenal cortex, 486–7
adrenal gland
  hyperplasia, 487, 488
  mass, incidental finding, 491
  neurofibroma, 491–2
  phaeochromocytoma, 319,
    490–1
  tumours, 487, 488, 489
adrenocorticotrophic hormone
  (ACTH), 486–7
adult polycystic kidney, 493–4
adult respiratory distress
  syndrome (ARDS), 67–8, 360,
  623

Advanced Trauma Life Support
  (ATLS) system
  approach, 599
  disability mnemonic, 601
ainhum, 168
airway maintenance, 26–7
  emergency access, 27
  endotracheal intubation, 26–7,
    602
  face-mask, 26
  laryngeal mask airway, 26
  manual emergency control, 26
airway obstruction/injury, 290,
    292, 311, 360, 361
  multiply injured, 600, 601–2
  postoperative, 66
Albright's syndrome, 638
alimentary tract
  ageing process, 104
  postoperative problems, 68–70
  see also gastrointestinal
Allen's test, 563
allergic rhinitis, 281
allergic skin responses, 191
alpha-1-antitrypsin deficiency,
    339
amaurosis fugax, 268, 547, 565
amblyopia, 265
amethocaine, 45
aminoglycosides, 18–19
amoebiasis, 149–51
amoeboma, 150
amyotrophic lateral sclerosis,
    666
anaemias
  aplastic, 175–6
  blood transfusion for severe,
    181
  of chronic disease/secondary,
    174–5
  clinical features, 169
  definitions, 168–9
  folate deficiency, 173–4, 740
  glucose-6-phosphate
    dehydrogenase deficiency,
    179–80
  haemolytic, 176–81, 474
  hereditary spherocytosis,
    176–7
  hypochromic microcytic, 169
  investigations, 169–70
  iron deficiency, 171
  macrocytic, 169, 172–6
  megaloblastic, 172–3
  normocytic, 170–1

normocytic normochromic,
    169
  pyruvate kinase deficiency, 180
  secondary, 174–5
  sickle-cell disease, 177–9
  sideroblastic, 174
  thalassaemias, 180–1, 474
  in tropics, 182
  vitamin B_{12} deficiency, 172–3
anaesthesia
  airway maintenance, 26–7
  allergy reactions, 31
  CNS effects, 30
  dangers and complications,
    29–32
  diathermy burns, 31, 32, 42
  endotracheal intubation, 26–7,
    31, 32
  epidural, 28, 31, 71–2
  hypothermia, 30
  induction, 27–8
  local, 28, 31, 45
  maintenance, 28
  medico-legal problems, 31
  metabolic effects, 30
  monitoring, 28–9
  musculoskeletal injuries, 31
  nerve injuries, 31, 32
  neuromuscular agents, 32
  patient assessment, 25
  physiological effects, 29–30
  postoperative complications,
    31
  premedication, 25–6
  pressure areas, 30, 32, 42
  prevention of complications,
    32
  principles, 24
  spinal, 28, 31, 71–2
  stages, 28
  surgical, 28
  ventilation during, 28
analgesia
  cancer pain, 107–8
  epidural, 47, 107
  pain management, 46–7
  patient-controlled, 46–7, 107
  peri-operative, 28
  pre-operative, 13, 25
  see also pain
analgesic ladder, 107
anaphylaxis, 31, 40, 191
anastomotic leak, 404, 405, 413
anencephaly, 219
aneurysmal bone cyst, 641

angina
  mesenteric, 545, 569
  nocturnal, 365
  pectoris, 365, 545
  unstable, 366, 367
angina (CCS) status, 365
angioneurotic oedema, 292
animal bites, 164–8, 192
ankle
  ruptured medial (deltoid)
    ligament, 729
  sprained, 729
  tuberculosis, 726
ankle-brachial pressure index,
  553
ankylosing spondylitis, 653–4
  juvenile, 657
Ann Arbor classification
  (Hodgkin's disease), 303
annular pancreas, 476
anorectal abscess, 446
anorectal atresia, 445
anorectal malformation, 445–6
anotia, 236
antacids, 25
anti-emetics, 25
anti-Jo 1 antibodies, 669
anti-oncogenes (tumour-
  suppressor genes), 183
anti-personnel mines, injuries
  from, 609–10
anti-reflux surgery, 419
anti-ulcer surgery, 429–30
antibiotics, peri-operative, 17–19
  culture sensitivities, 17, 19
  gut flora, 18
  local guidelines, 19
  resistant organisms, 18
  side-effects, 18–19
antibiotics, prophylactic use,
  25–6
anticardiolipin antibody, 568
anticholinesterase (edro-
  phonium) (Tensilon test), 668
anticoagulation, 76
  peri-operative, 15–16
antigen-binding fragments (Fab),
  116
antimicrosomal autoantibodies,
  314
antineutrophil cytoplasmic
  antibodies, 279, 566
antinuclear antibodies, 567, 652,
  774
antinuclear factor, 651, 774

antiphospholipid syndrome, 568
antiretroviral therapy, 129–30
antiseptic solutions, 42
antistaphylococcal antibodies,
  629, 630, 748
antithrombin III deficiency,
  567–8
antithrombotic agents, 25–6
antithyroglobulin autoantibodies,
  314
antivenom, 166, 167, 168
anuria, 60
anus
  abscess, 447
  anal stretch, 449
  carcinoma, 451–2
  covered, 445
  ectopic opening, 445
  fissure, 446
  fistula in ano, 447–8
  genital warts, 544
  haemorrhoids, 446, 448–50
  imperforate, 445
  pruritus ani, 449–50
  stenosis, 445
  warts, 127, 451
  see also anorectal
anxiety, 25
AO (Arbeitsgemeinschaft für
  Osteosynthesefragen) nail, 620
aorta, coarctation, 358
aortic aneurysm, 570–6
  clinical features, 571
  complications, 572
  Crawford classification, 571
  dissecting, 574
  endoluminal repair of
    abdominal, 572–3
  investigations, 571
  mycotic/inflammatory, 574–5
  ruptured abdominal, 573–4
  treatment, 571–2
aortic dissection (dissecting
  aortic aneurysm), 574–5
aortic occlusion, acute, 556
aortic regurgitation, 371–3
aortic root replacement, 372, 373
aortic stenosis, 369–70
aortic transection, 360, 363–4
aortic valve replacement, 370,
  372
Apert's syndrome, 256
aphasia, 547
aphthous ulcers, 274–5
  recurrent in HIV/AIDS, 126

aplastic anaemia, 175
apoptosis, 182–3
appendicitis, 402–3
appendix
    abscess, 403
    carcinoid tumours, 440
    mass (phlegmon), 403
Appley's grinding test, 715
apprehension sign, 681
arch support, 733, 734
argentaffinoma (midgut carcinoid), 440
Argyll Robertson pupil, 267
arm
    cubitus valgus, 682
    cubitus varus, 682–3
    forearm fracture, 689–90
    lymphoedema, 589
    'waiter's tip' position, 763
    see also elbow; hand; humerus; radius
arrhythmias, 73
    perioperative, 64
arterial injury, 578–9, 623
arterial switch, 390
arteriovenous fistulae, postoperative, 590
arteriovenous malformations, 590–1
arthritis
    juvenile chronic, 657
    septic, 658–60, 708
    suppurative, 629
    surgical management of shoulder, 676
    tuberculous, 660–1
arthrogryphoses, 673
ASA (American Society of Anaesthetists) scale (patient assessment), 25
ascariasis, 157–8
Asherman seal, 602
aspergillus granuloma, paranasal, 146
aspirin, 45, 96, 107
assessment, 11–12, 781–2
astigmatism, 263–4
astrocytoma, 223
ataxia, 663
atelectasis, 66–7
atherosclerosis, 104, 105, 544–6
athetosis, 663
atlas (C1) fracture, 751
atrial septal defect, 385–7
atrial switch, 390

auricular fibrillation (AF), 65
Austin–Flint murmur, 371
Austin–Moore hemi-arthroplasty, 712
axillary abscess, 336
axillary lymph nodes, see breast cancer
axillary nerve injury, 680, 766
axis (C2), fractured pedicle, 751
axonotmesis, 759–60

B lymphocytes, 115–16
back
    'log-roll' examination, 604
    non-organic pain, 759
    see also spine
bacterial (infective) endocarditis, 380–1
bacterial overgrowth, 94
bacterial parotitis, 294
bad news, breaking, 106
Baker's cyst, 649, 720
balanitis, 528–9
balanitis xerotica obliterans, 529
ballistic trauma, 605–10
    anti-personnel mines, 609–10
    blast injury, 608–9
    gunshot wounds, 605–8
Bankart lesion, repair, 681–2
Barlow's test, 703
barotrauma, 246–7
Barrett's oesophagus, 419
basophils, 115
Bassini herniorrhaphy, 393
bat ears, 237
Beau's lines, 189
Becker's muscular dystrophy, 671
Beck's triad, 383
Beckwith–Wiedermann syndrome, 391
Behçet's syndrome, 274, 275
Bell's palsy, 212, 235–6
Bence–Jones protein, 643
benign prostatic hypertrophy, 511–12, 514, 515
Bennet's fracture–dislocation, 697
beta-lactams, 18
bezoars, 426
biceps tendon rupture, 675–6
bile, 455, 464
bile duct
    carcinoma, 472–3
    gallstones, 468–9
bilharziasis (schistosomiasis), 151–2, 519–20

biliary drainage, 465
biliary strictures, 469–70
biliary tree, 464
    atresia, 464–5
    Caroli's disease, 465
    choledochal cyst, 465–6
    see also gallbladder
blackwater fever, 148
bladder
    acute cystitis, 514–15
    acute urinary retention, 508–9
    calculi, 515, 519
    chronic urinary retention,
        509–10
    colovesical fistula, 522–3
    contracted, 152
    cystocoele, 524
    diverticula, 515
    interstitial cystitis, 517–18
    recurrent cystitis, 515
    trauma, 526–7
    tuberculosis, 505, 516, 518
    vesicovaginal fistula, 523
    see also ureter; urethral; urinary
bladder carcinoma, 524–6
    squamous, 526
    TNM classification, 525
    transitional cell, 524
bladderworm, 162
blast injury, 608–9
bleeding time, 33
blepharitis, 248
blood
    film, 170
    functions, 35
    gases, 29
    patch, 47, 71
    pressure, 29
blood transfusion, 175, 180, 181,
        474
    acute haemolytic transfusion
        reaction, 39
    acute lung injury, 40
    acute normovolaemic
        haemodilution, 37
    anaphylactic reaction, 40
    cell salvage, 37
    collection, 36–7
    delayed haemolytic transfusion
        response, 40
    delivering blood, 37
    exchange, 181
    febrile non-haemolytic
        transfusion reaction, 40
    fibrinogen, 38

fresh frozen plasma, 36, 38
graft versus host reaction, 40
human albumin, 38
hyperkalaemia due to, 40
immunological problems,
    39–40
immunomodulatory effects, 40
increased cost, 41
indications, 35, 37–9
infective agents, 36, 41
iron overload, 40
leukodepletion, 36, 41
local thrombophlebitis, 40
monitoring during, 37
packed cells, 38, 40
plasma substitutes, 38
platelet antibodies, 40
platelet concentrates, 36, 38
predonated, 36–7
purpura, 40
recombinant activated factor
    VII, 39
refusal, 22, 38
screening, 36
severe anaemia, 181
storage, 37
typing, 36
urticarial transfusion reaction,
    40
wrong blood transfused, 39
Blount's disease, 714
blow-out fracture, 270–1
blue baby, 388
Boerhaave's syndrome, 415
boil (furuncle), 193
bone
    Brodie's abscess, 631
    chondrosarcoma, 645
    cyst
        aneurysmal, 641
        solitary, 639
    dwarfism, 636–7
    enchondroma, 640
    Ewing's tumour, 646
    fibrosarcoma, 645–6
    fibrous dysplasia, 638
    giant cell sarcoma, 646
    giant cell tumour, 641–2
    marble bone disease, 635–6
    multiple myeloma, 642–3
    natural repair process, 624
    necrosis in sickle-cell disease,
        629
    osteoarthritis, 627, 648–9,
        676, 709, 721

bone *cont.*
  osteochondroma, 639–40
  osteogenesis imperfecta, 637–8
  osteoid osteoma, 640–1
  osteomalacia, 634–5
  osteomyelitis, 628–30
  osteoporosis, 105, 631–2
  osteosarcoma, 43–4
  paediatric trauma, 616
  Paget's disease, 633–4
  primary hyperparathyroidism, 636
  rickets, 634–5
  scurvy, 632–3
  secondary neoplasia, 647–8
  von Recklinghausen's disease, 636
bone graft, 592, 596
bone marrow
  smear, 170
  transplant, 175, 178, 596
Boston brace, 742
Bouchard's nodes, 648
Boutonnière deformity, 650, 697
bowel
  colorectal carcinoma, 441–3, 599
  congenital megacolon, 435
  Crohn's disease, 435–7
  diverticular disease, 434–5
  polyps, 443–4
  radiation enteritis, 444
  tapeworms, 162–3
  ulcerative colitis, 437–40
  volvulus, 401–2
  see also gastrointestinal; small bowel
bowel obstruction
  advanced cancer, 109
  clinical features, 399
  definitions, 398–402
  investigations, 399
  pseudo-, 400
  treatment, 399–400
  tube caecostomy for irrigation, 453
Bowen's disease, 200
brachial plexus injury, 761–2
bradycardia, 64
bradykinin, 115
brainstem death, 23, 100–2, 593
  additional tests, 101–2
  clinical state, 100
  clinical tests, 100–1

legal time of death, 101
  preconditions, 100
  transplantation, 102
brainstem demyelination, 267, 664
brainstem stroke, tumour, 209, 211, 267
branchial cyst, fistula, sinus, 206, 306
breast
  abscess, 326–8
  benign changes, 322–3
  developmental anomalies, 320–1
  duct ectasia, 325
  duct papilloma, 324–5
  eczematous conditions, 325–6
  fat necrosis, 326
  fibroadenoma, 323–4
  granulomatous lobular mastitis, 325
  gynaecomastia, 321–2
  hypertrophy, 321
  involution, 323
  mammary fistula, 327–8
  periductal mastitis, 325
  phillodes tumour, 324
  radial scars, 327
  sclerosing adenosis, 327
  screening and assessment, 328–9
  superficial thrombophlebitis, 324
  tuberculosis, 328
breast carcinoma
  adjuvant, 333
  advanced, 335–6
  chemotherapy, 334, 335, 336
  clinical staging, 330–1
  endocrine therapy, 333–4, 336
  lymphoedema of arm, 589
  Nottingham Prognostic Index, 332
  primary, 329–30
  prognosis, 332
  radiotherapy, 333, 335, 336
  recurrence, 335
  in situ, 329
  surgery
    axillary, 331
    complications, 332
    prognosis, 332–3
    review of, 331–2
  surveillance, 334–5
'breast mouse', 324

breathing, paradoxical, 362, 395
Breslow's depth (malignant melanoma), 201
Bristow repair (shoulder dislocation), 682
broad beans ('favism'), 179
Brodie's abscess, 631
bronchial carcinoma, 340–5
  adenocarcinoma, 340
  bronchoalveolar, 340
  carcinoid, 340, 440
  complications, 344–5
  investigations, 342–3
  large-cell carcinoma, 340
  management, 343–4
    chemotherapy, 344
    complications, 344–5
    palliative, 344
    radiotherapy, 343–4
    surgical, 343
  metastases, 340–1
  non-small-cell lung cancer, 340
  paraneoplastic syndromes, 342
  prognosis, 344
  small-cell lung cancer, 340–1
  squamous cell carcinoma, 340
  TNM staging system (1997), 341
  treatment, 343–4
bronchial obstruction, 339
bronchiectasis, 338–40
bronchocavitary fistula, 337
bronchogenic cyst, 358
bronchopleural fistula, 338, 353
'bucket handle' tear, 714
Budd–Chiari syndrome, 459
Buerger's disease, 557–8
Buerger's sign, 553
bulbar palsy, 215–17
'bunions', 736
buprenorphine, 107
Burch colposuspension, 521
Burkitt's lymphoma, 132
burns, 55
  depth, 610–11
  diathermy, 31, 32, 42
  early management, 612–13
  first-degree, 610, 611, 613
  flash, 608
  investigation, 612
  laryngeal, 292
  Muir/Barclay fluid replacement formula, 613
  other injuries associated, 611–12
  second-degree, 610, 611, 613
  subsequent management, 613–14
  third-degree, 610, 611, 614
  total body surface area burnt, 611, 613
    paediatric, 616
burns unit, transfer to, 613
bursitis
  hip and thigh, 710
  iliopsoas, 710
  infrapatellar, 719
  prepatellar, 719
  semimembranosus, 720
  trochanteric, 710
bursitis anserina (breast-stroker's knee), 719
burst fracture, 752
Buruli ulcer, 135–6
Butchart staging system for malignant mesothelioma (1976), 355

c wave, 382
C-reactive protein (CRP), 114, 117
cachexia, 109
caderins, 183
caesarean section, 617–18
café au lait spots, 18, 202, 638
calabar swelling, 159
calamine lotion, 450
calcaneum
  fractured, 734–5
  knob, 726
  Sever's disease, 725
calcific tendinitis, acute, 675
calliper, 662, 667, 714, 726, 757
callosities, 192
Calot's triangle, 470
Campbell de Morgan spots, 199
cancer genes, 183
cancers
  carcinogenesis, 182–3, 184
  cutaneous manifestations, 190
  features, 182
  pain, 107–8
  paraneoplastic syndromes, 185, 342, 358
  presentation, 184–5
  spread, 184
  treatment, 186–7
  tumour assessment, 185
  tumour markers, 185
cancrum oris (noma), 136, 274

candidiasis, 197, 274, 276
  in HIV/AIDS, 125, 126, 127
cannula, 20
  failed, 75
  infection, 75
  thrombophlebitis, 75
  thrombosis, 75
capillary haemangiomas, 590
capitulum, fractured, 687
carbohydrate, daily requirement, 48
carbon monoxide poisoning, 29, 611, 612
carbuncle, 193
carcinogenesis, 182–3, 184
carcinoid syndrome, 439–40
cardiac catheterization, 378
cardiac index, 11
cardiac medication, peri-operative, 13
cardiac output, 11
cardiac problems
  postoperative, 64–5
  see also congenital heart disease; valve disease
cardiac stents, 548–9
cardiac tamponade, 360, 362, 382–4
cardiogenic shock (pump failure), 65
cardiorespiratory function, assessment, 11
cardiovascular system
  ageing process, 104
  fitness, 343
  ICU systems support, 91–2
caries, 272
Caroli's disease, 465
carotenaemia, 189
carotid artery disease, 546–52
  aneurysm, 210, 211, 551
  chemodectoma, 550–1
  clinical features, 547
  dissection, 549
  endarterectomy, 548
  injury, 580
  investigation, 547
  neurological deficits associated, 547
  prominent innominate artery, 551–2
  subclavian aneurysm, 551
  subclavian steal, 550
  vertebrobasilar artery disease, 549

carotid body tumour (chemodectoma), 550–1
carotid endarterectomy, 548
carotid-cavernous fistula, 260
carpal dislocation, 694
carpal tunnel syndrome, 690
carpometacarpal dislocation, 698
cartilage graft, 593
case notes, 3
cat-scratch disease, 302
cataracts, 263
Caterall's groups (Perthes' disease), 706
cat's eye, 259
cauda equina syndrome, 741
caval filter, 346
cavernous haemangioma, 258
cavernous sinus thrombosis, 257
CCS (Canadian Cardiovascular Society) angina status, 365
CD4, CD8 cells, 116
ced genes, 183
cell salvage, pre-operative, 37
cellulitis, 193
central retinal artery occlusion, 268–9, 547
central venous pressure (CVP), 91–2
cephalosporins, 19
cerebellar abscess, 213
cerebellopontine angle tumours, 213
cerebral palsy, 662–3
cerebral toxoplasmosis, 123–4
cerebrospinal fluid leak, postoperative, 71
ceruminomas, 239
cervical lymphadenopathy, 300–1
  acute inflammatory, 300–1
  rare causes, 302
  tuberculous lymphadenitis, 261–2
cervical pregnancy, 410
cervical spine injuries, 749–53
  atlas (C1) fracture, 751
  axis (C2) pedicle fracture, 751
  burst fractures, 752
  comminuted body fractures, 752
  dislocation/fracture–dislocation (C3–T1), 752–3
  hyperextension injury (C3–T1), 752
  investigations, 750

multiply injured, 600, 602
subluxations (C3–T1), 752
unilateral facet dislocation, 753
wedge compression (C3–T1), 752
whiplash, 750–1
cervical sympathetic chain (Horner's syndrome), 267–8, 761
chalazion (meibomian cysts), 249
chancroid, 138
Charcot–Marie–Tooth, 775
Charcot's joint, 662
Charcot's triad of symptoms, 472
Charing Cross bandage, 588
chemical cordectomy, 107
chemodectoma (carotid body tumour), 550–1
chemotherapy, 187
chest
  drains, 50
  flail, 360, 362
  sucking wound, 360, 361
  see also bronchial; lung; pleural; pulmonary; thoracic
Chevallet nasal fracture, 282
Chiari type II malformation, 221, 222
chlamydial infection
  conjunctivitis, 250–1
  genital, 138
  trachoma, 248–9
cholangiocarcinoma (bile duct carcinoma), 472–3
cholecystitis
  acalculous, 128, 466
  acute, 466–8
choledochal cysts, 465–6
choledocholithiasis (bile duct stones), 468–9
chondromalacia patellae, 718–19
chordoma, 758
choroid plexus melanoma, 258–9
Christmas disease (haemophilia B), 661
chromoblastomycosis, 147
chrondrosarcoma, 645
Chvostek's sign, 320
circoid aneurysms, 218
circumcision, 528
cirrhosis, 458–9
clam cystoplasty, 522
clavicle, fractured, 677–8
claw foot, 558, 771

claw hand, 763, 768
claw toe, 650, 733, 738
cleft lip and palate, 277
clergyman's knee (infrapatellar bursitis), 719
clinical consent
  anaesthesia, 21
  children and minors, 21–2
  competence, 21
  compulsory treatment, 21
  court application, 22
  emergency life-saving surgery, 22
  information given, 22–3
  organ donation, 23
  process, 21
  refusal or withdrawal, 23
  research, 23
clinical governance, 4
clinical skills, 778–80
clips, 50
club hand, 694
clubbing, 189
clubfoot (talipes equinovarus), 732
co-trimoxazole, 19
coagulation disorders, ICU-related, 96
coagulation pathway, 33, 115
coagulopathy, transplant-related, 595
Cobb's angle, 740
coccydynia, 747
Cock's peculiar tumour, 203
codeine, 45, 107
Codman's triangle, 644
coeliac disease (gluten enteropathy), 79, 275
cold sores, 197, 273–4
collar-stud abscess, 301
Colles' fracture, 692
colon
  polyps, 443–4
  trauma, 408
  washout, 398, 400
colorectal carcinoma, 441–3, 599
  Dukes' staging, 441
  investigations, 441–2
  syndromes, 443
  treatment, 442
colostomy, 452–3
  'double-barrel' (Paul–Mikulicz), 402, 408
colovesical fistula, 522–3
Commando operation, 287

Commission for Health Improvement (CHI), 784
common cold (acute rhinitis, coryza), 278
communication skills, 2, 781
compartment syndrome, 407, 622
    after limb ischaemia, 579–80
competence, 21
complement system
    proteins, 115
    deficiency, 94, 95
compression stockings, 16, 76, 581, 584, 586, 590
compulsory treatment, 21
cone shell stings, 168
confidentiality, 4, 780, 781
confusion, 110
    postoperative, 70–1
congenital aplastic anaemia (Fanconi's syndrome), 175
congenital cystic bronchiectasis, 338
congenital dislocation of hip, 703
congenital glaucoma, 253–4
congenital heart disease, 385–7
    atrial septal defect, 385–7
    patent ductus arteriosus, 387–8
    tetralogy of Fallot, 388–9
    transposition of great arteries, 389–90
    ventricular septal defect, 387
congenital intestinal atresias, 395–6
congenital megacolon (Hirschsprung's disease), 436
congenital nasolacrimal duct obstruction, 250
congenital proptosis, 256
congenital syphilis, 271, 279
congenital vesico-ureteric reflux, 516
coning, 209, 230, 267
conjunctivitis, 250–1
Conn's syndrome (primary hyperaldosteronism), 489
consciousness, altered, 71
consent, 783
contact lenses, 264
contact system, 115
Coomb's test, 177
cord demyelination, 664
cord transection, 756
Cori cycle, 78

corneal abrasions, 261
corneal foreign body, 261–2
corneal graft, 592, 593
coronary angiography, 367
coronary artery bypass graft surgery (CABG), 368
coronary artery stenosis, 364
coroner, 3
Corrigan's sign, 371
corticotropin-releasing factor (CRF), 486–7
coryza (common cold, acute rhinitis), 278
Cotrel–Dubousset fixation, 741
Courvoisier's law, 468, 472, 481
coxa vara, 705
cranial nerve palsies, 207–17
    abducent nerve (VI) and nucleus, 211
    accessory nerve (XI), 214–15
    bulbar and pseudobulbar (IX–XII), 215–17
    facial nerve (VII), 212–13
    glossopharyngeal nerve (IX), 214
    hypoglossal nerve (XII), 215
    oculomotor nerve (III) and nucleus, 209
    olfactory nerve (I), 207
    optic nerve (II) and interruption of pathway, 207–8, 267
    trigeminal nerve (V) and nucleus, 210–11
    trochlear nerve (IV) and nucleus, 209–10
    vagus nerve (X), 214
    vestibulocochlear nerve (VIII) and nucleus, 213
craniopharyngioma, 207
Crawford classification (thoraco-abdominal aneurysms), 571
creeping eruption (cutaneous larva migrans), 155
cretinism (neonatal hypo-thyroidism), 316–17, 391
Creutzfeld–Jacob disease, variant, 36, 41
Crohn's disease, 435–7
croup (laryngotracheo-bronchitis), 289
Crouzon's syndrome, 256
crush injury, 608
cryoprecipitate, 36
cubitus valgus, 682

cubitus varus ('gun-stock' deformity), 682–3
Cullen's sign, 477
Cushing's syndrome, 225, 488–9, 631
cutaneous larva migrans (creeping eruption), 155
cutaneous vasculitis, 193–4
cyanide poisoning, 612
cystic adventitial disease of popliteal artery, 560
cystic echinococcosis (hydatid disease), 161–2, 206, 461
cystic fibrosis, 339, 398
cystic hygroma, 300, 591
cystitis
  acute, 514–15
  interstitial, 517–18
  recurrent, 515
cystocoele, 524
cystogastrostomy, 480
cysts, 205–6
cytokines, 109, 114, 116
cytomegalovirus (CMV)
  in HIV/AIDS, 124–5, 126, 127
  iritis, 252

D-dimer, 33
dacryocystitis, 250
Dandy–Walker malformation, 221, 222
day case surgery
  disadvantages, 10–11
  hospital benefits, 8–9
  local guidelines, 9
  patient benefits, 8
  patient selection, 9
  procedure, choice of, 10
De Quervain's disease, 691
De Quervain's thyroiditis, 314–15
death
  at home, 111
  certification, 3, 102
  diagnosis, 111
  in hospital, 3, 80, 111
  managing process of, 111–12
  see also brainstem death
DeBakey classification (aortic dissection), 575
deep vein thrombosis (venous thromboembolism), 75–6, 583–5, 626
  postoperative prophylaxis, 16

delayed haemolytic transfusion response, 40
delirium, 105, 110
delirium tremens, postoperative, 71
dementia, 105, 110
demyelination
  brainstem, 664
  cord, 664
  retrobulbar, 664
dendritic cells, 116
dendritic ulcer, 253
dental abscess, 272
dental impaction, 273
dentigerous cysts, 272, 273
deoxyuridine suppression test, 173
Dercum's disease, 202
dermabrasion, 282
dermatitis (eczema), 190–1, 193, 586
dermatomyositis, 669–70
dermoid cyst, 191, 206, 247, 277
desferrioxamine infusion, 181
detrusor instability (urge incontinence), 521–2
dexamethasone suppression test, 488
dextrose solutions, 48, 58
diabetes insipidus, 58, 61, 225
diabetes mellitus, perioperative care, 14–15
diabetic foot, 558–9, 587, 662
diagnosis, 780
  differential, 2
diamorphine, 107
diaphragm
  air under, 69
  eventration, 395
  hernia, 394
  pus under, 70
  subphrenic abscess, 70, 405
  traumatic rupture, 394–5
diarrhoea
  infective, in HIV/AIDS, 127
  peri-operative, 20
diathermy burns, 31, 32, 42
diets
  elemental, 81
  polymeric, 81
diffuse axonal injury, 225
dihydrocodeine, 45
diphtheria, 284–5
diplegia, 663

disability
  ATLS system, 601
  Glasgow Coma Scale, 226, 604
    paediatric, 615
disc rupture, acute, 744–5
discharge plan, 3
discharge summary/letter, 3
disseminated intravascular
  coagulation (DIC), 96, 97
diverticular disease, 434–5
doctor–patient relationship, 2,
  781
documentation, 3–4, 780
Dohlman's operation, 289
double-stranded DNA antibody,
  774
dracunculiasis (guinea worm
  infection), 160–1
drains, drainage, 50–1
dressings, 50
Dressler's syndrome, 384
drinking, postoperative, 49
drug management, peri-
  operative, 12–20
  antibiotics, 17–19
  anticoagulation, 15–16
  bronchodilators, 13
  cardiac medication, 13
  diabetes, 14–15
  intra-abdominal infections,
    19–20
  jaundice, 16–17
  psychotherapeutic drugs, 13
  respiratory infections, 20
  urinary infections, 20
  ventilator-associated
    pneumonia, 20
Duchenne's muscular dystrophy,
  670–1
duct ectasia (periductal mastitis),
  325
duct papilloma, 324–5
ductal carcinoma in situ (DCIS),
  329, 332
Dukes' staging (colorectal
  carcinoma), 441, 442
duodenal atresia, 396, 424–5
duodenal trauma, 408
duodenal ulcer, chronic, 428–30
Dupuytren's contracture, 695
dwarfism, 636–7
dying patient, 110–12
  hospital vs home care, 111
  religious and cultural support,
    111

dysphagia, 416–17
dysphasia
  expressive, 547
  sensory, 547
dyspnoea (NYHA) status, 366
dystrophia myotonica, 671–2

ear
  accessory auricles, 237
  acoustic neuroma, 244–5
  acute mastoiditis, 241–2
  barotrauma, 246–7
  basal cell carcinoma, 239
  bat, 237
  cauliflower, 239
  ceruminomas, 239
  congenital deformities,
    236–7
  exostosis of external auditory
    canal, 239
  glomus jugulare, 213, 246
  glue, 242
  herpes zoster oticus, 244
  impacted wax, 239
  Menière's disease, 213, 245
  noise-induced hearing loss,
    246
  otitis externa, 237–8
  otitis externa malignans,
    238–9
  otitis media
    acute suppurative, 240–1
    chronic serous, 242
    chronic suppurative, 243
  otosclerosis, 240
  pre-auricular cysts and
    sinuses, 237
  presbycusis, 247
  Ramsay–Hunt syndrome,
    244
  squamous cell carcinoma,
    239
  tophi, 656
  traumatic rupture of tympanic
    membrane, 244
echocardiography, 91
ectopic pregnancy, 409–10
ectopic thyroid, 317
ectropion, 250
eczema (dermatitis), 190–1
  varicose, 586
  weeping, 193
edrophonium (anticholi-
  nesterase) (Tensilon test), 668
educational contract, 778

educational supervisor, 778, 779
Ehlers–Danlos syndrome, 228, 571, 574
Eisenmenger syndrome, 385, 387
elbow
  cubitus valgus, 682
  cubitus varus, 682–3
  dislocation, 688–9
  golfer's, 683
  pitcher's, 683
  pulled, 689
  tennis, 683
  see also humerus
elderly patient, 104–5, 744
electrocardiography (ECG), 12-lead, 29, 91, 367
elephantiasis, 158, 159, 539
elliptocytosis, 171
  hereditary, 177
embolectomy, 76
emergency admission, 8
emesis, see nausea and vomiting
empyema, 353–4, 467
enamel pearls, 272
enchondroma, 640
endocarditis, infective, 380–1
endotracheal intubation, 90, 311
  anaesthesia and, 26–7, 31, 32
  indications, 602
  paediatric, 614
    tube diameter, 614
enteral nutrition, 80–2, 93
  'elemental' diets, 81
  tube feeding, 81–2
enteric cyst, 358
entonox (oxygen 50%, nitrous oxide 50%), 45, 47
entropion, 250
enzyme-linked immunosorbent assay (ELISA) tests, 301
eosinophils, 115
epididymal cyst, 206, 540
epididymitis
  acute, 540–1
    caseous granulomatous, 506
  chronic, 541
epidural abscess, 47
epidural anaesthesia, 28, 31, 71–2
epidural analgesia, 47, 101
epidural (extradural) haematoma, 47, 226–8
epiglottitis, acute, 289–90
epiphyseal dysplasia, multiple, 637

epispadias, 527–8
epistaxis (nosebleed), 283
Erb's palsy, 763
erysipelas, 193
erythromycin, 19
erythroplakia, 274
erythroplasia of Queyrat, 200, 530
escharotomy, 613
ethical committee, 783
European Working Time Directive, 784–5
Euroscore, 368
euthyroid goitre, 307–8
evidence-based practice, 2, 5, 779
Ewing's tumour, 646–7
excision biopsy, 205
excoriation, 193
exercise test/stress ECG, 343, 366–7, 370
exomphalos (omphalocoele), 391
exophthalmic ophthalmoplegia, 210, 211, 309, 310
exophthalmos, 310
experimental design, 783
external fixation, 620
extracellular volume
  decreased, 56
  increased, 56–7
extradural (epidural) haematoma, 47, 226–8
eye
  amaurosis fugax, 268, 547, 565
  capillary haemangioma, 257–8
  carotid-cavernous fistula, 260
  cataracts, 263
  cat's eye, 259
  cavernous haemangioma, 258
  cavernous sinus thrombosis, 257
  central retinal artery occlusion, 268–9, 547
  choroid plexus melanoma, 258–9
  conjunctivitis, 250–1
  dacrocystitis, 250
  dendritic ulcer, 253
  field loss and blindness, 268–71
  fundal tumours, 258–60
  glaucoma, 253–6
  herpes zoster ophthalmicus, 125, 147, 247
  Horner's syndrome, 267–8
  hyphaema, 262

eye *cont.*
  iritis, 253
  keratitis, 253
  lacrimal gland tumours, 250
  macular degeneration, 270
  nasolacrimal duct obstruction, 250
  nystagmus, 266
  orbital cellulites, 256–7
    fungal, 257
  proptosis, 256
  pterygium, 252
  ptosis, 248
  pupillary response abnormalities, 266–7
  refractive errors, 263–4
  retinal detachment, 262, 268
  retinoblastoma, 259–60
  retro-ocular tumours, 257–8
  rhabdomyosarcoma, 258
  scleritis, 253
  strabismus, 264–5
  thyrotoxicosis, 308
  see also eye injuries; eyelids; optic
eye injuries
  corneal abrasion, 261
  foreign bodies, 261–2
  globe disruption, 262
  hyphaema, 262
  orbital fractures, 270–1
  panda sign, 220, 604
  retinal detachment, 262
eye test charts, 263
eyelids
  blepharitis, 248
  ectropion, 249, 250
  entropion, 249, 250
  Herbert's pits, 249
  Meibomian cysts, 249
  ptosis, 248
  styes, 249
  trachoma, 248–9
  trichiasis, 249

face and jaws
  alveolar fractures of mandible and maxilla, 234
  Bell's palsy, 235–6
  herpes zoster (shingles), 235
  mandibular fractures, 233, 234
  maxillary fractures, 232–3, 234
  paranasal sinuses, 232
  sinusitis, 231
  trigeminal neuralgia, 211, 234

face-mask, 26
facial nerve injury, 295
facial nerve palsy, 212–13
familial adenomatous polyposis, 443
Fanconi's syndrome (congenital aplastic anaemia), 175
fasting, 77–8
fat embolism, 623–4
fat necrosis, 326
fat-pad sign, 684
'favism', 179
febrile non-haemolytic transfusion reaction, 40
Felty's syndrome, 473
feminization, 487
femoral artery, false aneurysm, 576
femoral hernias, 392–3
femoral nerve injury, 770
femur
  condylar fracture, 724
  coxa vara, 705
  fracture-related blood loss causing shock, 619
  fractured neck, 711–12
  osteonecrosis of head, 709–10
  Perthes' disease, 706
  shaft fracture, 722–3
  slipped upper femoral epiphysis, 707
  subtrochanteric fracture, 712
  supracondylar fracture, 723
  see also hip
fentanyl patch, 47, 107
fetal trauma
  assessment, 617
  caesarean delivery, 617–18
  complications of blunt abdominal, 617
fetus, *see* pregnancy
fever (pyrexia)
  postoperative, 72–3
  see also sepsis
fibrin, 115
fibrinogen, 115
fibromuscular dysplasia, 569–60
fibrosarcoma, 645–6
fibrous dysplasia, 638
fibrous histiocytoma, 199
fibula
  fracture of shaft of tibia and, 726–7
  fracture–separation of distal epiphysis, 730

isolated fracture of shaft, 728
Pott's fracture, 730
recurrent dislocation of
    peroneal tendons, 731–2
filariasis, 158, 539–40, 589
finger
    apical abscess, 195
    Boutonnière deformity, 650,
        697
    Heberden's nodes, 650
    macrodactyly, 694
    mallet, 672, 696
    polydactyly, 694
    pulp abscess, 195
    swan-neck deformity, 650
    syndactyly, 694
    trigger, 695–6
    ulnar deviation, 650
    vibration white, 567
    whitlow, 699
    see also nails
fish stings, 167–8
fistula in ano, 447–8
fistulae, 206
    postoperative, 70
Fitz–Hugh–Curtis syndrome, 544
fixation
    external, 620
    internal, 620
flail chest, 360, 362
fluid balance, 47–8, 92–3
    assessment, 77
    daily requirement, 48
    lost from, 47–8, 55
    postoperative, 55–61
folate deficiency, 173–4, 740
Fontaine's grading (lower limb
    ischaemia), 552
foot
    anti-personnel mines, injury,
        611–12
    bunion, 736–7
    claw, 558, 771
    diabetic, 558–9, 587, 662
    drop, 771, 772
    equinus, 663
    Freiberg's disease, 736
    keratoderma
        blennorrhagicum, 657
    Kohler's disease, 735
    Madura, 145, 739–40
    malignant melanoma, 739
    Morton's metatarsalgia, 736
    pes cavus, 733
    pes planus, 733–4

plantar fasciitis, 739
postural equinovarus, 732
stress fracture of metatarsal,
    736
talipes equinovarus, 732
tarsal injuries, 735
tarsal tunnel syndrome, 735–6
'trash-foot', 556
valgus, 650
see also toe
forearm fracture, 689–90
foreign bodies
    bladder, 515
    eye, 261–2
    gastric, 426
    nasal, 283
four-glass test, 515–16
Fournier's (scrotal) gangrene,
    196, 538–9
fractures
    bumper, 772
    burst, 752, 755
    butterfly fragment, 618
    clinical features, 618–19
    closed, 618
    comminuted, 618
    complications, 622–6
        adult respiratory distress
            syndrome, 67
        arterial injury, 578
        compartment syndrome,
            407, 622
        delayed union, 624
        fat embolism, 623–4
        nerve injury, 759
    compound (open), 618
    epiphyseal, 621
    greenstick, 621
    Gustilo's classification, 618
    impacted, 620
    investigation, 619
    Le Fort classification, 232
    long bone and pelvic, 619
    malunion, 625–6
    natural repair process of bone,
        624
    non-union, 625
    oblique, 618
    pathological, 621–2
    Pott's, 729
    Salter–Harris, 730–1
    Smith's, 693
    spiral, 618
    stress (march), 736
    transverse, 618

fractures cont.
  treatment
    closed reduction, 619
    methods of holding
      reduction, 620
    open fractures, 620
    open (operative) reduction,
      619
    principles, 619
Freiberg's disease, 736
Freidreich's sign, 384
fresh frozen plasma (FFP), 36,
  38
Frey's syndrome, 295
Friedreich's ataxia, 775
Friedreich's sign, 384
Froment's sign, 768
frozen shoulder, 676
functional brace, 620
fundal tumours
  carotid–cavernous fistula, 260
  choroid plexus melanoma,
    258–9
  retinoblastoma, 259–60
fungal orbital cellulites, 257
furuncle (boil), 193

Gage's sign, 706
gait, intoe, 705
Galeazzi dislocation, 689
gallbladder, 464
  adenoma, 471
  carcinoma, 471
  empyema, 467
  fistulation, 468
  gangrene, 467
  mucocoele, 467
  sludge, 85
gallstone, 465–6, 468–9
  in bile duct, 468–9
  ileus, 469
  pancreatitis, 477, 478
gamekeeper's thumb, 697
ganglia, 203, 206
gangrene, 199
  dry/wet, 199
  Fournier's, 196, 538–9
  gallbladder, 467
  gas, 196, 199, 606–7
  Meleney's, 196
  synergistic, 196
  venous, 75
Garden's classification (femoral
  neck fracture), 712
Gardner's syndrome, 190

gas gangrene, 196, 199, 606–7
gas transfer factor, 343
gastric carcinoid tumours, 433,
  439–40
gastric foreign bodies, 426
gastric lymphomas, 432
gastric mucosa associated
  lymphoid tissue (MALT)
  lymphoma, 432
gastric physiology, 423
gastric surgery, for obesity,
  103–4, 433
gastric ulcer, 427–8
gastrinoma, 484–5
gastritis, 426–7
gastro-oesophageal reflux disease
  (acid reflux), 417–19
gastro-oesophageal varices,
  422–3, 459–60
gastrointestinal tract, 48–9
  postoperative problems,
    68–70
    adhesions, 69
    fistulae, 70, 206
    haemorrhage, 69
    nausea and vomiting, 68–9
    paralytic ileus, 69
    peritonism, 69
    peritonitis, 69–70
    subphrenic abscess, 70
gastroschisis, 390–1
gastrostomy, feeding, 452
Gaucher's disease, 709
generalized convulsive status
  epilepticus (GCSE), 97–8
genital chlamydia, 138
genital herpes, 138, 197, 544
genital ulcers, 138
genital warts, 197, 544
gentamicin, 19
genu recurvatum, 714
genu valgum (knock knee), 714
genu varum (bow leg), 714
giant cell sarcoma, 646
giant cell tumour, 641–2
gigantism (acromegaly), 225
Gil–Vernet pyelolithotomy, 502
gingivitis, chronic, 273
girdlestone pseudoarthrosis, 711
Glasgow Coma Scale (GCS),
  226, 604
  modified, in paediatric
    trauma, 615
glaucoma
  acute/closed-angle, 254

chronic simple/open-angle,
255–6
congenital, 253–4
glioblastoma, 223
global oxygen delivery index, 11
globe disruption, 262
glomus jugulare, 213, 246
glomus tumours, 199
glossitis, 276
glossopharyngeal nerve palsy,
214
glucagon, 476
glucagonoma, 483–4
glucocorticoids, 486
glucose-6-phosphate
dehydrogenase (G-6-PD)
deficiency, 179–80
glucose–alanine cycle, 78
glue ear (chronic serous otitis
media), 242
glycogen, 78
goitre
euthyroid, 307–8
malignant, 312–13
toxic nodular, 310
golfer's elbow, 683
gonorrhoea, 251–2, 514, 542
Goodsall's rule, 448
gout, 655–6, 684, 738
Gower's sign, 671
Gradenigo's syndrome, 210,
238
Gradenigo's triad, 241
graft rejection, 598–9
graft versus host transfusion
reaction, 40
granuloma inguinale, 138
granulomatous lobular mastitis,
325
Graves' disease, 309–10
Grawitz's tumour (renal cell
carcinoma, hypernephroma),
500–1
Grey Turner's sign, 477
grief counselling, 111
groin, hanging, 159
grommet insertion, 242, 245
Guedal airway, 602
Guillain–Barré syndrome, 215,
774
guinea worm infection
(dracunculiasis), 160–1
'gun-stock' deformity (cubitus
varus), 682–3
gunshot wounds, 605–8

Gustilo's classification
(compound fractures), 618
gynaecological emergencies
acute pelvic inflammatory
disease (PID), 543
ectopic pregnancy, 409–10
septic abortion, 411
torsion of ovarian pedicle,
cyst, 412
gynaecomastia, 321–2

haemangioma
capillary, 590
cavernous, 258
liver, 461
spinal, 757
strawberry, 590, 591
haemochromatosis, 455, 458
haemoconcentration, 56
haemodialysis, 496, 498
haemodilution, acute
normovolaemic, 37
haemofiltration, 118, 496
haemoglobins AS/SS, 177
haemolytic anaemias, 176–81
acquired autoimmune, 474
inherited, 176–81
haemopericardium, 383, 384
haemoperitoneum, 410
haemophilia A, 34, 661
haemophilia B (Christmas
disease), 34, 661
haemophilic arthropathy, 661–2
haemorrhage, postoperative, 55–6
haemorrhoidectomy, 449
haemorrhoids (piles), 448–9
sentinel, 446
haemostasis
disorders, 34–5
extrinsic system, 33
intrinsic system, 33
measures of, 33
normal, 32–3
haemothorax, large, 360, 361
Hageman factor, 115
hallux rigidus, 737
hallux valgus, 736
halo body cast, 750
hammer toe, 558, 737
hand
Bennet's fracture–dislocation,
697
capitulum fracture, 687
carpal dislocation, 694
carpal tunnel syndrome, 690

hand *cont.*
  carpometacarpal fractures, 698
  claw, 763, 768
  club, 694
  congenital abnormalities, 694
  De Quervain's disease, 691
  deep infections, 699
  Dupuytren's contracture, 695
  infections, 195
  interphalangeal dislocations, 698
  Keinbock's disease, 691–2
  macrodactyl, 694
  Madelung's deformity, 694
  metacarpal fractures, 698
  metacarpophalangeal dislocations, 698
  phalangeal fractures, 698
  polydactyl, 694
  radial club, 694
  rheumatoid arthritis, 649
  scaphoid fracture, 693–4
  syndactyl, 694
  tendon injury, 672
  trident, 636
  ulnar club, 694
  see also finger; thumb
hangman's fracture (fracture of pedicle of axis, C2), 751
Harrington fixation, 741
Hartmann's procedure, 435, 452
Hashimoto's thyroiditis, 313–15
head injury
  blast injury, 608
  diffuse axonal injury, 228
  Glasgow Coma Scale, 226, 604
  intracranial haematoma, 226–8
  multiply injured, 603–4
  paediatric trauma, 615
  raised intracranial pressure, 229–30
  skull fractures, 219–20
  subarachnoid haemorrhage, 228–9
  vegetative state, 230
  see also brainstem death
head lice, 198
headache
  postepidural, 47
  postoperative, 71
  in raised intracranial pressure, 229
Heaf/Mantoux tests, 302, 506
health service, 783–5

Health Trusts, 784
hearing aids, 240, 246, 247
hearing loss
  acoustic neuroma, 244–5
  age-related, 247
  barotrauma, 246
  Menière's disease, 245
  noise-induced, 146, 246
  presbycusis, 247
heart block, postoperative, 65
heart failure, 369, 377, 380, 381
heart/lung transplantation, 596
heart, *see* cardiac; congenital heart disease; valve disease
Heberden's nodes, 189, 650
heel cups, 734
heel-raise, 726
Heinz bodies, 179
Heller's operation (oesophago-cardiomyotomy), 414
helminthoma (oesophagostomiasis), 156–7
hemianopia
  bitemporal, 208
  homonymous, 208
heminephro-ureterectomy, 493
hemiplegia, 604
heparin
  peri-operative, 15
  postoperative, 16
hepatic adenoma, 460–1
hepatic encephalopathy, 457–8
hepatic iminodiacetic acid (HIDA) scan (radionuclide excretion scan), 464
hepaticojejunostomy, 465
hepatitis
  drug-induced, 128
  viral, 128, 457
hepatoblastoma, 462
hepatocellular carcinoma, 461–3
Herbert's pits, 249
hereditary elliptocytosis, 177
hereditary non-polyposis colon cancer syndromes, 443
hereditary spherocytosis, 176–7, 473–4
hereditary telangiectasia, 198
hernias, 50
  diaphragmatic, 394
  external, 392
  femoral, 392
  hiatus, 417–19

incisional, 393
inguinal, 392–3
inguinoscrotal, 392
internal, 392
irreducible, 392, 393
lumbar, 394
obturator, 392
para-oesophageal, 419
Richter, 392
Spigelian, 393
umbilical, 393
herniorrhaphy, 393
herpes simplex virus (HSV)
cold sores, 197
genital infection, 138, 197,
544
in HIV/AIDS, 125, 126, 127
herpes zoster (shingles), 197,
211, 212, 235
herpes zoster ophthalmicus,
125, 147, 247
herpes zoster oticus, 244
Hess test, 271
hiatus hernia, 417–19
clinical features, 418
complications, 419
rolling, 418
sliding, 417
treatment, 418–19
hydradinitis suppurativa, 194
hidradenoma (turban tumour),
200
high dependency unit (HDU),
99–100
high-risk patient
assessment and management,
11, 12
see also drug management,
peri-operative
Hill repair, 419
Hill–Sachs lesion (shoulder
dislocation), 681–2
hip
acetabular fractures, 701–2
bursitis, 710
coxa vara, 705
dislocation, 712–13
congenital, 703–4
irritable, 706
osteoarthritis, 709
rheumatoid arthritis, 649
septic arthritis, 708
snapping, 710
subluxation, 704–5
tuberculosis, 708

hip replacement, 709, 710, 711,
712
complications, 711
acute dislocation, 711
aseptic loosening, 711
chronic infection, 711
heterotopic bone formation,
711
hippocratic method (shoulder
reduction), 680
Hirschsprung's disease
(congenital megacolon), 436
histiocytosis X, 302
histioplasmosis, 339
history taking, 2, 780, 781
HIV and AIDS
acute HIV infection, 120
aetiology, 118
antiretroviral therapy, 129–30
bowel manifestations, 122
CDC classification (1992),
119–20
CNS disease, 123–4
cerebral toxoplasmosis,
123–4
meningitis, 123
primary CNS lymphoma,
124
progressive multifocal
leukoencephalopathy, 124
dermatological disease, 129
epidemiology, 118
gastrointestinal disease, 125–6
anal/peri-anal disorders,
127–8
CMV and HSV ulceration,
126, 127
HSV infection, 125
infective diarrhoea, 127
Kaposi's sarcoma, 125, 126,
127
oesophageal candidiasis, 126
oral candidiasis, 126
oral hairy leukoplakia, 125
pancreatitis, 127
recurrent aphthous
ulceration, 126
salivary glands, 126
warts, 125, 127
haematological disease, 129
hepatic/hepatobiliary disease
acalculous cholecystitis, 128
drug-induced hepatitis, 128
neoplastic liver disease, 129
other viral infections, 128

HIV and AIDS *cont.*
  hepatic/hepatobiliary disease
    cont.
    sclerosing cholangitis, 129
    viral hepatitis, 128
  investigations, 119
  musculoskeletal disease, 129
  natural history, 119
  neoplastic disorders, 122
    Kaposi's sarcoma, 122
    lymphoma, 122
  ophthalmologic disease, 123–5
    CMV retinitis, 124–5
    other conditions, 125
  pathogenesis, 119
  respiratory disease, 120–2
    bacterial pneumonia, 121–2
    P. carinii pneumonia, 120–1
    pulmonary tuberculosis,
      121
  symptomatic HIV disease
    (not AIDS), 120
HLA (major histocompatibility
  antigen) match, 593
Hodgkin's disease (lymphoma),
  302–3, 473, 599
Holmes–Adie pupil, 267
Homan's sign, 584
hookworm, 154–5
Horner's syndrome (cervical
  sympathetic chain), 267–8, 761
horseshoe kidney, 493
hospital admission, 8
hospital anxiety and depression
  scale, 110
housemaid's knee (prepatellar
  bursitis), 719
human albumin (4.5%), 38
human immunodeficiency virus
  (HIV), *see* HIV and AIDS
humerus
  bicondylar fracture, 685
  distal humeral epiphysis,
    fracture separation of entire,
    687
  fracture-related blood loss
    causing shock, 619
  lateral condylar epiphysis,
    fracture separation, 682,
    685–6
  medial condylar epiphysis,
    fracture separation, 686
  proximal, fractured, 679
  supracondylar fracture, 682,
    684–5

Hunner's ulcer (interstitial
  cystitis), 517–18
Hunter's syndrome, 637
Hurler's syndrome, 637
Hutchinson's freckle (lentigo
  maligna), 201
Hutchinson's incisors, 271
hydatid disease (cystic
  echinococcosis), 161–2, 206,
  461
hydrocephalus, 221–2
  communicating, 221
  obstructive, 221
hydrocoele, 541
hydronephrosis, 503–4
  infected, 505
hydroureter, 492, 503–4
hyperaldosteronism, primary, 489
hypercalcaemia, 359
hypercarbia, postoperative, 71
hypercoagulable states
  (thrombophilia/prothrombotic
  disorders), 567–8
hyperkalaemia, 41, 59–60
hypermetropia (long sight),
  263–4
hypernatraemia, 57, 58, 71
hypernephroma (Grawitz's
  tumour, renal cell carcinoma),
  500–1
hyperparathyroidism, 318–19
  primary, 636
hypersensitivity, delayed, 116
hypersplenism, 474
hyperthermia, malignant, 72–3
hyperthyroidism, 316
  neonatal, 310, 391
  recurrent, 311
hypertrophic pulmonary
  osteoarthropathy, 342
hypertrophic pyloric stenosis,
  424
hyperventilation, 62
hyphaema, 262
hypocalcaemia, 311
hypochloraemic alkalosis, 64
hypogammaglobulinaemia, 95,
  338
hypoglossal nerve palsy, 215
hypokalaemia, 58–9, 64
hypomagnesaemia, 59
hyponatraemia, 57–8, 71
hypoparathyroidism, 320
hypopyon, 261
hypospadias, 527

hypothalomopituitary axis, 487
hypothermia, 71, 73
  peri-operative, 30, 32
hypothyroidism, 311, 316–17
  neonatal, 316–17, 391
hypovolaemia, 55–6, 60, 360
hypoxia, 90
  postoperative, 66, 71
hysterectomy, 411

idiopathic thrombocytic
  purpura, 473
ileal atresia, 396
ileocystoplasty, 518
ileostomy, 452–3
iliopsoas bursitis, 710
imipenem, 19
immune system, 114–16
  cellular defences, 114–15
  humoral responses, 115
  innate immunity, 114–15
  reduced immunity and sepsis,
    94
  specific immunity, 115–16
immunodeficiency, acquired,
  94–5
immunoglobulin A deficiency, 338
immunosuppression, 592, 597–8
in-patient admission, 8
incisional hernia, 393
incisions, 49, 73
incontinence
  dribbling, 522
  stress, 520–1
  urge, 521–2
induction
  inhalation, 27–8
  intravenous, 27
infant polycystic kidney, 494
infections
  blood-transfusion-related, 41
  peri-operative, 19–20
infective (bacterial) endocarditis,
  380–1
inferior venal caval filters, 176
inflammatory bowel disease
  Crohn's disease, 435–7
  ulcerative colitis, 437–40
information technology (IT),
  3–4, 779
infrapatellar bursitis (clergyman's
  knee), 719
ingrowing toenail, 738
inguinal hernias, 392–3
inguinoscrotal hernias, 392–3

innominate artery, prominent,
  551–2
INR (international normalized
  ratio of prothrombin time), 33
insect bites, 192
insulin
  peri-operative, 14–15
  regulatory functions, 476
insulinoma, 481–2
integrity, 4
intensive care unit (ICU), 88–99
  acid–base balance, 93
  alimentary system, 93–4
  cardiovascular system, 91–2
  coagulation, 96
  controlled environment, 88–9
  fluid balance, 92–3
  follow-up, 99
  indications, 89
  metabolic acidosis, 93
  neurological system, 97–9
  patient assessment, 89
  respiratory system, 90–1
  sepsis, 94–5
  shock, 96–7
  staff, 88
  systems support, 89–90
interferons, 115
interleukins, 115, 117
internal fixation, 620
international normalized ratio of
  prothrombin time (INR), 33
interphalangeal dislocations, 698
intersex, 527
interstitial cystitis (Hunner's
  ulcer), 517–18
intestinal atresias, congenital,
  395–6
intestinal ischaemia, acute, 568–9
intestinal obstruction
  acute, in newborn, 395–8
  see also bowel obstruction
intoe gait, 705
intra-abdominal abscess, 405
intra-abdominal desmoid
  tumour, 454
intra-abdominal infections, peri-
  operative, 19–20
intracranial disorders
  abscess, 222–3
  acoustic neuroma, 225
  haematoma, 226–8, 266, 267
  hydrocephalus, 221–2
  intraventricular haemorrhage,
    208, 222

intracranial disorders *cont.*
  malignant tumours, 223–4
  meningioma, 224
  pituitary adenomas, 225
  raised pressure, 229–30
  schwannoma, 225
  subarachnoid haemorrhage,
    228–9
intraperitoneal haemorrhage,
  410
intussusception, 400–1
ionizing radiation, 188
iritis, 253
iron deficiency anaemia, 171–2
iron overload, 40
iron store, normal, 170
irritable hip, 706
ischaemic heart disease, 364–8
ischiorectal abscess, 447

Jaboulay's procedure, 541
Jaeger chart, 263
jaundice, peri-operative, 16–17
jaw
  wiring, 103, 433
  see also face and jaws
Jehovah's witness, 22, 38
jejunal atresia, 396
jejunostomy, feeding, 452
jellyfish stings, 168
joint mice, 718
joints and muscles
  ankylosing spondylitis, 653–4,
    657
  arthrogryphoses, 673
  cerebral palsy, 662–3
  Charcot's joint, 662
  dermatomyositis, 669–70
  gout, 655–6, 684, 738
  haemophilic arthropathy,
    661–2
  motor neurone disease, 216,
    217, 665–6
  multiple sclerosis, 207, 216,
    217, 664–5
  muscle tears, 670
  muscular dystrophies, 670–2
  myasthenia gravis, 359, 668
  osteoarthritis, 627, 648–9,
    676, 709, 721
  poliomyelitis, 666–7
  polymyalgia rheumatica, 653
  polymyositis, 669–70
  psoriatic arthropathy, 654–5
  pyomyositis, 670

Reiter's syndrome, 656–7
repetitive strain injury, 672
rhabdomyosarcoma, 673
rheumatoid arthritis, 649–50,
  657, 658, 677, 721
septic arthritis, 658–60, 708
Still's disease, 473, 657–8
systemic lupus erythematosus,
  474, 651–2
tendon injury, 672
tuberculous arthritis, 660
journals, 779
jugular venous pulse (JVP), 382
jumper's knee (patellar
  tendinitis), 719
juvenile chronic arthritis, 657

K (Kirschner) wire, 620
kala-azar (leishmaniasis), 148–9,
  281
Kaposi's sarcoma (KS), 133–4,
  201–2, 599
  in HIV/AIDS, 122, 125, 126,
    127, 133
Kartagener's syndrome, 339
keel repair, 393
Keinbock's disease, 691–2
Keller's operation, 737
keloid, 192
Kennedy syndrome, 215, 216
keratitis, 253
keratoacanthoma (molluscum
  sebaceum), 200
keratoderma blennorrhagicum,
  657
ketone bodies, 78
kidney
  absent, 492
  adult polycystic, 493–4
  Grawitz's tumour, 500
  horseshoe, 493
  hydronephrosis, 503–4
  hydroureter, 503–4
  infant polycystic, 494
  perinephric abscess, 504
  polycystic, of the newborn,
    494
  pyonephrosis, 505
  Wilms' tumour, 499–500
  see also renal; ureteric; urinary
Killian's dehiscence, 288, 288–9
Klippel–Feil syndrome, 677
Klumpke's palsy, 763
knee
  Baker's cyst, 649, 720

bursitis anserina, 719
chondromalacia patellae,
    718–19
chronic ligamentous
    instability, 717
genu recurvatum, 714
genu valgum, 714
genu varum, 714
infrapatellar bursitis, 719
ligament injury, 715–16
ligamentum patellae rupture,
    722
locking of, 649, 718
loose bodies, 178
meniscal cysts, 721
meniscal injury, 714–15
Osgood–Schlatter's disease,
    719
osteoarthritis, 721
osteochondritis dissecans,
    717–18
patellar dislocation, 720
patellar fracture, 722
patellar tendinitis, 719
prepatellar bursitis, 719
rectus femoris muscle rupture,
    721
rheumatoid arthritis, 721
semimembranosus bursitis,
    720
valgus, 650
knowledge base, 779
Kocher's manoeuvre, 680
Kohler's disease, 735
Krukenberg's tumour, 184
Kussmaul's sign, 384
kyphosis, 104, 105, 633, 635
    in elderly, 744
    osteoporosis, 632
    Scheurmann's, 743
    spinal tuberculosis, 749

lacrimal gland tumours, 250
Ladd's band, 397
Langer's lines, 49
laryngeal mask airway (LMA), 26
laryngeal nerve injury, 311
laryngeal web, 289
laryngitis, 289–90
    acute, 289
    chronic, 290
laryngocoele, 291–2
laryngomalacia, 289
laryngotracheobronchitis
    (croup), 289

larynx
    acute epiglottis, 289–90
    angioneurotic oedema, 292
    benign neoplasms, 291
    burns, 292
    carcinoma, 290–1
    leukoplakia, 291
    paralysis, 292–3
    singer's nodes, 291
    trauma, 293
lateral cutaneous nerve of thigh
    injury (meralgia
    paraesthetica), 770
Le Fort fractures I–III, 232
lead poisoning, 174
learning
    environment, 778
    partnership, 778
    self-directed, 778–9
leg
    lengthening, 637
    shin splints, 728
    soleus muscle tears, 725
    ulcers, 586–8
    see also ankle; calcaneum;
        fibula; knee; tibia
Leishman–Donovan bodies, 149
leishmaniasis (kala-azar), 148–9,
    281
lentigo maligna (Hutchinson's
    freckle), 201
leopard skin, 159
lepromatous neuropathy, 662,
    773
leprosy, 140, 252, 280, 662,
    773
Leriche's syndrome, 554
leukodepletion, 36, 41
leukoplakia, 275
    laryngeal, 291
    vocal cords, 291
leukotrienes, 114
lice, 198
Lichtenstein herniorrhaphy,
    393
lidocaine (lignocaine), 45, 47
ligamentum patellae (patellar
    ligament) rupture, 722
Light's criteria (1972), 351
limb injuries
    anti-personnel mines, 609–10
    blast, 608–9
    gunshot wounds, 606, 607,
        608
    multiply injured patient, 605

limb ischaemia
  acute upper, 560–2
  compartment syndrome after,
    579–80
  see also lower limb ischaemia
lipodermatosclerosis, 586
lipomas, 202
Lisfranc's (tarso-metatarsal)
  dislocation, 735
Little's area, 283
'lively' splint, 672, 767
liver, 461
  abscess, 461
  adaptation to starvation, 78
  cirrhosis, 458–9
  cysts, 461
  failure, 34, 455–6
  flukes, 152–3
  focal nodular hyperplasia,
    461
  haemangiomas, 461
  hydatid cysts, 461
  physiology, 454–5
  transplantation, 456, 462, 465,
    594–6
  trauma, 463–4, 606
  viral hepatitis, 457, 458
  see also hepatic
loa loa, 159
lobomycosis, 147
lobular carcinoma in situ
  (LCIS), 329, 331
lock-jaw (trismus), 196, 606
'log-roll' examination, 604
long thoracic nerve of Bell
  injury, 764
Looser's zone, 635
Lord's procedure, 541
lower limb
  acute ischaemia, 554–60
    aortic occlusion, 556
    Buerger's disease, 557–8
    diabetic foot, 558
    micro-embolism and 'trash-
      foot', 556–7
    see also popliteal artery
  chronic ischaemia, 552–4
    Leriche's syndrome, 554
  venous incompetence, 75
lumbar hernia, 394
lumps, differential diagnosis,
  204–6
lunate bone
  Keinbock's disease, 691–2
  prosthesis, 692

lung
  abscess, 337–8
  contusion, 360, 363
  fluke, 153–4
  gunshot wounds, 606
  see also bronchial; pleural;
    pulmonary; thoracic
lung cancer
  non-small-cell, 340
  resection, 343–5
  small-cell, 340–1
  see also bronchial cancer
lymphadenitis, tuberculous,
  301–2
lymphangiosarcomas, 202
lymphatic malformation, 590–1
lymphoedema, 588–90
  congenitalia, 589
  praecox, 589
  tarda, 589
lymphogranuloma venereum,
  138
lymphomas
  Burkitt's, 132
  gastric, 432
  in HIV/AIDS, 122, 124, 126
  Hodgkin's disease, 302–3,
    473, 599
  mediastinal, 357
  non-Hodgkin's disease, 122,
    127, 304–5, 473, 537, 757
  pharyngeal, 288
  testicular, 537
lymphoscintigraphy, 589
Lynch syndrome, 443

McBurney's point, 402
McMurray's test, 715
macrodactyly, 694
macrophages, 114
macular degeneration, 270
McVey herniorrhaphy, 393
Madelung's deformity, 694
Madura foot (mycetoma), 145,
  739–40
Maisonneuve fracture, 730
major histocompatibility antigen
  (HLA) match, 593
major histocompatibility
  complex (MHC), 116
malabsorption, 79–80
malaria, 147–8
malignant goitre, 312–13
malignant hypertension, 359
malignant hyperthermia, 72–3

malignant melanoma
  Breslow's depth, 201
  choroid plexus, 258–9
  cutaneous, 201
  foot, 739
  subungual, 201, 739
malignant neuropathy, 774
malingerer, 72
mallet finger, 672, 696
mallet thumb, 696
Mallory–Weiss syndrome, 69, 430–1
malnutrition, 109
malrotation, 396–7
MALT (gastric mucosa associated lymphoid tissue), 432
malunion, 625–6
mammary fistula, 327–8
mammography, 328–9
management, 2
  meetings, 4
  plan, 2, 780
  risk, 5
mandibular fractures, 233
  alveolar, 234
Mantoux/Heaf tests, 302, 506
marble bone disease, 635–6
march (stress) fracture, 736
Marfan's syndrome, 228, 371, 571, 574
Marjolin's ulcer, 201, 587, 588
mast cells, 115
mastectomy, 322, 328, 331–2
mastitis
  granulomatous lobular, 325
  periductal, 325
mastoiditis, acute, 241–2
maxillary fractures, 232–3
  alveolar fracture, 234
Mazzotti test, 159
mean cell haemoglobin concentration (MCHC), 170
mean cell haemoglobin (MCH), 170
mean cell volume (MCV), 169
Meary's angle, 733
Meckel's diverticulum, 397–8
meconium ileus, 398
median nerve injury, 769
mediastinal masses, 357–9
medical education, 778–9
medico-legal aspects, 3, 5, 31
Mediterranean anaemia (thalassaemias), 180–1, 474

Mediterranean lymphoma (primary upper small intestinal lymphoma, PUSIL), 31–2
medullary stroke, tumour, 210
medulloblastoma, 223
mega-oesophagus, 417
megacolon
  congenital, 436
  toxic, 438
megaloblastic anaemias, 172–3
meibomian cysts (chalazion), 249
Meleney's gangrene, 196
Ménière's disease, 213, 245
meningioma, 207, 224
meningitis, in HIV/AIDS
  bacterial, 123
  cryptococcal meningo-encephalitis, 123
  tuberculous, 123
meningitis, hydrocephalus arising, 221
meningocoele, 740
meningomyelocoele, 662, 740
meniscal cysts, 721
meniscal injury, 714–15
mental status schedule for cognitive impairment, 110
meralgia paraesthetica (lateral cutaneous nerve of thigh), 770
mesenteric adenitis, acute, 403
mesenteric ischaemia, chronic, 569
mesothelioma, malignant, 354–7
metabolic acidosis, 63, 93
metabolic alkalosis, 63–4
metacarpal fractures, 698
metacarpophalangeal dislocations, 698
metalloproteinases, 183
metastases, 184
metatarsal stress fracture, 736
methicillin-resistant Staphylococcus aureus (MRSA), 18
metronidazole, 19
micro-embolism, 117, 551, 556–7
microcephaly, 218–19
microtia, 236
microwave therapy, 512
middle-lobe syndrome, 339
midgut carcinoid (argentaffinoma), 440
milk–alkali syndrome, 64

Miller haemorrhoidectomy, 449
Milroy's disease, 589
Milwaukee brace, 742
Milwaukee shoulder, 677
minor surgery admission, 8
Mirizzi syndrome, 468
Mitchell's osteotomy, 737
mitral regurgitation, 376–8
mitral stenosis, 373–6
mitral valve repair, replacement, 375, 376, 379
mobility, 49
  postoperative, 49
molluscum sebaceum (keratoacanthoma), 200
Mondor's disease (superficial thrombophlebitis of breast), 324
Mongolian spot, 200
monocytes, 115
mononeuritis multiplex, 775
monospot test, 301
Monteggia dislocation, 689
Moon's molars, 271
Morgan haemorrhoidectomy, 449
morphine, 45, 46–7, 107
Morquio–Brailsford syndrome, 637
Morton's metatarsalgia, 736
motility factors, 183
motor neurone disease, 216, 217, 665–6
mouth
  aphthous ulcers, 274
  cancrum oris, 136, 274
  candidiasis, 274
  carcinoma, 275–6
  chronic gingivitis, 273
  cold sores, 197, 273–4
  dental impaction, 273
  dentigerous cysts, 273
  erythroplakia, 275
  leukoplakia, 274
  osteomas, 275
  plunging ranula, 307
  sublingual dermoid, 306
  syphilis, 274
  Vincent's angina, 273
  see also face and jaws; teeth; tongue
MRSA (methicillin-resistant Staphylococcus aureus), 18
mucoepidermoid carcinoma, 294–5

mucopolysaccharidoses, 637
mucormycosis, 257
Muir–Torre (Torre's) syndrome, 190
Muir/Barclay formula (intravenous fluid replacement), 613
multigated acquisition (MUGA) scanning (ventriculography), 91, 367
multiple endocrine neoplasia (MEN) type I, 225, 482
multiple endocrine neoplasia (MEN) type IIa/IIb, 312, 318, 319
multiple epiphyseal dysplasia, 637
multiple myeloma, 219, 642–3
multiple organ dysfunction syndrome (MODS), 117, 612
multiple sclerosis, 207, 216, 217, 664–5
multiply injured patient
  ballistic trauma, 605–10
    anti-personnel mines, 609–10
    blast injury, 608–9
    gunshot wounds, 605–8
  fetal assessment and management, 617–18
  initial assessment and resuscitation (ABCDE priority), 599–601
  paediatric, see paediatric trauma
  in pregnancy, 616–18
  second assessment and further management, 603–5
  see also burns
mumps, 293–4
Murphy's sign, 467
muscle
  relaxants, 28
  tears, 670
  see also joints and muscles
muscular dystrophies, 670–2
musculocutaneous nerve injury, 765
Mustard operation, 390
mutator genes, 183
myasthenia gravis, 359, 668
mycetoma, 145–6
  Madura foot, 739–40
mycosis fungoides, 202
myiasis, 164
myocardial contusion, 360, 363

myocardial infarction (MI), 343, 366
  postoperative, 65
myocardial ischaemia
  peri-operative prophylaxis, 12
  see also ischaemic heart disease
myocardial perfusion
  scintigraphy (thallium scan), 91, 367
myopathy, ICU-associated, 98–9
myopia (short sight), 263–4
myositis
  dermato-, 669–70
  poly-, 669
  pyo-, 670
myositis ossificans, 627
myotonia, 267, 671
myotonia congenitalia
  (Thomsen's disease), 672
myringotomy, 241, 242

naevi
  blue, 201
  compound, 200
  intradermal, 200
  junctional, 200
  spider, 198, 455
  strawberry, 590, 591
nails
  Beau's lines, 189
  clubbing, 189
  colour, 189
  deformity, 189
  glomus tumours, 199
  half-and-half, 189
  ingrowing toe, 189, 738
  onychogryphosis, 189, 738
  onycholysis, 189
  paronychia, 195, 699
  red moon bases, 189
  splinter haemorrhages, 189, 381, 551
  subungual lesions, 189
nappy rash, 450
nasal foreign body, 283
nasal fractures, 282–3
nasal polyposis, 281
nasolacrimal duct obstruction
  congenital, 250
  dacryocystitis, 250
nasopharyngeal carcinoma, 131, 286–7
National Clinical Assessment
  Authority (NCAA), 784
national guidelines, 2

National Institute of Clinical
  Excellence (NICE), 784
National Patient Safety
  Organization (NPSA), 784
natural killer (NK) cells, 115
nausea and vomiting, 423
  in dying patient, 108–9
  postoperative, 31, 46, 48–9, 68–9
navicular bone, osteochondritis, 735
neck
  branchial cyst, fistula, sinus, 306
  carotid body tumour, 550
  carotid and subclavian
    aneurysm, 551
  cervical lymphadenopathy, 261–2, 300–2
  cystic hygroma, 300, 591
  goitre, 307–8, 310, 312–13
  Hodgkin's disease, 302–3
  laryngocoele, 291–2
  multiple myeloma, 642
  multiply injured patient, 602, 604
  myeloma, 642
  non-Hodgkin's disease, 304–5
  pharyngocoele, 288
  plunging ranula, 306–7
  rhabdomyosarcoma of
    sternomastoid, 298
  secondary carcinoma, 305
  sternomastoid tumour of
    infancy, 298
  sublingual dermoid, 306
  superior vena cava syndrome, 299–300, 358
  thyroglossal cyst, sinus and
    fistula, 317
  tuberculous lymphadenitis, 301–2
necrolytic migratory erythema, 484
necrotizing fasciitis, 196
needle phobia, 26, 47
neonatal hyperthyroidism, 310, 391
neonatal hypothyroidism
  (cretinism), 316–17, 391
neonatal volvulus, 396–7
neoplasm, 205, see also cancers;
  tumour
nephrectomy, 500, 501, 502, 507
nephro-ureterectomy, 501

nephroblastoma (Wilms' tumour), 499–500
nerve palsies, 72
see also cranial nerve injuries; peripheral nerve injuries
nerve root transection, 756
neuralgia
post-herpetic, 247
trigeminal, 211, 234
neurofibroma, 202, 491–2
neurofibromatosis (von Recklinghausen's disease), 202
plexiform, 202
neurofibrosarcoma, 202
neurogenic tumour, 358
neurological injury
level of, and effects, 756
multiply injured patient, 604
neurological problems, postoperative, 70–2
neuromuscular anaesthetic agents, 32
neuropathy
ICU-associated, 98–9
see also peripheral neuropathy
neuropraxia, 756, 759–60
neurosyphilis, 253, 267
neurotmesis, 759–60
neutropenia, 95
neutrophils, 115
newborn, polycystic kidney, 493
NHS Trusts, 4–5
nipple, supernumerary, 321
Nissen fundoplication, 419
nitrogen balance, 77
NK (natural killer) cells, 115
noma (cancrum oris), 136, 274
non-accidental injury, 616
non-Hodgkin's disease (lymphoma), 122, 127, 304–5, 473, 537, 757
non-specific urethritis, 542
non-ST-elevation MI (NSTEMI), 366
non-steroidal anti-inflammatory drugs (NSAIDs), 44–5, 46
normocytic anaemia, 170–1
nose
acute rhinitis, 278
allergic rhinitis, 281
atresia of posterior apertures, 278
capillary haemangiomas, 590
dermoid cysts, 277
epistaxis, 283

leishmaniasis, 281
lepromatous involvement, 280
rhinophyma, 282
rhinoscleroma, 280
rhinosporidiosis, 281
septal haematoma, 283
simple chronic rhinitis, 278
sleep apnoea, 283–4
snoring, 283
Stewart's midline granuloma, 279
syphilitic gumma, 279
tuberculosis, 280
vasomotor rhinitis, 281–2
Wegener's granulomatosis, 278–9
yaws, 280
see also nasal
nosebleed (epistaxis), 283
Nottingham Prognostic Index (NPI), 332–3
NSTEMI (non-ST-elevation MI), 366
nutritional support
dying patient, 109
energy requirements, 77
enteral, 80–2, 93
feeding stomas, 452
indications, 77
nitrogen balance, 77
postoperative eating, 49
NYHA (New York Heart Association) dyspnoea status, 366
nystagmus, 213, 266
horizontal, 266
vertical, 266

ob gene, 102
obesity, 102–4, 284
associated problems, 103
drug therapy, 103
management, 103
morbid, 102
definition, 433
gastric surgery, 103–4, 433
overweight, 102
physiological changes, 103
obturator hernias, 392
octopus stings, 168
oculomotor nerve and nucleus palsy, 209, 267
odontomes, 272
odynophagia (pain on swallowing), 416–17

oesophageal patency, 413
oesophageal ring (Schatzki's ring), 421
oesophageal web (Plummer–Vinson syndrome), 420–1
oesophagitis, reflux, 417–19
oesophagocardiomyotomy (Heller's operation), 414
oesophagostomiasis (helminthoma), 156–7
oesophagus
    achalasia of cardia, 414
    atresia, 413
    Barrett's, 419
    carcinoma, 421–2
    chronic obstruction, 420
    diverticula, 358
    dysphagia, 416–17
    in HIV/AIDS, 126
    mega-, 417
    perforation, 414–15
    stenosis, 413
    varices, 422–3
olecranon
    bursitis, 684
    fracture, 688
olfactory nerve injury/palsy, 207, 609
oliguria, 60
omental patch, 428, 430
omphalocoele (exomphalos), 391
onchocerciasis (river blindness), 158–60
onychogryphosis, 189, 738
onycholysis, 189
opiates, opioids, 45, 107
opsonization, 115
optic nerve
    glioma, 258
    interruption of pathway, 207–8, 267
    meningioma, 258
    palsy, 207–8, 267
optimizing strategies, 12
oral candidiasis, 125, 274
oral hairy leukoplakia, 125
oral hypoglycaemic agents, perioperative, 14–15
orbital cellulitis, 256–7
    fungal, 257
orbital fractures, 270–1
orchidopexy, 534
orchitis, 541
organ donation, 3, 23, 102
    see also transplantation

oropharynx
    carcinoma, 287
    in HIV/AIDS, 125–6
Ortolani's test, 703
Osgood–Schlatter's disease, 719
Osler's nodes, 381
ossicles, adhesive otitis, 243
osteoarthritis, 648–9, 709
    knee, 721
    post-traumatic, 627, 648
    shoulder, 676
osteoblastoma, 757
osteochondritis, calcaneal, 725
osteochondritis dissecans, 717–18
osteochondroma, 639–40
osteogenesis imperfecta, 637–8
osteoid osteoma, 640–1
osteomalacia, 634–5
osteomas, 275
osteomyelitis
    acute, 628–9
    chronic, 630
    salmonella, 628
osteonecrosis, femoral head, 709–10
osteoporosis, 105, 631–2
osteosarcoma, 643–4
    parosteal, 644–5
otitis, adhesive, 243
otitis externa, 237–8
otitis externa malignans, 238–9
otitis media
    acute suppurative, 240–1
    chronic serous, 242
    chronic suppurative, 243
otosclerosis, 240
Otto pelvis (protrusio acetabuli), 702
ovarian pedicle or cyst, torsion, 208, 412
ovarian pregnancy, 410
ovarian tumour, 412
overhydration, 57
oxycodone, 45
oxygen consumption index, 11
oxygen saturation, 343
    mixed venous, 92
oxygenation, 29

packed cells, 38, 40
paediatric trauma, differences from adult management, 614–15
    abdominal blunt trauma, 616

paediatric trauma, differences
  from adult management *cont.*
  airway, 614
  breathing, 614
  burns, 616
  circulation, 614
  disability, 614
  exposure and environment,
    615
  head injury, 615
  non-accidental injury, 616
  skeletal injury, 610
  spinal cord injury, 615
Paget's disease
  bone, 633–4
  nipple, 326, 330
pain
  assessing severity, 43–4
  assessment, 43–4
  background, 46
  breakthrough, 46, 107
  cancer, 107–8
  'incident', 107
  management, 46–7
  morphine-resistant, 108
  non-drug methods, 108
  physiology, 44
  subjectivity, 43, 46
  visceral, 107
  see also analgesia
pain on swallowing
  (odynophagia), 416–17
painful arc syndrome, 674–5
palate
  cleft lip and, 277
  syphilitic gumma, 277
palliative care, 105–10
  breaking bad news, 106
  cachexia, 109
  cancer pain, 107–8
  emotional support, 106–7
  gastrointestinal symptoms,
    108–9
  malnutrition, 109
  mood changes, 109–10
  respiratory symptoms, 108
  team members, 106
Pancoast tumour, 267
pancreas
  annular, 476
  carcinoma, 480–1
  endocrine secretion, 476
  exocrine secretion, 475
  gastrinoma, 484–5
  glucagonoma, 483–4

insulinomas, 481–2
  pseudocyst, 206, 479–80
  transplant, 596
  trauma, 485–6
  VIPomas, 483–3
pancreatectomy, 479
pancreatitis
  acute, 476–8
  chronic, 478–9
  in HIV/AIDS, 127
pancreato-duodenectomy
  (Whipple's operation), 473,
    479, 481
panda sign, 220, 604
Papineau technique, 630
paracetamol (acetaminophen),
    44–5, 107
paralytic ileus, 69
paranasal aspergillus granuloma,
    146
paranasal fractures, 232
paranasal sinus carcinoma, 232
paraneoplastic syndromes, 185,
    342, 358
paraphimosis, 528
paraplegia, 604, 740–1
  management, 757
  Pott's, 749
parathyroid-like hormone
  secretion, 342
parenteral nutrition, 82–6, 93–4
  central, 83–4
  complications, 84–5, 86
  home, 85–6
  monitoring, 84
  peri-operative, 82
  peripheral vein, 83
  see also nutritional support
paronychia, 195, 699
parosteal osteosarcoma, 644
parotid gland, *see* salivary glands
pars interarticularis fracture, 754
Parsonnet score, 368
patella, bipartite, 722
patellar dislocation, 720
  recurrent, 720
patellar fractures, 722
  stellate, 722
  transverse, 722
patellar tendinitis ('jumper's
  knee'), 719
patent ductus arteriosus (PDA),
    387–8
patent foramen ovale (PFO), 385
patient identification, 41

patient–doctor relationship, 2, 781
patient-controlled analgesia (PCA), 46–7, 107
Paul–Mikulicz ('double-barrel') colostomy, 402, 408
Pavlik harness, 704
pectoral girdle, *see* shoulder joint and pectoral girdle
pediculosis pubis, 198
pelvic abscess, 70, 405
pelvic inflammatory disease (PID), 543–4
pelvis
   fractures, 699–701
      blood loss causing shock, 619
      stable (not involving pelvic ring), 700–1
      unstable (pelvic ring), 699–700, 701
   multiply injured, 604, 605
   Otto pelvis, 702
   see also femur; hip
pelviureteric carcinoma 501
pelviureteric junction obstruction, 499
penicillins, 19
penis
   balanitis xerotica obliterans, 529
   balantitis, 528–9
   carcinoma, 529–30
   epispadias, 527–8
   erythroplasia of Queyrat, 200, 530
   genital warts, 544
   hypospadias, 527
   paraphimosis, 528
   Peyronie's disease, 529
   phimosis, 528
   priapism, 530–1
   urethral injury, 531–3
   urethral strictures, 533
   see also testis and scrotum
pentose-phosphate shunt, 179
peptic ulcers, 64
percutaneous intervention (PCI), 368
pericardial cyst, 358
pericardiocentesis, 384
pericarditis, 384
pericardium
   cardiac tamponade, 382–4
   congenital defects, 384

cysts, 384
diverticula, 384
jugular venous pulse, 382
periductal mastitis (duct ectasia), 325
perinephric abscess, 504
   tuberculous, 504
periodontal cyst, 272
peripheral nerve injuries, 623, 759–73
   accessory nerve, 214–15, 760
   axillary nerve, 680, 766
   brachial plexus, 761–2
   cervical sympathetic chain, 761
   Erb's palsy, 763
   femoral nerve injury, 770
   general principles, 759–60
   Klumpke's paralysis, 763
   lateral cutaneous nerve of thigh, 770–1
   long thoracic nerve of Bell, 764
   median nerve injury, 769
   meralgia paraesthetica, 770
   musculocutaneous nerve, 765
   peroneal nerve, 72, 772
   radial nerve, 766–7
   saphenous nerve, 773, 783
   sciatic, 702, 770–1
   sciatic nerve, 770–1
   suprascapular nerve injury, 764–5
   sural nerve, 772–3, 783
   thoracodorsal nerve, 765–6
   tibial nerve, 771
   ulnar nerve, 72, 682, 767–8
peripheral neuropathy
   aetiology, 773
   Charcot–Marie–Tooth, 775
   clinical features, 774
   definition, 773
   Friedreich's ataxia, 775
   investigations, 774
   mononeuritis multiplex, 775
   treatment, 774–5
peripheral vein nutrition, 83
peritoneal dialysis, 498
peritoneal lavage, 406–7, 478
peritonism, 69, 410
peritonitis, 69–70, 403–5
peritonsillar abscess (quinsy), 285
Perkin's lines, 703
pernicious anaemia, 172–3

peroneal nerve injury, 72, 772
peroneal tendons, recurrent
    dislocation, 731–2
personal development, 778–85
    assessment, 781–2
    clinical skills, 779–80
    communication, 781
    education, 778–9
    EU directive, 785
    health service, 783–5
    knowledge base, 779
    postgraduate, 778–9
    research, 782–3
    teaching, 782
Perthes' disease, 706
pes cavus, 733
pes planus (flat foot), 733–4
pethidine, 107
Peustow operation, modified,
    479
Peyronie's disease, 529
phaeochromocytoma, 319,
    490–1
phaeohyphomycosis, 147
phagocytosis, 115, 116
phalangeal fractures, 698
Phalen's test, 690
pharyngeal pouch, 288–9
pharyngitis, acute, 284
pharyngocoele, 288
pharynx
    acute pharyngitis, 284
    acute tonsillitis, 285
    adenoidal hypertrophy, 286
    bifid uvula, 284
    chronic tonsillitis, 286
    diphtheria, 284–5
    lymphoma, 288
    nasopharyngeal carcinoma,
        286–7
    post-cricoid carcinoma, 287–8
    quinsy, 285
    retropharyngeal abscess, 286
    scarlet fever, 285
    tonsillar carcinoma, 287
    tuberculous tonsillitis, 286
    Vincent's angina, 284
phillodes tumour, 324
phimosis, 528
phlegmasia alba dolens, 585
phlegmasia caerulea dolens, 585
phlegmon (appendix mass), 403
phycomycoses, 146
physiological and operative
    severity score for the
enumeration of mortality and
    morbidity (POSSUM), 11
phytobezoars, 426
piles (haemorrhoids), 448–9
    sentinel, 446
Pilon fracture, 730
pilonidal abscess, sinus, 195
'pink tetralogy', 388
pinta, 137–8
pitcher's elbow, 683
pituitary adenomas, 207, 225,
    483, 488
    chromaffin, 483
placental abruption, 617
plantar fasciitis (policeman's
    heel), 739
plasma cells (memory B cells),
    116
plasma substitutes, 38
platelet activating factor (PAF),
    114
platelet concentrates, 36, 38, 40
platelet dysfunction
    iatrogenic, 96
    renal failure, 96
pleural effusion, 350–2
    causes, 350
    complications, 352
    investigations, 351–2
    Light's criteria (1972), 351
    malignant, 352
    physiology, 350
    recurrent, 352
    transudate/exudate, 352
    treatment, 352
pleural physiology, 347, 350
pleuritic pain, 351
pleurodesis, 349, 350, 352, 356
Plummer–Vinson syndrome
    (oesophageal web), 420–1
Plummer's disease, 308, 309
plunging ranula, 306–7
pneumatic compression devices,
    76
pneumonia
    aspiration, 217
    bacterial, 121–2
    P. carinii, 120
    postoperative, 67
    ventilator-associated, 20
pneumonitis, postoperative, 67
pneumothorax, 68, 347–50
    closed, 347
    open, 347
    recurrent, 348

secondary, 347
spontaneous, 347, 348
tension, 50, 68, 347–50, 360,
361, 600, 602
poikilocytosis, 171
Poland's syndrome, 321
policeman's heel (plantar
fasciitis), 739
poliomyelitis, 666–7
polyarteritis nodosa, 565–7
polycystic kidney, 493–4
polycythaemia, 189
polydactyly, 694
polymyalgia rheumatica, 653
polymyositis, 669–70
popliteal artery
aneurysm, 560
cystic adventitial disease, 560
entrapment, 559–60
port-wine stain, 590, 591
portal hypertension, 456, 459–60
positron emission tomography
(PET) scan, 342
POSSUM (physiological and
operative severity score for the
enumeration of mortality and
morbidity), 11
post-cricoid carcinoma, 287–8
post-gastrectomy syndromes, 430
post-herpetic neuralgia, 247
postgraduate education, 778–9
Postgraduate Medical Education
Training Board (PMETB),
778
postoperative adhesions, 69
postoperative care, 43–51
fluid balance, 47–8
gastrointestinal tract, 48–9
mobility, 49
pain and analgesia, 43–7
recovery area, 43
return to ward, 443
wound care, 49–51
postoperative complications,
54–76
postpericardiotomy syndrome,
384
postural equinovarus, 732
postvagotomy syndrome, 423
potassium, daily requirement, 48
Pott's disease of spine, 748–9
Pott's fracture, 730
Pott's paraplegia, 749
Pott's puffy tumour (skull
osteomyelitis), 231

pre-auricular cysts and sinuses,
237
pregnancy
cervical, 410
chronic gingivitis, 273
deep venous thrombosis, 585
ectopic, 409–10
fatty liver, 455
fetal assessment, 617–18
ovarian, 410
tetragenicity, 18
thyrotoxicosis, 310
trauma, 616–17
tubal, 409, 410
premedication, 25–6
prepatellar bursitis (housemaid's
knee), 719
presbycusis, 247
pressure areas, ulcers, 30, 32, 42,
192, 665
pressure monitoring 'bolt', 230
pressure overload, 369
priapism, 530–1
primary hyperaldosteronism
(Conn's syndrome), 489
primary hyperparathyroidism,
636
primary sclerosing cholangitis,
470
primary upper small intestinal
lymphoma (PUSIL)
(Mediterranean lymphoma),
131–2
progressive multifocal
leukoencephalopathy, 124
progressive muscular atrophy,
665–6
proptosis
congenital, 256
pulsating, 260
prostaglandins, 114
prostate carcinoma, 512–14
prostate stents, 512
prostate-specific antigen (PSA),
513
prostatitis, 515
protein C/S deficiency, 567–8
proteosomes, 116
prothrombotic disorders
(thrombophilia/hypercoagulable
states), 567–8
proto-oncogenes, 183
protocols, 2–3
protrusio acetabuli (Otto pelvis),
702

proximal humerus, fractured, 679
prune-belly syndrome, 516
pruritus, 190
pruritus ani, 449–50
pseudoarthrosis, girdlestone, 711
pseudobulbar palsy, 215–17
pseudocyst, 206
pseudoxanthoma elasticum, 228
psoas sign, 402
psoriasis, 191
  arthropathy, 654–5
psychological problems, 106–7, 109–10
pterygium, 252
ptosis, 248
pulmonary embolectomy, 347
pulmonary embolism, 68, 76, 345–7, 583
  complications, 350
  investigations, 348
  treatment, 349
pulmonary stenosis, 380
pulmonary venous drainage, partial anomalous, 385
pulpitis, 272
pulse
  pulsus paradoxus, 383
  'water hammer', 371
pulse oximetry, 28–9, 90
pupillary response abnormalities, 266–7
Putti–Platt repair (shoulder dislocation), 682
pyelonephritis, 516
pyloric stenosis, 64
  hypertrophic stenosis, 424
pyloromyotomy (Ramstedt's operation), 424
pyogenic discitis, 748
pyogenic granuloma, 198
pyogenic spondylitis, 748
pyomyositis, 143–4, 670
pyonephrosis, 505
pyruvate kinase deficiency, 180

quadrantanopia, homonymous, 208
quadriceps tear, 720
quantitative isotope perfusion scan, 343
quinolones, 19
quinsy (peritonsillar abscess), 285

radial club hand, 694
radial nerve injury, 766–7
radial scars, 327
radiation carcinogenesis, 184
radiation enteritis, 444
radionuclide excretion scan (hepatic iminodiacetic acid (HIDA) scan), 464
radiotherapy, 188
radius
  Colles' fracture, 692
  fracture of head, 687
  fracture of neck, 687–8
  Madelung's deformity, 694
  Smith's fracture, 693
raised intracranial pressure, 229–30
Ramsay–Hunt syndrome, 212, 213, 244
Ramstedt's operation (pyloromyotomy), 424
randomized controlled trial, 783
rashes, 193
Rastelli operation, 390
Ray amputation, 559
Raynaud's disease, phenomenon, syndrome, 551, 562, 565, 567, 652
recombinant activated factor VII (rFVIIa), 39
recovery area, 43
rectum
  examination in multiply injured, 605
  trauma, 409
  see also colorectal
rectus femoris rupture, 721
'red man syndrome', 19
'redcurrant jelly' stools, 401
reduction, fracture, 619–20
reduction mammoplasty, 321
Reed–Sternberg cells, 303
reflex sympathetic dystrophy (Sudek's atrophy), 626–7
reflux oesophagitis, 417–19
refractive errors, 63–4
Reiter's syndrome, 656–7
religion, 111
renal agenesis, 492
renal artery stenosis, 569–70
renal calculi, 501–3
renal cell carcinoma (Grawitz's tumour, hypernephroma), 500–1
renal cysts, simple, 494

renal failure, 34, 60, 494–8
    acute, 494–6
    chronic, 496–8
    ICU systems support, 92
renal tract trauma, 506–8, 604
renal transplantation, 498, 594,
    595
reperfusion syndrome, 595
repetitive strain injury, 672
research, 23, 782–3
respiratory acidosis, 62, 63, 360
respiratory alkalosis, 62–3
respiratory tract
    ageing process, 105
    dying patient, 108
    function tests, 342–3
    peri-operative infections, 20
    postoperative problems, 65–8
    thermal injury, 611, 612, 613
resuscitation protocol, 3
retinal detachment, 268
    traumatic, 262, 268
retinoblastoma, 259–60
retinopathy, micro-angiopathy,
    125
retro-ocular tumours, 207,
    257–8
retrobulbar neuritis, 664
retroperitoneal fibrosis, 506
retropharyngeal abscess, 286
Reye's syndrome, 455
rhabdomyosarcoma
    eye, 258
    hepatic, 462
    skeletal muscle, 673
    skin, 202
    sternomastoid, 298
rheumatic fever, 381–2
rheumatic heart disease, 373, 380
rheumatoid arthritis, 649–50
    juvenile, 657, 658
    knee, 721
    shoulder, 677
rheumatoid factor, 566, 651,
    652, 657, 658, 669, 774
rhinitis
    acute, 278
    allergic, 281
    simple chronic, 278
    vasomotor, 281–2
rhinophyma, 282
rhinoscleroma, 146, 280
rhinosporidiosis, 147, 281
rib fractures, 360, 364
Richter hernia, 392

rickets, 634–5
Riedel's thyroiditis, 314–15
ringworm (tinea), 197–9
risk management, 5
Risser's sign, 740
risus sardonicus, 196
river blindness (onchocerciasis),
    158–60
Robert Jones tendon transfer,
    733
Roos' test, 562
Rosvig's sign, 402
rotator cuff syndrome, 675
round worms, 154–61
Roux loop, 465

saddle embolism, 556
salivary glands, 293–7
    adenocarcinoma of minor, 288
    adenocystic carcinoma, 296
    bacterial parotitis, 294
    fistula, 295
    in HIV/AIDS, 126
    mucoepidermoid carcinoma,
        296–7
    mumps, 293–4
    parotidectomy, 295
    pleomorphic adenoma, 194–5,
        294–5
    plunging ranula, 307–8
    sialolithiasis, 297
    sublingual dermoid, 306
    swelling, causes of, 293
    Warthin's tumour, 295–6
salivary tumour, mixed, 294
Salter–Harris fractures (fracture–
    separation of distal tibial and
    fibular epiphyses), 730–1
Salter–Harris radiological
    classification (epiphyseal
    fractures), 621
saphenous nerve injury, 773, 783
sarcoidosis, 302
scabies, 198, 450
scalp
    basal cell carcinomas, 201
    circoid aneurysm, 218
    lipoma, 202
    meningocoele/meningo-
        encephalocoele, 740
    plexiform neurofibromas, 202
    sebaceous cysts, 203
    squamous cell carcinoma, 201
    temporal arteritis, 218, 564–5
    turban tumours, 200

scaphoid fracture, 693–4
scapula
  fracture, 678
  winging, 677
scarlet fever, 285
scars, 192
Schatzki's ring (oesophageal ring), 421
Scheuermann's kyphosis, 743
Schilling test (vitamin B_{12} absorption test), 172–3
schistosomiasis (bilharziasis), 151–2, 519–20
Schmorl's nodes, 743
schwannoma, 225
sciatic nerve injury, 702, 770–1
scissors stance, 663
scleritis, 253
scleroderma, 567
  pigmentosum, 200
sclerosing cholangitis
  in HIV and AIDS, 129
  primary, 470
scoliosis, 741–3
scorpion stings, 166–7
scrotum
  carcinoma, 538
  filariasis, 539–40, 589
  Fournier's gangrene, 196, 538–9
  haematocoele, 542
  varicocoele, 541–2
  see also testis and scrotum
scurvy, 631, 632
sea anemone/sea urchin stings, 168
sebaceous glands
  benign tumours, 200
  carcinoma, 202
  cysts, 203–4, 206
seborrhoeic keratosis (basal cell papilloma, senile wart), 203
sedation, 26, 70
semimembranosus bursitis, 720
Senning operation, 390
sentinel node biopsy, 332
sentinel pile, 446
sepsis, 88, 94–5
  management, 117–18
septic abortion, 411
septic arthritis, 658–60
  of hip, 708
septic shock, 116–17
Sever's disease (osteochondritis of the calcaneum), 725

sex hormones, 487
sexually transmitted diseases
  chlamydial, 138
  genital warts, 197, 544
  gonorrhoea, 251–2, 514, 542
  herpes, 138, 197, 544
  non-specific urethritis, 542
  pelvic inflammatory disease, 543–4
  syphilis, 27, 125, 138, 267
  warts, 125, 127, 197, 544
shin splints, 728
shingles (herpes zoster), 147, 197, 235, 244, 247
shivering, 73
shock, 96–7
  fracture-related blood loss, 619
  multiply injured, 600–1
  septic, 116–17
short bowel syndrome, 596
shoulder joint and pectoral girdle
  acromioclavicular dislocation, 678
  acute calcific tendinitis, 675
  biceps tendon rupture, 675
  dislocated, 679–82
    anterior, 679–80
    posterior, 680–1
    recurrent, 681–2
  fractured clavicle, 677–8
  frozen shoulder, 676
  Milwaukee shoulder, 677
  osteoarthritis, 676
  painful arc syndrome, 674
  proximal humerus fracture, 679
  rheumatoid arthritis, 677
  scapular fracture, 678
  Sprengel's deformity, 677
  sternoclavicular dislocation, 678
  winging of scapula, 677
  see also arm
Shouldice herniorrhaphy, 393
shrapnel, 608
shuttle walk test, 343
sialolithiasis, 297
sickle test, 178
sickle-cell disease, 177–9, 473, 474
  bone necrosis, 627–8
sickle-cell trait, 179
sideroblastic anaemia, 174
silicobezoars, 426

Simmonds' test, 725
singer's nodes, 291
sinus, 206
sinus venosus defect, 385
sinusitis, 231
Sjögren's syndrome, 652
skin
  associated diseases, 189
  basal cell carcinoma, 201
  basal cell papilloma, 203
  benign tumours, 199–203
  colour, 188
  congenital lesions, 191
  cysts, 203–4, 205–6
  degenerative lesions, 203–4
  fistulae, 206
  ganglia, 203
  infections, 192–4, 195–8
  leopard, 159
  lumps, 204–6
  malignant lesions, 201–2
  manifestations of malignancy,
      190
  nodules, 189
  pigmented naevi, 200
  premalignant lesions, 200–1
  pruritus, 190
  scars, 192
  sinuses, 206
  squamous cell carcinoma, 201
  squamous cell papilloma, 199
  tophi, 189
  trauma, 191–2
  ulcers, 204–6
  see also specific conditions and
      diseases
skin grafts, 193, 592
skin prick tests, 281
skull
  anencephaly, 219
  fractures, 207, 219–20, 604
  microcephaly, 218
  Paget's disease, 636
  Pott's puffy tumour, 231
  tumours, 219, 231
sleep apnoea, 283–4
slipped upper femoral epiphysis,
    707
small bowel
  gallstone ileus, 469
  transplant, 596
  trauma, 408
  tumours, 439
  see also bowel
Smith's fracture, 693

smoking, obesity and, 102
snake bites, 164–6
Snellen chart, 263
snoring, 283
sodium, daily requirement, 48
solar keratosis, 200
soleus muscle tear, 725
sparganosis, 163–4
sparganum, 163
specialist meetings, 4
spectacles (glasses), 264
spermatocoele, 540
spider bites, 166–7
spider naevi, 198, 455
Spigelian hernia, 393
spine
  acute disc rupture, 744–5
  ankylosing spondylitis, 653,
      657
  cauda equina syndrome, 741
  coccydynia, 747
  kyphosis in elderly, 744
  non-organic back pain, 759
  Pott's disease, 748–9
  pyogenic discitis, 748
  pyogenic spondylitis, 746
  Scheuermann's kyphosis, 743
  scoliosis, 741–3
  spondylolisthesis, 747
  spondylosis, 745–6
  stenosis, 746
  tuberculosis, 748–9
spina bifida, 740–1
  cystica, 740–1
  occulta, 740–1
spinal brace, 748
spinal fusion, 746
spinal injuries
  blast injury, 608
  management of paraplegia and
      tetraplegia, 757
  neurological, 756–7
  paediatric trauma, 615
  subluxations (C3–T1), 752
  thoracic, 753–4
spinal injuries, cervical, 602,
    749–53
  burst fractures, 752
  comminuted body fractures,
      752
  dislocation/fracture–dislocation
      (C3–T1), 752–3
  fracture of atlas (C1), 751
  fracture of pedicle of axis
      (C2), 751

spinal injuries, cervical *cont.*
　hyperextension injury
　　(C3–T1), 752
　unilateral facet dislocation,
　　753
　wedge compression (C3–T1),
　　752
　whiplash injury, 750–1
spinal injuries, thoracolumbar,
　754
　burst fracture, 755
　fracture–dislocations, 755
　jack-knife fracture, 755
　pars interarticularis fracture,
　　754
　transverse process fracture,
　　754
　wedge compression fracture,
　　755
spinal stroke, 572
spinal tumours
　chordoma, 758
　haemangioma, 757
　metastases, 758
　non-Hodgkin's lymphoma,
　　757
　osteoblastoma, 757
spirometry, 342
spleen
　functions, 473
　trauma, 474–5
splenomegaly, 473–4
splint, 'lively', 672, 767
splinter haemorrhages, 189, 381,
　551
spondyloepiphyseal dysplasia,
　637
spondylolisthesis, 747
spondylosis, 745–6
spray-on sealants, 50
Sprengel's deformity, 677
Stamey bladder neck suspension,
　521
Stamm incision, 452
star fish stings, 168
starvation, 47–8, 77–8, 93
　short-term, 78
Steindler's operation, 733
sternal fractures, 360, 364
sternoclavicular dislocation, 678
sternomastoid
　rhabdomyosarcoma, 298
　tumour of infancy, 298
Stewart's midline granuloma,
　279

Still's disease, 473, 657–8
stitches, 'butterfly', 50
stomach
　adenocarcinoma, 431–2
　bezoars, 426
　fibrosarcoma, 433
　in HIV/AIDS, 126
　leiomyosarcoma, 433
　Mallory–Weiss syndrome,
　　430–1
　neurofibrosarcoma, 433
　trauma, 407
　volvulus, 425
　Zollinger–Ellison syndrome,
　　484
　see also gastric
stomas
　complications, 453
　effluent, 452
　feeding, 452
　mucous fistula, 453
　permanent, 453
　siting of, 453
　temporary, 452
　tube caecostomy, 453
stool, 'redcurrant jelly', 401
strabismus, 211, 264–5
strawberry naevus, 590, 591
stress ECG/exercise test, 366–7
stress (gastric) ulcers, 427
stress incontinence, 520–1
stress (march) fracture, 736
stroke, 547
　spinal, 572
strongyloidiasis, 155–6
styes, 249
subarachnoid haemorrhage, 221,
　228–9
subarachnoid neurolysis, 107
subclavian aneurysm, 551
subclavian steal, 550
subdural haematoma, 226–8
sublingual dermoid, 306
sublingual gland, *see* salivary
　glands
submandibular gland, *see* salivary
　glands
subphrenic abscess, 70, 405
subtrochanteric fracture, 712
sucking chest wound, 360, 361
Sudek's atrophy (reflex
　sympathetic dystrophy), 626–7
sulphonamides, 19
superficial thrombophlebitis
　(Mondor's disease), 324

superior vena cava (SVC) syndrome, 299–300, 358
superior venal caval thrombosis, 86
supernumerary nipples, breast, 321
support brace, 742, 743
suprascapular nerve injury, 764–5
supraspinatus tear, 674
sural nerve injury, 772–3, 783
surgical procedures, 41–2
    antiseptic solution, 42
    medical students, 42
    operation notes, 42
    patient identification, 41
    positioning, 42
    safety, 41
    sterile techniques, 42
    trainees, 42
surgical sieve, 204–5
sutures, 50
Synacthen stimulation test, 487
syndactyly, 694
syndrome of inappropriate ADH secretion, 57–8, 342
syphilis, 125, 138, 267, 274
    congenital, 271, 279
    gumma of nose, 279
    gumma of palate, 277
syringomyelia, 210, 662
systemic inflammatory response, 116
systemic inflammatory response syndrome (SIRS), 114, 477
systemic lupus erythematosus, 474, 651–2
systemic sclerosis, 566, 567

T lymphocytes (T cells), 115–16
    deficiency and sepsis, 95
    graft rejection, 598
tachycardia, 64
Takayasu's arteriopathy, 563–4
talipes equinovarus (clubfoot), 732
talus fractures, 731
tapeworms (cestodes), 161–4
tarsal injuries, 735
tarsal tunnel syndrome, 735–6
tarso-metatarsal (Lisfranc's) dislocation, 735
task prioritization, 780
teaching, 782
teamwork, 4–5, 780

teeth
    abscess, 272
    absent, 271
    additional, 271
    caries, 272
    congenital syphilis, 271
    dentigerous cysts, 272, 273
    false, 32
    impaction, 273
    odontomes, 272
    wisdom, 273
teicoplanin, 19
telangiectasia, 198
telomerase, 183
temporal arteritis, 207, 564–5
tendon grafts, 672
tendon injury, 672
tendon lengthening, 662
tendon sheath infection, 195
tendon stretching exercises, 734
tendon transfer, 769
    Robert Jones, 733
tennis elbow, 683
tenosynovitis, 670
Tensilon test, 668
tension band wires, 722
tension pneumothorax, 50, 68, 347–50, 360, 361
    multiply injured, 600, 602
testis and scrotum
    acute epididymitis, 540–1
    chronic epididymitis, 541
    epididymal cyst, 206, 540
    filariasis, 539–40
    Fournier's gangrene, 196, 538–9
    haematocoele, 542
    hydrocoele, 541
    lymphoma, 537
    orchitis, 541
    prosthetic testis, 535
    seminoma, 535–6
    spermatocoele, 540
    teratoma, 536–7
    torsion, 534–5
    trauma, 542
    undescended testis, 533–4
tetanus, 196, 606–7
tetracycline, 19
tetralogy of Fallot, 388
tetraplegia, 663, 756–7
thalassaemias (Mediterranean anaemia), 180–1, 474
thallium scan (myocardial perfusion scintigraphy), 91, 367

Thomsen's disease (myotonia congenitalia), 672
thoracic injuries, 360–4
  airway obstruction/injury, *see* airway obstruction/injury
  aortic transection, 360, 363–4
  blast injury, 608
  cardiac tamponade, 360, 362, 382–4
  flail chest, 360, 362
  gunshot wounds, 606
  large haemothorax, 360, 361
  lung contusion, 360, 363
  multiply injured, 602, 604
  myocardial contusion, 360, 363
  paediatric trauma, 615
  pneumothorax, *see* pneumothorax
  rib fractures, 360, 364
  spinal, 753–4
  sternal fractures, 360, 364
  sucking chest wound, 360, 361
thoracic outlet compression syndrome (TOCS), 551, 562–3
thoracocentesis, 352
thoracodorsal nerve injury, 765–6
thoracolumbar spinal injuries, 755–6
thrombin time, 33
thrombocytic purpura, idiopathic, 473
thrombolysis, 346
thrombophilia (hypercoagulable states/prothrombotic disorders), 567–8
thrombophlebitis, 582–3
  blood-transfusion-related, 40
  cannula-related, 75
  superficial, of breast (Mondor's disease), 324
thromboplastin, 33
thrombosis, venous, 583–5
thumb
  Bennet's fracture–dislocation, 697
  fractured base, 697
  gamekeeper's, 697
  mallet, 696
thymoma, 357
thyroglossal sinus, cyst and fistula, 317
thyroid
  crisis, 311–12
  ectopic, 317
  goitre, 307–8, 310, 312–13
  solitary nodule, 315
thyroid antibodies, 308, 309, 314
thyroiditis
  De Quervain's, 314–15
  Hashimoto's, 313–14
  Riedel's, 314–15
thyrotoxicosis, 308–11
tibia
  fracture of shaft of fibula and, 726–7
  fracture–separation of distal epiphysis, 730
  fracture-related blood loss causing shock, 619
  isolated fracture of shaft, 728
  stress fracture, 728
  torsion, and intoe gait, 705
tibial nerve injury, 771
tibial plateau fracture, 724
tinea (ringworm), 197–8
Tinel's sign, 690
tissue factor/thromboplastin, 33
tissue oxygen availability, 11
TNM staging, 185
  bladder cancer, 525
  breast cancer, 330–1
  lung cancer (1997), 341
tobramycin, 19
toe
  ainhum, 168
  claw, 650, 733, 738
  gout, 656, 738
  hallux rigidus, 737
  hallux valgus, 736–7
  hammer, 558, 737
  'trash-foot', 556
toenail
  ingrowing, 189, 738
  keratoderma blennorrhagicum, 657
  onychogryphosis, 738
  subungual exostosis, 738
  subungual malignant melanoma, 201, 739
tolbutamide test (insulin secretagogues), 482
tongue
  carcinoma, 276–7
  glossitis, 276
  sublingual dermoid, 306
  wasting and weakness, 276
tonsillar carcinoma, 287

tonsillitis
  acute, 285
  chronic, 296
  tuberculous, 286
tonsoliths, 286
tophi, 656
Torre's (Muir–Torre) syndrome, 190
torticollis, 298
toxic adenoma, 310
toxic megacolon, 438
toxic nodular goitre, 310
toxoplasma chorioretinitis, 125
trachoma, 248–9
training portfolio, 778
tramadol, 45
transcutaneous electrical nerve stimulation (TENS), 108
transient ischaemia attack (TIA), 381, 545, 547
transplantation, 102, 592–9
  bone, 592, 596
  bone marrow, 175, 178, 596
  cartilage, 593
  complications, 595–7
  corneal, 592, 593
  criteria and procedure for donation, 3, 23, 102, 593
  donor and recipient screening, 593
  graft rejection, 598–9
  heart/lung, 596
  HLA match, 593
  immunosuppression, 597
  infection, 597–9
  liver, 456, 462, 465, 594–6
  malignancy in recipient, 599
  management of organ donor, 593–4
  monitoring transplant function, 597
  principles, 592–4
  renal, 498, 594, 595
  skin, 193, 592
transposition of great arteries, 389–90
transurethral resection of prostate (TURP), 512
'trash-foot', 556–7
treadmill stress test, 366
trematodes (liver flukes), 152–3
Trendelenburg tests, 581
Trethowan's sign, 707
triangle of Petit, 394
trichasis, 249

trichobezoars, 426
trick movements, 759
tricuspid valve disease, 380
trigeminal nerve and nuclear palsy, 210–11
trigeminal neuralgia, 211, 234
trigger finger, 695–6
triglycerides, 78
trimethoprim, 19
trismus (lock-jaw), 196, 606
trochlear nerve and nucleus palsy, 209–10
tropical splenomegaly syndrome, 473, 474
tropical ulcer, 134–5
tropical/subtropical diseases, 130–64
  actinomycosis, 144, 739
  amoebiasis, 149–51
  animal bites/stings, 164–8
  ascariasis, 157–8
  bladderworm, 162
  bowel tapeworms, 162–3
  Burkitt's lymphoma, 132–3
  Buruli ulcer, 135
  cancrum oris, 136–7, 274
  chromoblastomycosis, 147
  cutaneous larva migrans, 155
  dracunculiasis, 160–1
  elephantiasis, 158, 159, 539
  filariasis, 158–60, 539–40, 589
  hookworm, 154–5
  hydatid disease, 161–2, 206, 461
  Kaposi's sarcoma, 133–4
  leishmaniasis, 148–9, 281
  leprosy, 140, 140–1, 252, 280, 662, 773
  liver flukes, 152–3
  loa loa, 159
  lobomycosis, 147
  lung flukes, 153–4
  malaria, 147–8
  Mediterranean lymphoma, 131
  mycetoma, 145–6, 739–40
  myiasis, 164
  nasopharyngeal cancer, 131
  oesophagostomiasis, 156–7
  onchocerciasis, 158–60
  oropharyngeal cancer, 130–1
  paranasal aspergillus granuloma, 146
  phaeohyphomycosis, 147
  phycomycoses, 146

tropical/subtropical diseases *cont.*
  pinta, 137–8
  pyomyositis, 143–4
  rhinoscleroma, 146
  rhinosporidiosis, 147, 281
  schistosomiasis, 151–2,
    519–20
  sparganosis, 163–4
  strongyloidiasis, 155–6
  tropical ulcer, 134
  tuberculosis, 142–3
  typhoid, 138–40
  veld sore, 136
  yaws, 137, 280
Trotter's triad, 287
Trousseau's sign, 190, 320
tube caecostomy (bowel
  irrigation), 453
tube feeding, 81–2, 93
tuberculosis, 142–3, 339
  ankle joint, 726
  arthritis, 660–1
  bladder, 505, 516, 518
  breast, 328
  hip, 708
  in HIV/AIDS, 121, 123
  lymphadenitis, 301–2
  nasal, 280
  perinephric abscess, 504
  spine, 748–9
  tonsillitis, 286
  urinary tract, 505–6
tumour, 205
  angiogenesis, 183
  assessment, 185
  markers, 185
  see also cancers
tumour necrosis factor alpha,
  114, 117
tumour-suppressor genes (anti-
  oncogenes), 183
turban tumour (hidradenoma),
  200
tympanic rupture, 244
tympanosclerosis, 243
'Type A' personality, 545
typhoid, 138–40

ulcerative colitis, 437–8
ulcers
  biopsy, 205
  differential diagnosis, 204–6
ulna
  club hand, 694
  Madelung's deformity, 694

ulnar nerve injury, 72, 682,
  767–8
umbilical hernia, 393
union
  delayed, 624
  mal-, 625–6
  non-, 625
  normal process, 624
uraemic syndrome, 498
ureter
  calculi, 501–2
  duplex, 492–3
  hydro-, 492
urethral injury, 531–3, 604–5
urethral strictures, 514, 515, 533
urethritis, non-specific, 542
urethrocoele, 524
urge incontinence (detrusor
  instability), 521–2
urinary catheterization, 60
urinary tract
  peri-operative infection, 20
  postoperative infection, 60–1
  schistosomiasis, 519–20
  tuberculosis, 505–6
urine
  acute retention, 508–9
  chronic retention, 509–10
  failure to pass, 60
  output, 29, 55, 60–1
urinoma, 507
urticarial transfusion reaction, 40
uvula, bifid, 284

v wave, 382
vagus nerve palsy, 214
valve disease
  aortic regurgitation, 371–3
  aortic stenosis, 369–70
  endocarditis, 380–1
  mitral regurgitation, 376–9
  mitral stenosis, 373–6
  pulmonary stenosis, 380
  rheumatic fever, 381–2
  tricuspid disease, 380
valvotomy, 375, 376
vancomycin, 19–20
VAP (ventilator-associated
  pneumonia), 20
varicella zoster retinitis, 125
varicocoele, 541–2
varicose eczema, 586
varicose veins, 580–2
vascular graft infection, 576–8
vascular injury, 578–9

vascular malformations, 590–1
vasculitic disorders, 563–7
    Raynaud's disease/
        phenomenon/syndrome,
        551, 562, 565–7, 652
    scleroderma, 567
    Takayasu's arteriopathy, 563–4
    temporal arteritis, 207, 564–5
    thrombophilia, 567–8
    vibration white finger, 567
vasculitis, cutaneous, 193–4
vasomotor rhinitis, 281–2
VATS (video-assisted
    thorascopic surgery), 349
vegetative state, 230
    persistent, 100
vein reflux, perforating, 586
veld sore, 136
Velpeau chest bandage, 679
vena caval filter, 585
venous gangrene, 75
venous insufficiency, chronic,
    585–6
venous malformation, 198, 590–1
venous thromboembolism (deep
    vein thrombosis), 75–6,
    583–5, 626
    postoperative prophylaxis, 16
ventilation
    indications, 90
    methods of, 90–1
ventilation–perfusion scan, 346
ventilator-associated pneumonia
    (VAP), 20
ventricular septal defect (VSD),
    387
ventriculography (multigated
    acquisition scanning, MUGA
    scan), 91, 367
verrucae, see warts
vertebrobasilar artery disease,
    208, 549
vertical banded gastroplasty,
    104, 433
vesico-ureteric reflux, 516–17
vesicovaginal fistula, 523
vestibulo-occular reflex, 101
vestibulocochlear nerve and
    nucleus palsy, 213
vibration white finger, 567
video-assisted thorascopic
    surgery (VATS), 349
Vincent's angina, 273, 284
Vincent's organisms, 284
VIPomas, 482–3

viral hepatitis, 457, 458
Virchow's triad, 583
virilism, 47
visual field loss and blindness,
    268–70
    optic nerve/pathway palsy,
        208, 267
visually evoked response, 664
vitamin B_{12} absorption test
    (Schilling test), 172–3
vitamin B_{12} deficiency anaemia,
    172–3
vitamin C deficiency, 632, 714
vitamin D deficiency, 634, 714
vitamin K, peri-operative, 15,
    16–17
vocal cord tumours, 290–1
Volkmann's contracture, 580,
    684, 727
volvulus
    bowel, 401–2
    stomach, 425
vomiting (emesis), see nausea
    and vomiting
Von Hippel–Lindau syndrome,
    500
Von Recklinghausen's disease
    (neurofibromatosis), 202
    of bone, 636
    plexiform, 202
Von Rosen's lines, 703
Von Rosen's malleable splint,
    704
Von Willebrand's disease, 34
Von Willebrand's factor, 117

'waiter's tip' position, 763
walking plaster, 559
ward, return to, 43
Warthin's tumour, 295–6
warts (verrucae), 197
    anal, 127, 451
    genital, 197, 544
    in HIV/AIDS, 125, 127
    senile, 203
Waterhouse–Friderichsen
    syndrome, 487
wedge compression fractures,
    752, 755
wedge resection, 343, 344–5
Wegener's granulomatosis,
    278–9, 565–7
whiplash injury, 750–1
Whipple's operation (pancreato-
    duodenectomy), 473, 479, 481

whitlow, 699
Wilms' tumour
  (nephroblastoma), 499–500
Wilson's disease
  (haemochromatosis), 455,
  458
worm infestations
  bladderworm, 162
  bowel tapeworms, 162–3
  dracunculiasis, 160–1
  elephantiasis, 158–60
  filariasis, 158, 158–60,
    539–40, 589
  guinea worm, 160–1
  hookworm, 154–5
  hydatid disease, 161–2, 206,
    461
  loa loa, 159
  onchocerciasis, 158–60
  round worm, 154–61
  sparganosis, 163–4
  tapeworm, 161–4
wounds
  ballistic, 605–10
  sucking chest, 360, 361
  surgical
    care, 49–51
    infections, 73–4

wrist
  carpal dislocation, 694
  carpal tunnel syndrome, 690
  Colles' fracture, 692
  De Quervain's disease, 691
  'dinner-fork' deformity, 692
  drop, 767
  ganglion, 203, 691
  Keinbock's disease, 691
  scaphoid fracture, 693–4
  Smith's fracture, 693
  see also hand
wuchereria infection, 158–60

x-descent, 382
X-linked bulbar palsy, 217
X-linked impaired renal tubular
  phosphate reabsorption, 634
X-linked motor neuropathy,
  216–17

y-descent, 382
yaws, 137–8, 280

Zadik's operation, 738
Zancolli's operation, 768
Zenker's diverticulum, 288–9
Zollinger–Ellison syndrome, 484